Pre-eclampsia
Etiology and Clinical Practice

Pre-eclampsia is one of the leading causes of death and disability in mothers and babies. Over four million women worldwide will develop the disorder every year. This book, written by an international team of experts, focuses on both the scientific basis of pre-eclampsia and its management. The basic science section contains up-to-date reviews of the most exciting research developments in pre-eclampsia. The clinical chapters provide a comprehensive review of the pertinent literature, highlighting recent data and new ideas or developments in current management. There is a section in each chapter (where relevant) that deals with practical management, giving clinicians a formulated treatment plan that they can implement directly. The book will be of interest to all professionals interested in the reproductive sciences, and to obstetricians and physicians with an interest in pre-eclampsia.

Fioan Lyall is Professor of Maternal and Fetal Health at the University of Glasgow. She is Chief Editor of the journal *Hypertension in Pregnancy*.

Michael Belfort is Professor of Obstetrics and Gynecology at the University of Utah. He is also Director of Perinatal Research and Co-director of Fetal Surgery at the Hospital Corporation of America in Nashville.

Pre-eclampsia

Etiology and Clinical Practice

Fiona Lyall

University of Glasgow

Michael Belfort

University of Utah

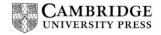
CAMBRIDGE
UNIVERSITY PRESS

CAMBRIDGE UNIVERSITY PRESS

Cambridge, New York, Melbourne, Madrid, Cape Town, Singapore, São Paulo

Cambridge University Press
The Edinburgh Building, Cambridge CB2 2RU, UK

Published in the United States of America by Cambridge University Press, New York

www.cambridge.org
Information on this title: http://www.cambridge.org/052183189X

First published 2007

Printed in the United Kingdom at the University Press, Cambridge

A catalogue record for this publication is available from the British Library

Library of Congress Cataloging-in-Publication data
Lyall, F.
Pre-eclampsia: etiology and clinical practice/Fiona Lyall and Michael Belfort.
    p. ; cm.
Includes bibliographical references.
ISBN-13: 978-0-521-83189-5 (hardback)
ISBN-10: 0-521-83189-X (hardback)
1. Preeclampsia. I. Belfort, Michael A., 1958- II. Title.
[DNLM: 1. Pre-Eclampsia- -etiology. 2. Pre-Eclampsia- -therapy. WQ 215 L981p2007]

RG575.5.L93 2007
618.3'6132- -dc22

                            2007002767

ISBN-13   978-0-521-83189-5 hardback
ISBN-10   0-521-83189-X hardback

For my mother,
Patricia Stratton Wilson Belfort,
1932–2006
MB

For my mother, Margaret Stewart Malcolm
Struthers Lyall (1935–1997) and my father,
Alexander George Lyall.
FL

Contents

Contributors

John Anthony
University of Cape Town
Department of Medicine
Division of Hypertension
Cape Town, ZA-7925
South Africa

John Aplin
Division of Human Development
Faculty of Medicine
University of Manchester
St Mary's Hospital
Manchester M13 0JH
UK

Michael Belfort
Department of Obstetrics and Gynecology
University of Utah Health Sciences Center
Salt Lake City, Utah
USA

Fiona Broughton Pipkin
Academic Division of Obstetrics & Gynecology
Maternity Unit, City Hospital
Nottingham NG5 1PB
UK

Graham Burton
Department of Anatomy
University of Cambridge
Downing Street
Cambridge CB2 3DY
UK

Lavenia Carpenter
Department of Obstetrics and Gynecology
University of Cincinnati College of Medicine
P.O. Box 670526
231 Albert Sabin Way
Cincinnati, OH 45267
USA

Kristin Coppage
Department of Obstetrics and Gynecology
University of Cincinnati
231 Albert Sabin Way
M/L 0526
Cincinnati, OH 45267-0526
USA

Jonathan Coutts
The Queen Mother's Hospital
Yorkhill
Glasgow G3 8SJ, UK

Ian Crocker
Division of Human Development
Faculty of Medicine
University of Manchester
St Mary's Hospital
Manchester M13 0JH
UK

James Cross
Genes and Development Research Group
Department of Biochemistry and Molecular Biology
Faculty of Medicine
University of Calgary
HSC Room 2279
3330 Hospital Drive NW
Calgary, Alberta T2N 4N1
Canada

F. Gary Cunningham
Department of Obstetrics and Gynecology
UT Southwestern Medical Center
5323 Harry Hines Blvd.
Dallas, TX 75390
USA

J. M. Davison
Obstetrics & Gynaecology
4th Floor, Leazes Wing
Royal Victoria Infirmary
Newcastle upon Tyne NE1 4LP

Gus Dekker
Women's and Children's Division
Lyell McEwin Health Service
Northern Campus University of Adelaide
Haydown Road
Elizabeth Vale, SA 5112
Australia

Gary Dildy
Department of Obstetrics and Gynecology
Louisiana State University School of Medicine
1542 Tulane Avenue
New Orleans, LA 70112
USA

Tracey Glanville
Leeds Teaching Hospital Trust
St James University Hospital
Beckett Street
Leeds LS9 7TF
UK

Myriam Hanssens
Department of Obstetrics and Gynaecology
University Hospital Gasthuisberg
Herestraat 49
B3000 Leuven, Belgium

Susan Hiby
Department of Pathology
Tennis Court Road
University of Cambridge
Cambridge CB2 1QP
UK

J. Hornbuckle
Centre for Reproduction, Growth and Development
University of Leeds
UK

Carl Hubel
Magee-Womens' Research Institute
204 Craft Avenue
Pittsburgh, PA 15213
USA

Tai-Ho Hung
Department of Anatomy
Downing Street
Cambridge CB2 3DY, UK

Berthold Huppertz
Institute of Cell Biology, Histology and Embryology,
Medical University of Graz,
Harrachgasse 21/7
8010 Graz
Austria

Eric Jauniaux
Academic Department of Obstetrics and Gynaecology
University College London
89–96 Chenies Mews
London WC1E 6HX, UK

Peter Kaufmann
Department of Anatomy
University Hospital RWTH Aachen
Wendlingweg 2
D-52057 Aachen
Germany

Fiona Lyall
Maternal and Fetal Medicine Section
Institute of Medical Genetics
University of Glasgow
Yorkhill
Glasgow G3 8SJ
UK

Ashley Moffett
Department of Pathology
Tennis Court Road
University of Cambridge
Cambridge CB2 1QP
UK

Leslie Myatt
Department of Obstetrics and Gynecology
University of Cincinnati College of Medicine
P.O. Box 670526
231 Albert Sabin Way
Cincinnati, OH 45267
USA

Catherine Nelson-Piercy
10th floor, Directorate Office
North Wing
Guy's and St. Thomas' NHS Foundation
Lambeth Palace Road
London SE1 8EH
UK

Muna Noori
Division of SORA
Imperial College London
Chelsea and Westminster Hospital
309 Fulham Road
London SWIO 9WH
UK

Robyn North
Department of Obstetrics and Gynaecology
University of Auckland
Private Bag 92019
New Zealand

Errol Norwitz
Yale University School of Medicine
Department of Obstetrics, Gynecology and
   Reproductive Sciences
Yale-New Haven Hospital
333 Cedar Street
New Haven, CT 06520-8063
USA

Joong Shin Park
Department of Obstetrics and Gynecology
Seoul National University College of Medicine
Seoul 110-744
Korea

Jeffrey Phelan
959 East Walnut Street
Suite 200
Pasadena, CA 91106
USA

Robert Pijnenborg
Department of Obstetrics and Gynaecology
University Hospital Gasthuisberg
Herestraat 49
B3000 Leuven, Belgium

Lucilla Poston
Maternal and Fetal Research Unit
Department of Women's Health
St Thomas' Hospital
Lambeth Palace Rd
London SE1 7EH
UK

Maarten T. M. Raijmakers
Máxima Medisch Centrum
Department of Clinical Chemistry
PO Box 7777
5500 MB Veldhoven
The Netherlands

Chris W. G. Redman
Nuffield Department of Obstetrics and Gynaecology
John Radcliffe Hospital
Oxford OX3 9DU
UK

Annemarie Reinders
Nieuweweg 47
7241 ES LOCHEM
The Netherlands

Jose Rivers
Department of Anesthesiology
Suite 1003
6550 Fannin Street
Houston, TX 77030
USA

Jim Roberts
Magee-Womens' Research Institute
204 Craft Avenue
Pittsburgh, PA 15213
USA

Pierre Yves Robillard
Neonatology
Center Hospitalier Sud-Reunion
BP 350 97488
Saint-Pierre cedex
Reunion
France

Stephen Robson
Surgical and Reproductive Sciences
3rd Floor Leech Building
Medical School
Newcastle upon Tyne NE2 4HH
UK

Ian L. Sargent
Nuffield Department of Obstetrics and Gynaecology
John Radcliffe Hospital
Oxford OX3 9DU
UK

Mina Savvidou
Harris Birthright Research Centre for Fetal Medicine
Kings College Hospital
Denmark Hill
London SE9 5RS
UK

Andrew Shennan
Maternal and Fetal Research Unit
Department of Women's Health
St Thomas' Hospital
London SE1 7EH
UK

Baha Sibai
Department of Obstetrics & Gynecology
University of Cincinnati,
Cincinnati, OH 45221
USA

Gordon Smith
Department of Obstetrics and Gynaecology
Cambridge University
Rosie Maternity Hospital
Cambridge CB2 2SW
UK

Marie Smith
Obstetrics & Gynaecology
4th Floor, Leazes Wing
Royal Victoria Infirmary
Newcastle upon Tyne NE1 4LP
UK

Maya Suresh
Department of Anesthesiology
Suite 1003
6550 Fannin Street
Houston, TX 77030
USA

Diane Twickler
University of Texas
SouthWestern Medical Center
Department of Radiology
5323 Harry Hines Blvd
Dallas, TX 75390
USA

F. André Van Assche
Department of Obstetrics and Gynaecology
University Hospital Gasthuisberg
Herestraat 49
B3000 Leuven, Belgium

Michael Varner
University of Utah School of Medicine
50 North Medical Drive,
Salt Lake City, UT 84132
USA

Lisbeth Vercruysse
Department of Obestetrics and Gynaecology
University Hospital Gasthuisberg
Herestraat 49
B3000 Leuven, Belgium

Isobel Walker
Department of Haematology
Glasgow Royal Infirmary
Glasgow G4 0SF
UK

James Walker
Leeds Teaching Hospital Trust
St James University Hospital
Beckett Street
Leeds LS9 7TF
UK

Kenneth Ward
Department of Obstetrics and Gynecology
Kapiolani Hospital
1319 Punahou Street, Room 824
Honolulu, HI 96826, USA

David Williams
Institute for Women's Health
University College London
Elizabeth Garrett Anderson Hospital
Huntley Street
London WC1E 6DH
UK

Stacy Zamudio
UMD-New Jersey Medical School
Department of Obstetrics, Gynecology and
    Women's Health
185 South Orange Ave MSB £-505
Newark, NJ 07103-2714
USA

Preface

Pre-eclampsia complicates 2–3% of primigravid pregnancies and 5–7% of nulliparous women. It is one of the leading causes of death and disability of mothers and babies. Over four million women will develop the disorder worldwide every year. This book, written by scientists and clinicians who are internationally recognized as experts in their respective fields, focuses on both the scientific basis of pre-eclampsia along with management.

The basic science section contains up-to-date reviews and theories focused on the most exciting research developments in pre-eclampsia. The clinical chapters provide a comprehensive review of the pertinent literature highlighting recent data and work that suggest new ideas or changes in current management. There is a section in each chapter (when appropriate) that deals with management on a practical level so that the clinician (residents/registrars/consultants) will be able to take away a formulated treatment plan that they can implement directly.

The book will be of interest to scientists and students interested in reproductive sciences as well as medical students, obstetricians and physicians with an interest in pre-eclampsia.

PART I

Basic Science

Trophoblast invasion in pre-eclampsia and other pregnancy disorders

Robert Pijnenborg, Lisbeth Vercruysse, Myriam Hanssens and F. André Van Assche

Trophoblast invasion is a major feature of hemo-chorial placentation, notably in the human where this invasion is exceptionally deep compared with the few other primate species studied so far (Ramsey *et al.*, 1976). It is assumed that pre-eclampsia/eclampsia, which occurs almost exclusively in the human species, is in some way associated with problems related to this deep invasion. So far, only a few case reports have been published suggesting a similar complication in pregnant gorillas (Baird, 1981; Thornton and Onwude, 1992). Unfortunately nothing is known about trophoblast invasion in this species.

It is now common knowledge that during pregnancy extensive vascular alterations take place in the spiral arteries which supply maternal blood to the placenta. In this chapter we will first sketch briefly the historical context of the discovery of structural changes in placental bed spiral arteries and the role of invading extravillous trophoblast. The importance of this "physiological change" of spiral arteries is highlighted by its restricted occurrence in pre-eclampsia, and there-fore we will discuss next the evidence for impaired trophoblast invasion preceding the onset of clinical symptoms of pre-eclampsia. In the third part the structural features of invaded and non-invaded spiral arteries will be described in some detail, and finally we will evaluate the occurrence of physio-logical changes and vascular lesions in other disorders of pregnancy.

Impaired physiological change in spiral arteries

Although pre-eclampsia/eclampsia has been recognized for a long time in history as an important pregnancy complication (Lindheimer *et al.*, 1999), a possible histopathological basis for this condition was only identified in the late 1960s. The idea that maternal perfusion of the placenta is disturbed in pre-eclampsia is an old one, and was based on the regular occurrence of placental infarcts in such cases (reviewed by Robertson *et al.*, 1967). Searching for associated vascular pathologies, atherosclerosis-like lesions were described in spiral arteries of decidual fragments attached to delivered placentae, and the term "acute atherosis" was introduced for the characteristic lesion of fibrinoid necrosis and accumulated foam cells (Hertig, 1945; Zeek and Assali, 1950). Following the suggestion that a reduced uterine blood flow in primigravidae predisposes to pre-eclampsia, attempts were made to measure maternal placental flow in normal and pre-eclamptic pregnancies, using a variety of techniques (reviewed by MacGillivray, 1983). Of all the early placental flow studies, the highest impact was made by the demonstration of Browne and Veall (1953) of reduced maternal blood flow in the placenta of hypertensive pregnancies. This paper provided the primary inspiration for histological work on the placental bed in the hope of identifying a pathogenic basis for the disturbed flow. It was felt that restricting oneself to vascular structures within decidual fragments attached to delivered placentas was not appropriate and therefore, for the first time, placental bed biopsies including myometrium and decidua were collected during Cesarean section (Dixon and Robertson, 1958). While looking for atherosclerotic lesions in these biopsies, however, other vascular alterations were discovered, and this was totally unexpected.

During the initial studies of placental bed biopsies it soon became obvious that in uncomplicated pregnancies normal arteries were virtually absent from both decidua and myometrium. Instead, unusual structures were observed of apparently vascular origin, which could be identified as spiral arteries only by tracing them to their origin from the radial arteries deep in the myometrium (Brosens et al., 1967). In specimens from normal pregnancies these vascular alterations, referred to as "physiological changes" to indicate that they are not pathological, consisted of the replacement of the smooth muscle wall by a fibrinoid matrix material with embedded cells (Figure 1.1a). Although the nature of the embedded cells was unknown at that time, it was postulated that they were derived from invasive trophoblast. Surprisingly, however, in specimens obtained from pre-eclamptic pregnancies recognizable arterial structures could be found readily in the inner myometrium, and it was speculated that in such cases the restricted occurrence of physiological changes was caused by inadequate trophoblast invasion, confined to the decidual segments of the spiral arteries (Brosens et al., 1972). These histological observations provided the structural basis for a new insight in maternal flow regulation to the placenta. Indeed, the physiological changes involve a loss of the musculo-elastic vascular components resulting in substantial dilatation, thus allowing an uninterrupted maternal blood supply to the placenta. It was postulated that, in the absence of vascular smooth muscle, such vessels can no longer respond to vasoactive agents. In pre-eclampsia, on the other hand,

non-converted arteries remain muscular and narrow, and maternal blood flow to the placenta must therefore be reduced. Some of these unchanged vessels may develop acute atherosis, but an important conclusion of these studies was that it is not the atherotic lesion, which occurs in only a minority of spiral arteries (Khong and Robertson, 1992), which is the main pathological defect, but the absence of physiological changes.

Meanwhile, evidence was obtained to support the hypothesis that embedded cells in physiologically changed spiral arteries are trophoblastic in nature. The presence of endovascular cells in lumina of spiral arteries had been reported in occasional first-trimester pregnancy specimens as early as 1870 by Friedländer (quoted by Boyd and Hamilton, 1970). Much later, a histological continuity was demonstrated between endovascular cells and extravillous trophoblast (Hamilton and Boyd, 1960; Harris and Ramsey, 1966). A more extensive quantitative study of trophoblast invasion in whole pregnant uteri from 8 to 18 weeks was then undertaken, which highlighted the existence of two spatial pathways, interstitial and endovascular (Pijnenborg et al., 1980, 1981, 1983). The process of interstitial trophoblast invasion of both the decidua basalis and the inner myometrium starts at the center of the implantation site and spreads toward the placental bed margins. During the early second trimester this invasion process often results in a ring-like trophoblast distribution with lower cell counts at the center of the placental bed. The interstitial mononuclear trophoblastic cells show progressive clustering and subsequently fuse to multinuclear giant cells, which are thought to be no longer invasive. Some of the interstitial trophoblastic cells may surround spiral arteries and take up a perivascular position. While during the first few weeks of pregnancy mononuclear interstitial trophoblast cells are likely to enter the spiral artery lumina in the superficial decidual compartment near the placental–decidual junction, there is no direct evidence of a direct transmural invasion of interstitial cells into the spiral arteries deeper in the myometrial compartment. On the

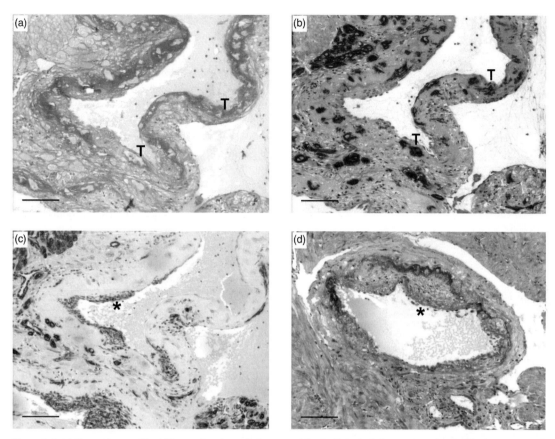

Figure 1.1 (a) Term placental bed biopsy showing spiral artery with physiological change near the decidual–myometrial junction, characterized by replacement of the smooth muscle layer by fibrinoid (darkly stained) with embedded trophoblastic cells (T). PAS staining (bar = 100 μm). (b) Same vessel. Cytokeratin immunostaining, revealing darkly stained trophoblast (T). (c) Same vessel. α-Actin immunostaining, showing replacement of the original vascular smooth muscle by fibrinoid. Streaks of intima thickening (*) stain for actin because of the presence of myofibroblasts. (d) Spiral artery with partial physiological change, showing intimal thickening (*) at the side of trophoblast invasion. PAS staining (bar = 100 μm).

contrary, histological continuity suggests an endovascular migration pathway from decidual to myometrial segments of spiral arteries, with myometrial segments being invaded from 15 weeks onwards. In the original studies a time interval of at least 1 month was found between endovascular trophoblast invasion of decidual and myometrial segments, respectively (Pijnenborg *et al.*, 1983). Based on these observations the existence of two successive waves of endovascular invasion, with a temporary halt at the decidual–myometrial junction, was postulated. In recent years this two-wave hypothesis has been criticized, mainly based on studies of first-trimester placental bed biopsies (Robson *et al.*, 2001). Since biopsy material, in contrast to complete hysterectomy specimens, does not allow judgment of the actual depth of invasion and associated changes, this question needs to be re-examined.

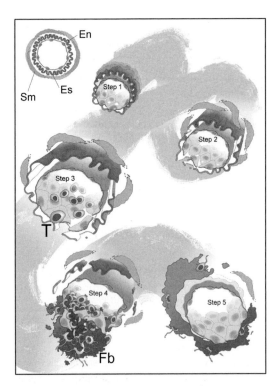

Figure 1.2 Diagrammatic representation of the different steps in spiral artery remodeling. Step 1 shows endothelial (En) vacuolization. Step 2 involves early media (Sm) disorganization and weakening of the elastica (Es), which is associated with beginning dilatation of the vessel. In step 3, endovascular trophoblast (T) appears in the arterial lumen. The next two steps are depicted as a partial physiological change. In step 4, endovascular trophoblast becomes incorporated into the vessel wall, a process associated with fibrinoid (Fb) deposition. The original smooth muscle layer and elastica is replaced by this fibrinoid material, while the embedded trophoblast acquires a "spidery" shape. The final step (5) involves endothelial repair and occasional intimal thickening (left).

In the myometrium as well as in the decidua, interstitial invasion precedes endovascular invasion. The associated spiral artery changes involve a series of steps, summarized diagrammatically in Figure 1.2 (more extensively reviewed by Pijnenborg et al., 2006). As a first step, early changes, involving vacuolation of endothelium and media, develop spontaneously, i.e. independent of the presence of the trophoblast. This first step is not restricted to the placental bed, and may therefore be associated with the decidualization process (decidua-associated early vascular remodeling). The second step leads to further media disorganization as shown by a widening of intercellular spaces resulting in a loosely structured and disrupted muscle coat. This early vascular remodeling is correlated with the presence of an interstitial trophoblast, which therefore may induce extracellular matrix changes by secretion of matrix-degrading enzymes (interstitial trophoblast-associated early vascular remodeling). As a third step, endovascular trophoblast appears in the lumina of those vessels which have undergone the early remodeling. The fourth step involves the mural incorporation of this luminal trophoblast, which must therefore penetrate the vascular endothelium. It is often stated that at this stage the trophoblast replaces the endothelium, but there are indications that the latter is never completely lost and that trophoblast may penetrate the endothelium via intercellular gaps (J. N. Bulmer, personal communication, 2003). On the other hand, there is evidence that the trophoblast is able to induce endothelial apoptosis, at least in an in vitro explant model (Ashton et al., 2005). Mural incorporation of the trophoblast is associated with the deposition of fibrinoid material, which starts to accumulate between trophoblastic cells while they are still in a luminal position (Pijnenborg, 1996). The fibrinoid with incorporated endovascular trophoblast then effectively replaces the vascular smooth muscle layer, as can be demonstrated by the absence of elastica and actin immunostaining. A remarkable feature of the fibrinoid-embedded endovascular trophoblast is that it remains mononuclear, in contrast to the interstitial trophoblast. Furthermore, these trophoblasts also show a characteristic "spidery" shape because of the presence of irregular cell extensions, which is in marked contrast to the smooth outlines of the non-fibrinoid-embedded interstitial trophoblast. The fifth and final step in the development of the "physiological changes" involves the repair of the maternal endothelium, which may be associated with intimal thickening by proliferation of myo-intimal cells of maternal origin. Since endovascular trophoblast invasion only starts after the second step of interstitial trophoblast-related initial vascular remodeling, the full physiological changes of steps four and five will develop first in the spiral arteries at the center of the placental bed, gradually moving to the more peripheral areas. Spiral artery changes therefore follow the same spatial progression through the placental bed area as the interstitial trophoblast invasion. The time course of the successive steps in the physiological change of individual spiral arteries is not known.

At the time of the first histological mapping of trophoblast invasion, all the evidence had to be derived from morphological continuities on serial histological sections using standard staining techniques such as hematoxylin and eosin (H & E) and periodic acid Schiff (PAS), because appropriate immunohistochemical technology was not yet available. Later immunohistochemical studies on early specimens largely confirmed the previously described patterns of invasion (Bulmer *et al.*, 1984; Kam *et al.*, 1999; Lyall, 2002; Robson *et al.*, 2002). Extrapolating to pre-eclampsia, it was assumed that absence of physiological changes in spiral arteries indicates a failure of the trophoblast to properly invade the spiral arteries. This also implied that, if impairment of trophoblast invasion is indeed a primary cause of pre-eclampsia, the disease must originate in early pregnancy.

Observations of restricted physiological conversion of spiral arteries in pre-eclampsia have been confirmed by many investigators over several years (Frusca *et al.*,1989; Gerretsen *et al.*, 1981; Hanssens *et al.*, 1998; Hustin *et al.*, 1983; Khong *et al.*, 1986; Lyall *et al.*, 2001b; Meekins *et al.*, 1994a; Moodley and Ramsaroop, 1989; Pijnenborg *et al.*, 1991; Sheppard and Bonnar, 1981). However, the originally proposed decidual/myometrial dichotomy, thought to reflect the two time-related waves of endovascular trophoblast invasion, was countered by the observation that restricted physiological change did not exclusively involve the myometrial

segments of the spiral arteries, but that also some of the decidual segments might show defective change (Khong *et al.*, 1986). The actual location of the spiral arteries in central or peripheral areas of the placental bed is probably an important determinant for the likelihood of failed conversion of decidual segments (Brosens, 1988).

While searching for functional correlates of the extensive vascular changes or their absence in spiral arteries, maternal placental flow patterns were studied using Doppler imaging techniques. A correlation between the resistance index of the uterine arterial circulation and the depth of physiological changes in the placental bed was indicated for the first time in a review article by McParland and Pearce (1988), and has since then been confirmed by other investigators (Aardema *et al.*, 2001; Lin *et al.*, 1995; Olofsson, 1993; Sagol *et al.*, 1999; Voigt and Becker, 1992). Flow patterns can also be obtained from individual spiral arteries. Matijevic and colleagues (1995) evaluated blood flow through central and lateral spiral arteries at 17–20 weeks, revealing lower resistance and pulsatility indices in the central arteries known to undergo physiological change at that period of gestation (Pijnenborg *et al.*, 1983). In the third trimester, women with pre-eclampsia show significantly higher impedance to flow in the spiral arteries than normotensive controls (Matijevic and Johnston, 1999). These findings therefore provide a strong support for the original hypothesis that defects in the uterine vasculature underlie impaired maternal placental blood flow.

Evidence for impaired trophoblast invasion in pre-eclampsia

Although the current understanding of trophoblast invasion patterns would imply that defective physiological change in pre-eclampsia must be the consequence of failed invasion during the first trimester, there is little direct evidence to support this view. Indeed, the absence of a trophoblast in third-trimester biopsies may result either from defective invasion, or from trophoblastic cell death induced after normal invasion in the first trimester. The fate of the two respective trophoblast invasion pathways – interstitial and endovascular – has to be reviewed separately.

Interstitial trophoblast invasion in the decidual and myometrial stroma precedes the endovascular migration into the spiral arteries. Although it is often stated that pre-eclampsia is characterized by an overall shallow invasion by trophoblast as a consequence of a failed integrin shift in the cell columns at the tips of the anchoring villi (Damsky et al., 1992; Zhou et al., 1993), this idea is not really consistent with placental bed histology. Indeed, the cell columns generate precursors of both interstitial and endovascular trophoblasts, and high numbers of interstitial trophoblasts are regularly seen in the myometrium of pre-eclamptic patients in the third trimester. Therefore, whether or not this interstitial invasion is disturbed in pre-eclampsia is not immediately clear. Initial attempts to quantify interstitial invasion by cell counts in normal and pre-eclamptic pregnancies provided highly variable results and did not reveal a significant difference (Pijnenborg et al., 1998a). A significantly decreased interstitial invasion of the myometrium was demonstrated by application of image analysis technology (Naicker et al., 2003). Since the data did not indicate absence of myometrial invasion, the term "impaired interstitial invasion" should be preferred to "shallow invasion." There are no data concerning more or less impairment of interstitial invasion in peripheral or central areas of the placental bed, which might indicate interference with the spatial spreading of invasion.

We may wonder how far impaired interstitial invasion has demonstrable effects on the invaded maternal tissue. Theoretically, such a massive invasion could have a major effect on both the anatomical and the physiological coherence of the myometrium, at least in early pregnancy when millions of cells are invading this area. It is well known now that an invasive trophoblast produces a variety of proteolytic enzymes which may induce major alterations in the extracellular matrix composition of the surrounding tissue (Huppertz et al., 1998). Furthermore, interstitial trophoblastic cells also contain steroid-converting enzymes, suggesting a local endocrine function which may possibly influence myometrial tissue growth and function (Brosens, 1977). We mentioned above that interstitial trophoblast invasion in the myometrium is related to early vascular remodeling of spiral arteries, including disorganization of the vascular smooth muscle layer, which precedes endovascular invasion (Pijnenborg et al., 1981, 1983). It was thereby postulated that early vascular disorganization might provide an essential trigger for subsequent endovascular invasion. A possible hypothesis is therefore that the early vascular remodeling is inhibited in women destined to become pre-eclamptic, and that failed or impaired interstitial trophoblast invasion might be a likely cause of this defect. However, smooth muscle disorganization is regularly observed in third-trimester myometrial spiral arteries in pre-eclampsia which had not undergone physiological change. This finding might imply that the early vascular remodeling, which is related to interstitial trophoblast invasion, may develop normally in pre-eclamptic women even if this invasion is impaired, but we should refrain from extrapolating too readily the observations in near-term placental bed biopsies to the first trimester. Gerretsen and colleagues (1983) reported that in pre-eclampsia spiral arteries without physiological changes were regularly surrounded by high numbers of multinucleated giant cells, and postulated that these invading trophoblasts had precociously differentiated to giant cells and were thereby prevented from traversing the vessel walls. Gerretsen therefore believed that also in the myometrial compartment all the endovascular trophoblast is derived from perivascular interstitial trophoblast, and, as stated earlier, in this we disagree (Pijnenborg et al., 2006). Alternatively, one could postulate that in the situation described by Gerretsen et al. the giant cells lost their capacity to induce the early vascular remodeling necessary to allow endovascular migration prematurely. In other studies, however, perivascular giant cell clustering in pre-eclampsia was not shown to be such a regular event, and therefore the hypothesis of Gerretsen *et al.* has to be treated with caution (Meekins *et al.*, 1994a).

The endovascular invasion pathway is of highest interest, since restriction in physiological changes of spiral arteries with absence of a fibrinoid-embedded endovascular trophoblast is the main defect in pre-eclampsia. An intriguing finding was that in the previously studied series of 8–18 weeks pregnant hysterectomy specimens one post-15 weeks specimen did not show endovascular trophoblast in the myometrial segments of spiral arteries, while interstitial trophoblast invasion was normal (Pijnenborg *et al.*, 1983). Of course, retrospective prediction of the development of pre-eclampsia if the pregnancy would have been allowed to continue is pointless, and without further information from other collections of first-trimester specimens, one should refrain from drawing definite conclusions from this single aberrant case.

A different possible scenario is that of a normal invasion during the first trimester, followed by the destruction of the trophoblast at a later stage. In occasional specimens endovascular trophoblast invasion is associated with marked infiltration by inflammatory cells (Figures 1.4a,b). Increased apoptosis of extravillous trophoblast has been reported in pre-eclampsia (DiFederico *et al.*, 1999), occurring mainly in the immediate surroundings of blood vessels associated with increased macrophage infiltrations (Reister *et al.*, 2001). These observations can also be related to the occasional findings of trophoblastic cell remnants in noninvaded atherotic spiral arteries in pre-eclampsia (Hanssens *et al.*, 1998; Meekins *et al.*, 1994a) (Figure 1.4d). A major inflammatory cytokine produced by macrophages is tumor necrosis factor (TNF-)α, which is potentially cytotoxic to trophoblast, as demonstrated by in vitro experiments (Yui *et al.*, 1994). Histological observations in near-term placental bed biopsies indicate higher local expression of this cytokine in pre-eclamptic patients, showing immunohistochemical localization in inflammatory cells including the foam cells of atherotic spiral arteries (Pijnenborg *et al.*, 1998b). These findings may be related to the elevated serum concentrations of TNF-α in pre-eclampsia (Keith *et al.*, 1995). Of course, it is to be expected that cytotoxic cytokines may affect interstitial as well as endovascular trophoblast. It is clear that the question of trophoblastic cell killing and the role of maternal cell-derived cytotoxic cytokines will be an important research topic in the coming years.

Histopathology of the spiral arteries in pre-eclampsia

In the previous paragraphs spiral artery histology near term, as resulting from trophoblast action on the arterial wall, was presented as a black-and-white picture: either a trophoblast had invaded the arteries and these had undergone physiological changes, or a trophoblast had not invaded and the vessels had maintained their "normal" vascular architecture, except for the occasional development of atherosis. Such black-and-white schemes do not always represent the reality. To begin with, physiological changes may not involve the whole circumference and may be restricted to only a limited sector of a vessel. Such a situation has been referred to as *"partial"* change. Sometimes only a few isolated trophoblastic cells can be seen in the arterial wall. In vessels with partial invasion we can obtain a good idea of the local effects of the endovascular trophoblast on vessel wall structure. In such cases the complete removal of media smooth muscle and elastica and its replacement by trophoblast and fibrinoid are immediately obvious, in contrast to the non-invaded sectors of the spiral artery (Figures 1.3a–d). The presence of PAS-positive fibrinoid, which is associated with endovascular invasion from early stages onwards, is thereby very helpful for delineating the extent of physiological change as induced by early endovascular invasion.

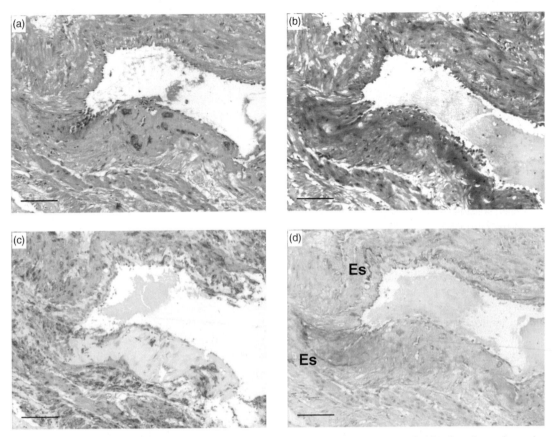

Figure 1.3 (a) Myometrial spiral artery near term showing partial physiological change. Trophoblast invasion and vascular incorporation is restricted to the lower side of the vessel. Cytokeratin immunostaining (bar = 100 µm). (b) Same artery, showing fibrinoid deposition at the lower side of the vessel. PAS staining. (c) Same artery, showing α-actin immunostaining. Smooth muscle cells have disappeared from the invaded area of the vessel wall. (d) Same artery, showing elastica (Es) staining. No elastica is present at the lower side of the vessel. Orcein staining.

As explained in a previous section, the invaded spiral arteries of the third trimester show restoration of the maternal endothelial layer, which must have been penetrated by a trophoblastic cells previously. In this matter there is confusion in the recent literature, as it is often mentioned that the endovascular trophoblast replaces the endothelium, and it is then usually understood that this is the case until the end of pregnancy. Because of the histological features of physiologically changed spiral arteries such "*endothelial replacement*" can at the most be a temporary situation, restricted to the first or early second trimester. Another matter of confusion is the claim that the trophoblast may express endothelial cell markers during its endovascular invasion (Zhou *et al.*, 1997a), which may thereby be an important factor in the so-called endothelial replacement. Expression of vascular endothelial markers by trophoblast could not be confirmed by other investigators, however (Lyall *et al.*, 2001a; Pijnenborg *et al.*, 1998a), and also a possible defective expression in pre-eclamptic women needs further confirmation (Zhou *et al.*, 1997b).

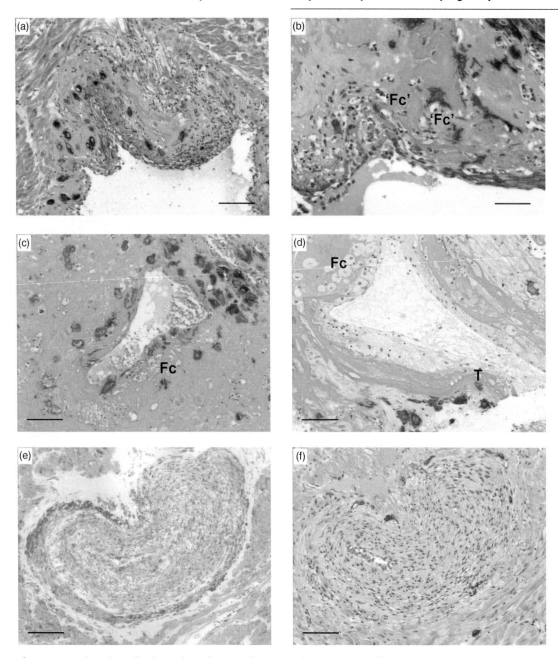

Figure 1.4 (a) Physiologically changed spiral artery, showing marked leukocytic infiltration. Cytokeratin immunostaining (bar = 100 μm). (b) Same vessel, showing swelling of infiltrated leukoytes, which are probably being converted into foam cells ("Fc") (bar = 50 μm). (c) Physiologically changed spiral artery near the basal plate. A few foam cells (Fc) are present between intramural trophoblastic cells. Cytokeratin immunostaining (bar = 100 μm). (d) Spiral artery with acute atherosis, containing foam cells (Fc) within a necrotic wall. Remnants of trophoblast (T) are present within the necrotic wall. Cytokeratin immunostaining (bar = 100 μm). (e) Myometrial spiral artery without physiological change, showing muscular hyperplasia. α-Actin immunostaining (bar = 100 μm). (f) Same vessel. Perivascular trophoblastic cells are present, presumably derived from the interstitial pathway of invasion. Cytokeratin immunostaining.

The process of endothelial repair may be associated with different degrees of *intimal thickening*, which involves proliferation of fibroblasts and the appearance of myo-intimal cells. Since the latter are immunopositive for α-actin, the occurrence of such cells may confuse inexperienced histologists who expect complete disappearance of smooth muscle in physiologically changed spiral arteries (Figures 1.1a–c). Physiologically changed vessels with thick intimal cushions can be found in decidual and myometrial spiral artery segments in normal pregnancies, but also in decidual invaded arteries in pre-eclamptic women. There is no evidence for a higher incidence of intimal thickening in decidual spiral arteries in pre-eclamptic compared to normal pregnancies, precluding more extensive maternal repair responses in pre-eclampsia (Hanssens *et al.*, 1998). In some situations intimal thickening, comprising the whole circumference of the vessel, may be so intense, even in normal pregnancies, that it leads to a narrowing of the vascular lumen, giving the false impression of a pathological lesion. A consistent observation is that with partial or isolated physiological change, intimal cushions are almost always overlying vascular sectors containing invaded trophoblast and fibrinoid (Figure 1.1d).

In the absence of trophoblast and physiological changes, spiral arteries retain an essentially normal architecture, in the sense that there is an intact medial smooth muscle layer. Nevertheless, as mentioned before, subtle changes have been noted to occur in such vessels (Pijnenborg *et al.*, 1991). One such feature is the occurrence of *endothelial vacuolation*. Furthermore, the media often shows *disorganization*, resulting in a loosely structured rather than a tightly packed muscle layer. Occasionally, the media may even become split into two layers, which may be separated by a "hyaline" substance, which may reflect alterations in the extracellular matrix. In addition, marked *medial hyperplasia* may occur, which may lead to extreme narrowing or even a virtual obliteration of the arterial lumen (Figures 1.4e,f). It is not clear at what gestational age these changes take place,

which are obviously not associated with the trophoblast-related physiological change. As suggested in the previous section, media disorganization may reflect the early spiral artery remodeling preceding endovascular invasion in the first trimester, which is related to the presence of an interstitial trophoblast (Pijnenborg *et al.*, 1983). It is possible, but hard to prove, that completely unaltered vessels at term are those that did not respond to interstitial trophoblast in the first trimester, but of course early changes may have become reversed later in pregnancy. Media hyperplasia is usually thought to result from increased blood pressure, and is therefore likely to occur more frequently in chronic hypertensive women. Endothelial vacuolation is a feature not exclusively related to the placental bed, as it also occurs in the decidua vera (Pijnenborg *et al.*, 1983). It has been argued recently that the decidualization process, which forms a necessary prelude to a well-developing pregnancy, should not be viewed exclusively as a feature of the endometrial stroma, but also involves vascular alterations such as endothelial vacuolization or early media disorganization in the inner myometrium. Indeed, there is evidence that the inner myometrium differs structurally and functionally from the outer myometrium, showing different responsiveness to steroid hormones, and therefore rather forms a functional unit with the decidua (Brosens *et al.*, 2002). It has been speculated that in some women early decidual changes of the inner myometrium may be defective from the very beginning, and thus determine pregnancy outcome from the implantation period onwards. The observation that pre-eclamptic women show a higher degree of clustering of separate spiral arteries (Starzyk *et al.*, 1997) may indeed reflect defective decidualization resulting from ineffective extracellular matrix changes and/or disturbed myometrial growth response to steroid hormones. It will not be easy, however, to distinguish systemic steroid effects from the local effects of interstitially invading trophoblast.

A completely different pathological event is the development of *acute atherosis*. Atherosclerotic-like fibrinoid necrosis with infiltration of lipid-laden foam cells represents the histopathological characteristics of this lesion, which in pregnancy-induced hypertension develops over a shorter time period than the typical hypertension-related vasculopathies in non-pregnant women. Various plasma proteins have been shown to accumulate in atherotic spiral artery walls, suggesting excessive vascular leakage. There is marked deposition of fibrin, showing analogy with the "plasmatic vasculosis" described by Lendrum (1963) in diseased kidneys. Other plasma protein accumulations such as immunoglobulins, complement components (Kitzmiller and Benirschke, 1973; Labarrere, 1988) and fibronectin (Pijnenborg *et al.*, 1992) have been detected in such vessels. Meekins and colleagues (1994b) pointed out that lipoprotein(A) deposition is an early indicator of atherotic change, but can also be found at low concentrations in normal-looking physiologically changed spiral arteries. The pathogenesis of acute atherosis is still unknown, but an immunological element has often been suspected. Robertson and colleagues (1967) pointed out the histological resemblance of acute atherosis to vascular lesions in rejected kidney allografts, which would suggest some similarity with a delayed maternal hypersensitivity response, possibly directed to fetal antigens. Infiltration of macrophage-derived foam cells sometimes occurs in physiologically changed spiral arteries containing mural trophoblasts (McFadyen *et al.*, 1986; Meekins *et al.*, 1994a) (Figure 1.4c) and, vice versa, cytokeratin-positive cell remnants, doubtless of trophoblastic origin, are occasionally found in the wall of atherotic arteries (Hanssens *et al.*, 1998; Meekins *et al.*, 1994a) (Figure 1.4d). On the other hand, acute atherosis also occurs in spiral arteries in the decidua vera, thus in the absence of trophoblasts (Robertson *et al.*, 1986), and this will need further investigation. Atherotic vessels in the placental bed are associated with infarction in the overlying placental regions (Brosens and Renaer, 1972). Extensive placental infarction could seriously interfere with proper placental function. It is, however, important to remember that acute atherosis only occurs in a relatively small number of placental bed spiral arteries (Khong and Robertson, 1992), and that placental infarctions are usually restricted in extent, so that the negative effects can normally be met by the high reserve capacity of the placenta. In our own collection of placental bed biopsies of pre-eclamptic women the incidence of acute atherosis in a biopsy containing at least one spiral artery is on average 30% (Pijnenborg *et al.*, unpublished results). Another aspect of possible importance is the depth of atherosis in the placental bed: in the majority of cases this lesion is found within the spiral arteries of the decidua basalis only, while an extension to the myometrium seems to be indicative for a more severe situation, as shown in the next section.

Vascular defects in different disorders of pregnancy

In the years immediately following the discovery of failed physiological changes in pre-eclampsia, it was assumed that this histopathological defect could be considered as pathognomonic for the disease. It was thereby thought that in other hypertensive disorders, such as essential or chronic hypertension, trophoblast invasion occurred normally, as long as no pre-eclampsia was superimposed on the pre-existing hypertension (Brosens, 1977). The finding that the physiological change of spiral arteries could also be impaired in intrauterine growth restriction without hypertension, was initially somewhat of a surprise and led to animated debates between different investigators (Brosens *et al.*, 1977; Robertson *et al.*, 1986; Sheppard and Bonnar, 1976, 1981). Especially the occurrence of acute atherosis, another putative pathognomonic feature, in non-hypertensive cases of intrauterine growth restriction (IUGR) was under discussion. One of the difficulties was how to distinguish true foam cells from senescent trophoblasts with lipid changes, and in the long run this problem could only be solved after the introduction of immunohistochemical staining techniques. Later reports confirmed restricted physiological change in spiral arteries associated with non-hypertensive IUGR (Gerretsen *et al.*, 1981; Khong *et al.*, 1986), with occasional occurrence of acute atherosis (Hanssens *et al.*, 1998; Khong, 1991).

An issue we always return to is the need for properly defining the patient populations under study, and particularly to distinguish the different categories of pregnancy-associated hypertension. Part of the problem is, of course, the ignorance of the real nature and underlying causes of the disease, and the uncertainty whether the hypertension-related symptoms represented only one or different diseases. Based upon a more extensive classification system (Davey and MacGillivray, 1988) a study on placental bed biopsies from a wide range of patients was performed (Pijnenborg *et al.*, 1991). In this series, acute atherosis was indeed limited to cases of proteinuric hypertension (classical pre-eclampsia as well as pre-eclampsia superimposed on chronic hypertension), confirming previous claims. Unexpectedly, in women with chronic hypertension (without superimposed pre-eclampsia) several cases with non-invaded spiral arteries, i.e. without physiological changes, were found. Various degrees of hyperplasia of the vascular smooth muscle layer were observed in all categories of hypertensive women. Unfortunately, the group of non-proteinuric gestational hypertensives was under-represented in this particular study. In a different series it was shown later that acute atherosis is not really restricted to pre-eclampsia, and can also occur in non-proteinuric pregnancy-induced hypertension (Hanssens *et al.*, 1998). In a small series, Frusca and colleagues (1989) found inadequate physiological change in three out of five chronic hypertensive women, one of them showing acute atherosis. A separate, more recently defined category of hypertensive pregnancy is the so-called HELLP (hemolysis, elevated liver enzymes and low platelets) syndrome. It is to be expected that in such cases histopathological findings overlap with observations in "classical" pre-eclampsia (Aardema *et al.*, 2001). In our own series, 7 out of 10 HELLP cases showed acute atherosis, which is a much higher incidence than observed in pre-eclampsia, and also the incidence of atherosis in myometrial segments (5 out of 10 cases) was unexpectedly high, compared with 8% in the pre-eclamptic group (unpublished results). These observations are compatible with the concept that the HELLP syndrome forms part of severe pre-eclampsia. It could be speculated that extension of this lesion over a longer distance of a vessel may compromise vascular function even further, also leading to an increased release of cytotoxic cytokines into the blood and surrounding tissues.

Defects in placental bed development have also been described in other groups of patients, including women with antiphospholipid antibody syndrome. Placentas of such cases may show severe infarction, and acute atherosis was observed in the attached decidual fragments (De Wolf *et al.*, 1982; Magid *et al.*, 1998). However, the only systematic study so far on placental bed biopsies from this particular group of patients showed higher concentrations of inflammatory cells, but absence of atherosis (Stone *et al.*, 2006). Recently, disturbed invasion and defective physiological changes were also found in cases of pre-term pre-labor rupture of membranes, but less frequently than in pre-eclampsia (Kim *et al.*, 2002). In diabetic women without hypertension, atherotic lesions with foam cells were described by Emmrich and colleagues (1975). In contrast, Björk and colleagues (1984) mentioned "intramural fibrosis" as the only placental bed lesion in diabetes without hypertension, but their illustrated case is clearly an example of intimal thickening, described above as a normal event. Also Pinkerton (1963) and Khong (1991) failed to detect obvious placental bed defects in such women. Also in a recent study, Jauniaux and Burton (2006) only noted disturbed spiral artery conversion in diabetic pregnancies which were complicated by chronic hypertension or pre-eclampsia. Finally, it has to be mentioned that also in some apparently normal pregnancies with normal fetal growth, defective physiological changes and pathologic lesions, even including atherosis, have been observed (Aardema *et al.*, 2001; Hanssens *et al.*, 1998).

In summary, the results of all these studies indicate that the former black-and-white picture has been replaced by the more subtle concept of a spectrum of histopathological changes that may occur throughout different disorders of pregnancy. Such a concept is also more in line with present ideas on the complexity of pregnancy-associated diseases (Brown *et al.*, 2000), which may represent different patterns of maternal pathophysiological response to early implantation or placentation defects (Roberts and Lain, 2002). In an extreme situation, when the mother cannot cope with defective early placentation, spontaneous early miscarriage would occur. Indeed, specimens of spontaneous miscarriage often show defective trophoblast invasion and physiological change in spiral arteries (Hustin *et al.*, 1990; Khong *et al.*, 1987), and this has also been shown to be the case for early pregnancy losses in women with antiphospholipid syndrome (Sebire *et al.*, 2002).

Conclusions

The discovery of physiological changes in spiral arteries and its defect in pre-eclampsia provided a major advance in the understanding of pre-eclampsia and pregnancy-associated hypertension in general. These findings highlighted the importance of trophoblast invasion, an aspect of placentation which until then was merely regarded as a curiosity without obvious meaning. Extensive clinical studies led to the realization that pregnancy-induced hypertension is a complex process, which usually finds its cause in early pregnancy, but may depend on different maternal physiological responses. This may be reflected by the variable patterns of histopathological change in the placental bed, illustrating a spectrum of arterial changes in different pregnancy complications,

rather than a black-and-white picture of pathognomonic well-defined lesions. Advance in the field needs a double approach, requiring on the one hand better clinical and physiological characterization of patients, and on the other hand a better understanding of the cellular aspects of placentation and trophoblast invasion.

Acknowledgment

We are grateful to Tom Pijnenborg for producing an artistic representation of the physiological change of spiral arteries in Figure 1.2.

REFERENCES

Aardema, M. W., Oosterhof, H., Timmer, A., van Rooy, I. and Aarnoudse, J. G. (2001). Uterine artery Doppler flow and uteroplacental vascular pathology in normal pregnancies and pregnancies complicated by pre-eclampsia and small for gestational age fetuses. *Placenta*, **22**, 405–11.

Ashton, S. V., Whitley, G. StJ., Dash, P. R., Wareing, M., Crocker, I. P., Baker, P. N. and Cartwright, J. E. (2005). Uterine spiral artery remodeling involves endothelial apoptosis induced by extravillous trophoblasts through Fas/FasL interactions. *Arterioscler. Thromb. Vasc. Biol.*, **25**, 102–8.

Baird, J. N. Jr. (1981). Eclampsia in a lowland gorilla. *Am. J. Obstet. Gynecol.*, **141**, 345–6.

Björk, O., Persson, B., Stangenberg, M. and Vaclavinkova, V. (1984). Spiral artery lesions in relation to metabolic control in diabetes mellitus. *Acta Obstet. Gynecol. Scand.*, **63**, 123–7.

Boyd, J. D. and Hamilton, W. J. (1970). *The Human Placenta*. Cambridge: W. Heffer.

Brosens, I. A. (1977). Morphological changes in the utero-placental bed in pregnancy hypertension. *Clin. Obstet. Gynaecol.*, **4**, 573–93.

Brosens, I. A. (1988). The utero-placental vessels at term – the distribution and extent of the physiological changes. *Trophoblast Res.*, **3**, 61–7.

Brosens, I. and Renaer, M. (1972). On the pathogenesis of placental infarcts in pre-eclampsia. *J. Obstet. Gynaec. Br. Cwlth*, **79**, 794–9.

Brosens, I., Robertson, W. B. and Dixon, H. G. (1967). The physiological response of the vessels of the placental bed to normal pregnancy. *J. Path. Bact.*, **93**, 569–79.

Brosens, I. A., Robertson, W. B. and Dixon, H. G. (1972). The role of spiral arteries in the pathogenesis of preeclampsia. In *Obstetrics and Gynecology Annual*, ed. R. M. Wynn. New York: Appleton-Century-Crofts, pp. 177–91.

Brosens, I., Dixon, H. G. and Robertson, W. B. (1977). Fetal growth retardation and the arteries of the placental bed. *Br. J. Obstet. Gynaecol.*, **84**, 656–63.

Brosens, J. J., Pijnenborg, R. and Brosens, I. (2002). The myometrial junctional zone spiral arteries in normal and abnormal pregnancies. *Am. J. Obstet. Gynecol.*, **187**, 1416–23.

Brown, M. A., Hague, W. M., Higgins, J., *et al.* (2000). The detection, investigation and management of hypertension in pregnancy: full consensus statement. *Aust. N. Z. J. Obstet. Gynaecol.*, **40**, 139–55.

Browne, J. C. M. and Veall, N. (1953). The maternal placental blood flow in normotensive and hypertensive women. *J. Obstet. Gyn. Br. Emp.*, **60**, 141–8.

Bulmer, J. N., Billington, W. D. and Johnson, P. M. (1984). Immunohistologic identification of trophoblast populations in early human pregnancy with the use of monoclonal antibodies. *Am. J. Obstet. Gynecol.*, **148**, 19–26.

Damsky, C. H., Fitzgerald, M. L. and Fisher, S. J. (1992). Distribution patterns of extracellular matrix components and adhesion receptors are intricately modulated during first trimester cytotrophoblast differentiation along the invasive pathway, in vivo. *J. Clin. Invest.*, **89**, 210–22.

Davey, D. A. and MacGillivray, I. (1988). The classification and definition of the hypertensive disorders of pregnancy. *Am. J. Obstet. Gynecol.*, **158**, 892–989.

De Wolf, F., Carreras, L. O., Moerman, P., Vermylen, J., Van Assche, A. and Renaer, M. (1982). Decidual vasculopathy and extensive placental infarction in a patient with repeated thromboembolic accidents, recurrent fetal loss, and a lupus anticoagulant. *Am. J. Obstet. Gynecol.*, **142**, 829–34.

DiFederico, E., Genbacev, O. and Fisher, S. J. (1999). Preeclampsia is associated with widespread apoptosis of placental cytotrophoblasts within the uterine wall. *Am. J. Pathol.*, **155**, 293–301.

Dixon, H. G. and Robertson, W. B. (1958). A study of the vessels of the placental bed in normotensive and hypertensive women. *J. Obstet. Gyn. Br. Emp.*, **65**, 803–9.

Emmrich, P., Birke, R. and Gödel, E. (1975). Beitrag zur Morphologie der myometrialen und dezidualen Arterien bei normalen Schwangerschaften, EPH-Gestosen und mütterlichem Diabetes mellitus. *Path. Microbiol.*, **43**, 38–61.

Frusca, T., Morassi, L., Pecorelli, S., Grigolato, P. and Gastaldi, A. (1989). Histological features of uteroplacental vessels in normal and hypertensive patients in relation to birthweight. *Br. J. Obstet. Gynaecol.*, **96**, 835–9.

Gerretsen, G., Huisjes, H. J. and Elema, J. D. (1981). Morphological changes of the spiral arteries in the placental bed in relation to pre-eclampsia and fetal growth retardation. *Br. J. Obstet. Gynaecol.*, **88**, 876–81.

Gerretsen, G., Huisjes, H. J., Hardonk, M. J. and Elema, J. D. (1983). Trophoblast alterations in the placental bed in relation to physiological changes in spiral arteries. *Br. J. Obstet. Gynaecol.*, **90**, 34–9.

Hamilton, W. J. and Boyd, J. D. (1960). Development of the human placenta in the first three months of gestation. *J. Anat.*, **94**, 297–328.

Hanssens, M., Pijnenborg, R., Keirse, M. J. N. C., Vercruysse, L., Verbist, L. and Van Assche, F. A. (1998). Renin-like immunoreactivity in uterus and placenta from normotensive and hypertensive pregnancies. *Eur. J. Obstet. Gynecol. Reprod. Biol.*, **81**, 177–84.

Harris, J. W. S. and Ramsey, E. M. (1966). The morphology of human uteroplacental vasculature. *Contrib. Embryol.*, **38**, 43–58.

Hertig, A. T. (1945). Vascular pathology in the hypertensive albuminuric toxaemias of pregnancy. *Clinics*, **4**, 602–14.

Huppertz, B., Kertschanska, S., Demir, A. Y., Frank, H.-G. and Kaufmann, P. (1998). Immunohistochemistry of matrix metalloproteinases (MMP), their substrates, and their inhibitors (TIMP) during trophoblast invasion in the human placenta. *Cell Tissue Res.*, **291**, 133–48.

Hustin, J., Foidart, J. M. and Lambotte, R. (1983). Maternal vascular lesions in pre-eclampsia and intrauterine growth retardation: light microscopy and immunofluorescence. *Placenta*, **4**, 489–98.

Hustin, J., Jauniaux, E. and Schaaps, J. P. (1990). Histological study of the materno-embryonic interface in spontaneous abortion. *Placenta*, **11**, 477–86.

Jauniaux, E. and Burton, G. J. (2006). Villous histomorphometry and placental bed biopsy investigation in type I diabetic pregnancies. *Placenta*, **27**, 468–74.

Kam, E. P. Y., Gardner, L., Loke, Y. W. and King, A. (1999). The role of trophoblast in the physiological change in decidual spiral arteries. *Hum. Reprod.*, **14**, 2131–8.

Keith, J. C. Jr., Pijnenborg, R., Spitz, B., Hanssens, M. and Van Assche, F. A. (1995). Assessment of differential serum cytotoxicity in gestational hypertension using a fibrosarcoma cell line and the MTT assay. *Hypertens. Pregnancy*, **14**, 81–90.

Khong, T. Y. (1991). Acute atherosis in pregnancies complicated by hypertension, small-for-gestational-age infants, and diabetes mellitus. *Arch. Pathol. Lab. Med.*, **115**, 722–5.

Khong, T. Y. and Robertson, W. B. (1992). Spiral artery disease. In *Immunological Obstetrics*, ed. C. B. Coulam, W. P. Faulk and J. McIntyre. New York, Norton, pp. 492–501.

Khong, T. Y., De Wolf, F., Robertson, W. B. and Brosens, I. (1986). Inadequate maternal vascular response to placentation in pregnancies complicated by pre-eclampsia and by small-for-gestational age infants. *Br. J. Obstet. Gynaecol.*, **93**, 1049–59.

Khong, T. Y., Liddell, H. S. and Robertson, W. B. (1987). Defective haemochorial placentation as a cause of miscarriage: a preliminary study. *Br. J. Obstet. Gynaecol.*, **94**, 649–55.

Kim, Y. M., Chaiworapongsa, T., Gomez, R., *et al.* (2002). Failure of physiologic transformation of the spiral arteries in the placental bed in preterm premature rupture of membranes. *Am. J. Obstet. Gynecol.*, **187**, 1137–42.

Kitzmiller, J. L. and Benirschke, K. (1973). Immunofluorescent study of placental bed vessels in pre-eclampsia of pregnancy. *Am. J. Obstet. Gynecol.*, **115**, 248–51.

Labarrere, C. A. (1988). Acute atherosis. A histopathological hallmark of immune aggression? *Placenta*, **9**, 95–108.

Lendrum, A. C. (1963). The hypertensive diabetic kidney as a model of the so-called collagen diseases. *Canad. Med. Ass. J.*, **88**, 442–52.

Lin, S., Shimizu, I., Suehara, N., Nakayama, M. and Aono, T. (1995). Uterine artery Doppler velocimetry in relation to trophoblast migration into the myometrium of the placental bed. *Obstet. Gynecol.*, **85**, 760–5.

Lindheimer M. D., Roberts, J. M., Cunningham, F. G. and Chesley, L. (1999). Introduction, history, controversies, and definitions. In *Chesley's Hypertensive Disorders in Pregnancy*, eds. M. D. Lindheimer, J. M. Roberts and F. G. Cunningham. Stamford, CT: Appleton & Lange, pp. 3–41.

Lyall, F. (2002). The human placental bed revisited. *Placenta*, **23**, 555–62.

Lyall, F., Bulmer, J. N., Duffie, E., Cousins, F., Theriault, A. and Robson, S. C. (2001a). Human trophoblast invasion and spiral artery transformation. The role of PECAM-1 in normal pregnancy, preeclampsia, and fetal growth restriction. *Am. J. Pathol.*, **158**, 1713–21.

Lyall, F., Simpson, H., Bulmer, J. N., Barber, A. and Robson, S. C. (2001b). Transforming growth factor-β expression in human placenta and placental bed in third trimester normal pregnancy, preeclampsia, and fetal growth restriction. *Am. J. Pathol.*, **159**, 1827–38.

MacGillivray, I. (1983). *Pre-eclampsia, the Hypertensive Disease of Pregnancy*. London: WB Saunders Company Ltd, pp. 78–82.

Magid, M. S., Kaplan, C., Sammaritano, L. R., Peterson, M., Druzin, M. L. and Lockshin, M. D. (1998). Placental pathology in systemic lupus erythematosus: a prospective study. *Am. J. Obstet. Gynecol.*, **179**, 226–34.

Matijevic, R. and Johnston, T. (1999). In vivo assessment of failed trophoblastic invasion of the spiral arteries in pre-eclampsia. *Br. J. Obstet. Gynaecol.*, **106**, 78–82.

Matijevic, R., Meekins, J. W., Walkinshaw, S. A., Neilson, J. P. and McFadyen I. R. (1995). Spiral artery blood flow in the central and peripheral areas of the placental bed in the second trimester. *Obstet. Gynecol.*, **86**, 289–92.

McFadyen, I. R., Price, A. B. and Geirsson, R. T. (1986). The relation of birthweight to histological appearances in vessels of the placental bed. *Br. J. Obstet. Gynaecol.*, **93**, 476–81.

McParland, P. and Pearce, J. M. (1988). Doppler blood flow in pregnancy. *Placenta*, **9**, 427–50.

Meekins, J. W., Pijnenborg, R., Hanssens, M., McFadyen, I. R. and Van Assche, A. (1994a). A study of placental bed spiral arteries and trophoblast invasion in normal and severe pre-eclamptic pregnancies. *Br. J. Obstet. Gynaecol.*, **101**, 669–74.

Meekins, J. W., Pijnenborg, R., Hanssens, M., Van Assche, A. and McFadyen, I. R. (1994b). Immunohistochemical detection of lipoprotein(a) in the wall of placental bed spiral arteries in normal and severe pre-eclamptic pregnancies. *Placenta*, **15**, 511–24.

Moodley, J. and Ramsaroop, R. (1989). Placental bed morphology in black women with eclampsia. *S. Afr. Med. J.*, **75**, 376–8.

Naicker, T., Khedun, S.M., Moodley, J. and Pijnenborg, R. (2003). Quantitative analysis of trophoblast invasion in pre-eclampsia. *Acta Obstet. Gynecol. Scand.*, **82**, 722–9.

Olofsson, P. (1993). A high uterine artery pulsatility index reflects a defective development of placental bed spiral arteries in pregnancies complicated by hypertension and fetal growth retardation. *Eur. J. Obstet. Gynecol. Reprod. Biol.*, **49**, 161–8.

Pijnenborg, R. (1996). The placental bed. *Hypertens. Pregnancy*, **15**, 7–23.

Pijnenborg, R., Anthony, J., Davey, D.A., *et al.* (1991). Placental bed spiral arteries in the hypertensive disorders of pregnancy. *Br. J. Obstet. Gynaecol.*, **98**, 648–55.

Pijnenborg, R., Bland, J.M., Robertson, W.B. and Brosens, I. (1983). Uteroplacental arterial changes related to interstitial trophoblast migration in early human pregnancy. *Placenta*, **4**, 397–414.

Pijnenborg, R., Bland, J.M., Robertson, W.B., Dixon, G. and Brosens, I. (1981). The pattern of interstitial trophoblastic invasion of the myometrium in early human pregnancy. *Placenta*, **2**, 303–16.

Pijnenborg, R., Dixon, G., Robertson, W.B. and Brosens, I. (1980). Trophoblastic invasion of human decidua from 8 to 18 weeks of pregnancy. *Placenta*, **1**, 3–19.

Pijnenborg, R., McLaughlin, P.J., Vercruysse, L., *et al.* (1998b). Immunolocalization of tumor necrosis factor-α (TNF-α) in the placental bed of normotensive and hypertensive human pregnancies. *Placenta*, **19**, 231–9.

Pijnenborg, R., Vercruysse, L., Ballegeer, V., *et al.* (1992). The distribution of fibronectin in the placental bed in normotensive and hypertensive human pregnancies. *Trophoblast Res.*, **6**, 343–50.

Pijnenborg, R., Vercruysse, L. and Hanssens, M. (2006). The uterine spiral arteries in human pregnancy: facts and controversies. *Placenta*, **27**, 939–58.

Pijnenborg, R., Vercruysse, L., Verbist, L. and Van Assche, F.A. (1998a). Interaction of interstitial trophoblast with placental bed capillaries and venules of normotensive and pre-eclamptic pregnancies. *Placenta*, **19**, 569–75.

Pinkerton, J.H.M. (1963). The placental bed arterioles in diabetes. *Proc. R. Soc. Med.*, **56**, 1021–2.

Ramsey, E.M., Houston, M.L. and Harris, J.W.S. (1976). Interactions of the trophoblast and maternal tissues in three closely related primate species. *Am. J. Obstet. Gynecol.*, **124**, 647–52.

Reister, F., Frank, H.-G., Kingdom, J.C.P., *et al.* (2001). Macrophage-induced apoptosis limits endovascular trophoblast invasion in the uterine wall of preeclamptic women. *Lab. Invest.*, **81**, 1143–52.

Roberts, J.M. and Lain, K.Y. (2002). Recent insights into the pathogenesis of pre-eclampsia. *Placenta*, **23**, 359–72.

Robertson, W.B., Brosens, I. and Dixon, H.G. (1967). The pathological response of the vessels of the placental bed to hypertensive pregnancy. *J. Path. Bact.*, **93**, 581–92.

Robertson, W.B., Khong, T.Y., Brosens, I., De Wolf, F., Sheppard, B.L. and Bonnar, J. (1986). The placental bed biopsy: review from three European centres. *Am. J. Obstet. Gynecol.*, **155**, 401–12.

Robson, S.C., Ball, E., Lyall, F., Simpson, H., Ayis, S. and Bulmer, J. (2001). Endovascular trophoblast invasion and spiral artery transformation: the 'two wave' theory revisited. *Placenta*, **22**, A.25.

Robson, S.C., Simpson, H., Ball, E., Lyall, F. and Bulmer, J.N. (2002). Punch biopsy of the human placental bed. *Am. J. Obstet. Gynecol.*, **187**, 1349–55.

Sagol, S., Özkinay, E., Öztekin, K. and Özdemir, N. (1999). The comparison of uterine artery Doppler velocimetry with the histopathology of the placental bed. *Aust. N.Z.J. Obstet. Gynaec.*, **39**, 324–9.

Sebire, N.J., Fox, H., Backos, M., Rai, R., Paterson, C. and Regan, L. (2002). Defective endovascular trophoblast invasion in primary antiphospholipid antibody syndrome-associated early pregnancy failure. *Hum. Reprod.*, **17**, 1067–71.

Sheppard, B.L. and Bonnar, J. (1976). The ultrastructure of the arterial supply of the human placenta in pregnancy complicated by fetal growth retardation. *Br. J. Obstet. Gynaecol.*, **83**, 948–59.

Sheppard, B.L. and Bonnar, J. (1981). An ultrastructural study of utero-placental spiral arteries in hypertensive and normotensive pregnancy and fetal growth retardation. *Br. J. Obstet. Gynaecol.*, **88**, 695–705.

Starzyk, K.A., Salafia, C.M., Pezzullo, J.C., *et al.* (1997). Quantitative differences in arterial morphometry define the placental bed in preeclampsia. *Hum. Pathol.*, **28**, 353–8.

Stone, S., Pijnenborg R., Vercruysse, L., *et al.* (2006). The placental bed in pregnancies complicated by primary antiphospholipid syndrome. *Placenta*, **27**, 457–67.

Thornton, J.G. and Onwude, J.L. (1992). Convulsions in pregnancy in related gorillas. *Am. J. Obstet. Gynecol.*, **167**, 240–1.

Voigt, H.J. and Becker, V. (1992). Doppler flow measurements and histomorphology of the placental bed in uteroplacental insufficiency. *J. Perinat. Med.*, **20**, 139–47.

Yui, J., Garcia-Lloret, M., Wegmann, T. G. and Guilbert, L. J. (1994). Cytotoxicity of tumor necrosis factor-alpha and gamma-interferon against primary human placental trophoblasts. *Placenta*, **15**, 819–35.

Zeek, P. M. and Assali, N. S. (1950). Vascular changes in the decidua associated with eclamptogenic toxemia of pregnancy. *Am. J. Clin. Path.*, **20**, 1099–109.

Zhou, Y., Damsky, C. H., Chiu, K., Roberts, J. M. and Fisher, S. J. (1993). Preeclampsia is associated with abnormal expression of adhesion molecules by invasive cytotrophoblasts. *J. Clin. Invest.*, **91**, 950–60.

Zhou, Y., Damsky, C. H. and Fisher, S. J. (1997b). Preeclampsia is associated with failure of human cytotrophoblasts to mimic a vascular adhesion phenotype. *J. Clin. Invest.*, **99**, 2152–64.

Zhou, Y., Fisher, S. J., Janatpour, M. J., *et al.* (1997a). Human cytotrophoblasts adopt a vascular phenotype as they differentiate. A strategy for successful endovascular invasion? *J. Clin. Invest.*, **99**, 2139–51.

2

Development of the utero-placental circulation: purported mechanisms for cytotrophoblast invasion in normal pregnancy and pre-eclampsia

Fiona Lyall

Introduction: the placental bed

The placental bed underlies the fetal placenta and includes the decidua basalis and the underlying myometrium containing the uterine spiral arteries. In order to establish human hemochorial placentation and to provide a progressive increase in blood supply to the growing fetus, the placental bed spiral arteries must undergo considerable alterations. These physiological modifications are thought to be brought about by the interaction of invasive cytotrophoblast with the spiral artery vessel wall. Failure of spiral artery transformation is thought to play an important role in the sequence of events which gives rise to pre-eclampsia. The mechanisms that control human trophoblast invasion in normal, let alone abnormal pregnancy, are still poorly understood. This is partly due to difficulties in obtaining "true" placental bed biopsies.

Much of the information on the early physiological changes within the placental bed comes from unique studies on intact hysterectomy specimens (Pijnenborg et al., 1981) Details of trophoblast invasion during late pregnancy and in pregnancies complicated by pre-eclampsia and fetal growth restriction is principally derived from the study of placental bed biopsies taken at the time of Cesarean section. Placental bed biopsies may not be representative of the whole placental bed. To help circumvent this problem, multiple biopsies combined with large numbers of cases should help to provide a more representative picture. The entire blood vessel will not be present in a single biopsy, thus limiting our interpretation of what is happening along its full length. Great care must be taken in distinguishing between veins and transformed spiral arteries, and mistakes can easily be made. The methods of sampling the placental bed along with advantages, pitfalls and success rates have recently been reviewed elsewhere (Lyall, 2002). Due to the difficulties in obtaining placental bed biopsies, many investigators have relied on in vitro models of trophoblast invasion. While in vitro models can be extremely useful in dissecting out some of these processes, the invasive process is no longer occurring in its natural environment and may be open to artefacts. Thus the interpretation of such studies must be tempered with a degree of caution. The mechanisms underlying normal and failed trophoblast invasion appear to be complex. Evidence to date suggests that these will involve several factors. In this chapter the mechanisms which control the invasion of trophoblast into the decidua and myometrium are reviewed. Along with this is a review of the purported mechanisms underlying failed spiral artery transformation. Particular emphasis has been placed on topics which, in the author's opinion, have been where the most exciting developments have been made.

Extravillous trophoblast

Extravillous trophoblast (EVT) is made up of all trophoblasts found outside the villi. EVT are primarily mononuclear cells, although syncytial or multinucleated cells are also found, mainly in the deeper parts of the junctional zone. EVT are found in the chorionic plate, the smooth chorion, cell islands, cell columns, the basal plate, the placental septa and in the walls and lumen of uteroplacental vessels. EVT is a highly migratory, proliferative and invasive population of cells which emerge from tips of anchoring villi. Trophoblast invasion of the uterus involves attachment of the cells to the extracellular matrix, degradation of the matrix and subsequent migration. It is a tightly controlled process regulated by decidual cells, the trophoblast cells themselves and many diffusible factors within the placental bed.

Trophoblast invasion during normal pregnancy and pre-eclampsia

The basic changes that occur as cytotrophoblasts invade the uterus has been covered in much more detail in the chapter by Dr. Pijnenborg. EVT proliferate from the tips of anchoring chorionic villi to form a shell lining the uterine cavity. Two populations of EVT can be identified. Interstitial cytotrophoblasts invade the decidual stroma and superficial myometrium (Pijnenborg et al., 1981, 1983). The second population of EVT are endovascular cytotrophoblasts, which invade the lumen of the spiral arteries (Robertson et al., 1986). This process of trophoblast invasion leads to the transformation of the normally small muscular arteries into distended flaccid vessels. Myometrial arteries from women with pre-eclampsia often fail to show evidence of physiological change (Brosens et al., 1972; Pijnenborg et al., 1991). Decidual arteries also often show abnormalities (Khong et al., 1986; Meekins et al., 1994). The result of these defective vascular changes is that blood flow into the intervillous space is dramatically reduced in pre-eclampsia.

Markers of trophoblast

To study the mechanisms controlling trophoblast invasion it is important to be able to identify proliferating and/or extravillous trophoblast. Proliferation markers used include Ki-67, MIB-1, antibodies against proliferating cell nuclear antigen (PCNA) or ^{3}H-thymidine (Bulmer et al., 1988; King and Blankenship, 1993; Kohnen et al., 1993; Kosanke, 1994; Mühlhauser et al., 1993). Cytokeratins are related to differentiation and proliferation of epithelial cells and this appears to include trophoblast cells. Thus cytokeratin antibodies are often used to identify EVT (Mühlhauser et al., 1993). These studies have shown that trophoblasts express different cytokeratins according to their state of differentiation and development.

Trophoblast invasion: the extracellular matrix and cell adhesion molecules

Cell adhesion molecules (CAMs) expressed on the surface of invasive cytotrophoblasts interact with the extracellular matrix (ECM) in the decidua to control invasion. The ECM of tissues is composed of a variety of proteins and polysaccharides assembled into an organized meshwork and are mainly produced by cells within the matrix (Alberts et al., 1994; Birk et al., 1991; Kreis and Vale, 1993). In most connective tissues, matrix molecules are secreted by fibroblasts or overlying epithelial sheets. The two main classes of molecules that make up the matrix are (i) polysaccharide chains of the glycosaminoglycan (GAG) class and (ii) fibrous proteins of two functional types: those which are mainly structural, e.g. collagen and elastin, and those which mainly play a role in attachment, e.g. fibronectin and laminin.

Cell adhesion molecules

The adhesion of cells to each other, to other cell types and to the ECM relies on the expression of CAMs and their ligands. At implantation, the trophoectoderm attaches to the uterine epithelial surface and CAMs play a major role. Interstitial and intravascular invasion of maternal tissue by trophoblast requires a new repertoire of CAM expression. Understanding the part played by adhesion molecules in pregnancy is paramount because pre-eclampsia as well as several pregnancy-associated disorders including fetal growth restriction, miscarriage and infertility problems have been linked to abnormalities in expression of particular CAMs and/or their ligands (Lyall, 1998). The majority of CAMs fall into one of four families: the immunoglobulin superfamily, the integrins, the selectins and the cadherins.

The cadherins include E-, N-, P-, R-, B- and VE-cadherins. The integrins bind to extracellular matrix proteins (fibronectin, fibrinogen, laminin, collagen, thrombospondin, vitronectin and von Willebrand factor) and to members of the immunoglobulin superfamily such as intercellular adhesion molecule (ICAM)-1, 2 and 3, and vascular cell adhesion molecule (VCAM). All integrins are made up of two subunits, α and β. The $\alpha\beta$ pairing determines the binding specificities. The immunoglobulin family can act as calcium-independent intercellular adhesion molecules, signal-transducing receptors, or both. This family includes platelet endothelial cell adhesion molecule (PECAM-1), VCAM-1 and ICAM-1, 2 and 3. Although interactions between identical and non-identical family members are common amongst members of the immunoglobulin super-family, non-members have also been identified as ligands. These include LFA-1 and Mac-1 which bind ICAM-1 and VLA-4 and $\alpha 4\beta 7$ which bind VCAM-1. Additional receptors include components of the ECM including collagen, heparin and heparan sulfate. Selectins are a group of cell adhesion molecules that bind to carbohydrates expressed on cells. The three members of this family, E-, P- and L-selectin, are involved in leukocyte extravasation.

Cytotrophoblast invasion and cell adhesion molecules

Cytotrophoblast invasion is analogous to tumor progression. It is accompanied by a reduction in proliferation as well as expression of specific proteinases (Fisher *et al.*, 1989; Vicovac and Aplin, 1996). All highly invasive cells have altered expression of CAM phenotypes and matrix-degrading enzymes (Alexander and Werb, 1991). This is also the case for invasive cytotrophoblast.

In vivo studies suggest cytotrophoblast invasion is associated with switching of integrins and altered extracellular matrix expression

Much of the information on the mechanisms of human trophoblast invasion has come from studies on placental bed biopsies; these contain basal decidua and underlying myometrium with one or more uteroplacental (spiral) arteries. Immunohistochemical approaches have been used to study adhesion molecules and ECM components on first-trimester implantation sites. It is important to note that adhesion by integrins can also be mediated by switching from high- to low-affinity states without altered expression (Mould *et al.*, 1995). Such studies suggest that marked changes in the expression of adhesion molecules and ECM components occur in parallel to the spatial distribution of cytotrophoblasts from the chorionic villi through to the uterine wall; however, the exact timing of these changes is unknown.

In the villi, where cytotrophoblasts exist as an epithelial monolayer anchored to the trophoblast basement membrane, trophoblast cells express integrin ECM receptors typical of many polarized epithelia (Carter *et al.*, 1990; Larjava *et al.*, 1990). $\alpha6/\beta4$ is the major integrin expressed by cytotrophoblasts in villi (Aplin, 1993; Burrows *et al.*, 1994; Damsky *et al.*, 1992, 1994; Korhonen *et al.*, 1991), while about a third of villous cytotrophoblasts weakly express $\alpha3/\beta1$. Within cell columns, where cytotrophoblasts are no longer associated with the basement membrane, fibronectin and collagen IV are no longer expressed. There is also a selective down-regulation of laminin production by cytotrophoblast (Church *et al.*, 1997; Damsky *et al.*, 1992; Leivo *et al.*, 1989). The $\alpha3$ integrin is no longer detectable; however, $\alpha6/\beta4$ remains intensely expressed (Damsky *et al.*, 1992). Absence of proteins may also be due to the activity of matrix-degrading enzymes.

In the distal regions of the columns, cellular fibronectin (A^+B^+) and collagen IV expression increases (Damsky *et al.*, 1992), moreover, onco-fetal fibronectin can be found (Feinberg and Kliman, 1993). The source of these is probably the cytotrophoblast. Matching the increase in fibronectin is a marked increase in the $\alpha5/\beta1$ subunits of the fibronectin receptor on cytotrophoblast cells (MacCalman and Chen, 1998), while the laminin receptor $\alpha6/\beta4$ decreases (Aplin, 1993; Damsky *et al.*, 1992), although one study identified $\alpha6$ in at least some cytotrophoblasts infiltrating the decidua (Aplin *et al.*, 1990).

Within the placental bed cytotrophoblast cells exist as single cells or clusters of cells. Here they express $\alpha1/\beta1$ and $\alpha5/\beta1$ integrins (Damsky *et al.*, 1992). In this area, decidual cells express $\alpha1/\beta1$ and $\alpha6/\beta1$ integrins (Damsky *et al.*, 1992) and they interact primarily with matrix associated with maternal cells, i.e. fibronectin A^+B^+, collagen IV and laminins A ($\alpha1$), B1 ($\beta1$), B2 ($\gamma1$) and M ($\alpha2$). Different from the basal layer of stem cells, secretion of the ECM is not polarized but appears all over the surface of the cells (Castellucci *et al.*, 1991; Huppertz *et al.*, 1996). The matrix is no longer homogenous but shows a patchy mosaic pattern. Collagen IV laminin, heparan sulfate, fibronectins and vitronectins can be detected but not collagens I, III, VI or fibrin.

In vitro studies also suggest that invasion is associated with switching of integrin repertoires

Studies have been performed on cytotrophoblasts isolated from first-trimester human placentas. The cells are plated onto a porous filter coated with a reconstituted basement membrane material, matrigel. The isolated cytotrophoblasts attach, migrate and form aggregates and then penetrate the matrigel (Damsky *et al.*, 1994). Cytotrophoblasts within the matrigel produce ECM molecules characteristic of those produced by cells about to enter the uterine wall, i.e. fibronectin, type IV collagen and laminins A ($\alpha1$), B1 ($\beta1$) and B2 ($\gamma1$). The integrin pattern also generally matches that seen in vivo, i.e. strong immunostaining for $\beta1$, $\alpha1$ and $\alpha5$ subunits while $\beta4$ and $\alpha6$ immunostaining is markedly reduced (Damsky *et al.*, 1994).

Antibody perturbation studies suggest that cytotrophoblast–fibronectin and cytotrophoblast–collagen/laminin interactions appear to have opposing effects (Damsky *et al.*, 1994; Librach *et al.*, 1991a). $\alpha1/\beta1$-laminin/collagen interactions promote invasion whereas $\alpha5/\beta1$–fibronectin interactions restrain invasion. Late gestation cytotrophoblasts, which have a greatly decreased invasive capacity, are unable to upregulate $\alpha1/\beta1$, providing further evidence that $\alpha1/\beta1$, is important for invasion. Studies to identify the mechanisms involved in cytotrophoblast invasion have also been performed using villous tissue co-cultured with decidua parietalis (Vicovac *et al.*, 1995). In this model, contact with the decidua stimulates formation of columns. The columns show similar alterations to those seen in vivo, including induction of $\alpha5/\beta1$ and loss of $\alpha6/\beta4$. However, not all studies agree; one study has shown that blocking $\alpha5/\beta1$ inhibits trophoblast invasion in vitro (Irving and Lala, 1995). Differences in findings may reflect unknown differences in experimental conditions.

Invading cytotrophoblast cells express endothelial CAMs

More recent studies have suggested that cytotrophoblast cells that invade spiral arteries switch their adhesion molecule repertoire so as to mimic an endothelial phenotype (Zhou et al., 1997a). Immunohistochemistry performed on chorionic villi and placental bed biopsies demonstrated the following: in second-trimester tissue, of the αv integrins, αv/β5 was detected on cytotrophoblast on chorionic villi and αv/β6 was detected at sites of column formation and on the first cell layers. However, αv/β3 expression was enhanced on cytotrophoblasts that had invaded the uterine wall and maternal vasculature but was weak on villous cytotrophoblast or initial layers of the cell columns.

E-cadherin expression is intense on cytotrophoblasts in contact with one another and on syncytiotrophoblasts. It is reduced on cytotrophoblasts in cell columns near the uterine wall and on cytotrophoblasts within the decidua or maternal blood vessels (MacCalman et al., 1995; Winterhager et al., 1996; Zhou et al., 1997a). Paradoxically, E-cadherin expression is intense in cytotrophoblast in all locations in term placentae, a time when cytotrophoblast invasion is minimal. A marked reduction in E-cadherin expression occurs during synctialization (Coutifaris et al., 1991). Antibodies against E-cadherin blocked formation of the syncytium. VE-cadherin is present on endothelium of fetal blood vessels, absent on villous cytotrophoblast but present on cytotrophoblasts on cell columns and in the decidua and on unmodified maternal vessels (Zhou et al., 1997a). Cytotrophoblasts in maternal blood vessels express VE-cadherin strongly. Parallel in vitro studies largely supported these findings.

Zhou et al. (1997a) reported that VCAM-1, PECAM-1 and E-selectin are expressed during cytotrophoblast invasion. Neither VCAM-1 or PECAM-1 were expressed on villous cytotrophoblasts but were expressed on cytotrophoblast within the uterine wall, on endovascular cytotrophoblasts and on maternal endothelium. Studies by Coukos et al. (1998) have shown that on first-trimester implantation sites only, interstitial EVT and endovascular trophoblast immunostain positively for PECAM-1. Cytotrophoblasts in cell columns express the α4 subunit of the VCAM-1 receptor and in vitro data support the possibility that this pair could be involved in cytotrophoblast–cytotrophoblast or cytotrophoblast–endothelial interactions during endovascular invasion (Zhou et al., 1997a). A number of papers report different findings. Three studies (Divers et al., 1995; Lyall et al., 2001a; Pijnenborg et al., 1998) found that while villous endothelial cells and endothelial cells of spiral arteries were PECAM-positive, all cytotrophoblast cells in villous tissue and cytotrophoblast in the placental bed and associated with spiral arteries were PECAM-negative. Since spiral arteries are re-endothelialized in the third trimester, one possibility for these differences is that PECAM-positive cells lining spiral arteries are being mistaken for cytotrophoblast cells but may be endothelial in origin. In early pregnancy NCAM-positive EVT cells are abundant in all parts of the basal plate, including intraluminal trophoblast cells in the rhesus monkey (King and Blankenship, 1995). These findings have been confirmed in humans (King and Loke, 1988). ICAM-1 is expressed on maternal endothelial cells, large granular lymphocytes, macrophages, interstitial trophoblast around uteroplacental vessels and intravascular trophoblast (Burrows et al., 1994).

Cytotrophoblast invasion, CAMs and pre-eclampsia

Pre-eclampsia is associated with failed trophoblast invasion. Immunocytochemical studies have shown that pre-eclampsia is associated with abnormal expression of integrins by invasive cytotrophoblasts. Zhou et al. (1993) reported that in pre-eclampsia cytotrophoblasts in floating villi, in contrast to normal pregnancy, failed to down-regulate α6β4 and up-regulate α1β1 in distal columns and in the uterine wall. Expression of cytotrophoblast-associated ECM appeared to be generally unaltered. In pre-eclampsia, cytotrophoblasts were reported to not express the same repertoire of endothelial CAMs as those from normal pregnancies (Zhou *et al.*, 1997a, 1997b). Pre-eclampsia was associated with differences in all three αV family members. In pre-eclampsia, fewer villous cytotrophoblast cells were positive for β5. In pre-eclampsia, αvβ6 staining was increased and extended beyond the columns into the superficial decidua. In pre-eclampsia, αvβ3 immunostaining was absent. Also in pre-eclampsia, cytotrophoblast E-cadherin expression remained strong on invasive cytotrophoblast and VE-cadherin was not detected on any cytotrophoblast in the placental bed. Finally, this group have studied CAMs associated with leukocyte migration in pre-eclampsia cases. VCAM-1 was not expressed by decidual cytotrophoblasts and PECAM-1 expression was not present in column or decidual cytotrophoblasts. The expression of E-selectin in pre-eclampsia was not reported.

Others have not been able to confirm all these findings. Divers *et al.* (1995) reported no differences in integrin expression in the amniochorion and the placental basal plate of women with pre-eclampsia and normal pregnancies. Furthermore, others (Lyall *et al.*, 2001a; Pijnenborg *et al.*, 1998) failed to identify PECAM-1 on cytotrophoblasts in placental bed biopsies taken from normal or pre-eclampsia cases. Further studies are required before this can be resolved unequivocally.

Labarrere and Faulk (1995) reported that endovascular EVT of decidual vessels were ICAM-1-negative in normal pregnancies. However, in pre-eclampsia and fetal growth restriction in spiral arteries which did contain endovascular trophoblast, the cells were ICAM-1-positive. These vessels were surrounded by numerous macrophages and T lymphocytes, suggesting ICAM-1 up-regulation may be mediated by cytokines released from the surrounding inflammatory cells.

In a recent study of EVT in placental tissue collected from normal pregnancies and pregnancies complicated by fetal growth restriction, VCAM-1, α2β1, α3β1 and α5β1 expression on EVT were all reported to be reduced in the fetal growth restriction group when compared with the controls (Zygmunt *et al.*, 1997). ICAM-3 was also expressed on EVT and expression was upregulated in the EVT of fetal growth restriction placentae. No differences were noted for ICAM-1, ICAM-2, α4β1 and α6β1.

The nitric oxide synthase/nitric oxide pathway and trophoblast invasion

Human placental syncytiotrophoblasts express endothelial eNOS but not inducible iNOS. eNOS is also expressed on villous endothelial cells and NO produced from these cells is believed to be an important vasodilator within the placental vasculature (Lyall, 2003). Pijnenborg *et al.* (1983) suggested that interstitial cytotrophoblast close to spiral arteries may produce vasoactive mediators. Nanaev *et al.* (1995) reported that guinea pig interstitial trophoblast expressed eNOS and iNOS. Their results suggested, at least in the guinea pig, that local production of NO by invading cytotrophoblasts may be an important mediator of spiral artery transformation. The studies of Lyall *et al.* (1999) on placental/decidual tissue revealed that while syncytiotrophoblasts were eNOS-positive, the cytotrophoblast cells of cell columns were eNOS-negative. Examination of placental bed specimens showed positive eNOS staining on the spiral artery vessel endothelium but cytokeratin-positive interstitial cytotrophoblast never showed eNOS immunostaining. None of the trophoblast cells within the vessels expressed eNOS. With regard to iNOS, no expression was found either on cytotrophoblasts within cytotrophoblast cell columns, in cytotrophoblast cell islands, interstitially or as they surrounded blood vessels. These findings strongly suggest that cytotrophoblast-derived NO is not responsible for dilatation of the spiral arteries during human placentation. Finally, there were no differences in NOS expression on invasive cytotrophoblasts within the placental bed of cases complicated by pre-eclampsia or fetal growth restriction. Direct comparison of the animal studies with results in humans is difficult because human placentation differs from the guinea pig and cell columns do not exist in rodents. Furthermore, the NOS isoforms expressed in the guinea pig differ from humans.

The carbon monoxide/hemeoxygenase pathway and trophoblast invasion

Carbon monoxide (CO) is produced by heme-oxygenase (HO), an enzyme that cleaves heme, to produce biliverdin and CO (Maines, 1988, 1993; Zakhary et al., 1996). CO, like nitric oxide, produces the second messenger cGMP. HO consists of three homologous isoenzymes: HO-1 is inducible and HO-2 is constitutive. HO-1 is expressed in the spleen and liver, where it is responsible for the destruction of heme from red blood cells. HO-1 can be induced by numerous stimuli. The actions of HO-1 rid cells of pro-oxidants. HO-2 is widely distributed throughout the body. It has been proposed that HO-2 and eNOS may have complimentary and co-ordinated physiological roles (Verma et al., 1993). HO-3 has little activity. CO acts as a neurotransmitter, inhibits platelet aggregation and is a vascular smooth muscle relaxant (Maines 1988, 1993; Verma et al., 1993; Zakhary et al., 1996). The similarities between NO and CO effects led to investigations as to whether CO may contribute to spiral artery dilatation or placental blood flow (Lyall et al., 2000). In the first trimester, HO-2 was primarily localized to the trophoblast layer and only occasionally was light staining noted on endothelial cells. Trophoblast immunostaining was reduced in third-trimester samples compared with both first- and second-trimester samples. In contrast, endothelial immunostaining was greater in second- compared to first-trimester samples and greater in third- compared to second-trimester

samples. Functional studies where HO-2 activity was blocked in the isolated perfused placenta showed that HO-2 inhibition increased placental perfusion pressure.

HO-2 on syncytiotrophoblast may have similar roles to those proposed for eNOS: NO produced by syncytiotrophoblast has at least three physiological targets: the intervillous space, autocrine effects on trophoblast function, and paracrine interactions with villous core components. Nitric oxide inhibits platelet aggregation and leukocyte adhesion while modulating the immune response. Similar effects by CO produced by syncytiotrophoblast would benefit both maternal blood flow through the intervillous space and the avoidance of immune recognition of the feto-placental allograft. The same group subsequently reported that placental endothelial HO-2 expression was significantly reduced in pregnancies complicated by pre-eclampsia and fetal growth restriction but HO-1 was unaffected (Barber et al., 2001). Thus the reduction in HO-2 expression on endothelial cells in pre-eclampsia and fetal growth restriction could contribute to the reduction of blood flow. Within the placental bed all EVT were positive for HO-2. No differences in HO-2 or HO-1 immunostaining on extravillous cytotrophoblast within the placental bed in pre-eclampsia or fetal growth restriction. The expression of HO-2 by invasive cytotrophoblasts opens the possibility that CO could be produced from these cells and contribute to spiral artery dilatation. The expression of HO-1 was very low in all the cells in the placenta and placental bed, supporting the notion that HO-1 is expressed at low levels in the human placenta.

Matrix metalloproteinases and their tissue inhibitors

Matrix metalloproteinases (MMPs) are a family of proteolytic enzymes which play a pivotal role in invasion processes by degrading basement membranes and ECM components (Nawrocki et al., 1997). The MMPs are secreted into the

ECM as inactive proforms and therefore must be cleaved to be activated. There are four main groups of MMPs (Hulboy *et al.*, 1997). Collagenases (e.g. MMP-1, MMP-8, MMP-13), which primarily degrade fibrillar collagens I, II and III; gelatinases (e.g. MMP-2, MMP-9), which primarily degrade denatured collagens (gelatin) and collagen IV; stromelysins (e.g. MMP-3, MMP-7, MMP-10, MMP-11, MMP-12) have a much wider range of substrates, including fibronectin, laminin, elastin, proteoglycans and collagens III, IV, V and IX; and membrane-type matrix metalloelastases (e.g. MMP-14, MMP-15, MMP-16, MMP-17) are located at cell surfaces and their substrate specificities are unclear, although they appear to activate progelatinase-A. Natural inhibitors of MMPs can be divided into plasma (α macroglobulins) and tissue inhibitors (TIMPs) (Hulboy *et al.*, 1997). There are four tissue inhibitors of MMPs (TIMPs): TIMP-1 inhibits all activated MMPs and both latent and activated MMP-9; TIMP-2 blocks activity of all active MMPs. TIMPs-3 and 4 are less well-characterized.

Human implantation requires that trophoblast cells become highly invasive, a process analogous to tumor invasion (Lala and Graham, 1990) but trophoblast invasion is tightly regulated. The trophoblast cells must break through the maternal ECM. This requires the degradation of the matrix and is thought to involve several MMPs and TIMPs. Normal invasion is achieved by a balance between secretion of MMPs by trophoblasts and decidual cells and their inhibition by TIMPs produced by the same cells. Abnormalities in these processes could lead to excessive invasion, such as in placenta accreta, invasive moles or choriocarcinoma or restricted invasion as in early pregnancy failure, pre-eclampsia and fetal growth restriction.

MMPs and TIMPs in normal pregnancy

Cultured trophoblast secretes MMP-1. Both protein and mRNA for MMP-1 are found in trophoblast columns and invading trophoblast. MMP-1 protein is present on invasive trophoblast in the second and third trimester. MMP-1 staining was more intense in deeply invaded trophoblast where cells are more in contact with decidual tissue rich in interstitial collagens (Huppertz *et al.*, 1998a; Vettraino *et al.*, 1996).

Cultured first-trimester cytotrophoblast cells secrete MMP-2 and MMP-9 and this secretion appears to be linked to surface integrin expression (Bischof *et al.*, 1991, 1995a; Emonard *et al.*, 1990; Librach *et al.*, 1991b). Blocking MMP-9 in vitro inhibited invasion while inhibitors of MMP-1 had no effect (Librach *et al.*, 1991b). Cytokines such as IL-1β, leukemia inhibitory factor (LIF) and corti-costeroids may regulate MMP release and invasion (Bischof *et al.*, 1995b; Librach *et al.*, 1994). Studies on leukocytes obtained from first-trimester decidua have also shown that all populations of leucocytes secrete both MMP-2 and MMP-9 (Shi *et al.*, 1995). Studies on first-trimester placentae have confirmed that MMP-2 is present in all types of trophoblast and decidual cells (Autio-Harmainen *et al.*, 1992; Fernandez *et al.*, 1992). MMP-2 and -9 are expressed in early invasive trophoblast (Hurskainen *et al.*, 1996; Polette *et al.*, 1994) but not at term (Polette *et al.*, 1994). MMP-3 is expressed in the placenta and EVT express MMP-3 over the entire invasive pathway (Vettraino *et al.*, 1996). Invading trophoblasts express MMP-11 in the first trimester while anchoring cells of columns and decidual cells do not. Expression is reduced in the third trimester (Maquoi *et al.*, 1997). MMP-14 has been observed in columns and infiltrating EVT in decidual membranes and decidual cells in the first and third trimester (Nawrocki *et al.*, 1996). The parallel expression of MMP-2 by EVT in cell islands, anchoring villi and in invading tropho-blasts, as well as some decidual cells, suggests that these cells may use the MMP-14 pathway to activate MMP-2 (Bjorn *et al.*, 1997).

In vitro cytotrophoblast cells express primarily TIMP-3 and highest levels were expressed on invasive cells and with MMP-9 expression (Bass *et al.*, 1997). In vivo studies suggest TIMPs appear to be largely restricted to decidual cells;

Nawrocki *et al.* (1997) reported that TIMP-1, 2 and 3 were expressed in first-trimester decidual cells and that TIMP-1 and TIMP-3 were up-regulated in the third trimester. Ruck *et al.* found TIMP-2 expression in cell columns (Ruck *et al.*, 1997) and others have found TIMP-1, 2 and 3 expressed in cell columns and decidualized stromal cells of early placenta (Hurskainen *et al.*, 1996). Huppertz *et al.* (1998b) reported that TIMP-1 and TIMP-2 were expressed in EVT throughout pregnancy, although proliferative EVT were negative for TIMP-2. In vitro both TIMP-1 and TIMP-2 completely inhibit cytotrophoblast invasion (Librach *et al.*, 1991b). In summary, the evidence above supports MMP-1, MMP-2, MMP-3, MMP-7, MMP-9, MMP-11 and TIMPs-1–3 involvement in normal trophoblast invasion of decidua. There are inconsistencies in the literature on decidual invasion, a lack of accurate gestational dates and an absence of data on myometrial invasion.

MMPs and TIMPs in pre-eclampsia

There is much less known about pre-eclampsia. The inactive MMP-9 is the principle MMP secreted from cytotrophoblast cultures prepared from cases of pre-eclampsia whereas the active form is more abundant in uncomplicated pregnancies (Lim *et al.*, 1997). Purified cytotrophoblast cells from the cases of pre-eclampsia showed reduced invasive potential and failed to modulate expression of MMP-9. In vivo data are also limited; a study of two placenta with attached decidua reported that in pre-eclampsia, MMP-7 was expressed in cytotrophoblasts and syncytiotrophoblasts, decidual cells and EVT while in normal pregnancy cytotrophoblast and syncytial staining was absent at term and only present in early pregnancy (Vettraino *et al.*, 1996). MMP-1 expression is reduced in decidual endothelial cells prepared from women with pre-eclampsia. The authors suggested that this may inhibit endovascular invasion by cytotrophoblasts.

Transforming growth factor-βs and trophoblast invasion in normal pregnancy and pre-eclampsia

Transforming growth factor-βs (TGF-βs) are members of a large superfamily of cytokines (Pepper, 1997). The TGF family is composed of three related proteins, TGF-β1, 2 and 3. TGF-βs act through receptors designated types I, II and III. TGF-β, produced primarily by the decidua, may regulate trophoblast invasion (Lala and Hamilton, 1996). Expression of TGF-β3 in placental villous tissue was reported to be low at 5–6 weeks' gestation, peaking at 7–8 weeks' gestation and virtually undetectable by 9 weeks (Caniggia *et al.*, 1999). Interpretation of these findings is not straightforward for several reasons (Simpson *et al.*, 2002). Simpson *et al.* examined the expression of TGF-β1, 2 and 3 in placental bed biopsies and placentae from 7–19 weeks' gestation. TGF-β1 protein was undetectable using Western blot analysis but RT-PCR confirmed the presence of TGF-β1 mRNA in placental homogenates between 7 and 19 weeks' gestation. TGF-β2 was produced in both the placenta and placental bed, where it was localized mainly to cytotrophoblast islands and decidua. Villous trophoblast was consistently negative. Much lower levels of TGF-β3 were present in placental homogenates. Immunolocalization studies showed little reactivity for TGF-β3 in placenta. Levels of TGF-β1, TGF-β2 and TGF-β3 did not change between 7 and 19 weeks of pregnancy. These results suggest that TGF-β2, but not TGF-β1 or TGF-β3, may play a role in trophoblast invasion. Specifically, a dramatic reduction in trophoblast TGF-β3 expression at the time of the first or second wave of trophoblast invasion was not found.

Interpretation of early immunohistochemical studies of TGF-β in the human placenta is confounded by the use of antibodies which are not specific for individual isoforms (Lysiak, 1995; Selick *et al.*, 1994; Vuckovic *et al.*, 1992). More recent studies, including the one by Simpson *et al.*, used antibodies specific for each isoform.

Comparison of studies is further confounded by the variability of techniques used for tissue preparation. Many studies have reported results only for total TGF protein, much of which is latent. Incorporation of an ELISA immunoassay, which measures only bioactive forms, is therefore likely to yield more functionally relevant information.

There is evidence that TGF-β can regulate trophoblast invasion in vitro, although the data are not consistent (Bass et al., 1994; Caniggia et al., 1999; Graham et al., 1992). It is not clear why in vitro data are not consistent between groups but the discrepancies may be related to the cell preparation techniques or the culture conditions employed.

Caniggia et al. (1999) reported that TGF-β3 is over-expressed in the placenta of pre-eclampsia patients and that this may be responsible for failed trophoblast invasion. In the same study it was also shown that explants from pre-eclampsia placentas failed to show outgrowth or invasion. However, interpretation of these data is not straightforward since interstitial migration of EVT into the decidua and myometrium proceeds normally in pre-eclampsia. Others have used immunohistochemistry, Western blot analysis and ELISA to examine the expression of TGF-β1, TGF-β2 and TGF-β3 in placenta and placental bed of pregnancies complicated by pre-eclampsia, fetal growth restriction and matched control pregnancies (Lyall et al., 2001b). No changes in expression of either isoform were found in placenta or placental bed in pre-eclampsia or fetal growth restriction compared with normal pregnancy. These data are not consistent with over-expression of TGF-β3 being responsible for failed trophoblast invasion in pre-eclamspia or fetal growth restriction.

Oxygen tension and trophoblast invasion in normal pregnancy and pre-eclampsia

Oxygen tension at the feto-maternal interface may, at least in part, be responsible for some of the changes associated with cytotrophoblast proliferation and invasion. There is no real blood flow into the intervillous space prior to 10 weeks' gestation (Hustin and Schapps, 1987). Thereafter, with dissolution of the trophoblast plugs, intervillous blood flow increases. Oxygen pressure in the intervillous space increases from 17.9 ± 6.9 mmHg at $8-10$ weeks' gestation to 60.7 ± 8.5 mmHg at $12-13$ weeks' gestation as a result of remodeling of the spiral arteries (Rodesch et al., 1992).

Pre-eclampsia and fetal growth restriction have been reported to be associated with placental hypoxia, although this is controversial (Kingdom and Kaufmann, 1997). Oxygen concentration can alter the expression of many different proteins. In vitro, cytotrophoblasts from first- and second-trimester placentae grown under hypoxic conditions (2% oxygen) fail to up-regulate the integrin $\alpha 1\beta 1$ (just as in pre-eclampsia) but do up-regulate $\alpha 5\beta 1$ (Genbacev et al., 1996).

Isolated first-trimester cytotrophoblast cultured on an ECM in 20% oxygen will invade the matrix (Fisher et al., 1989). First-trimester villi which have been explanted onto matrigel and cultured in 20% oxygen form new invasive sites at the tips of the explants (Aplin et al., 1999; Genbacev et al., 1997; Vicovac and Aplin, 1996), while those cultured in 2% oxygen are maintained in a proliferative, non-invasive immature state (Caniggia et al., 2000a, 2000b; Genbacev et al., 1997; Zhou et al., 1998). Cytotrophoblasts cultured in low oxygen do not undergo the switch in integrin receptors normally found as the invasive phenotype is acquired (Genbacev et al., 1997). Several studies have examined other responses of trophoblasts to low oxygen including increased production of inflammatory cytokines, vascular endothelial growth factor (VEGF), PAI-1 and syncytialization (Alsat et al., 1996; Benyo et al., 1997; Taylor et al., 1997).

The effects of oxygen are mediated by transcription factors such as hypoxia inducible factor 1 (HIF-1α), a nuclear protein which activates gene transcription in response to low concentrations of oxygen (Semenza, 1998). Caniggia et al. (2000) reported that placental expression of TGF-β3 paralleled that of HIF-1α. Expression of mRNA for both decreased at 9–12 weeks' gestation. A similar reduction in HIF-1α and TGF-β3 was found in explants cultured with increasing oxygen concentrations. Inhibition of HIF-1α inhibited expression of TGF-β3 mRNA, reduced trophoblast proliferation and triggered MMP-9 expression and α1 integrin expression, markers of trophoblast invasion phenotype. Just as for TGF-β3, the authors reported that pre-eclampsia placentae overexpressed HIF-1α. Rajakumar and Conrad (2000) found that HIF-1α mRNA was expressed at a constant level in all placenta across gestation, whereas HIF-2α mRNA increased significantly with gestational age. HIF-1α and -2α proteins decreased significantly with gestational age. The regulation of these transcription factors by oxygen was studied using placental villous explants. HIF-1α and -2α proteins, but not mRNA, was induced by hypoxia in the placental villous explants. The authors suggested that physiological hypoxia contributes to the increased expression of HIF-1α and -2α proteins in early placentas and that regulation of these transcription factors by hypoxia in the human placenta occurs at the level of protein and not mRNA. The reasons for the difference in the two studies of mRNA results are not yet clear. Subsequent studies have shown that the TGF-β3 gene has the potential to be directly regulated by HIF (Schaffer et al., 2003). HIF-1α and 2-α proteins are both over-expressed in pre-eclampsia (Rajakumar et al., 2001a, 2001b). The same group then showed that placental explants obtained form cases of pre-eclampsia did not down-regulate HIIF-1 proteins following exposure to hypoxia and reoxygenation, whereas cases from uncomplicated pregnancies did. Studies on true placental bed biopsies have not been performed. However, a final word of caution in interpretation of the above data is warranted; Janatpour et al. (1999) reported that expression of HIF-1α was dramatically up-regulated in standard (20%) oxygen conditions, whereas culturing the cells in hypoxic (2% oxygen) conditions slightly diminished expression of HIF-1α. Clearly, with oxygen concentration being implicated as a key regulator

of trophoblast invasion, further studies in this area are required.

HLA-G

HLA-G is an unusual class 1B major histocompatibility antigen expressed by EVT and may protect cells from natural killer cell lysis (Chumbly et al., 1994; Moffett and Loke, 2004). See also the chapter by Dr. Moffett. Cytotrophoblast cells which invade the decidua express HLA-G. In culture, purified cytotrophoblasts upregulate HLA-G as they become invasive (McMaster et al., 1995). Expression of HLA-G protein by EVT is reported to be reduced in pre-eclampsia (Colbern et al., 1994; Goldman-Wohl et al., 2000; Hara et al., 1996). Thus there may be a link between HLA-G expression and failed trophoblast in pre-eclampsia (O'Brien et al., 2000). Lim et al. (1997) have shown that cultured villous cytotrophoblasts obtained from normal pregnancies up-regulate HLA-G as they differentiate in vitro, whereas cytotrophoblasts prepared from cases complicated by pre-eclampsia did not express HLA-G. The authors suggested that reduced HLA-G expression may be due to an alteration in the interaction between invasive cytotrophoblast and maternal immune cells in pre-eclampsia. Expression of HLA-G may also allow trophoblasts to evade cell damage by interleukin-2, a cytotoxic cytokine in decidual tissue (Hamai et al., 1999). Recently, increased frequency in expression of the HLA-G G5 spliceform was found in placentae of cases of pre-eclampsia (Emmer et al., 2004) and the authors suggested this may also play a role in failed trophoblast invasion.

Apoptosis

This article would not be complete without mentioning apoptosis. Apoptosis (programmed cell death) is a physiological and pathological process which regulates the number of cells in tissues (Thompson, 1995). Because apoptotic cells are degraded in a short time (1–2 h), small changes in the number of apoptotic cells in a tissue may have important biological significance. Little is known about apoptotic events in the placental bed of women with pre-eclampsia. One study (DiFederico et al., 1999) showed that normal control samples showed almost no apoptosis but between 15 and 50% of cytotrophoblasts within the uterine wall of women with pre-eclampsia were positive. The same cells did not express Bcl-2, a survival factor normally expressed by these cells. The authors suggested that programmed cell death in these cells may account for some of the symptoms of pre-eclampsia. In contrast, Kadyrov et al. (2003) found, in their study of placental bed biopsies, that the number of apoptotic EVT was reduced in pre-eclampsia compared with normal pregnancy. Further studies in this area are required.

Conclusions

While some aspects of trophoblast invasion resemble tumor invasion, the striking difference between the two is that trophoblast invasion of the uterus is tightly controlled by a plethora of factors expressed within the decidua and on the trophoblasts themselves. These include CAMs and the ECM, proteinases and their inhibitors, growth factors, cytokines and others. Abnormalities in any one of these mechanisms may have the potential to lead to impaired cytotrophoblast invasion. The precise mechanisms are still poorly understood and require further investigation. Only by understanding these pathological mechanisms can future strategies for therapeutic targets be developed.

REFERENCES

Alberts, B., Bray, D., Lewis, J., Raff, M., Roberts, K. and Watson, J. (1994). *Molecular Biology of the Cell.* New York: Garland Publishing Inc.

Alexander, C. and Werb, Z. (1991). Extracellular matrix degradation. In *Cell Biology of the Extracellular Matrix*, ed. E. Hay. New York: Plenum Press, pp. 255–302.

Alsat, E., Wyplosz, P., Malassine, A., et al. (1996). Hypoxia impairs cell fusion and differentiation process in human cytotrophoblast in vitro. *J. Cell Physiol.*, **168**, 346–53.

Aplin, J. D. (1993). Expression of integrin α6β4 in human trophoblast and its loss from extravillous cells. *Placenta*, **14**, 203–15.

Aplin, J. D., Charlton, A. K. and Ayad, S. (1990). The role of matrix macromolecules in the invasion of decidua by trophoblast. *Trophoblast Res.*, **4**, 139–58.

Aplin, J. D., Haigh, T., Jones, C. J. P., Church, H. J. and Vicovac, L. J. (1999). Development of cytotrophoblast columns from explanted first trimester placental villi: role of fibronectin and integrin α5β1. *Biol. Reprod.*, **60**, 828–38.

Autio-Harmainen, H., Hurskainen, T., Niskasaari, K., Hoyhtya, M. and Tryggvason, K. (1992). Simultaneous expression of 70 kilodalton type IV collagenase and type IV collagen alpha 1 (IV) chain genes by cells of early human placenta and gestational endometrium. *Lab. Invest.*, **67**, 191–200.

Barber, A., Robson, S. C., Myatt, L., Bulmer, J. N. and Lyall, F. (2001). Hemeoxygenase expression in human placenta and placental bed: reduced expression of placenta endothelial HO-2 in preeclampsia and fetal growth restriction. *FASEB J.*, **15**, 1158–68.

Bass, K. E., Li, H. X., Hawkes, S. P., et al. (1997). Tissue inhibitor of metalloproteinase-3 expression is upregulated during human cytotrophoblast invasion in vitro. *Dev. Genetics*, **21**, 61–7.

Bass, K. E., Morrish, D. W., Roth, I., et al. (1994). Human cytotrophoblast invasion is upregulated by epidermal growth factor. Evidence that paracrine factors modify this process. *Dev. Biol.*, **164**, 560–1.

Benyo, D. F., Miles, T. M. and Conrad, K. P. (1997). Hypoxia stimulates cytokine production by villous explants from the human placenta. *J. Clin. Endo. Metabol.*, **82**, 1582–8.

Birk, D. E., Silver, F. H. and Trelstad, R. L. (1991). Matrix assembly. In *Cell Biology of Extracellular Matrix*, ed. E. Hay. New York: Plenum Press, pp. 221–54.

Bischof, P., Friedli, E., Martell, M. and Campana, A. (1991). Expression of extracellular matrix degrading metalloproteinases by cultured human cytotrophoblast cells – effects of cell adhesion and immunopurification. *Am. J. Obstet. Gynecol.*, **165**, 1791–801.

Bischof, P., Haenggeli, L. and Campana, A. (1995a). Gelatinase and oncofetal fibronectin secretion is dependent on integrin expression on human cytotrophoblasts. *Human Reprod.*, **10**, 734–42.

Bischof, P., Haenggeli, L. and Campana, A. (1995b). Effect of leukemia inhibitory factor on human cytotrophoblast differentiation along the invasive pathway. *Am. J. Reprod. Immunol.*, **34**, 225–30.

Bjorn, S. F., Hastrup, N., Lund, L. R., Dano, K., Larsen, J. F. and Pyke, C. (1997). Co-ordinated expression of MMP-2 and its putative activator, MT1-MMP in human placentation. *Mol. Hum. Reprod.*, **3**, 713–23.

Brosens, I. A., Robertson, W. B. and Dixon, H. G. (1972). The role of the spiral arteries in the pathogenesis of pre-eclampsia. In *Obstet Gyn Ann*, ed. R. M. Wynn, vol. 4. New York: Appleton-Century-Crofts, pp. 177–91.

Bulmer, J. N., Morrison, L. and Johnson, P. M. (1988). Expression of the proliferation markers Ki67 and transferrin receptor by human trophoblast populations. *J. Reprod. Immunol.*, **14**, 291–302.

Burrows, T. D., King, A. and Loke, Y. W. (1994). Expression of adhesion molecules by endovascular trophoblast and decidual endothelial cells – implications for vascular invasion during implantation. *Placenta*, **15**, 21–33.

Caniggia, I., Grisaru-Gravnosky, S., Kuliszewsky, M., Post, M. and Lye, S. J. (1999). Inhibition of TGFBβ3 restores the invasive capability of extravillous trophoblasts in preeclamptic pregnancies. *J. Clin. Invest.*, **103**, 1641–50.

Caniggia, I., Mostachfi, H., Winter, J., *et al.* (2000a). Hypoxia-inducible factor-1 mediates the biological effects of oxygen on human trophoblast differentiation through TGF-β3. *J. Clin. Invest.*, **105**, 577–87.

Caniggia, I., Winter, J., Lye, S. J. and Post, M. (2000b). Oxygen and placental development during the first trimester: implications for the pathophysiology of pre-eclampsia. *Placenta*, **21**, S25–30.

Carter, W. G. P., Kaur, S. G., Gil, P. J. and Wayer, E. A. (1990). Distinct functions for α3β1 in focal adhesions and α6/β4 bullous pemphigoid antigen in a new stabilising anchoring contact (SAC) of keratinocytes: relation to hemidesmosomes. *J. Cell Biol.*, **111**, 3141–54.

Castellucci, M., Classen-Linke, I., Munlhauser, J., Kaufmann, P., Zardi, L. and Chiquet-Ehrismann, R. (1991). The human placenta: a model for tenascin expression. *ImmunoHistochem.*, **95**, 449–58.

Chumbly, G., King, A., Robertson, K., Holmes, N. and Loke, Y. W. (1994). Resistance of HLA-G and HLA-A2 transfectants to lysis by decidual NK cells. *Cell Immunol.*, **155**, 312–22.

Church, H. J., Richards, A. J. and Aplin, J. D. (1997). Laminins in decidua, placenta and choriocarcinoma cells. *Trophoblast Res.*, 143–62.

Colbern, G. T., Chiang, M. H. and Main, E. K. (1994). Expression of the nonclassic histocompatibility antigen HLA-G by preeclamptic placenta. *Am. J. Obstet. Gynecol.*, **170**, 1244–50.

Coukos, G., Makrigiannakis, A., Amin, K., Albelda, S. M. and Coutifaris, C. (1998). Platelet endothelial cell adhesion molecule-1 is expressed by a subpopulation of human trophoblasts: a possible mechanism for trophoblast–endothelial interaction during haemochorial placentation. *Mol. Hum. Reprod.*, **4**, 357–67.

Coutifaris, C., Kao, L. C., Sehdev, H. M., *et al.* (1991). E-cadherin expression during the differentiation of human trophoblasts. *Development*, **113**, 767–77.

Damsky, C. H., Fitzgerald, M. L. and Fisher, S. J. (1992). Distribution patterns of extracellular matrix components are intricately modulated during first trimester cytotrophoblast differentiation along the invasive pathway, in vivo. *J. Clin. Invest.*, **89**, 210–22.

Damsky, C. H., Librach, C., Lim, K.-H., *et al.* (1994). Integrin switching regulates normal trophoblast invasion. *Development*, **120**, 3657–66.

DiFederico, E., Genbacev, O. and Fisher, F. J. (1999). Preeclampsia is associated with widespread apoptosis of placental cytotrophoblasts within the uterine wall. *Am. J. Pathol.*, **155**, 293–301.

Divers, M. J., Bulmer, J. N., Miller, D. and Lilford, R. J. (1995). Beta 1 integrins in third trimester human placentae: no differential expression in pathological pregnancy. *Placenta*, **16**, 245–60.

Emmer, P. M., Joosten, I., Schut, M. H., Zusterzeel, P. L. M., Hendriks, J. C. M. and Steegers, E. A. P. (2004). Shift in expression of HLA-G mRNA spliceforms in pregnancies complicated by preeclampsia. *J. Soc. Gyn. Invest.*, **11**, 220–6.

Emonard, H. P., Christiane, Y., Smet, M., Grimaud, J. A. and Foidart, J. M. (1990). Type IV and interstitial collagenolytic activities in normal and malignant trophoblast cells are specifically regulated by the extracellular matrix. *Invasion Metastasis*, **10**, 170–7.

Feinberg, R. F. and Kliman, H. J. (1993). Tropho-uteronectin (TUN): a unique oncofetal fibronectin deposited in the extracellular matrix of the tropho-uterine junction and regulated in vitro by cultured human trophoblast cells. *Troph. Res.*, **7**, 167–81.

Fernandez, P. L., Merino, M. J., Nogales, F. F., Charonis, A. S., Stetler Stevenson, W. G. and Liotta, L. (1992). Immunohistochemical profile of basement membrane proteins and 72-kilodalton type-IV collagenase in the implantation placental site – an integrated view. *Lab. Invest.*, **66**, 572–9.

Fisher, S. J., Cui, T. Y., Zhang, L., *et al.* (1989). Adhesive and degradative properties of human placental cytotrophoblast cells in vitro. *J. Cell. Biol.*, **109**, 891–902.

Genbacev, O., Joslin, R., Damsky, C. H., Polliotti, B. M. and Fisher, S. J. (1996). Hypoxia alters early gestation human cytotrophoblast differentiation/invasion in vitro and models the placental defects that occur in preeclampsia. *J. Clin. Invest.*, **97**, 540–50.

Genbacev, O., Zhou, Y., Ludlow, J. W. and Fisher, S. J. (1997). Regulation of human placental development by oxygen tension. *Science*, **277**, 1669–72.

Goldman-Wohl, D. S., Ariel, I., Greenfield, C., *et al.* (2000). Lack of human leucocyte antigen-G expression in extravillous trophoblast is associated with preeclampsia. *Mol. Hum. Reprod.*, **6**, 88–95.

Graham, C. H., Lysiak, J. J., McCrae, K. R. and Lala, P. K. (1992). Localization of transforming growth factor-B at the human fetal–maternal interface: role in trophoblast growth and differentiation. *Biol. Reprod.*, **46**, 561–72.

Hamai, Y., Fujii, T., Yamashita, T., *et al.* (1999). The expression of human leukocyte antigen-G on trophoblasts abolishes the growth-suppressing effect of interleukin-2 towards them. *Am. J. Reprod. Immunol.*, **41**, 153–8.

Hara, N., Fujii, T., Yamashita, T., Kozuma, S., Okai, T. and Taketani, Y. (1996). Altered expression of human leukocyte antigen (HLA-G) on extravillous trophoblasts in preeclampsia: immunohistological demonstration with Anti-HLA-G specific antibody '87G' and anti-cytokeratin antibody 'CAM5.2'. *Am. J. Reprod. Immunol.*, **36**, 349–538.

Hulboy, D. L., Rudolf, L. A. and Matrisisan, L. M. (1997). Matrix metalloproteases as mediators of reproductive function. *Mol. Hum. Reprod.*, **3**, 27–45.

Huppertz, B., Kertschanska, S., Frank, H. G., Gaus, G., Funayama, H. and Kaufmann, P. (1996). Extracellular matrix components of placental extravillous trophoblast: immunocytochemistry and ultrastructural distribution. *Histochem. Cell Biol.*, **106**, 291–301.

Huppertz, B., Kertschanska, S., Demir, A., Frank, H. G. and Kaufmann, P. I. (1998a). Immunohistochemistry of matrix metalloproteinases (MMP), their substrates and their inhibitors (TIMP) during trophoblast invasion in the human placenta. *Cell Tiss. Res.*, **291**, 133–48.

Huppertz, B. S., Kertschanska, S., Demir, A., Frank, H. G. and Kaufmann, P. (1998b). Production of membrane-type matrix metalloproteinase-1 (MT-MMP-1) in early human placenta: a possible role in placental implantation. *Cell Tiss. Res.*, **291**, 133–48.

Hurskainen, T., Hoyhtya, M., Tuuttila, A., Oikarinen, and Autio-Harmainen, H. (1996). mRNA expressions of TIMP-1, -2 and -3 and 92-kD type IV collagenase in early human placenta studied by in situ hybridization. *J. Histochem. Cytochem.*, **44**, 1379–88.

Hustin, J. and Schapps, J. P. (1987). Echocardiographic and anatomic studies of the maternotrophoblastic border during the 1st trimester of pregnancy. *Am. J. Obstet. Gynecol.*, **157**, 62–168.

Irving, J. A. and Lala, P. K. (1995). Functional role of cell surface integrins on human trophoblast cell migration: regulation by TGFβ, IGF-II and IGFBP-1. *Exp. Cell Res.*, **217**, 419–27.

Janatpour, M. J., Utset, M. F., Cross, J. C., *et al.* (1999). A repertoire of differentially expressed transcription factors that offers insight into mechanisms of human cytotrophoblast differentiation. *Dev. Gen.*, **25**, 146–57.

Kadyrov, M., Schmitz, C., Black, S., Kaufmann, P. and Huppertz, B. (2003). Pre-eclampsia and maternal anaemia display reduced apoptosis and opposite invasive phenotypes of extravillous trophoblast. *Placenta*, **24**, 540–48.

Khong, T. Y., De Wolf, F., Robertson, W. B. and Brosens, I. (1986). Inadequate maternal vascular response to placentation in pregnancies complicated by preeclampsia and by small-for-gestational age infants. *Br. J. Obstet. Gynaecol.*, **93**, 1049–59.

King, B. F. and Blankenship, T. N. (1993). Expression of proliferating cell nuclear antigen (PCNA) in developing macaque placentas. *Placenta*, **14**, A36.

King, B. F. and Blankenship, T. N. (1995). Neural cell adhesion molecule is present on macaque intra-arterial cytotrophoblast. *Placenta*, **16**, A36.

King, A. and Loke, Y. W. (1988). Differential expression of blood-group-related carbohydrate antigens by trophoblast subpopulations. *Placenta*, **9**, 513–21.

Kingdom, J. C. P. and Kaufmann, P. (1997). Oxygen and placental villous development: origins of fetal hypoxia. *Placenta*, **18**, 613–21.

Kohnen, G., Kosanke, G., Korr, H. and Kaufmann, P. (1993). Comparison of various proliferation markers applied to human placental tissue. *Placenta*, **14**, A38.

Korhonen, M., Ylanne, J., Laitnen, L., Cooper, H. N., Quaranta, V. and Virtanenen, I. (1991). Distribution of the α1–α6 integrin subunits in human developing and term placenta. *Lab. Invest.*, **65**, 347–56.

Kosanke, G. (1994). *Proliferation, Wachstum und Differenzierung der Zottenbäume der menschlichen Placenta*. Aachen: Verlag Shaker.

Kreis, T. and Vale, R. (1993). *Guidebook to the Extracellular Matrix and Adhesion Proteins*. Oxford: Oxford University Press.

Labarrere, C. and Faulk, W. P. (1995). Intercellular adhesion molecule-1 (ICAM-1) and HLA-DR antigens are expressed on endovascular cytotrophoblasts in abnormal pregnancies. *Am. J. Reprod. Immunol.*, **33**, 47–53.

Lala, P. K. and Graham, C. H. (1990). Mechanisms of trophoblast invasiveness and their control: the role of proteases and protease inhibitors. *Cancer Metastasis Rev.*, **9**, 369–79.

Lala, P. K. and Hamilton, G. S. (1996). Growth factors, proteases and protease inhibitors in the maternal–fetal dialogue. *Placenta*, **17**, 545–55.

Larjava, H., Peltonen, J., Akiyama, S., Gralnik, H., Uitto, J. and Yamada, K. M. (1990). Novel functions for β1 integrins in keratinocyte cell–cell interactions. *J. Cell Biol.*, **111**, 803–185.

Leivo, I. P. L., Wahlström, T. and Engvall, E. (1989). Expression of merosin, a tissue specific basement membrane protein, in the intermediate trophoblast cells of choriocarcinoma and placenta. *Lab. Invest.*, **60**, 783–90.

Librach, C. L., Feigenbaum, S. L., Bass, K. E., *et al.* (1994). Interleukin-1 beta regulates human cytotrophoblast invasion in vitro. *J. Biol. Chem.*, **269**, 125–31.

Librach, C. L., Fisher, S. J., Fitgerald, M. L. and Damsky, C. H. (1991a). Cytotrophoblast–fibronectin and cytotrophoblast–laminin interactions have distinct roles in cytotrophoblast invasion. *J. Cell Biol.*, **115**, 6a.

Librach, C. L., Werb, Z., Fitzgerald, M. L., *et al.* (1991b). 92-kD type IV collagenase mediates invasion of human trophoblasts. *J. Cell Biol.*, **113**, 437–49.

Lim, K. H., Zhou, Y., Janatpour, M., *et al.* (1997). Human cytotrophoblast differentiation/invasion is abnormal in pre-eclampsia. *Am. J. Path.*, **151**, 1809–18.

Lyall, F. (1998). Cell adhesion molecules: their role in pregnancy. *Fetal Mat. Med. Rev.*, **10**, 21–44.

Lyall, F. (2002). The human placental bed revisited. *Placenta*, **23**, 555–62.

Lyall, F. (2003). Development of the uteroplacental circulation: the role of carbon monoxide and nitric oxide in trophoblast invasion and spiral artery transformation. *Microscop. Res. Tech.*, **60**, 402–11.

Lyall, F., Barber, A., Myatt, L., Bulmer, J. N. and Robson, S. C. (2000). Hemeoxygenase expression in human placenta and placental bed implies a role in regulation of trophoblast invasion and placental function. *FASEB J.*, **14**, 208–19.

Lyall, F., Bulmer, J. N., Duffie, E., Cousins, F., Theriault, E. A. and Robson, S. C. (2001a). Human trophoblast invasion and spiral artery transformation. The role of PECAM-1 in normal pregnancy, pre-eclampsia and fetal growth restriction. *Am. J. Pathol.*, **158**, 1713–21.

Lyall, F., Robson, S. C., Bulmer, J. N., Kelly, H. and Duffie, E. (1999). Human trophoblast invasion and spiral artery transformation: the role of nitric oxide. *Am. J. Pathol.*, **154**, 1105–14.

Lyall, F., Simpson, H., Robson, S. C., Bulmer, J. N. and Barber, A. (2001b). Transforming growth factor β expression in human placenta and placental bed in normal pregnancy, preeclampsia and fetal growth restriction. *Am. J. Pathol.*, **159**, 1827–38.

Lysiak, J. J., Hunt, J., Pringle, G. A. and Lala, P. K. (1995). Localization of transforming growth factor beta and its natural inhibitor decorin in the human placenta and decidua throughout gestation. *Placenta*, **16**, 221–31.

MacCalman, C. D. and Chen, G. T. C. (1998). Type 2 cadherins in the human endometrium and placenta: their putative roles in human implantation and placentation. *Am. J. Reprod. Immunol.*, **39**, 96–107.

MacCalman, C. D., Omigbodum, A., Bronner, M. P. and Struass, J. F. (1995). Identification of the cadherins present in human placenta. *J. Soc. Gynecol. Invest.*, **2**, 146.

Maines, M. D. (1988). Heme oxygenase: function, multiplicity, regulatory mechanisms and clinical applications. *FASEB J.*, **2**, 2257–568.

Maines, M. D. (1993). Carbon monoxide: an emerging regulator of cGMP in the brain. *Mol. Cell. Neurosci.*, **4**, 389–97.

Maquoi, E., Polette, M., Nawrocki, B., *et al.* (1997). Expression of stromelysin-3 in the human placenta and placental bed. *Placenta*, **18**, 277–85.

McMaster, M. T., Librach, C. L., Zhou, Y., *et al.* (1995). Human placental HLA-G expression is restricted to differentiated cytotrophoblasts. *J. Immunol.*, **154**, 3771–8.

Meekins, J. W., Pijnenborg, R., Hanssens, M., McFadyen, I. R. and Van Assche, A. (1994). A study of placental bed spiral arteries and trophoblast invasion in normal and severe pre-eclamptic pregnancies. *Br. J. Obstet. Gynaecol.*, **101**, 669–74.

Mould, P., Garratt, A. N., Askari, J. A., Akiyama, S. K. and Humphries, M. J. (1995). Identification of a novel anti-integrin monoclonal antibody that recognises a ligand-induced binding site epitope on the β1 subunit. *FEBS Lett.*, **363**, 118–22.

Moffett, A. and Loke, Y. W. (2004). The immunological paradox of pregnancy: a reappraisal. *Placenta*, **25**, 1–8.

Mühlhauser, J., Crescimanno, C., Kaufmann, P., Höfler, H., Zaccheo, D. and Castellucci, M. (1993). Differentiation and proliferation patterns in human trophoblast revealed by c-erbB-2 oncogene product and EGR-R. *J. Histochem. Cytochem.*, **41**, 165–73.

Nanaev, A. K., Chwalisz, K., Frank, H. G., Kohnen, G., Hegele-Hartung, C. and Kaufmann, P. (1995). Physiological dilation of uteroplacental arteries in the guinea pig depends on nitric oxide synthase of extravillous trophoblast. *Cell Tiss. Res.*, **282**, 407–21.

Nawrocki, B., Polette, M., Marchand, V., *et al.* (1996). Membrane-type matrix metalloproteinase-1 expression at the site of human implantation. *Placenta*, **17**, 565–72.

Nawrocki, B., Polette, M., Maquoi, E. and Birembaut, P. (1997). Expression of matrix metalloproteinases and their inhibitors during human placental development. *Troph. Res.*, **10**, 97–113.

O'Brien, M., Dausset, J., Carosella, E. D. and Moreau, P. (2000). Analysis of the role of HLA-G in preeclampsia. *Hum. Immunol.*, **61**, 1126–31.

Pepper, M. S. (1997). Transforming growth factor-beta: vasculogenesis and vessel wall integrity. *Cytok. Growth Factor Rev.*, **8**, 21–4.

Pijnenborg, R., Anthony, J., Davey, D. A., *et al.* (1991). Placental bed spiral arteries in the hypertensive disorders of pregnancy. *Br. J. Obstet. Gynaecol.*, **98**, 648–55.

Pijnenborg, R., Bland, J. M., Robertson, W. B., Dixon, G. and Brosens I. (1981). The pattern of interstitial trophoblast invasion in early human pregnancy. *Placenta*, **2**, 303–16.

Pijnenborg, R., Bland, J. M., Robertson, W. B. and Brosens, I. (1983). Uteroplacental arterial changes related to interstitial trophoblast migration in early human pregnancy. *Placenta*, **4**, 397–414.

Pijnenborg, R., Vercruysse, L., Verbist, L. and Van Assache, F. A. (1998). Interaction of interstitial trophoblast with placental bed capillaries and venules of normotensive and pre-eclamptic pregnancies. *Placenta*, **19**, 569–75.

Polette, M., Nawrocki, B., Pintiaux, B., *et al.* (1994). Expression of gelatinases A and B and their tissue inhibitors by cells of early and term human placenta and gestational endometrium. *Lab. Invest.*, **71**, 838–46.

Rajakumar, A. and Conrad, K. P. (2000). Expression, ontogeny, and regulation of hypoxia-inducible transcription factors in the human placenta. *Biol. Rep.*, **63**, 559–69.

Rajakumar, A., Whitelock, K. A., Weissfeld, L. A., Daftary, A. R., Markovic, N. and Conrad, K. P. (2001a). Selective overexpression of the hypoxia-inducible transcription factor, HIF-2 alpha, in placentas from women with preeclampsia. *Biol. Reprod.*, **64**, 499–506.

Rajakumar, A., Whitelock, K. A., Weissfeld, L. A., Daftary, A. R., Markovic, N. and Conrad, K. P. (2001b). Erratum. *Biol. Reprod.*, **64**, 1019–20.

Robertson, W. B., Khong, T. Y., Brosens, I., De Wolf, F., Sheppard, B. L. and Bonnar, J. (1986). The placental bed biopsy: review from three European centres. *Am. J. Obstet. Gynecol.*, **155**, 401–12.

Rodesch, F., Simon, P., Donner, C. and Jauniaux, E. (1992). Oxygen measurements in endometrial and trophoblastic tissues during early pregnancy. *Obstet. Gynecol.*, **80**, 283–5.

Ruck, P., Marzusch, K., Krober, S., Horny, H.-P., Dietl, H. and Kaiserling, E. (1997). The distribution of tissue inhibitor of metalloproteinases-2 (TIMP-2) in decidua and trophoblast of early human pregnancy. *Troph. Res.*, **10**, 115–21.

Schaffer, L., Scheid, A., Spielmann, P., *et al.* (2003). Oxygen-regulated expression of TGF-beta 3, a growth factor involved in trophoblast differentiation. *Placenta*, **24**, 941–50.

Selick, C. E., Horowitz, G. M., Gratch, M., Scott Jr, R. T., Navot, D. and Hofmann, G. E. (1994). Immunohistochemical localization of transforming growth factor-β in human implantation sites. *J. Clin. Endocrinol. Metabol.*, **78**, 592–6.

Semenza, G. L. (1998). Hypoxia-inducible factor-1 and the molecular physiology of oxygen homeostasis. *J. Lab. Clin. Med.*, **131**, 207–14.

Shi, W. L., Mognetti, B., Campana, A. and Bischof, P. (1995). Metalloproteinase secretion by endometrial leukocyte subsets. *Am. J. Reprod. Immunol.*, **34**, 299–310.

Simpson, H., Robson, S. C., Bulmer, J. N., Barber, A. and Lyall, F. (2002). Transforming growth factor β expression in human placenta and placental bed during early pregnancy. *Placenta*, **23**, 44–58.

Taylor, C. M., Stevens, H., Anthony, F. W. and Wheeler, T. (1997). Influence of hypoxia on vascular endothelial growth factor and chorionic gonadotrophin production in trophoblast derived cell lines; JEG, Jar and BeWo. *Placenta*, **18**, 451–8.

Thompson, C. B. (1995). Apoptosis in the pathogenesis and treatment of disease. *Science*, **267**, 1456–62.

Verma, A., Hirsch, D. J., Glatt, C. E., Ronnett, G. V. and Snyder, S. H. (1993). Carbon monoxide: a putative neural messenger. *Science*, **259**, 381.

Vettraino, I. M., Roby, J., Tolley, T. and Parks, W. C. (1996). Collagenase-1, stromelysin-1 and matrilysin are expressed within the placenta during multiple stages of human pregnancy. *Placenta*, **17**, 557–63.

Vicovac, L. and Aplin, J. (1996). Epithelial–mesenchymal transition during trophoblast differentiation. *Acta Anat.*, **156**, 202–16.

Vicovac, L., Jones, C. S. and Aplin, J. D. (1995). Trophoblast differentiation during formation of anchoring in a model of the early human placenta in vitro. *Placenta*, **16**, 41–56.

Vuckovic, M., Genbacev, O. and Kumar, S. (1992). Immunolocalization of transforming growth factor beta in 1st and 3rd trimester human placenta. *Pathobiology*, **60**, 149–50.

Winterhager, E., von Ostau, C., Grümmer, R., Kaufmann, P. and Fisher, S. J. (1996). Connexin and E-Cadherin Expression während der Differenzierung des humanen Trophoblasten. *Ann. Anat.*, **178**, 41.

Zakhary, R., Gaine, S. P., Dinerman, J. L., Ruat, M., Flavahan, N. A. and Snyder, S. H. (1996). Hemeoxygenase 2: endothelial and neuronal localization and role in endothelium-dependent relaxation. *Proc. Natl Acad. Sci. USA*, **93**, 795–8.

Zhou, Y., Damsky, C. H., Chiu, K., Roberts, J. M. and Fisher, S. J. (1993). Preeclampsia is associated with abnormal expression of adhesion molecules by invasive cytotrophoblasts. *J. Clin. Invest.*, **91**, 950–60.

Zhou, Y., Damsky, C. H. and Fisher, S. J. (1997b). Preeclampsia is associated with failure of human cytotrophoblasts to mimic a vascular adhesion phenotype. *J. Clin. Invest.*, **99**, 2152–64.

Zhou, Y., Fisher, S. J., Janatpour, M., Genbacev, O., Dejana, E. and Wheelock, M. (1997a). Human cytotrophoblasts adopt a vascular phenotype as they differentiate. A strategy for successful endovascular invasion? *J. Clin. Invest.*, **99**, 2139–51.

Zhou, Y., Genbacev, O., Damsky, C. H. and Fisher, S. J. (1998). Oxygen regulates human cytotrophoblast differentiation and invasion: implications for endovascular invasion in normal pregnancy and in pre-eclampsia. *J. Reprod. Immunol.*, **39**, 197–213.

Zygmunt, M., Boving, B., Wienhard, J., *et al.* (1997). Expression of cell adhesion molecules in the extravillous trophoblast is altered in IUGR. *Am. J. Reprod. Immunol.*, **38**, 295–301.

3

In vitro models for studying pre-eclampsia

John D. Aplin and Ian P. Crocker

Introduction

Profound morphological changes occur during the comparatively short life span of the placenta (Benirschke and Kaufmann, 2000; Fox, 1997). Most of these can be related directly to functional requirements; establishing support for fetal development and growth, maintaining an immunological barrier and adjusting maternal physiology to meet the demands of pregnancy. Histology and ultrastructure present snapshots of cell and tissue behavior, but not an account of cellular interactions or pathological mechanisms. Appropriate and robust in vitro models are therefore essential in bridging the gap between structure and function, as they can accommodate mechanistic questions and offer scope for the design and testing of possible therapeutic interventions. Models should mimic cell responses in vivo and go at least part way to reflecting physiological events within the placenta. Experimental levels range from tissue perfusion to explant and cell culture. Recently, genomic, transcriptomic, proteomic and computational biology approaches have become available to complement and extend in vitro methodologies. To appreciate how these models have been applied to studying pre-eclampsia, and the scope of the in vitro methods currently available, it is convenient to divide the placenta into structurally and functionally distinct compartments, i.e. the chorionic villus and the placental bed. In turn, we have subdivided these into individual cellular components, namely those of the trophoblast, vasculature and stroma.

Villus components

Cytotrophoblast and syncytiotrophoblast in primary culture

Cytotrophoblast cells of the human placenta are the precursors of all other trophoblast phenotypes. As such, a variety of methods have been employed for their purification. Most current isolation methods are derived from the classic work of Thiede in the 1960s and since then, a consensus has emerged regarding the preparation of a relatively pure, viable population of cytotrophoblasts from both early and late gestational tissue. Of the enzymes available, trypsin has consistently proved the most reliable for cytotrophoblast isolation. Most current procedures use serial digestion (Hall *et al.*, 1977). In general, a successful digestion requires conditions to be as mild and treatment as brief as possible, to minimize disturbances in stromal and non-cytotrophoblast compartments. For first-trimester tissue, cytotrophoblasts released under mild conditions originate largely from the adherent cell columns and are therefore not true villous trophoblasts (see later section). On the whole, first-trimester villous cytotrophoblasts require more stringent enzymatic conditions.

Further purification of cytotrophoblasts from proteolytic digests is required and a range of techniques is available (Hemmings and Guilbert, 2002; Karl *et al.*, 1992; Kliman *et al.*, 1986; Sacks *et al.*, 2001; Tarrade *et al.*, 2001a; Yui *et al.*, 1994). Most employ protease-resistant cell surface antigens, such as CD45, CD9, MHC-class I, or MHC-class II, to mark mesenchymal or immune cells and separate them from the dissociated cytotrophoblasts. The presence of MHC-class I and CD9 on extravillous cytotrophoblasts and their absence from villous trophoblasts is useful in distinguishing these populations (Copeman *et al.*, 2000; Hirano *et al.*, 1999).

Following immuno-purification, a frequently encountered problem is contamination with syncytial fragments, i.e. resealed syncytial vesicles containing zero, one or more nuclei. Being mainly non-adherent, these can be removed by routine culturing, but fluorescence activated cell sorting (FACS) is increasingly employed to maximize purity and viability. Using this method, non-viable cells can be eliminated through propidium iodide resistance and syncytial fragments removed by recognition of exteriorized phospatidylserine (Guilbert *et al.*, 2002). More recently, positive immunoselection using antibody C76/18 to hepatocyte growth factor activator inhibitor 1 has been used to derive pure populations of cytotrophoblast cells, devoid of both syncytial fragments and extravillous cytotrophoblast elements (Potgens *et al.*, 2003). Trophoblast populations can be confirmed by cytokeratin-7 immunostaining (Blaschitz *et al.*, 2000; Haigh *et al.*, 1999).

Unlike their in vivo counterparts, isolated cytotrophoblasts are unable to proliferate in culture. Term villous cells differentiate in vitro, initially adhering to the culture surface before migrating, aggregating and fusing within 24–96 h. Immunostaining with antibodies to actin, cytokeratin or the desmosomal protein desmoplakin are all useful methods for distinguishing mononucleate from multinucleate cells (Crocker *et al.*, 2001b; Parast *et al.*, 2001). Functionally, the multinucleate cells synthesize and secrete hCG, hPL, leptin,

progesterone and estrogens and these can be used to verify the extent of differentiation in culture (Douglas and King, 1990). Although they share certain characteristics with their in vivo syncytiotrophoblast counterpart, developing into a polarized epithelial sheet with apical microvilli (Bloxam *et al.*, 1997), it is difficult to achieve full confluency, an important limitation for syncytiotrophoblast transport studies. Their morphological and biochemical differentiation can become uncoupled in vitro as evidenced by production of hCG by mononucleate cells (Kao *et al.*, 1988). They rarely contain more than 10–20 nuclei and in certain respects are more reminiscent of placental bed giant cells than villous syncytiotrophoblast.

In vitro, environmental stimuli can be applied to primary trophoblasts to investigate responses to either normal or aberrant placental conditions. Examples of these studies are numerous and include the actions of oxygen (Kilani *et al.*, 2003), cytokines (Crocker *et al.*, 2001a) and growth factors (Crocker *et al.*, 2001b). The issues surrounding oxygen and the appropriate levels for culturing are currently debated (Kilani *et al.*, 2003). It is generally agreed that the oxygen tension in the intervillous space is approximately 45–50 mmHg at term (Soothill *et al.*, 1986) and that levels may be as low as 18 mmHg in early gestation (Jauniaux *et al.*, 2003a). There is an emerging consensus that levels of ambient oxygen should be reduced to 6–8% to simulate physiological conditions in late pregnancy with lower levels (2–3%) required to simulate first-trimester conditions and avoid oxidative stress (Jauniaux *et al.*, 2003b). Co-cultures between cell types can be performed to define interactions between trophoblasts, endothelial cells (Cockell *et al.*, 1997), fibroblasts (Lacey *et al.*, 2002) and leukocytes (von Dadelszen *et al.*, 1999).

Undoubtedly, multinucleate trophoblast in culture has proved a useful model in studies of villous transport, particularly in systems that depend upon, or are affected by, intracellular metabolites. One-sided uptake across the microvillous membrane can be achieved using a basic syncytiotrophoblast monolayer. However, investigating the syncytiotrophoblast basal membrane, or transtrophoblast transfer in either direction, requires a two-sided approach. This can be achieved by culture on filters, typically nitrocellulose, polyester or gelatin-coated microporous polycarbonate (Bloxam et al., 1997). Using these models, the directional transfer of immunoglobulin G and glucose has been demonstrated and system A amino acid transporter and the Na(+)/H(+) exchanger activities measured. As the polarized status of cultured syncytiotrophoblast has been questioned, a more accepted approach is the preparation of syncytial microvillous or basal membrane vesicles from fresh tissue (Sibley et al., 1998). Using this method, domain variation between plasma membrane distributions of transporters has been observed.

Limitations of primary cell isolates include paucity of numbers, variations occasioned by changing batches of enzyme, inability to stimulate proliferation, uncontrolled differentiation, contamination and a limited lifespan in vitro. Cell lines, generated from normal or choriocarcinoma tissue, provide more stable, long-lived and homogenous populations, which overcome many of these culture anomalies. However, methods employed to extend lifespan (i.e. transfection or spontaneous immortalization/transformation) alter the regulation of cell division and impact upon differentiation (including relatively low rates of cell fusion) and gene expression. Typical human trophoblastic cell lines are SGHPL-4 and -5, derived from first-trimester placenta through transfection with early region SV40, and the choriocarcinoma cell lines, BeWo, JEG and JAR which have been widely used in secretion, fusion, invasion and transport studies (Cartwright et al., 1999; Dutta-Roy, 2000; Kudo et al., 2003). These cell lines have been extensively characterized and differ in numerous important respects from primary cell isolates (Shiverick et al., 2001). The overriding consideration is to recognize both their strengths and limitations. It is hoped that with the development of methods to isolate and propagate mouse trophoblast stem cells

(Tanaka et al., 1998) and the demonstration that human embryonic stem (ES) cells can be stimulated to differentiate into trophoblast by treatment with bone morphogenetic protein 4 (BMP-4), a member of the TGF-beta superfamily, the availability of early trophoblast lineages will allow improved studies of the early developmental origins of pregnancy pathology.

Explant models of the villous pathway

Cytotrophoblast cells in primary culture are useful for studying aspects of trophoblast regulation and interactions, but suffer the disadvantages of not fully achieving the in vivo phenotype and of being divorced from potentially important interactions with other components of the placental villus. Explant cultures of chorionic villous fragments escape some of these limitations. A comparison of short-term dual perfusion with explants revealed a severe and rapid loss of trophoblast viability in explants with better survival during perfusion (Di Santo et al., 2003). However, when fragments of chorionic villous tissue are dissected from the placenta and maintained for up to 11 days in culture, syncytiotrophoblast degeneration (during the first 48 h) and sloughing from the villous surface, is followed by renewal with differentiation and fusion of underlying viable cytotrophoblasts (Siman et al., 2001). Syncytial degeneration/regeneration can be easily monitored by the liberation of hCG (human chorionic gondatrophin), which dramatically falls with syncytial loss and then rises exponentially as the fresh syncytiotrophoblast emerges (Watson et al., 1995). Studies are presently ongoing to assess the extent to which this new trophoblastic layer mimics syncytiotrophoblast in vivo (Siman et al., 2001). Reducing the concentration of magnesium ions to 0.7 mM is reported to yield improved preservation of the native syncytium in explants (Huppertz et al., 2003). Unlike isolated cytotrophoblasts, this model readily accommodates cell proliferation. The syncytiotrophoblast life cycle can be influenced by conditions pertaining to the pre-eclamptic placenta. Thus, for example, severe hypoxia increases trophoblast necrosis in term tissue explants (Huppertz *et al.*, 2003). Moreover, explanted fragments taken from these placentae have shown alterations in aspects of cell proliferation, differentiation and apoptosis (Mayhew *et al.*, 2003).

Villous mesenchymal cells

Pre-eclampsia may invoke, or even arise from, alterations to the phenotype of placental cells other than trophoblasts. Cells resident in the villous mesenchyme may have a profound influence on trophoblast phenotype (Garcia-Lloret *et al.*, 1994; Lacey *et al.*, 2002; Tanaka *et al.*, 1998). They include fibroblasts, vascular cells and immune cells, and although there are to date rather few reports in the literature, for completeness short descriptions of their isolation and use in vitro are included.

Placental fibroblasts

A variety of methods for the isolation of fibroblasts from villous mesenchyme have been described and compared (Garcia-Lloret *et al.*, 1994; Haigh *et al.*, 1999). Villous extracellular matrix (ECM) is produced by these cells. First-trimester cells synthesize higher amounts of several ECM components than term cells. Production of the ECM components collagen IV and fibronectin increases with lower oxygen partial pressure (Chen and Aplin, 2003) and, correspondingly, basement membrane thickness increases in vivo in hypoxia.

Placental endothelial cells

The fetal endothelial monolayer is responsible for regulating vascular tone, micro-vascular coagulation and angiogenesis. Placental endothelial cells, unlike those from maternal vascular beds, have only recently been characterized and have yet to be used extensively in vitro (Dye *et al.*, 2001). Much of our previous knowledge of these cells in the fetal–placental circulation has come from studies using cultured human umbilical vein endothelial cells (HUVECs). However, it is increasingly recognized that HUVECs differ both phenotypically and functionally with their intra-placental microvascular counterparts (Dye *et al.*, 2003). Small endothelial aggregates can be isolated from placental microvessels by sequential enzymatic digestion, followed by positive selection using magnetic microbeads coated with anti-thrombomodulin antibodies (Kacemi *et al.*, 1996). When placed in culture these microvascular cells stain positively for von Willebrand factor and can incorporate acetylated low-density lipoproteins (Kacemi *et al.*, 1996). Isolating, maintaining and growing these cells is notoriously difficult, and the human placental endothelial cell line, HPEC-A1, has been derived to overcome these problems (Schutz *et al.*, 1997). With functional changes in placental endothelium implicated in pathological pregnancies, future studies of their properties are anticipated.

Placental macrophages

Macrophages can be found within the fetal villi from week 4 until term. Their role in the placenta is still largely unclear. They can express class II major histocompatibility complex (MHC) antigens and Fc receptors and, when activated, can produce various potent cytokines and interleukins. In addition to phagocytic activity, there is evidence for their involvement in (i) substrate transport across the stroma, (ii) the regulation of angiogenesis, and (iii) fetal immunological defence. Their position in the stroma, close to both fetal vessels and placental trophoblasts, makes them likely candidates for involvement in regulatory functions during placental development and placental physiology. Presently, very few experimental data exist regarding their interactions with other cells of the placenta.

Villous macrophages may be isolated by treating small pieces of villous tissue with pronase, followed by selective adherence of the released cells to tissue culture plastic (Khan *et al.*, 2000).

Immunocytochemistry with anti-CD68 may be used to determine the degree of purity and in some cases Ficoll and Percoll gradient centrifugation and negative selection of trophoblast with anti-epidermal growth factor (EGF)-receptor-coated Dynabeads have been used to improve purity (Wetzka *et al.*, 1997). Isolated placental macrophages, termed Hofbauer cells, produce prostaglandin E2 (PGE2) and thromboxane (TXA2) following stimulation with lipopolysaccharide (LPS) (Wetzka *et al.*, 1997). Notably, these paracrine mediators, which are important in both pre-eclampsia and labor, can be affected by oxygen exposure. To date, the properties of Hofbauer cells obtained from pre-eclamptic placentae have been little studied.

Placental fibroblasts and macrophages are capable of producing both CSF-1 and GM-CSF, cytokines that regulate macrophage survival, growth and activation (Garcia-Lloret *et al.*, 1994; Khan *et al.*, 2000). Studies in vitro suggest that macrophage secretions can influence trophoblast differentiation (Khan *et al.*, 2000).

Extravillous trophoblast

Cytotrophoblasts proliferate to form columns at anchoring sites where peripheral villi make contact with the maternal decidual interstitium (Aplin *et al.*, 1998). Large numbers of extravillous cytotrophoblasts detach from the distal columns and migrate into interstitial and endovascular locations in the placental bed (Pijnenborg *et al.*, 1981). Migration proceeds as far as the inner third of the myometrium in normal pregnancy, but is shallower in pre-eclampsia, where there are also a lesser proportion of interstitial apoptotic cells (Kadyrov *et al.*, 2003; Kaufmann *et al.*, 2003; Naicker *et al.*, 2003). Trophoblast-mediated remodeling of the myometrial segments of maternal spiral arteries is impaired in pre-eclampsia, where endovascular cytotrophoblasts are largely absent from the vessel walls (Meekins *et al.*, 1994; Naicker *et al.*, 2003). Migration continues from the early

post-implantation stages of pregnancy up to week 20, after which cell columns diminish in size and there is a progressively increasing incidence of large polygonal or dendritic trophoblast and multinucleate giant cells in the placental bed (Kemp *et al.*, 2002). The formation of these cells appears to be a terminal differentiation step, and many of them show apoptotic features.

Though most attention has been focused on factors that might impair or retard cell migration, the present state of knowledge leaves open the possibility that poor trophoblast invasion might result from other causes: fewer anchoring sites, fewer cells entering the extravillous lineage, impairment to the extravillous differentiation program, restriction of the escape of cells from the distal columns, elevated rates of terminal differentiation to placental bed giant cells, altered apoptosis of extravillous cells or specific inhibition of access of interstitial cells to spiral arteries in the myometrium. Thus, for example, it is noteworthy that mice lacking one allele of the *p57kip2* gene, which is expressed in trophoblast and antagonizes cyclin-dependent kinases, have features of pre-eclampsia (Kanayama *et al.*, 2002). A higher proliferation index (Redline and Patterson, 1995) and lower rate of trophoblast apoptosis (Kadyrov *et al.*, 2003) have been observed in extravillous cells in pre-eclampsia. There is also evidence that maternal macrophages can trigger apoptosis in trophoblast, and may be more abundant in peri-arterial regions in pre-eclamptic myometrim (Kaufmann *et al.*, 2003). Unraveling the causes of impaired invasion of trophoblast in pre-eclampsia will therefore depend on a careful combination of appropriate in vitro models with observations made in vivo.

In vitro models include choriocarcinoma cell lines, trophoblast lines derived by transformation of various types of primary isolate with viral oncogenes such as SV40 large T (Choy and Manyonda, 1998; Choy *et al.*, 2000; Fukushima *et al.*, 2003; Logan *et al.*, 1992), trophoblast hybridomas obtained after fusion with HGPRT-resistant choriocarcinoma cells and selection

(Frank *et al.*, 2000), primary cytotrophoblast isolates from first-trimester or term tissue, villous tissue explants, and co-cultures in which trophoblast interaction with maternal or fetal cells can be examined.

The use of either trophoblast cell preparations or explanted villous tissue in principle allows evaluation of the relative influence of the intrinsic placental developmental program as against the maternal environment (Aplin, 1991). For studies of the extravillous lineage, first-trimester cells should be used as cytotrophoblast derived from third-trimester placenta show much lower migratory activity. The irreversible exit of trophoblast from the cell cycle with differentiation is fundamental to their life cycle, so continued proliferation is a key objection to the use of tumor and transformed cell lines. It is a truism that all such cells display patterns of gene expression that differ from normal trophoblast. Data obtained with these models must therefore be interpreted with caution and are not discussed here further.

Numerous investigators have examined the effect of varying ambient oxygen concentration on third-trimester trophoblast gene expression and behavior in vitro. However, since the first-trimester placenta develops in a state of physiological hypoxia, it may not be clear whether the resulting data are pertinent to the earlier developmental stage, or the late gestation organ pathology of preeclampsia, or both. It is not our intention here to review the effect of hypoxic or hyperoxic conditions on trophoblast, but selected examples are given.

Primary extravillous cytotrophoblast cultures

Trophoblast can be isolated from first-trimester villous tissue using protocols adapted from those used in term tissue as discussed above (Librach *et al.*, 1991; Tarrade *et al.*, 2001a). Treatment with DNAse and trypsin releases trophoblasts and

further purification is effected by percoll gradient centrifugation. Residual CD45-positive leukocytes or CD9-positive stromal cells can be removed by negative selection, for example using antibody-conjugated magnetic beads. Obtaining viable mononuclear cytotrophoblasts from term tissue requires syncytial disruption, whereas first-trimester cell preparations, made with minimal tissue shearing, are relatively enriched in cells from cytotrophoblast columns that remain attached to the peripheral villi at separation and are generally lacking in overlying syncytium. Differential display has been used to identify genes that are expressed in the first-trimester pool and not at term, and the observation of selective expression of the corresponding mRNA in cytotrophoblast columns reflects the relative enrichment of these cells in the starting isolates (Huch *et al.*, 1998).

Cells that are already committed to the extravillous lineage at isolation are likely to be post-mitotic, polyploid (Zybina *et al.*, 2002), and distinguishable by surface phenotype (Damsky *et al.*, 1994; Vicovac and Aplin, 1996). Since the column contains a gradient of cells from the undifferentiated ones at the base to those that already bear the hallmarks of interstitial extravillous trophoblast at the periphery, a mixed population of cells bearing features of different stages of extravillous differentiation is released. The cells can be further purified by panning or flow cytometry, selecting for extravillous markers such as integrin alpha 1 or HLAG or using negative selection of CD45-positive immune cells. In addition, depending on the degree of syncytial disruption in the protocol, some villous cytotrophoblasts are present. Some of these cells are likely to find fusion partners during the first few days in vitro, generating a variable proportion of multinucleate trophoblast.

Isolated cytotrophoblasts exit the cell cycle within approximately the first 24 h in vitro, although this can be prolonged by culture in low oxygen. There are many reports in the literature of cytotrophoblast preparations that incorporate thymidine at later time points, and this can probably be accounted for by polyploidization or the increasing influence of contaminating fibroblasts, which while initially at a low level, may proliferate. Thus, cell proliferation assays should be interpreted with caution. They can be performed in situ so that each cell can be concurrently identified by marker expression. As with term villous trophoblasts, it is useful (Haigh et al., 1999) to monitor the purity of the cell population obtained using the intermediate filament markers cytokeratin-7 (present on tropho-blasts but not fibroblasts or blood cells) and vimentin (present on most contaminating cells but not trophoblast). One should note that a figure of, for example, 98% cytokeratin-7 positive cells at isolation can rapidly alter with fibroblast prolifera-tion, and that trans-filter migration assays can enrich a small proportion of non-trophoblast cells. Thus cellular phenotype should be confirmed at the end of the experiment.

Cytotrophoblast survival is anchorage-dependent, with apoptosis occurring at a high rate in suspension. Furthermore, these cells do not adhere efficiently to tissue culture plastic, and a surface containing matrigel is preferred for optimal adhesion and continuing viability. Primary first-trimester cytotrophoblasts have been used effec-tively to study various molecular systems in migration. Thus, for example, a combined role for MMP9 and plasminogen activator in cytotrophoblast invasion was suggested by assays of the migration of first-trimester cytotrophoblasts across matrigel-coated filters and its inhibition by specific blocking reagents (Librach et al., 1991). PPARgamma/RXRalpha heterodimers are expressed in extravillous trophoblast in vivo and agonist ligands similarly inhibit trans-filter migration (Tarrade et al., 2001b).

Studies of the properties of primary trophoblasts obtained from normal and pre-eclamptic tissue show interesting differences. Thus, for example, cells from pre-eclamptic placentas show a lower rate of attachment to matrix proteins than control cells and reduced rates of cell fusion (Pijnenborg et al., 1996). This indicates a cell-autonomous impairment of function, but does not indicate

whether this has arisen from an abnormality intrinsic to the trophoblast, or as the result of changes that occurred during the exposure of the cells to the abnormal environment of the pre-eclamptic pregnancy. Since the symptoms of pre-eclampsia appear only in the third trimester, it has not been possible to compare the properties of cultured cytotrophoblasts obtained during the period of extravillous cell migration from normal and pre-eclamptic pregnancies. Microarray analy-sis of whole placental mRNA has revealed differ-ences between pre-eclamptic and normal tissues (Reimer et al., 2002), but the multicellular origin of these libraries is an important impediment to data interpretation. Microarrays have also allowed characterization of gene expression changes as primary trophoblast isolates differentiate in vitro (Aronow et al., 2001), and this approach is likely to yield new insights into trophoblast-specific gene expression alterations in pre-eclampsia.

Primary cultured cytotrophoblasts have lost an environmental constraint that is no doubt of importance to their behavior, that is, the highly directional, asymmetric environment of the maternal–fetal interface, with the placental stroma in one direction and the decidua in the other. They have also lost their normal intercellular contact with adjacent trophoblast. Their utility comes in assessing the cell-autonomous contribution of the placenta to diseases such as pre-eclampsia. Where differences are evident, however, it is important to bear in mind that these could either be truly autonomous (programmed de novo into the trophoblast lineage) or could alternatively have arisen from a cellular memory, created in vivo in response to an environmental signal.

Co-culture models

Cytotrophoblast has been co-cultured with decid-ual cells, macrophages, NK cells or vascular endothelial cells to examine the intercellular inter-actions that occur in the placental bed. Decidual endothelial cells have been isolated by pronase/ trypsin digestion followed by positive selection on magnetic beads conjugated to Ulex europaeus lectin (UEA1) (Gallery et al., 1991). The observation that decidual endothelial cells from pre-eclamptic pregnancies express a lower level of MMP-1 than control cells from normal gestations led to the suggestion that reduced MMP action may be important in relation to reduced trophoblast invasion of maternal vessels in pre-eclampsia (Gallery et al., 1999). Trans-filter co-culture of term cytotrophoblast with decidual endothelial cells resulted in reduced latent MMP-9 secretion and reduced cytotrophoblast migration (Campbell et al., 2003).

Co-culture of cytotrophoblasts with macro-phages has shown that the latter are capable of stimulating apoptosis, though experiments were carried out with a trophoblast hybridoma cell line (Reister et al., 2001). Thus an excessive number, or inappropriately activated population, of macrophages in the placental bed has been postulated to impair the viability of the extravillous trophoblast population in pre-eclampsia, with a suggested mechanism of tryptophan depletion combined with TNF alpha secretion.

Explant models

First-trimester mesenchymal villi explanted on a three-dimensional (gel) substrate of collagen I or matrigel attach and within 24 h column-like structures outgrow from the villous tips. These can be shown to contain pure cytotrophoblast. An initial burst of proliferation over the first approximately 24 h creates a pool of cells that, over the following few days, grows out as one or several invasion fronts (Aplin et al., 1999; Vicovac and Aplin, 1996). The assay can be adapted to a trans-filter format with migrating cells counted at the distal side. If the ambient oxygen is reduced to 2%, cells remain in cycle up to 36 h, and differentiation has been reported to be retarded, with a reduced expression of the extravillous trophoblast markers, integrin alpha 1 and alpha 5 (Genbacev et al., 1996). cAMP has been shown to enhance the expression of melanoma cell adhesion

molecule (MCAM) in extravillous trophoblast in explant culture (Higuchi et al., 2003). The emerging extravillous cytotrophoblasts can be treated with antisense oligonucleotides and this approach has been used to demonstrate that TGF-beta-mediated signaling inhibits the development of cells in the extravillous trophoblast lineage (Caniggia et al., 2000), leading to the hypothesis that over-production of TGF-beta3 may account for the disturbance of extravillous trophoblast behavior in pre-eclampsia (Caniggia et al., 1999).

This assay format preserves the spatial relation-ship between the villous trophoblast and its underlying mesenchyme, and has been used to demonstrate a paracrine relationship in which IGFs, derived from the mesenchyme and the trophoblast itself, both stimulate cell migration (Lacey et al., 2002). The fact that columns develop at all is instructive, indicating that decidual signals other than a permissive ECM are not required for this step in differentiation. However, the number of cells detaching at the periphery of the columns and migrating as single cells into the surrounding ECM is much smaller than seen in vivo. It is interesting in this light to note that in ectopic (tubal) implantation sites, the cytotrophoblast columns are longer (Goffin et al., 2003). Both these observations imply that a decidual signal stimulates cells to detach from the distal column and escape into the stroma. An effect indicative of environmental influence on migration efficiency is also evident in tubal implantation sites in which higher incidences of viable implants are at the mesosalpingeal side. It appears that cytotropho-blast colonization of the stroma is greater in the mesometrial plane, that is, in the direction of the arterial supply. Furthermore, a greater fraction of extravillous cells remains in cycle as compared with eutopic implants (Kemp et al., 1999, 2002).

When first-trimester mesenchymal villous tissue is co-cultured in contact with parietal decidua, column formation is stimulated at the villous tips (Vicovac et al., 1995). Extensive de novo interstitial colonization is not observed directly from the columns, but the cells migrate into small arteries, cause disruption of the walls and then invade the surrounding decidual stroma (Dunk *et al.*, 2003).

Vessel invasion models

A vessel explant model has been developed in which uninvaded spiral arteries are dissected from myometrial tissue obtained at Cesarian section or hysterectomy and first-trimester cytotrophoblasts introduced either intraluminally, with the aid of a pressure myograph, or interstitially, by tying off the vessel and mounting it in a fibrin gel containing primary cytotrophoblasts (Cartwright *et al.*, 2002). Omental vessels have been used as controls. Attachment of trophoblast to the endothelium is observed and apoptosis of endothelial cells follows by a Fas ligand-dependent mechanism (Ashton *et al.*, 2005). Trophoblast migration into arterial walls is 5–10-fold more efficient at 20% ambient oxygen concentration than at 2%, and occurs more efficiently into uterine than into omental vessels (Crocker *et al.*, 2005). This model has also been used to demonstrate that endovascular trophoblasts trigger apoptosis in spiral arterial smooth muscle cells, again by a Fas ligand-dependent mechanism (Harris *et al.*, 2006). Introduction of culture medium from human first-trimester cytotrophoblasts into rat mesenteric resistance arteries also alters vasomotor behavior (Gratton *et al.*, 2001).

Gene arrays and proteomics

Differential transcriptomic analyses have been reported using tissue from different gestational ages (Hemberger *et al.*, 2001), cytotrophoblasts following different treatment regimes, or placental tissue biopsies derived from normal and pre-eclamptic pregnancies. Studies at several time points during trophoblast differentiation in culture led to the idea of 'categorical reprogramming' of genes during cytotrophoblast differentiation (Handwerger and Aronow, 2003) and the up-regulation of pre-eclamptic susceptibility genes, like those associated with the interleukin and TNF receptor superfamilies (Reimer *et al.*, 2002).

Such studies identify candidate genes for functional study in experimental models.

More recently, interest has been directed toward the differential analysis of proteomes in normal and pre-eclamptic placental tissue, and normal and pre-eclamptic maternal plasma (Kalionis and Moses, 2003; Myers *et al.*, 2004; Page *et al.*, 2002). A proteomic analysis has also been reported of the effects of varying oxygen concentration on first-trimester cytotrophoblast in primary culture (Hoang *et al.*, 2001). With potential implications in screening and therapeutic targeting and advances in automation, proteomics will undoubtedly be further applied to in vitro models of placental function and will play an increasing role in the understanding of pregnancy complications, such as pre-eclampsia.

REFERENCES

Aplin, J.D. (1991). Implantation, trophoblast differentiation and haemochorial placentation: mechanistic evidence in vivo and in vitro. *J. Cell Sci.*, **99**(4), 681–92.

Aplin, J.D., Haigh, T., Jones, C.J., Church, H.J. and Vicovac, L. (1999). Development of cytotrophoblast columns from explanted first-trimester human placental villi: role of fibronectin and integrin alpha5beta1. *Biol. Reprod.*, **60**, 828–38.

Aplin, J.D., Haigh, T., Vicovac, L., Church, H.J. and Jones, C.J. (1998). Anchorage in the developing placenta: an overlooked determinant of pregnancy outcome? *Hum. Fertil. (Camb.)*, **1**, 75–9.

Aronow, B.J., Richardson, B.D. and Handwerger, S. (2001). Microarray analysis of trophoblast differentiation: gene expression reprogramming in key gene function categories. *Physiol. Genomics*, **6**, 105–16.

Ashton, S.V., Whitley, G.S., Dash, P.R., *et al.* (2005). Uterine spiral artery remodeling involves endothelial apoptosis induced by extravillous trophoblasts through Fas/FasL interactions. *Arterioscler. Thromb. Vasc. Biol.*, **25**(1), 102–8.

Benirschke, K. and Kaufmann, P. (2000). *Pathology of the Human Placenta*. New York: Springer Verlag.

Blaschitz, A., Weiss, U., Dohr, G. and Desoye, G. (2000). Antibody reaction patterns in first trimester placenta: implications for trophoblast isolation and purity screening. *Placenta*, **21**, 733–41.

Bloxam, D. L., Bax, B. E. and Bax, C. M. (1997). Culture of syncytiotrophoblast for the study of human placental transfer. Part II: Production, culture and use of syncytiotrophoblast. *Placenta*, **18**, 99–108.

Campbell, S., Rowe, J., Jackson, C. J. and Gallery, E. D. (2003). In vitro migration of cytotrophoblasts through a decidual endothelial cell monolayer: the role of matrix metalloproteinases. *Placenta*, **24**, 306–15.

Caniggia, I., Grisaru-Gravnosky, S., Kuliszewsky, M., Post, M. and Lye, S. J. (1999). Inhibition of TGF-beta 3 restores the invasive capability of extravillous trophoblasts in preeclamptic pregnancies. *J. Clin. Invest.*, **103**, 1641–50.

Caniggia, I., Mostachfi, H., Winter, J., *et al.* (2000). Hypoxia-inducible factor-1 mediates the biological effects of oxygen on human trophoblast differentiation through TGFbeta(3). *J. Clin. Invest.*, **105**, 577–87.

Cartwright, J. E., Holden, D. P. and Whitley, G. S. (1999). Hepatocyte growth factor regulates human trophoblast motility and invasion: a role for nitric oxide. *Br. J. Pharmacol.*, **128**, 181–9.

Cartwright, J. E., Kenny, L. C., Dash, P. R., *et al.* (2002). Trophoblast invasion of spiral arteries: a novel in vitro model. *Placenta*, **23**, 232–5.

Chen, C. P. and Aplin, J. D. (2003). Placental extracellular matrix: gene expression, deposition by placental fibroblasts and the effect of oxygen. *Placenta*, **24**, 316–25.

Choy, M. Y. and Manyonda, I. T. (1998). The phagocytic activity of human first trimester extravillous trophoblast. *Hum. Reprod.*, **13**, 2941–9.

Choy, M. Y., St Whitley, G. and Manyonda, I. T. (2000). Efficient, rapid and reliable establishment of human trophoblast cell lines using poly-L-ornithine. *Early Pregnancy*, **4**, 124–43.

Cockell, A. P., Learmont, J. G., Smarason, A. K., Redman, C. W., Sargent, I. L. and Poston, L. (1997). Human placental syncytiotrophoblast microvillous membranes impair maternal vascular endothelial function. *Br. J. Obstet. Gynaecol.*, **104**, 235–40.

Copeman, J., Han, R. N., Caniggia, I., McMaster, M., Fisher, S. J. and Cross, J. C. (2000). Posttranscriptional regulation of human leukocyte antigen G during human extravillous cytotrophoblast differentiation. *Biol. Reprod.*, **62**, 1543–50.

Crocker, I. P., Barratt, S., Kaur, M. and Baker, P. N. (2001a). The in-vitro characterization of induced apoptosis in placental cytotrophoblasts and syncytiotrophoblasts. *Placenta*, **22**, 822–30.

Crocker, I. P., Strachan, B. K., Lash, G. E., Cooper, S., Warren, A. Y. and Baker, P. N. (2001b). Vascular endothelial growth factor but not placental growth factor promotes trophoblast syncytialization in vitro. *J. Soc. Gynecol. Invest.*, **8**, 341–6.

Crocker, I. P., Wareing, M., Ferris, G. R. *et al.* (2005). The effect of vascular origin, oxygen and tumour necrosis factor alpha on trophoblast invasion of matenal arteries in vitro. *J. Pathol.*, **206**, 476–85.

Damsky, C. H., Librach, C., Lim, K. H., *et al.* (1994). Integrin switching regulates normal trophoblast invasion. *Development*, **120**, 3657–66.

Di Santo, S., Malek, A., Sager, R., Andres, A. C. and Schneider, H. (2003). Trophoblast viability in perfused term placental tissue and explant cultures limited to 7–24 hours. *Placenta*, **24**, 882–94.

Douglas, G. C. and King, B. F. (1990). Differentiation of human trophoblast cells in vitro as revealed by immunocytochemical staining of desmoplakin and nuclei. *J. Cell Sci.*, **96**, 131–41.

Dunk, C., Petkovic, L., Baczyk, D., Rossant, J., Winterhager, E. and Lye, S. (2003). A novel in vitro model of trophoblast-mediated decidual blood vessel remodeling. *Lab. Invest.*, **83**(12), 1821–8.

Dutta-Roy, A. K. (2000). Transport mechanisms for long-chain polyunsaturated fatty acids in the human placenta. *Am. J. Clin. Nutr.*, **71**, 315S–22S.

Dye, J. F., Jablenska, R., Donnelly, J. L., *et al.* (2001). Phenotype of the endothelium in the human term placenta. *Placenta*, **22**, 32–43.

Dye, J. F., Vause, S., Johnston, T., *et al.* (2003). Characterization of cationic amino acid transporters and expression of endothelial nitric oxide synthase in human placental microvascular endothelial cells. *FASEB J.*, **3**, 3.

Fox, H. (1997). Aging of the placenta. *Arch. Dis. Child. Fetal. Neonatal Ed.*, **77**, F171–5.

Frank, H. G., Gunawan, B., Ebeling-Stark, I., *et al.* (2000). Cytogenetic and DNA-fingerprint characterization of choriocarcinoma cell lines and a trophoblast/choriocarcinoma cell hybrid. *Cancer Genet. Cytogenet.*, **116**, 16–22.

Fukushima, K., Miyamoto, S., Komatsu, H., *et al.* (2003). TNFalpha-induced apoptosis and integrin switching in human extravillous trophoblast cell line. *Biol. Reprod.*, **68**, 1771–8.

Gallery, E. D., Campbell, S., Arkell, J., Nguyen, M. and Jackson, C. J. (1999). Preeclamptic decidual microvascular endothelial cells express lower levels of matrix metalloproteinase-1 than normals. *Microvasc. Res.*, **57**, 340–6.

Gallery, E. D., Rowe, J., Schrieber, L. and Jackson, C. J. (1991). Isolation and purification of microvascular endothelium from human decidual tissue in the late phase of pregnancy. *Am. J. Obstet. Gynecol.*, **165**, 191–6.

Garcia-Lloret, M. I., Morrish, D. W., Wegmann, T. G., Honore, L., Turner, A. R. and Guilbert, L. J. (1994). Demonstration of functional cytokine-placental interactions: CSF-1 and GM-CSF stimulate human cytotrophoblast differentiation and peptide hormone secretion. *Exp. Cell Res.*, **214**, 46–54.

Genbacev, O., Joslin, R., Damsky, C. H., Polliotti, B. M. and Fisher, S. J. (1996). Hypoxia alters early gestation human cytotrophoblast differentiation/invasion in vitro and models the placental defects that occur in preeclampsia. *J. Clin. Invest.*, **97**, 540–50.

Goffin, F., Munaut, C., Malassine, A., *et al.* (2003). Evidence of a limited contribution of feto-maternal interactions to trophoblast differentiation along the invasive pathway. *Tiss. Antig.*, **62**, 104–16.

Gratton, R. J., Gandley, R. E., Genbacev, O., McCarthy, J. F., Fisher, S. J. and McLaughlin, M. K. (2001). Conditioned medium from hypoxic cytotrophoblasts alters arterial function. *Am. J. Obstet. Gynecol.*, **184**, 984–90.

Guilbert, L. J., Winkler-Lowen, B., Sherburne, R., Rote, N. S., Li, H. and Morrish, D. W. (2002). Preparation and functional characterization of villous cytotrophoblasts free of syncytial fragments. *Placenta*, **23**, 175–83.

Haigh, T., Chen, C., Jones, C. J. and Aplin, J. D. (1999). Studies of mesenchymal cells from 1st trimester human placenta: expression of cytokeratin outside the trophoblast lineage. *Placenta*, **20**, 615–25.

Hall, C. S., James, T. E., Goodyer, C., Branchaud, C., Guyda, H. and Giroud, C. J. (1977). Short term culture of human midterm and term placenta: parameters of hormonogenesis. *Steroids*, **30**, 569–80.

Handwerger, S. and Aronow, B. (2003). Dynamic changes in gene expression during human trophoblast differentiation. *Recent Prog. Horm. Res.*, **58**, 263–81.

Harris, L. K., Keogh, R. J., Wareing, M., *et al.* (2006). Invasive trophoblasts stimulate vascular smooth muscle cell apoptosis by a Fas ligand-dependent mechanism. *Am. J. Pathol.*, **169**, 1853–74.

Hemberger, M., Cross, J. C., Ropers, H. H., Lehrach, H., Fundele, R. and Himmelbauer, H. (2001). UniGene cDNA array-based monitoring of transcriptome changes during mouse placental development. *Proc. Natl Acad. Sci. USA*, **98**, 13,126–31.

Hemmings, D. G. and Guilbert, L. J. (2002). Polarized release of human cytomegalovirus from placental trophoblasts. *J. Virol.*, **76**, 6710–17.

Higuchi, T., Fujiwara, H., Egawa, H., *et al.* (2003). Cyclic AMP enhances the expression of an extravillous trophoblast marker, melanoma cell adhesion molecule, in choriocarcinoma cell JEG3 and human chorionic villous explant cultures. *Mol. Hum. Reprod.*, **9**, 359–66.

Hirano, T., Higuchi, T., Ueda, M., *et al.* (1999). CD9 is expressed in extravillous trophoblasts in association with integrin alpha3 and integrin alpha5. *Mol. Hum. Reprod.*, **5**, 162–7.

Hoang, V. M., Foulk, R., Clauser, K., Burlingame, A., Gibson, B. W. and Fisher, S. J. (2001). Functional proteomics: examining the effects of hypoxia on the cytotrophoblast protein repertoire. *Biochemistry*, **40**, 4077–86.

Huch, G., Hohn, H. P. and Denker, H. W. (1998). Identification of differentially expressed genes in human trophoblast cells by differential-display RT-PCR. *Placenta*, **19**, 557–67.

Huppertz, B., Kingdom, J., Caniggia, I., *et al.* (2003). Hypoxia favours necrotic versus apoptotic shedding of placental syncytiotrophoblast into the maternal circulation. *Placenta*, **24**, 181–90.

Jauniaux, E., Gulbis, B. and Burton, G. J. (2003a). Physiological implications of the materno-fetal oxygen gradient in human early pregnancy. *Reprod. Biomed. Online*, **7**, 250–3.

Jauniaux, E., Hempstock, J., Greenwold, N. and Burton, G. J. (2003b). Trophoblastic oxidative stress in relation to temporal and regional differences in maternal placental blood flow in normal and abnormal early pregnancies. *Am. J. Pathol.*, **162**, 115–25.

Kacemi, A., Challier, J. C., Galtier, M. and Olive, G. (1996). Culture of endothelial cells from human placental microvessels. *Cell Tissue Res.*, **283**, 183–90.

Kadyrov, M., Schmitz, C., Black, S., Kaufmann, P. and Huppertz, B. (2003). Pre-eclampsia and maternal anaemia display reduced apoptosis and opposite invasive phenotypes of extravillous trophoblast. *Placenta*, **24**, 540–8.

Kalionis, B. and Moses, E. (2003). Advanced molecular techniques in pregnancy research: proteomics and genomics – a workshop report. *Placenta*, **24**, S119–22.

Kanayama, N., Takahashi, K., Matsuura, T., *et al.* (2002). Deficiency in p57Kip2 expression induces preeclampsia-like symptoms in mice. *Mol. Hum. Reprod.*, **8**, 1129–35.

Kao, L. C., Caltabiano, S., Wu, S., Strauss, J. F. 3rd and Kliman, H. J. (1988). The human villous cytotrophoblast: interactions with extracellular matrix proteins, endocrine function, and cytoplasmic differentiation in the absence of syncytium formation. *Dev. Biol.*, **130**, 693–702.

Karl, P. I., Alpy, K. L. and Fisher, S. E. (1992). Serial enzymatic digestion method for isolation of human placental trophoblasts. *Placenta*, **13**, 385–7.

Kaufmann, P., Black, S. and Huppertz, B. (2003). Endovascular trophoblast invasion: implications for the pathogenesis of intrauterine growth retardation and preeclampsia. *Biol. Reprod.*, **69**, 1–7.

Kemp, B., Kertschanska, S., Handt, S., Funk, A., Kaufmann, P. and Rath, W. (1999). Different placentation patterns in viable compared with nonviable tubal pregnancy suggest a divergent clinical management. *Am. J. Obstet. Gynecol.*, **181**, 615–20.

Kemp, B., Kertschanska, S., Kadyrov, M., Rath, W., Kaufmann, P. and Huppertz, B. (2002). Invasive depth of extravillous trophoblast correlates with cellular phenotype: a comparison of intra- and extra-uterine implantation sites. *Histochem. Cell Biol.*, **117**, 401–14.

Khan, S., Katabuchi, H., Araki, M., Nishimura, R. and Okamura, H. (2000). Human villous macrophage-conditioned media enhance human trophoblast growth and differentiation in vitro. *Biol. Reprod.*, **62**, 1075–83.

Kilani, R. T., Mackova, M., Davidge, S. T. and Guilbert, L. J. (2003). Effect of oxygen levels in villous trophoblast apoptosis. *Placenta*, **24**, 826–34.

Kliman, H. J., Nestler, J. E., Sermasi, E., Sanger, J. M. and Strauss, J. F. 3rd. (1986). Purification, characterization, and in vitro differentiation of cytotrophoblasts from human term placentae. *Endocrinology*, **118**, 1567–82.

Kudo, Y., Boyd, C. A., Kimura, H., Cook, P. R., Redman, C. W. and Sargent, I. L. (2003). Quantifying the syncytialisation of human placental trophoblast BeWo cells grown in vitro. *Biochim. Biophys. Acta*, **1640**, 25–31.

Lacey, H., Haigh, T., Westwood, M. and Aplin, J. D. (2002). Mesenchymally-derived insulin-like growth factor 1 provides a paracrine stimulus for trophoblast migration. *BMC Dev. Biol.*, **2**, 5.

Librach, C. L., Werb, Z., Fitzgerald, M. L., *et al.* (1991). 92-kD type IV collagenase mediates invasion of human cytotrophoblasts. *J. Cell Biol.*, **113**, 437–49.

Logan, S. K., Fisher, S. J. and Damsky, C. H. (1992). Human placental cells transformed with temperature-sensitive simian virus 40 are immortalized and mimic the phenotype of invasive cytotrophoblasts at both permissive and nonpermissive temperatures. *Cancer Res.*, **52**, 6001–9.

Mayhew, T. M., Ohadike, C., Baker, P. N., Crocker, I. P., Mitchell, C. and Ong, S. S. (2003). Stereological investigation of placental morphology in pregnancies complicated by pre-eclampsia with and without intrauterine growth restriction. *Placenta*, **24**, 219–26.

Meekins, J. W., Pijnenborg, R., Hanssens, M., McFadyen, I. R. and van Asshe, A. (1994). A study of placental bed spiral arteries and trophoblast invasion in normal and severe pre-eclamptic pregnancies. *Br. J. Obstet. Gynaecol.*, **101**, 669–74.

Myers, J., Macleod, M., Reed, B., Harris, N., Mires, G. and Baker, P. (2004). Use of proteomic patterns as a novel screening tool in pre-eclampsia. *J. Obstet. Gynaecol.*, **24**, 873–4.

Naicker, T., Khedun, S. M., Moodley, J. and Pijnenborg, R. (2003). Quantitative analysis of trophoblast invasion in preeclampsia. *Acta Obstet. Gynecol. Scand.*, **82**, 722–9.

Page, N. M., Kemp, C. F., Butlin, D. J. and Lowry, P. J. (2002). Placental peptides as markers of gestational disease. *Reproduction*, **123**, 487–95.

Parast, M. M., Aeder, S. and Sutherland, A. E. (2001). Trophoblast giant-cell differentiation involves changes in cytoskeleton and cell motility. *Dev. Biol.*, **230**, 43–60.

Pijnenborg, R., D'Hooghe, T., Vercruysse, L. and Bambra, C. (1996). Evaluation of trophoblast invasion in placental bed biopsies of the baboon, with immuno-histochemical localisation of cytokeratin, fibronectin, and laminin. *J. Med. Primatol.*, **25**, 272–81.

Pijnenborg, R., Robertson, W. B., Brosens, I. and Dixon, G. (1981). Review article: trophoblast invasion and the establishment of haemochorial placentation in man and laboratory animals. *Placenta*, **2**, 71–91.

Potgens, A. J., Kataoka, H., Ferstl, S., Frank, H. G. and Kaufmann, P. (2003). A positive immunoselection method to isolate villous cytotrophoblast cells from first trimester and term placenta to high purity. *Placenta*, **24**, 412–23.

Redline, R. W. and Patterson, P. (1995). Pre-eclampsia is associated with an excess of proliferative immature intermediate trophoblast. *Hum. Pathol.*, **26**, 594–600.

Reimer, T., Koczan, D., Gerber, B., Richter, D., Thiesen, H. J. and Friese, K. (2002). Microarray analysis of differentially expressed genes in placental tissue of pre-eclampsia: up-regulation of obesity-related genes. *Mol. Hum. Reprod.*, **8**, 674–80.

Reister, F., Frank, H. G., Kingdom, J. C., *et al.* (2001). Macrophage-induced apoptosis limits endovascular trophoblast invasion in the uterine wall of preeclamptic women. *Lab. Invest.*, **81**, 1143–52.

Sacks, G. P., Clover, L. M., Bainbridge, D. R., Redman, C. W. and Sargent, I. L. (2001). Flow cytometric measurement of intracellular Th1 and Th2 cytokine production by human villous and extravillous cytotrophoblast. *Placenta*, **22**, 550–9.

Schutz, M., Teifel, M. and Friedl, P. (1997). Establishment of a human placental endothelial cell line with extended life span after transfection with SV40 T-antigens. *Eur. J. Cell Biol.*, **74**, 315–20.

Shiverick, K. T., King, A., Frank, H., Whitley, G. S., Cartwright, J. E. and Schneider, H. (2001). Cell culture models of human trophoblast II: trophoblast cell lines – a workshop report. *Placenta*, **22**, S104–6.

Sibley, C. P., Birdsey, T. J., Brownbill, P., *et al.* (1998). Mechanisms of maternofetal exchange across the human placenta. *Biochem. Soc. Trans.*, **26**, 86–91.

Siman, C. M., Sibley, C. P., Jones, C. J., Turner, M. A. and Greenwood, S. L. (2001). The functional regeneration of syncytiotrophoblast in cultured explants of term placenta. *Am. J. Physiol. Regul. Integr. Comp. Physiol.*, **280**, R1116–22.

Soothill, P. W., Nicolaides, K. H., Rodeck, C. H. and Campbell, S. (1986). Effect of gestational age on fetal and intervillous blood gas and acid–base values in human pregnancy. *Fetal Ther.*, **1**, 168–75.

Tanaka, S., Kunath, T., Hadjantonakis, A. K., Nagy, A. and Rossant, J. (1998). Promotion of trophoblast stem cell proliferation by FGF4. *Science*, **282**, 2072–5.

Tarrade, A., Lai Kuen, R., Malassine, A., *et al.* (2001a). Characterization of human villous and extravillous trophoblasts isolated from first trimester placenta. *Lab. Invest.*, **81**, 1199–211.

Tarrade, A., Schoonjans, K., Pavan, L., *et al.* (2001b). PPARgamma/RXRalpha heterodimers control human trophoblast invasion. *J. Clin. Endocrinol. Metab.*, **86**, 5017–24.

Vicovac, L. and Aplin, J. D. (1996). Epithelial–mesenchymal transition during trophoblast differentiation. *Acta Anat. (Basel)*, **156**, 202–16.

Vicovac, L., Jones, C. J. and Aplin, J. D. (1995). Trophoblast differentiation during formation of anchoring villi in a model of the early human placenta in vitro. *Placenta*, **16**, 41–56.

von Dadelszen, P., Hurst, G. and Redman, C. W. (1999). Supernatants from co-cultured endothelial cells and syncytiotrophoblast microvillous membranes activate peripheral blood leukocytes in vitro. *Hum. Reprod.*, **14**, 919–24.

Watson, A. L., Palmer, M. E., *et al.* (1995). Human chorionic gonadotrophin release and tissue viability in placental organ culture. *Hum. Reprod.*, **10**, 2159–64.

Wetzka, B., Clark, D. E., Charnock-Jones, D. S., Zahradnik, H. P. and Smith, S. K. (1997). Isolation of macrophages (Hofbauer cells) from human term placenta and their prostaglandin E2 and thromboxane production. *Hum. Reprod.*, **12**, 847–52.

Yui, J., Garcia-Lloret, M., Brown, A. J., *et al.* (1994). Functional, long-term cultures of human term trophoblasts purified by column-elimination of CD9 expressing cells. *Placenta*, **15**, 231–46.

Zybina, T. G., Kaufmann, P., Frank, H. G., Freed, J., Kadyrov, M. and Biesterfeld, S. (2002). Genome multiplication of extravillous trophoblast cells in human placenta in the course of differentiation and invasion into endometrium and myometrium. I. Dynamics of polyploidization. *Tsitologiia*, **44**, 1058–67.

4

Endothelial factors

Muna Noori, Mina Savvidou and David Williams

Introduction

Vascular tone is influenced by the autonomic nervous system, intrinsic vascular smooth muscle reflexes and the endothelium (Figure 4.1). The endothelium is the cell layer lining the internal surface of blood vessels and in a person weighing 70 kg, covers an area of approximately $700\,m^2$ and weighs between 1 and 1.5 kg (Luscher and Barton, 1997). The endothelium is responsible for an extensive array of highly specialized, homeostatic functions. It plays an important role in the control of blood pressure, blood flow, angiogenesis, coagulation, fibrinolysis, vessel patency, and local inflammatory responses. These functions are achieved through the release of endothelium-derived relaxing and contracting factors, thromboregulatory molecules, growth factors, and neutrophil adhesion molecules (Petty and Pearson, 1989) (Table 4.1). Impaired endothelial function contributes substantially to cardiovascular disorders such as hypertension, atherosclerosis and pre-eclampsia.

Stimulation of endothelial receptors activates pathways within the endothelium that mediate either relaxation or constriction of the underlying vascular smooth muscle. Endothelial responses are triggered by acetylcholine (ACh), serotonin (5-HT), angiotensin II (AngII), vasopressin (AVP), histamine, bradykinin and several other vasoactive hormones (Hill *et al.*, 2001; Lincoln and Burnstock, 1990; Vanhoutte and Rimele, 1983). Endothelial-derived vasoactive factors influence vascular smooth muscle tone through prostaglandins, which are both vasodilatory (prostacyclin) and vasoconstrictor (thromboxane) (Moncada *et al.*, 1976; Mombouli and Vanhoutte, 1999), endothelins, which are predominantly vasoconstrictor (Bagnall and Webb, 2000), endothelial-derived hyperpolarizing factor (EDHF), which is predominantly vasodilator (Chen *et al.*, 1988; Garland *et al.*, 1995), but still not fully characterized, and nitric oxide, which is a vasodilator (Palmer *et al.*, 1987; Vallance *et al.*, 1989).

The vascular endothelium plays an important role in the cardiovascular adaptation to pregnancy and in the pathogenesis of pre-eclampsia. This chapter outlines the major functions of the endothelium in health and disease, how it adapts during healthy pregnancy and how endothelial dysfunction mediates many of the features of the multi-organ syndrome, pre-eclampsia.

Endothelial-derived vaso-active factors

Endothelium-derived relaxing factors

Stimulation of intact endothelial cells by circulating neurotransmitters, hormones and substances derived from platelets and the coagulation system causes the release of a substance that induces relaxation of the underlying vascular smooth muscle (Furchgott and Zawadzki, 1980). Furthermore, mechanical forces such as shear stress, which are generated by changes in blood flow, induce endothelium-dependent vasodilatation, an important adaptive response during exercise.

Table 4.1. Endothelial-derived factors and their functions

Endothelium-derived factors	Effects
Nitric oxide	Control of vascular tone (vasodilatation)
	Inhibition of platelet aggregation
	Regulation of myocardial contractility
	Regulation of endothelial–leukocyte interactions
	Regulation of endothelial integrity
	Regulation of vascular cell proliferation
Prostacyclin (Prostaglandin I_2)	Vasodilatation
Hyperpolarizing factor(s)	Vasodilatation
Endothelin-1	Vasoconstriction
Thromboxane A_2; prostaglandin H_2	Vasoconstriction
Angiotensin II	Vasoconstriction
Urotensin II	Vasoconstriction
VEGF; sFlt-1	Control of angiogenesis
tPA; PAI-1	Regulation of fibrinolysis
Cytokines (IL-1, IL-6, CSFs)	Lymphocyte activation
	Local and systemic inflammation
	Acute phase response
	Hemopoiesis
Chemotactic factors (IL-8)	Leukocyte recruitment and activation
PDGF	Smooth muscle cell proliferation

VEGF, vascular endothelial growth factor; sFlt-1, soluble fms-like tyrosine kinase; tPA, tissue plasminogen activator; PAI-1, plasminogen activator inhibitor-1; IL-1, interleukin-1; IL-6, interleukin-6; CSF, colony stimulating factor; IL-8, interleukin-8; MCP-1, monocyte chemotactic protein-1; PDGF, platelet-derived growth factor.

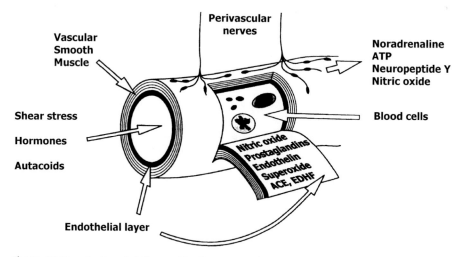

Figure 4.1 Vascular tone is influenced by the autonomic nervous system, intrinsic vascular smooth muscle reflexes and the endothelium.

Nitric oxide

In 1980, Furchgott and Zawadzki first postulated the existence of an endothelium-derived relaxing factor (EDRF). The identity of the factor within the endothelium that mediated vascular relaxation was later found to be nitric oxide (NO) (Furchgott, 1988; Ignarro *et al.*, 1988; Palmer *et al.*, 1987).

Nitric oxide is synthesized from one of the guanidine-nitrogen atoms of the amino acid L-arginine, by the enzyme, nitric oxide synthase (NOS) (Palmer *et al.*, 1988), yielding L-citrulline as a byproduct. NO is a potent vasodilator, and acts on vascular smooth muscle through the second messenger cyclic guanyl monophosphate (cGMP). It is highly labile, with a half-life of 10–60 s and is rapidly metabolized to nitrite and nitrate before being excreted in the urine (Moncada and Higgs, 1993; Figure 4.2).

Nitric oxide synthase

Nitric oxide has many biological roles and dysregulation of its production has been implicated in the pathogenesis of a range of cardiovascular disorders, including hypertension, atherosclerosis, and pre-eclampsia. Nitric oxide is synthesized in a wide variety of tissues and cell types as well as vascular endothelial cells including platelets, macrophages, and neurones. The enzyme that is responsible for its production, nitric oxide synthase (NOS), exists in three identified isoforms: neuronal (nNOS; Type I), inducible (iNOS; Type II), and constitutive endothelial (eNOS; Type III), all of which are involved in controlling vascular tone (Fostermann *et al.*, 1994). While eNOS and nNOS are present in healthy cells, iNOS expression becomes evident only in the presence of infection or inflammation.

There is continuous basal release of NO from the vascular endothelium, which serves to regulate vascular tone (Vallance *et al.*, 1989). Endothelial NOS is activated by raised intracellular calcium and the subsequent binding of calcium/calmodulin. This process can be triggered by ACh, bradykinin (BK), thrombin, and adenosine 5′-triphosphate (ATP), which all increase levels of intracellular free calcium (Furchgott and Vanhoutte, 1989; Moncada, 1992).

The role of estrogen in stimulating NOS activity

Estrogen is a potent vasoactive hormone that causes rapid vasodilation in a number of vascular beds. Circulating estrogen levels rise gradually

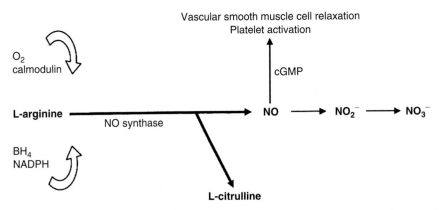

BH$_4$, tetrahydrobiopterin; NADPH, nicotinamide adenine dinucleotide phosphate; cGMP, cyclic guanosine 3, 5-monophosphate; NO, nitric oxide; NO$_2^-$, nitrite; NO$_3^-$, nitrate

Figure 4.2 NO metabolism.

from the time of conception to reach levels at term that are 250-fold higher than found in the non-pregnant state (Chapman *et al.*, 1998). There is much evidence to suggest that estrogen mediates vasodilatation and increases uterine artery blood flow through NO derived from the uterine artery endothelium (Magness *et al.*, 1997; Vangoni *et al.*, 1998).

The mechanism by which estrogen modulates NO production has not been elucidated fully, but it is known that there are 11 copies of an incomplete (half palindromic motif) estrogen response element (ERE) on the endothelial NOS gene 5′ flanking "promotor" region (Robinson *et al.*, 1994). In other genes, these "half motifs" interact to form a complete ERE and the occupied estrogen receptor may similarly activate eNOS by binding to these regions. There is evidence to suggest the presence of an estrogen receptor on the plasma membrane of an endothelial cell or vascular smooth muscle cell (Russell *et al.*, 2000a), which is likely to mediate the prompt "nongenomic" responses to estradiol. The immediate release of NO is inhibited by a specific estrogen receptor antagonist (ICI 182,780). The observation that estrogens stimulate endothelial cells to rapidly produce heat shock protein 90 (hsp90), activate calcium-independent NOS (Russell *et al.*, 2000b) and mitogen-activated protein kinases (MAPK; signal transduction molecules) are features of the "nongenomic" response of endothelial cells exposed to shear stress. Estrogens may stimulate flow-mediated dilatation by "priming" these pivotal endothelial pathways to respond to shear stress.

Two estrogen receptors have been identified, ERα and ERβ, both of which are expressed in human vascular endothelium, vascular smooth muscle cells (Farhat *et al.*, 1996; Mendelsohn and Karas, 1994) and the myometrium (Gargett *et al.*, 2002). In the vascular endothelium, eNOS protein and/or mRNA expression has been reported to be increased by estrogen stimulation (MacRitchie *et al.*, 1997; Yang *et al.*, 2000). Increasing evidence suggests, however, that initiation of vasodilatation in response to estrogen is mediated by increased

activity of eNOS rather than increased production of eNOS itself (Vangoni *et al.*, 1998). Furthermore, acute administration of estrogen stimulates rapid production of endothelial-derived NO without altering eNOS expression (Chen *et al.*, 2004) and the mRNA synthesis blockade does not affect estrogen-induced uterine blood flow (Penney *et al.*, 1981).

There is much evidence to support a role for estrogen mediating vasodilatation through increased NOS activity. First, infusion of 17β-estrodiol to oophorectomized animals results in a tenfold increase in uterine blood flow within 90–120 min (Killam *et al.*, 1973), which is antagonized by an NOS inhibitor (Weiner *et al.*, 1994a). Estrogen rapidly activates eNOS to produce NO in uterine artery endothelial cells in vitro (Chen *et al.*, 2004). Flow-mediated dilatation (FMD; an index of NO-mediated endothelial function – discussed below) has been shown to be significantly higher during the luteal phase of the menstrual cycle, when estrogen levels are at their highest (Hashimoto, 1995) and during pregnancy (Cockell and Poston, 1997b).

Inhibitors of nitric oxide synthase

There are several analogs of L-arginine that competitively inhibit NOS. These include two naturally occurring NOS inhibitors, N^G-monomethyl-L-arginine (L-NMMA) and N^G,N^G-dimethyl-L-arginine (asymmetric dimethylarginine; ADMA). The stereoisomer of ADMA is symmetric dimethylarginine (SDMA), which does not inhibit NOS (Vallance *et al.*, 1992). In human plasma ADMA is present at ten times the concentration of naturally occurring L-NMMA (Vallance *et al.*, 1992). L-NMMA inhibits NOS in cultured vascular endothelial cells (Palmer *et al.*, 1988) and increases mean arterial pressure in animals (Rees *et al.*, 1989). When infused into the brachial artery in humans, it halves basal blood flow and attenuates the dilator response to ACh (Vallance *et al.*, 1989).

ADMA is generated in endothelial cells by proteolysis of proteins that have undergone

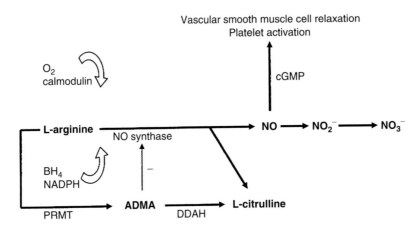

PRMT, Protein-arginine methyltransferase; ADMA, Asymmetric dimethylarginine;
DDAH, Dimethylarginine dimethylaminohydrolase

Figure 4.3 Nitric oxide and ADMA metabolism.

methylation by protein-arginine methyltrans-ferases (PRMTs) (Figure 4.3). Isolation of ADMA and SDMA in human urine led to the assumption that renal excretion was the sole means of elimination of methylarginines (Kakimoto and Akazawa, 1970). However, the urinary concentration of SDMA was found to be 30 times greater than that of ADMA, suggesting an alternative pathway of ADMA elimination (McDermott et al., 1976). ADMA is selectively metabolized to L-citrulline and dimethylamine by the enzyme dimethylarginine dimethylaminohydrolase (DDAH), which exists in two isoforms DDAH I and II (Leiper et al., 1999). DDAH I is expressed mainly in the brain and kidney whereas DDAH II is found predominantly in heart, kidney and placenta. DDAH II is more highly expressed in fetal compared with adult tissues (Tran et al., 2000). DDAH is therefore important in regulating NOS activity via its actions on ADMA (Leiper and Vallance, 1999).

Elevated ADMA levels have been found in a number of pathological states, including athero-sclerosis (Miyazaki et al., 1999), hypertension (Goonasekera et al., 1997), renal failure (Vallance et al., 1992) and pre-eclampsia (Fickling et al., 1993). DDAH activity is suppressed by oxidative stress, which may explain the higher ADMA levels evident in these disease states. Overexpression of DDAH I results in increased NOS activity in vitro and in vivo (Dayoub et al., 2003). DDAH is therefore an important indirect regulator of NOS activity and may represent a new therapeutic target for increasing NOS activity.

Prostacyclin

Prostacyclin, also known as prostaglandin I_2 (PGI₂), is produced primarily by vascular endothelial cells. It is derived from arachidonic acid and its formation relies on the cyclo-oxygenase (COX) system (Vane, 1983). Prostacyclin is a potent vasodilator and increases cyclic 3'-5'-adenosine monophosphate (cAMP) in smooth muscle and platelets. It acts via a G-protein coupled cell-surface receptor, termed IP, as well as a nuclear receptor, the peroxisomal proliferator-activated receptor α (PPAR α). These receptors are thought to mediate both the anti-platelet and vasodilatory effects of PGI₂ in the vasculature (Marx et al., 2003). Nitric oxide and prostacyclin act synergistically to inhibit platelet aggregation and promote endothelial-derived vasodilatation.

Endothelium-derived hyperpolarizing factor

Inhibition of both nitric oxide synthesis and cyclo-oxygenase does not result in complete inhibition of endothelium-dependent vasodilatation (Ashworth et al., 1996; Kenny et al., 2002a; Knock and Poston, 1996). An additional endothelium-derived mediator that hyperpolarizes vascular smooth muscle is known as endothelium-derived hyperpolarizing factor (EDHF). Hyperpolarization of the smooth muscle has been attributed to an increase in conductance to potassium (K^+) ions, whereby increased K^+ efflux results in a more negative resting membrane potential and hyperpolarization.

The chemical nature of EDHF is disputed; the various candidates include potassium ions (Edwards et al., 1998), a cytochrome oxidase P450-derived metabolite of arachidonic acid (Hecker et al., 1994), one of the epoxyeicosatrienoic acids (EETs) and an endogenous cannabinoid (Feletou and Vanhoutte, 1988; Randall et al., 1996). It has been suggested that myoendothelial gap junctions may play a role in EDHF-type responses (Kenny et al., 2002b). These gap junctions may provide sites for the electronic conduction of hyperpolarization from endothelial cells to smooth muscle cells (Coleman et al., 2001), or the preferential transfer of a chemical factor (Feletou and Vanhoutte, 1988). However, as myoendothelial gap junctions are much smaller than other gap junctions, many of the suggested candidates for EDHF would be unable to pass through. It is possible that electrical and mechanical mechanisms, modulated by other chemical factors, may be responsible (Edwards et al., 2000).

Mechanical forces

The capacity of blood vessels to respond to physical stimuli confers the ability to self-regulate vascular tone and to adjust blood flow and distribution in response to changes in the local environment. Nitric oxide is released by endothelial cells in response to shear stress through a number of mechanisms. Rapid release occurs via a combination of Ca^{2+}, K^+ and Cl^- ion channel activation (Resnick et al., 2000), fast release occurs as a result of phosphorylation (Kuchan and Frangos, 1994), whilst slow release occurs as a result of increased eNOS transcription (Resnick et al., 2000).

Endothelium-derived contracting factors

Endothelial cells can also mediate contraction of underlying vascular smooth muscle cells (Luscher and Vanhoutte, 1990). Endothelium-derived contracting factors include endothelin-1, vasoconstrictor prostanoids such as thromboxane A_2, prostaglandin H_2, and components of the renin–angiotensin system such as angiotensin II.

Endothelins

The endothelins are a family of 21 amino acid peptides that are produced by endothelial cells (Yanagisawa et al., 1988). There are three recognized endothelins, endothelin-1 (ET-1), endothelin-2 (ET-2) and endothelin-3 (ET-3), although only ET-1 has been shown to be released by human endothelial cells (Masaki, 1989). Endothelin-1 causes vasodilatation at low concentrations but marked and sustained vasoconstriction at higher concentrations. Endothelin-1 is released from endothelial cells in response to a variety of stimuli, including adrenaline and hypoxia (Boulanger and Luscher, 1990). Like NO, ET-1 also has a short half-life, which suggests a locally active vasoregulatory function. It is important in the maintenance of basal vessel tone and is present in low concentrations in healthy individuals (Davenport et al., 1990).

Endothelin receptors in humans include the ET_A and ET_{B2} receptors on vascular smooth muscle, which mediate vasoconstriction. In contrast, the ET_{B1} receptor results in NO-dependent vasodilatation. ET-1-mediated vasoconstriction occurs through a calcium-dependent pathway. Activation of the ET_A receptor by ET-1 stimulates the release of arachidonic acid, which in turn may stimulate the synthesis of other endothelium-dependent vasoactive factors, including PGI_2 and thromboxane A_2 (TxA_2). Therefore, ET-1 plays a role in stimulating other vasoactive factors, as well as its own vasoconstrictive properties (Molnar and Hertelendy, 1995).

Prostaglandin H₂ and thromboxane A₂

Prostaglandin H_2 and TxA_2 are both arachidonic acid metabolites that are secreted by endothelial cells in smaller amounts compared with PGI_2. They diffuse to adjacent vascular smooth muscle cells where they cause calcium-dependent vasoconstriction. Thromboxane A_2 and prostaglandin H_2 activate thromboxane receptors in vascular smooth muscle and platelets, thereby counteracting the effects of NO and prostacyclin in both types of cell. Thromboxane A_2 is predominantly produced by platelets, where it promotes platelet aggregation.

Angiotensin II

The renin–angiotensin system is partially regulated within the endothelium. Angiotensin-converting enzyme (ACE), which converts inactive angiotensin I (AngI) to active angiotensin II (AngII), is expressed on the endothelial cell membrane. Angiotensin II activates endothelial receptors, which stimulate the production of ET-1 and other mediators, such as plasminogen activator inhibitor-1 (PAI-1), which promotes thrombogenesis (Vaughan et al., 1995).

More recently, the serine protease, chymase, has also been found to convert AngI into AngII – this enzyme is also expressed by vascular endothelial cells. The actions of AngII are mediated by two receptors, AT_1 and AT_2 (Wang et al., 1999). AT_1 receptors are known to be responsible for the majority of physiological actions of AngII in humans, such as vasoconstriction, mitogenesis and aldosterone release. AT_2 receptors were discovered more recently and their role remains unclear, although they have been found to suppress coronary cell proliferation and neointima formation following balloon injury.

Mediators of endothelial damage

Reactive oxygen species

Toward the end of normal pregnancy, maternal plasma levels of cholesterol and triglyceride increase by 50–100%, respectively (Potter and Nestel, 1979). Women with pre-eclampsia have even higher lipid levels (Hubel et al., 1996), which can result in increased levels of lipid oxidation products (Chirico et al., 1993), which are toxic to vascular endothelium (see related chapters).

Reactive oxygen species (ROS), such as the superoxide anion (O_2^-), are produced as a consequence of NO metabolism in the vessel wall, and suppress endothelium-dependent vasodilatation (Freeman et al., 1995). Endothelial NOS is also capable of producing oxygen free radicals from L-arginine. Superoxide anions are converted to hydrogen peroxide (H_2O_2) in a reaction catalyzed by the enzyme superoxide dismutase (SOD), which is an important cellular defense mechanism against free radical damage. There are three known isoenzymes of SOD – a cytosolic, mitochondrial and an extracellular form (ecSOD), the latter form of which predominates in the vessel wall. Superoxide anions react rapidly with NO to form peroxynitrite ($ONOO^-$). Levels of $ONOO^-$ in the body are usually kept low by the actions of SOD.

Adhesion molecules

Adhesion molecules, which mediate cell–cell interactions, belong to four major families – selectins, selectin ligands, integrins and members of the immunoglobulin family (Xu et al., 1994). Elevated adhesion molecule expression is evident in a number of pathological states including atherosclerosis, inflammation, and pre-eclampsia. Their role is to promote adhesion of circulating cells to the endothelium. For example, neutrophils will be signaled to gather at the site of inflammation and platelets at the site of endothelial damage to generate thrombosis.

Fibronectin – a marker of endothelial dysfunction

Fibronectins are a family of high-molecular-weight extracellular matrix glycoproteins that exist in the plasma, extracellular fluid and many body tissues. The predominant isoform is circulating fibronectin (plasma fibronectin), which is derived from hepatocytes. The cellular isoform of fibronectin (cFN) is present in endothelial cells and the endothelial cell matrix and is generated by alternative post-transcriptional processing of the fibronectin gene product. Under normal circumstances, cFN exists in low concentrations in circulating plasma but in clinical conditions characterized by endothelial injury it is elevated. Women with pre-eclampsia have higher circulating levels of cFN compared with those who have normotensive pregnancies (Sudd et al., 1999). Elevated circulating maternal levels of cFN are evident several months prior to the onset of clinical disease (Chavarria et al., 2002; Taylor et al., 1991) and may therefore be a useful predictor of pre-eclampsia. Cellular fibronectin levels are also raised in cord blood in the blood of infants of pre-eclamptic women (Davidge et al., 1996).

The role of the endothelium in clotting

In addition to producing vasoactive mediators, the endothelium has an important role in the control of thrombus formation. Nitric oxide and PGI_2 inhibit platelet activation, adhesion, and aggregation (Moncada et al., 1977; Moncada, 1982). The endothelium also produces a number of other anticoagulant factors, including thrombomodulin, protein S, endothelial surface heparin sulfate, in addition to von Willebrand factor (vWF), which promotes thrombosis. In healthy endothelium, the overall effect of these factors is to prevent thrombosis, whereas if the endothelium is damaged, thrombogenesis prevails.

Endothelial cells secrete tissue plasminogen activator (t-PA), a powerful thrombolytic, which is counteracted by plasminogen activator inhibitor-1 (PAI-1). These are both important in the control of fibrinolysis. PAI-1 expression is enhanced following vascular injury and in conditions associated with thrombosis (Kitching et al., 2003; Schafer et al., 2003).

The endothelium and healthy pregnancy

Adaptive cardiovascular changes of healthy pregnancy

The maternal cardiovascular system undergoes profound physiological changes during pregnancy (Williams, 2003). Blood flow to each maternal organ changes at different stages and by different amounts (Figure 4.4). Ultimately, the aim of these gestational changes is to ensure that the mother can meet the metabolic demands of the growing conceptus. The mechanisms of these widespread and variable cardiovascular changes are incompletely understood.

One of the earliest manifestations of this adaptive response is a fall in peripheral vascular resistance. Peripheral vasodilatation is evident from as early as 5 weeks gestation and is almost complete by 16 weeks (Robson et al., 1989). By the end of the first trimester, peripheral vascular resistance has fallen by 40% compared with non-pregnant women. By 24 weeks gestation, cardiac output will have increased by 45% above non-pregnant levels due to an increase in stroke volume and heart rate, and a fall in systemic vascular resistance (Easterling et al., 1987; Robson et al., 1989). Consequently, blood supply to several maternal organs increases dramatically. By 24 weeks, renal perfusion increases by 80% (Davison, 1984), and by term, blood flow to the skin of the hands and feet will have increased by over 200% and uterine artery blood flow by 1000%. Conversely, hepatic and cerebral blood flow remains virtually unaltered (Figure 4.3).

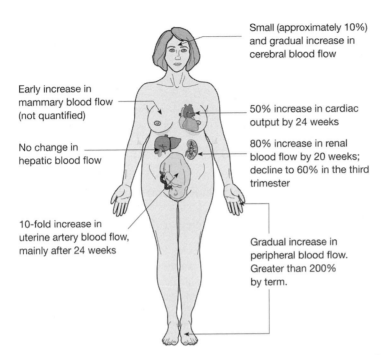

Small (approximately 10%) and gradual increase in cerebral blood flow

Early increase in mammary blood flow (not quantified)

No change in hepatic blood flow

10-fold increase in uterine artery blood flow, mainly after 24 weeks

50% increase in cardiac output by 24 weeks

80% increase in renal blood flow by 20 weeks; decline to 60% in the third trimester

Gradual increase in peripheral blood flow. Greater than 200% by term.

Figure 4.4 The distribution of blood flow to maternal organs during pregnancy (from Williams, 2003).

Studies in pregnant baboons (Phippard *et al.*, 1986) and pregnant women (Chapman *et al.*, 1998) suggest that despite this increase in renal blood flow, the relatively under-filled peripheral and renal vasculature stimulates the renin–angiotensin–aldosterone system, which leads to a rise in plasma volume of 1.2–1.5 L (Brown and Gallery, 1994). Stroke volume plateaus at 16 weeks whilst heart rate continues to rise gradually until 32 weeks (Robson *et al.*, 1989). Despite the increase in intravascular volume, the fall in systemic vascular resistance leads to a fall in diastolic blood pressure, which reaches its lowest level at 22–24 weeks gestation, then rises to reach pre-pregnancy levels by term. Systolic blood pressure is not significantly altered during healthy pregnancy (Halligan *et al.*, 1993).

Endothelial factors in healthy pregnancy

The mechanism for the primary reduction in total peripheral vascular resistance in normal pregnancy is multifactorial and results from alterations in endothelial-derived vasoactive substances interacting with changes in the autonomic nervous system (Poston and Williams, 2000). Animal studies provide considerable evidence that increased NOS activity contributes to the generalized vasodilatation and attenuated response to exogenous vasoconstrictors characteristic of pregnancy (Conrad *et al.*, 1993; Weiner *et al.*, 1994b). In vivo studies of the L-arginine–nitric oxide pathway during human pregnancy and pre-eclampsia are more challenging.

Evidence for increased nitric oxide synthase activity in healthy pregnancy

Cyclic guanosine monophosphate (cGMP)

Circulating levels of cGMP, the second messenger for NO, has been used as a surrogate marker for NOS activity. Studies on pregnant rats have demonstrated an increase in both plasma and urinary cGMP levels as renal blood flow increases with advancing gestation (Conrad and Vernier, 1989). Renal vasodilatation and hyperfiltration is abolished by inhibition of NOS (Danielson and Conrad, 1995).

In human pregnancy, there is agreement that urinary concentrations of cGMP increase early in pregnancy and remain elevated until term (Chapman et al., 1998; Kopp et al., 1977). Cyclic-GMP clearance increases as early as the sixth week of gestation, in parallel with a fall in plasma cGMP levels that remain low throughout pregnancy (Chapman et al., 1998). Others have found slight or significant increases in plasma cGMP during normal pregnancy, remaining high until term (Boccardo et al., 1996; Schneider et al., 1996). Platelets do not appear to contribute to excessive NO production in pregnancy (Boccardo et al., 1996).

Cyclic GMP concentrations in plasma or urine are only an indirect indication of NOS activity as responses to atrial natriuretic peptide (ANP) are also mediated through cGMP. In a meta-analysis of 53 studies it was concluded that the circulating concentration of ANP did not rise until the third trimester (Castro et al., 1994). This is long after the increase in urinary cGMP, which coincides with the gestational increase in renal blood flow and glomerular filtration rate (Dunlop, 1981; Roberts et al., 1996). It is possible that increased NOS activity has a role in renal vasodilatation during healthy human pregnancy, but it cannot be concluded from the measurement of cGMP alone that increased NOS activity plays a role in the gestational fall in systemic vascular resistance.

Oxidation products of nitric oxide, nitrite and nitrate

Several investigators have measured the serum concentration of nitrite (NO_2^-) and nitrate (NO_3^-), or their product, NO_x, during healthy pregnancy. However, most have ignored the confounding problem that concentrations of these NO metabolites are sensitive to dietary nitrogen intake. Not surprisingly, studies of normotensive pregnant women on uncontrolled nitrogen diets have shown either increased (Seligman et al., 1994) or unchanged (Curtis et al., 1995; Smarason et al., 1997) plasma NO metabolites in comparison with non-pregnant women. In one study, plasma NO_x levels were measured after a 12–15 h fast, and found to be significantly elevated in normotensive pregnancy (from before 12 weeks gestation until term) compared with non-pregnant women (Nobunaga et al., 1996). In another carefully controlled study, guanidino [N^{15}]L-arginine was infused into five healthy pregnant volunteers after being on a nitrate-free diet for the preceding week and a 12 h fast pre-infusion. Arginine flux and nitrite/nitrate pool turnover were higher in early compared with late pregnancy, suggesting NO production is higher in early pregnancy (Goodrum et al., 1996).

Stimulated nitric oxide synthase activity in vitro

Much of the evidence favoring an increase in endothelial NO synthesis in the vasculature in pregnancy is derived from studies of small arteries in animals, in which a significant reduction in the EC_{50} for ACh or methacholine has repeatedly been observed. Although indicative of enhanced NO synthesis, conclusive proof is not always available, as selective inhibition of NOS has not been attempted often. The reduced responsiveness to constrictor agonists observed in some small artery preparations from pregnant animals, using NOS inhibitors, has sometimes been attributed to enhanced NO synthesis. Perhaps the most convincing evidence for an increase in NOS activity comes from a study of small rat arteries, which has shown an increase in expression of eNOS in pregnancy (Xu et al., 1996). These confusing and often conflicting studies of NO in the vasculature in animal pregnancy were covered in great detail in a comprehensive review by Sladek et al. (1997).

Limited availability of human tissue is an obvious drawback to investigation in human pregnancies. However, small arteries may be obtained from subcutaneous fat, omentum and myometrium by biopsy at Cesarean section. The development of a variety of techniques for reproducible investigation of small artery tension and diameter has greatly facilitated studies in human tissue, as small biopsies may provide adequate material for experiment.

The blood flow to the skin is greatly enhanced in human pregnancy and investigation of the cutaneous circulation provides insight into pregnancy-induced mechanisms of vasodilatation. Small subcutaneous arteries (250–300 µm) obtained from subcutaneous fat at Cesarean section relaxed in response to the endothelium-dependent vasodilator ACh to the same extent as similar arteries from non-pregnant women (McCarthy et al., 1994). Interestingly, the NO synthase inhibitor, L-NMMA, failed to completely inhibit relaxation to ACh, and indomethacin had little effect. The residual relaxation to ACh in the presence of the NOS inhibitor was greater in the arteries from pregnant women and suggests the presence of an additional endothelium-derived hyperpolarizing factor (Gerber et al., 1998). Pre-constricted small subcutaneous arteries from normotensive pregnant women have enhanced relaxation to another endothelial vasodilator bradykinin (BK), compared with non-pregnant women (Knock and Poston, 1996). Inhibition of NOS and COX produced a similar degree of residual BK-induced relaxation in both groups. This suggests that pregnancy may induce an alteration in the signal transduction pathway for BK (Knock and Poston, 1996).

In contrast, using arteries from the omental circulation, Pascoal and Umans (1996) concluded that neither ACh- nor BK-mediated vasodilatation was different in arteries from term pregnant women and non-pregnant women, although pregnancy was associated with an increase in a novel component of BK-mediated relaxation, possibly a hyperpolarizing factor (Pascoal and Umans, 1996).

However, small myometrial arteries from pregnant women respond well to ACh and this relaxation is greater than relaxation to ACh in omental arteries from term pregnant women, perhaps indicating that enhanced receptor-mediated relaxation may contribute to increased myometrial blood flow in pregnancy (Kublickiene et al., 1997a). Taken together, these studies show little consensus regarding the role of agonist-stimulated NO synthesis in vasodilatation of pregnancy, perhaps because of the different vascular beds studied.

There is more agreement that flow-mediated NO synthesis is raised in the resistance vasculature in human pregnancy. Subcutaneous arteries from pregnant women demonstrate an increased response to flow compared with those from non-pregnant women, which was totally inhibited by the NOS inhibitor L-NAME (Cockell et al., 1997). This substantiated earlier work in arteries from pregnant rats (Cockell and Poston, 1997a; Learmont et al., 1996) showing enhanced flow-mediated dilatation. Using the same technique, NO-mediated responses to flow have been observed in small myometrial arteries from women at term (Kublickiene et al., 1997b).

Nitric oxide synthase activity in vivo

In vivo functional studies provide the most compelling evidence that NO synthase is upregulated in the maternal circulation during normal pregnancy. Infusion of the NO synthase inhibitor, L-NMMA, into the brachial artery causes a greater reduction in hand and forearm blood flow of pregnant compared with non-pregnant women (Anumba et al., 1999; Williams et al., 1997). In the hand, the increased efficacy of L-NMMA was observed during early pregnancy (9–15 weeks), a time when there was not yet a measurable increase in hand blood flow. This suggests that a mechanism other than shear stress mediates the gestational increase in NO generation. Furthermore, in late pregnancy (36–41 weeks), L-NMMA returned the elevated hand blood flow back to non-gravid levels, implicating a major role for NO in the peripheral vasodilatation of healthy pregnancy (Williams *et al.*, 1997).

L-NMMA has also been shown to induce a non-sustained venoconstriction in hand veins of healthy women in the early puerperium, but not in the same women 12–16 weeks postpartum (Ford *et al.*, 1996). Normally, in the non-gravid state, infusion of L-NMMA, at a dose that maximally inhibits bradykinin does not produce venoconstriction of hand veins (Vallance *et al.*, 1989). Isolated endothelial cells from hand veins of pregnant women have been shown to respond to adenine triphosphate (ATP) with a large transient increase in intracellular Ca^{2+} (Mahdy *et al.*, 1998). This response was significantly greater in endothelial cells isolated from the hand veins of healthy pregnant women compared to non-pregnant and pre-eclamptic women (Mahdy *et al.*, 1998). However, the extrapolation of evidence from the venous circulation to peripheral vascular control must be interpreted with caution.

Endothelium-dependent vasodilatation can be assessed non-invasively using measurement of flow-mediated dilatation (FMD) of the brachial artery (Celermajer, 1992). High-frequency ultrasonographic imaging of the brachial artery allows measurement of vessel diameter before and after cuff inflation around the forearm to supra-systolic levels for a period of time (usually 300 mmHg for 5 min). Cuff deflation results in a reactive hyperemic response, which is mediated by endothelium-dependent NO. The degree of vasodilatation is an index of systemic endothelial vasomotor function (Anderson, 1995). Endothelium-independent vasodilatation can be assessed using the same technique following administration of sublingual nitroglycerin (GTN). Using this technique, Dorup *et al.* (1999) showed significantly increased resting blood flow and brachial artery diameter in the second and third trimesters of normal pregnancy compared to non-pregnant controls. The degree of FMD was greater in pregnant compared with non-pregnant women, and increased as pregnancy progressed. This supports the hypothesis that maternal endothelial-derived NOS activity is enhanced during pregnancy and is likely to contribute to the decrease in peripheral vascular resistance that occurs in pregnancy. Using the same technique of brachial artery FMD, Savvidou *et al.* (2000) confirmed an increase in FMD between 10 and 30 weeks gestation compared with non-pregnant controls, but observed a fall in FMD to pre-pregnancy levels after 30 weeks. This reduction in endothelium-dependent vasodilatation coincides with the rise in maternal blood pressure to pre-pregnancy levels in the third trimester.

Endothelium-derived hyperpolarizing factor

A number of studies have suggested that prostaglandin and NO-independent but endothelium-dependent mechanisms of relaxation are enhanced in human pregnancy (McCarthy *et al.*, 1994; Pascoal and Umans, 1996). Acetylcholine-induced vasodilatation that persists despite inhibition of cyclo-oxygenase and NO synthase is greater in pregnant compared with virgin rats. In both groups, elevation of the potassium concentration in the organ bath totally abolished any remaining relaxation, which is strongly indicative of a role for enhanced synthesis of EDHF.

Endothelin

The plasma concentration of ET-1 is not affected by normal pregnancy and is very low or undetectable in maternal plasma (Wolff *et al.*, 1997). However, ET-1 causes potent constriction of myometrial arteries from pregnant (Wolff *et al.*, 1993) and non-pregnant women (Fried and Samuelson, 1991). ET-1 may therefore play a role in the regulation of uteroplacental blood flow.

Endothelial dysfunction and thrombosis

Normal pregnancy is characterized by low grade, chronic intravascular coagulation within both the maternal and utero-placental circulation, perhaps as a pre-emptive measure against the anticipated hemorrhage associated with childbirth (Lestky, 1995). There is evidence that clotting factors, particularly fibrinogen, are increased (Bonnar, 1987) and that fibrinolysis is depressed (Kruitthof et al., 1987). However, more recent studies suggest that fibrinolysis increases in order to compensate for the procoagulant state of normal pregnancy (Sorensen et al., 1995). Some elements of endothelial function are directly involved in promoting a procoagulant state in healthy pregnancy. During the third trimester, plasma levels of endothelium-derived von Willebrand factor are elevated, which promotes coagulation and platelet adhesion (Sorensen et al., 1995). Furthermore, there is a gestational increase in endothelium production of plasminogen activator inhibitor (PAI-1) and t-PA, with the effect of both inhibition and promotion of fibrinolysis, respectively. The t-PA and PAI-1 ratio remains unchanged in healthy pregnancy (Sorensen et al., 1995). Thrombin generation is also increased in normal pregnancy, as are circulating levels of fibrin degradation products (FDP) (de Boer et al., 1989; Sorensen et al., 1995), although the ratio of thrombin to FDP remains unchanged. The procoagulant state of the endothelium therefore appears to be compensated by upregulation of the fibrinolytic system (Bremme et al., 1992; Sorensen et al., 1995).

Circulating angiogenic factors

Vascular endothelial growth factor

The vascular endothelial growth factor (VEGF) family of proteins include VEGF-A, VEGF-B, VEGF-C, VEGF-D and placental growth factor (PGF). VEGF is an important growth factor in the placenta where it regulates angiogenesis (Ahmed et al., 1995; Zhou et al., 2002). VEGF-A is expressed in the syncytiotrophoblast cells and along with VEGF-C is also present in the cytotrophoblast. VEGF interacts through three different receptors: VEGFR-1 (flt-1), VEGFR-2 (KDR/flk-1), and VEGFR-3 (flt-4), which mediate different functions

within endothelial cells. VEGFR-1 is a soluble receptor, and has been localized to the placental trophoblast. VEGFR-1 and 3 are expressed on invasive cytotrophoblast cells in early pregnancy. VEGFR-1 is present in serum from pregnant women but only in small concentrations from non-pregnant females or males. Anti-VEGFR-1 reactivity has been demonstrated in the first cell layers of the cytotrophoblast column, which indicates a likely autocrine or paracrine effect that activates VEGF receptors in close proximity to the maternal extracellular matrix (Ahmed et al., 1995; Dunk and Ahmed, 2001).

Soluble fms-like tyrosine kinase 1 (sFlt-1)

Soluble Flt-1 is a circulating anti-angiogenic protein that acts by adhering to the receptor-binding domains of placental growth factor (PlGF) and VEGF, thus preventing interaction with endothelial cell surface receptors and resulting in endothelial dysfunction. During healthy pregnancy, sFlt-1 levels are low until the end of the second trimester, and PlGF levels are high, thus creating a pro-angiogenic state. As pregnancy advances, s-Flt1 levels gradually increase and the balance shifts to attenuate placental growth.

Pre-eclampsia

Whereas healthy maternal endothelium is crucial for the physiological adaptation to normal pregnancy, widespread endothelial dysfunction is an integral part of the multi-organ involvement of pre-eclampsia (Roberts and Redman, 1993). Women with pre-existing medical disorders that are characterized by endothelial dysfunction, such as hypertension and diabetes, are at increased risk of pre-eclampsia. Indeed, many of the risk factors for cardiovascular disease (all except smoking) are also risk factors for pre-eclampsia. Poor placental implantation also plays an important but not yet fully defined role toward maternal endothelial dysfunction.

Endothelial factors in pre-eclampsia

Markers of endothelial dysfunction

Healthy endothelial cells maintain vascular integrity, prevent platelet adhesion and influence the tone of underlying vascular smooth muscle. Once damaged, these functions lead to increased capillary permeability, platelet thrombosis and increased vascular tone (Flavahan and Vanhoutte, 1995). These features are found in pre-eclampsia and suggest that the maternal syndrome is, at least in part, an endothelial disorder (Roberts *et al.*, 1989). Evidence of endothelial cell damage prior to clinical manifestation of pre-eclampsia can be demonstrated by the presence of markers of endothelial cell activation. Specifically, levels of fibronectin (Ballegeer *et al.*, 1989) and Factor VIII-related antigen are elevated early in pregnancies that result in pre-eclampsia (Roberts and Redman, 1993). Morphological evidence of endothelial damage in pre-eclampsia can be seen in the glomerular capillaries (endotheliosis) and in the utero-placental arteries – a vasculopathy known as acute atherosis (Poston and Williams, 2000)

Nitric oxide in pre-eclampsia

Chronic inhibition of NO synthesis with L-NMMA in pregnant rats results in hypertension, proteinuria and fetal growth restriction, a syndrome mimicking pre-eclampsia (Yallampali and Garfield, 1993). Simultaneous infusion of L-arginine has been shown to reverse the hypertension and growth restriction (Molnar *et al.*, 1994; Yallampali and Garfield, 1993). It would be expected that endothelial dysfunction in pre-eclampsia would lead to impaired NOS activity. Due to methodological limitations, however, human studies have not reached a consensus on how NOS activity is altered during pre-eclampsia.

Cyclic GMP and NO metabolites

Measurement of NO metabolites in urine and plasma is fraught with methodological limitations and therefore, not surprisingly, studies in pre-eclamptic women have shown no change (Cameron *et al.*, 1993; Curtis *et al.*, 1995), an increase (Nobunaga *et al.*, 1996; Smarason *et al.*, 1997), or a fall in circulating or urinary NO metabolites, compared with normotensive controls (Seligman *et al.*, 1994). Such differences are also likely to reflect variations of nitrogen in the diet. In a study in which volunteers were starved for 12–15 h in an attempt to control for dietary nitrogen there was a correlation between systolic blood pressure and increasing plasma concentrations of NO_x (Nobunaga *et al.*, 1996).

Stimulated NO synthesis in vitro

There are many aspects of endothelial dysfunction that culminate in the development of pre-eclampsia, the abnormal relaxation to agonists representing just one endothelial cell defect. In small subcutaneous arteries, sensitivity to both ACh (McCarthy *et al.*, 1994) and to BK is reduced in women with pre-eclampsia compared with normotensive pregnant women (Knock and Poston, 1996).

Using omental vessels from women with pre-eclampsia, Pascoal *et al.* (1998) found relaxation to ACh was totally absent whilst responses to BK were unaffected when compared to normotensive controls. Studies using small myometrial arteries from pre-eclamptic women showed that relaxation to BK was completely absent, whereas normotensive controls relaxed well (Ashworth *et al.*, 1997). Other studies using similar vessels showed that maximal responses to ACh were reduced in pre-eclamptic women (Kublickiene *et al.*, 1998). Whilst these studies generally agree that endothelium-dependent dilatation is impaired in women with pre-eclampsia, the role of NO in these mechanisms remains equivocal. Knock and Poston (1996) and Kublickiene *et al.* (1998) have suggested that the blunting of responses to endothelium-dependent dilators is due to reduced NO synthesis, but Pascoal *et al.* (1998) have suggested that the defect is NO-independent.

Isolated arteries from subcutaneous fat of normotensive pregnant women relaxed in response to flow-induced shear stress, but the same vessels from pre-eclamptic women did not. This lack of response was unchanged by the presence of a NOS inhibitor (Cockell and Poston, 1997a). These findings suggest that increased NO synthesis contributes to vasodilatation of healthy pregnancy which appears to be reduced in pre-eclamptic women. More recently, vasodilator responses to bradykinin in small myometrial arteries isolated from pregnant, non-pregnant, and pre-eclamptic women have been shown to be similar in terms of sensitivity and magnitude (Kenny *et al.*, 2002b). This illustrates the heterogeneity of responses by different vessels to different vasoactive substances under different experimental conditions.

In vivo studies of nitric oxide activity in pre-eclampsia

It remains unclear as to whether systemic NO production is altered in women with pre-eclampsia. Using forearm venous occlusion plethysmography, Anumba *et al.* (1999) found that responses to an endothelium-dependent NO-mediated vasodilator (serotonin) were blunted to a similar extent during both normotensive and pre-eclamptic pregnancies. They also demonstrated that vascular smooth muscle sensitivity to exogenous NO (GTN) is unaltered in normal pregnancy or pre-eclampsia.

Asymmetric dimethylarginine (ADMA)

During the first half of normotensive pregnancy the gestational fall in blood pressure is accompanied by a fall in the circulating concentration of ADMA, an endogenous NO synthase inhibitor (Fickling *et al.*, 1993; Holden *et al.*, 1998). Plasma ADMA levels are significantly higher in women with pre-eclampsia than gestationally matched normotensive controls (Fickling *et al.*, 1993; Holden *et al.*, 1998).

In a recent study, Savvidou *et al.* (2003) showed that women with bilateral uterine artery notches at 24 weeks gestation had markedly elevated ADMA levels compared with those who have a normal uterine artery waveform. Impaired brachial artery FMD at 23–25 weeks gestation was also evident up to 10 weeks prior to the onset of clinical signs and symptoms of pre-eclampsia. In women who later developed pre-eclampsia, ADMA levels were inversely correlated with FMD (Figure 4.5). These findings suggest that ADMA may provide a biochemical link between elevated placental vascular resistance and maternal endothelial dysfunction. At the concentrations reached in women with uterine artery notches, ADMA is able to inhibit synthesis of NO from L-arginine and attenuate endothelium-dependent vasodilatation (Calver *et al.*, 1993; Vallance *et al.*, 1992).

In this study, women with uterine artery notches had a selective elevation of ADMA but not its stereoisomer, SDMA, implicating impaired activity of DDAH, the enzyme that metabolizes ADMA. Preliminary work indicates that DDAH II, like eNOS, is highly expressed in the placenta, and it has been hypothesized that reduced DDAH II activity from the hypoperfused placenta could limit metabolism of ADMA. Increased concentrations of ADMA might attenuate the physiological vasodilatation of pregnancy and contribute to the development of pre-eclampsia. As only some women with high ADMA levels developed PET, its occurrence may be linked genetically to polymorphisms of eNOS. It has been shown that in early pregnancy, FMD is modulated by carriage of the Glu298Asp polymorphism of eNOS, which has been linked to pre-eclampsia (Yoshimura *et al.*, 2000).

Endothelin in the maternal circulation in pre-eclampsia

Studies in isolated omental (Vedernikov *et al.*, 1995; Wolff *et al.*, 1996a) and myometrial arteries

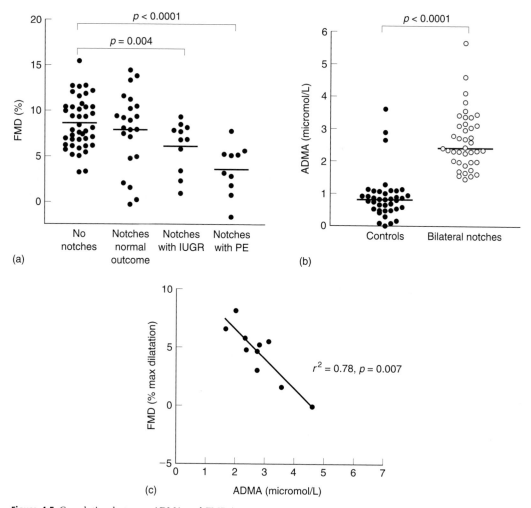

Figure 4.5 Correlation between ADMA and FMD in women who later developed pre-eclampsia.

(Wolff *et al.*, 1996b) have shown similar responses to ET-1 in arteries from normal and pre-eclamptic women, suggesting that enhanced sensitivity to ET-1 is unlikely to contribute to vasoconstriction of the maternal vasculature. One report suggests urinary excretion of ET-1 is reduced in women with pre-eclampsia (Clark *et al.*, 1997) and as ET-1 is natiuretic, could be implicated as a cause of sodium retention. More recently, Ajne *et al.* (2003) analyzed levels of endothelin converting enzyme (ECE), that catalyzes ET-1 synthesis from its precursor, as a marker of ET-1 production.

They found enhanced ECE activity in the plasma of a small number of pre-eclamptic women compared with normal pregnant women, which may indicate enhanced ET-1 production in pre-eclampsia. Further studies are necessary for further clarification of their findings.

Prostanoids in the maternal circulation in pre-eclampsia

Prostaglandins are now known to play an important role in the adaptive changes associated with normal pregnancy, with inadequate synthesis being a likely contributory factor to the development of pre-eclampsia (Davidge, 2001). In contrast to normal pregnancy, pre-eclampsia is associated with relative underproduction of PGI_2 and the over-abundance of TxA_2 (Fitzgerald et al., 1990). A reduction in the PGI_2/TxA_2 ratio increases the likelihood of hypertension (Granger et al., 2001).

The imbalance between these opposing prostanoids formed the rationale for investigations of "low dose aspirin" therapy for prevention of pre-eclampsia. Whereas aspirin in excess of $150\,mg\,day^{-1}$ inhibits both PGI_2 and TxA_2, low or intermittent doses lead to preferential inhibition of TxA_2 biosynthesis (Ritter et al., 1989), and could redress the imbalance between these prostanoids in pre-eclampsia. Selectivity for TxA_2 may lie in differential access of aspirin to platelet cyclo-oxygenase in the portal circulation (Pederson and Fitzgerald, 1984) with pre-systemic metabolism preventing access of aspirin to the systemic vasculature and placenta and/or the differential affinity of aspirin for cyclo-oxygenase in platelets (Patrignani et al., 1982). Also platelets, being anuclear, lack the capacity to regenerate cyclo-oxygenase, whereas endothelium can regenerate the enzyme and so maintain PGI_2 production (Ritter et al., 1989). The potential benefit of aspirin had also been highlighted by the reduced risk of pre-eclampsia in women at high risk of pre-eclampsia (Coomerasamy et al., 2003). Post hoc analysis of the CLASP Trial has shown a 15% reduction in recurrent pre-eclampsia for women who had early (prior to 32 weeks gestation), severe pre-eclampsia (CLASP, 1994).

More recently, Mills et al. (1999) conducted a multicentered prospective study to examine changes in PGI_2 and TxA_2 levels through pregnancy. They found reduced PGI_2 production rather than increased TxA_2 production occurred many months prior to the onset of clinical disease and speculated that aspirin trials were likely to have been less successful than hoped, because increased TxA_2 synthesis was not the primary abnormality. A decreased ratio of $PGF_{1\alpha}:TxB_2$ is evident in

pregnant women who go on to develop pre-eclampsia (Chavarria et al., 2003). These findings suggest early platelet activation and endothelial dysfunction. They also demonstrated a positive correlation between TxB_2 levels and cFN (Chavarria et al., 2002).

Effect of sera from pre-eclamptic women on cultured endothelial cells

Whether the vascular changes that occur in pre-eclampsia arise as a result of intrinsic vascular dysfunction or are mediated by circulating factors, or a combination of both, remains unresolved. Several experiments have shown changes to different types of cultured endothelial cells (human umbilical vein (HUVEC)), human decidual tissue (animal and fetal cells) following exposure to plasma or sera of varying concentrations from normal pregnant or pre-eclamptic women. Initial studies implied a possible circulating factor in the sera of pre-eclamptic women that was cytotoxic to endothelial cells (Rogers et al., 1988). However, more recent studies on HUVEC have shown that pre-eclamptic serum is not cytotoxic (Endersen et al., 1995). The suggestion that pre-eclampsia was associated with reduced PGI_2 synthesis prompted investigators to determine whether a blood-borne factor or factors could inhibit endothelial PGI_2 production. Results from various studies have been conflicting and are likely to represent differences in experimental methodology.

Circulating angiogenic factors in pre-eclampsia

VEGF has been proposed to play a part in the pre-eclamptic process. Initial studies showed serum levels of VEGF to be elevated in pre-eclampsia and suggested a role in endothelial cell activation (Baker et al., 1995). More recently, VEGF and VEGFR expression have been shown to be down-regulated in severe pre-eclampsia (Lyall et al., 1997; Zhou et al., 2002). This suggests impaired vascular development in the placenta and supports the hypothesis that the VEGF system has an important

regulatory role in the process of trophoblastic invasion. Reduced endothelium-dependent relaxation
of blood vessels incubated in pre-eclamptic serum
in the presence of anti-VEGF antibody suggests a
role for low concentrations of VEGF in the pathogenesis of pre-eclampsia (Brockelsby *et al.*, 1999).

Soluble Flt-1 (sFlt-1), which binds VEGF,
increases in the serum of women with pre-
eclampsia (Koga *et al.*, 2003; Maynard *et al.*, 2003;
Tsatsaris *et al.*, 2003) as concentrations of circulating free PlGF and VEGF decrease, even prior to the
onset of the clinical syndrome (Polliotti *et al.*, 2003;
Taylor *et al.*, 2003). A pre-eclamptic-like state with
hypertension, proteinuria and glomerular endotheliosis was induced in pregnant rats by administering
exogenous sFlt-1 (Maynard *et al.*, 2003). Moreover,
cancer patients treated with VEGF-signaling inhibitors have developed hypertension and proteinuria
(Kabbinavar *et al.*, 2003; Yang *et al.*, 2003). Thus,
excess sFlt-1 may indeed play an important role in
the pathogenesis of pre-eclampsia.

In a cross-sectional study, sFlt-1 levels were
shown to increase about 5 weeks prior to the onset
of pre-eclampsia (Levine *et al.*, 2004). In women
destined to develop early-onset pre-eclampsia and
intra-uterine growth restriction, there was a greater
variation in sFlt-1 and PlGF levels, supporting a
role for abnormal placental angiogenesis in the
aetiology of pre-eclampsia.

During pregnancy, another antiangiogenic
protein, soluble endoglin (a co-receptor for transforming growth factor β_1 and β_3) is released into the
maternal circulation from the placenta. Circulating
soluble endoglin levels increase 2–3 months before
the onset of pre-eclampsia (Levine *et al.*, 2006). This
rise in soluble endoglin concentration was usually
accompanied by an increased ratio of sFlt-1: PlGF
ratio. Combined together rising levels of these two
values strongly predicts the future onset of pre-
eclampsia (Levine *et al.*, 2006).

Abnormalities of the uterine vasculature

In normal pregnancy, the most striking change to a
maternal artery occurs within the small spiral
arteries within the uterus (see chapters by Lyall
and Pijnenborg), but in women who develop pre-
eclampsia, cytotrophoblast invasion of the spiral
arteries is incomplete and high-resistance vessels
that retain their muscular wall persist until term.
Prior to any clinical symptoms or signs, Doppler
ultrasound of uterine arteries at 20–24 weeks gestation can aid in the identity of women with high-
resistance vessels at risk of pre-eclampsia. The
presence of a diastolic "notch" at 24 weeks gestation, which is thought to reflect a systolic wave
"bouncing off" the high-resistance vascular bed,
may predict 30–50% of women who will go on to
develop pre-eclampsia (Bower *et al.*, 1993; Savvidou
et al., 2003).

The sympathetic nervous system in pre-eclampsia

It has been suggested that the pathological increase
in vascular tone evident in pre-eclampsia occurs
secondary to changes in the autonomic nervous
system. Women with pre-eclampsia have been
found to have increased sympathetic nerve activity
in muscle–nerve fascicles of the peroneal nerve
(Schobel *et al.*, 1996) and higher plasma noradrenaline levels compared with normotensive women
(Manyonda *et al.*, 1998). In this latter study, tyrosine
hydroxylase activity and mRNA levels were greater
in placental tissue from pre-eclamptic compared
with normotensive pregnancies. It is proposed that
excessive noradrenaline breaks down more triglyceride to free fatty acids, which are then oxidized to
lipid peroxides that are cytotoxic to endothelial cells
(Manyonda *et al.*, 1998). However, systemic blockade of the autonomic nervous system with tetraethylammonium chloride (TEAC) or high spinal
anesthesia causes a dramatic fall in blood pressure
in normotensive pregnant women, but is much less
effective in women with pre-eclampsia (Assali
and Prystowsky, 1950). Despite the potential non-
specificity of this method, this unique study would
suggest that the hypertension of pre-eclampsia is
mediated by a factor independent of the autonomic
nervous system.

Link between the endothelium and immune factors in pre-eclampsia

Pre-eclampsia is likely to result from an interaction between immunological, cardiovascular and metabolic factors. Defective cytotrophoblast invasion of the maternal spiral arteries leads to reduced uteroplacental perfusion and hence placental ischemia/hypoxia. Placental ischemia results in the release of a variety of factors including inflammatory cytokines and reactive oxygen species that cause maternal endothelial dysfunction.

Neutrophils and platelets are activated in normal pregnancy and further activated in pre-eclampsia (Greer et al., 1989; Zemel et al., 1990). Activated neutrophils adhere to endothelium and mediate vascular damage by the release of proteases and reactive oxygen radicals. Neutrophil adhesion to the endothelium is mediated through the expression of cell adhesion molecules on the endothelial cell surface. During endothelial cell activation, expression of certain cell adhesion molecules is increased on both neutrophils and the endothelium. Neutrophil adhesion is much more marked in women with pre-eclampsia, as they have increased expression of certain cell adhesion molecules compared with healthy normotensive pregnant women (Barden et al., 1997). Specifically, vascular endothelial cell adhesion molecule (VCAM-1) and E-selectin circulate in higher concentrations in women with pre-eclampsia than in normotensive pregnant women (Lyall et al., 1994). The stimulus to neutrophil activation remains unknown, but pro-inflammatory cytokines can activate neutrophils and simultaneously increase expression of cell adhesion molecules on endothelial cells (Lyall and Greer, 1996). Furthermore, placental debri in the form of apoptotic fragments of syncytiotrophoblast, which are found in increased concentrations in the maternal circulation of women with pre-eclampsia may be the stimulus to an inflammatory response (Redman et al., 1999).

Cytokines are produced by leukocytes, vascular endothelial cells, smooth muscle cells and placental trophoblasts, which suggests an important role for inflammation in pre-eclampsia (Conrad and Benyo, 1997). The cytokines TNF-α and IL-1 are major pro-inflammatory cytokines and have been shown to induce alterations in endothelial cells, including endothelial activation and expression of adhesion molecules that are vital for the recruitment of inflammatory cells into the vessel wall (Pober and Cotran, 1990). They also stimulate chemoattractant cytokines such as monocyte chemotactic protein-1 (MCP-1) and IL-8 (Mantovani, 1997), as well as IL-6, which in turn stimulates hepatic production of acute phase reactants.

Elevated TNF-α levels may cause endothelial dysfunction both directly and indirectly. Leukocyte TNF-α gene expression and circulating levels of TNF-α are enhanced in pre-eclamptic patients compared with normotensive and non-pregnant women (Chen et al., 1996; Kupfermine et al., 1994). TNF-α can generate reactive oxygen species, inhibit NOS, favor synthesis of TXA$_2$ over prostacyclin, change endothelial cells from an anti-hemostatic to a pro-coagulant state and activate transcription of VCAM-1 (Chen et al., 1996). On the basis of its biological properties therefore, TNF-α is a strong candidate for mediating endothelial damage in pre-eclampsia. Recent reports suggest that serum concentrations of IL-2, IL-6 and TNF-α are significantly higher in the first and second trimesters in pregnant women who go on to develop pre-eclampsia compared to controls. Thus defective immunological processes are likely to exist prior to the onset of clinical disease (Sacks et al., 1998; Williams et al., 1999).

Conclusion

The control of vascular tone is multifactorial. The autonomic nervous system, intrinsic vascular smooth muscle reflexes and the endothelium all play a role in maintaining blood flow to an organ. Defects in one parameter are counterbalanced by another, making it difficult to understand the primary pathology. Prospective studies in healthy and diseased pregnancy will help our understanding of cardiovascular change during pregnancy and in those women who go on to develop pre-eclampsia.

One of the most important adaptations made by the endothelium during healthy pregnancy is increased nitric oxide synthase (NOS) activity, which is stimulated by the gestational increase in estradiol levels. During pregnancy, maternal organs vary in their degree of vasodilatation, possibly reflecting the variable expression of eNOS in their vasculature. Blood flow to the uterus in particular increases secondary to increased NOS activity. A healthy endothelium also prevents hemostasis and inflammatory activity. When the endothelium is damaged, the vasodilatory, anti-thrombotic and anti-inflammatory roles of the endothelium are attenuated. This leads to reduced maternal organ blood flow due to vasoconstriction, microthrombi and local inflammation, all of which are present in affected organs during pre-eclampsia.

The risk factors for pre-eclampsia (all except smoking) are similar to those for cardiovascular disease in later life. It is clear therefore that some women who go on to develop pre-eclampsia have pre-existing endothelial dysfunction. They are vulnerable to even a mild inflammatory stress or increased antiangiogenic response. The source of this anti-endothelial stress appears to be a poorly implanted placenta, but may also involve a hormone-induced metabolic state that is damaging to the endothelium. Further understanding of the clinical spectrum of pre-eclampsia will allow us to customize anti-pre-eclampsia prophylaxis according to maternal and possibly paternal phenotype.

REFERENCES

Ahmed, A., Li, X. F., Dunk, C., *et al.* (1995). Co-localization of vascular endothelial growth factor and its Flt-1 receptor in human placenta. *Growth Factors*, **12**, 235–43.

Ajne, G., Wolff, K., Fyhrquist, F., *et al.* (2003). Endothelin converting enzyme (ECE) activity in normal pregnancy and pre-eclampsia. *Hypertens. Pregn.*, **22**, 215–24.

Anumba, D. O. C., Robson, S. C., Boys, R. J. and Ford, G. A. (1999). Nitric oxide activity in the peripheral vasculature during normotensive and preeclamptic pregnancy. *Am. J. Physiol.*, **277**, H848–54.

Ashworth, J. R., Warren, A. Y., Baker, P. N. and Johnson, I. R. (1996). Endothelium-dependent relaxation in omental and myometrial resistance arteries in pregnant and non-pregnant women. *Am. J. Obstet. Gynecol.*, **175**, 1307–12.

Ashworth, J. R., Warren, A. Y., Baker, P. N. and Johnson, I. R. (1997). Loss of endothelium-dependent relaxation in myometrial resistance arteries in pre-eclampsia. *Br. J. Obstet. Gynecol.*, **104**, 1152–8.

Assali, N. S. and Prystowsky, H. (1950). Studies on autonomic blockade. I. Comparison between the effects of tetraethylammonium chloride (TEAC) and high selective spinal anesthesia on blood pressure of normal and toxemic pregnancy. *J. Clin. Invest.*, **29**, 1354–66.

Bagnall, A. J. and Webb, D. J. (2000). The endothelin system: physiology. In *Vascular Endothelium in Human Physiology and Pathophysiology*, eds. P. J. T. Vallance and D. J. Webb. The Netherlands: Harwood Academic Publishers.

Baker, P. N., Krasnow, J., Roberts, J. M. and Yeo, K. T. (1995). Elevated serum levels of vascular endothelial growth factor in patients with pre-eclampsia. *Obstet. Gynecol.*, **86**, 815–21.

Barden, A., Graham, D., Beilin, L. J., *et al.* (1997). Neutrophil CD11B expression and neutrophil activation in pre-eclampsia. *Clin. Sci.*, **92**, 37–44.

Boccardo, P., Soregaroli, M., Aiello, S., *et al.* (1996). Systemic and fetal–maternal nitric oxide synthesis in normal pregnancy and pre-eclampsia. *Br. J. Obstet. Gynaecol.*, **103**, 879–86.

Bonnar, J. (1987). Haemostasis and coagulation disorders in pregnancy. In *Haemostasis and Thrombosis*, eds. A. L. Bloom and D. P. Thomas. Edinburgh: Churchill Livingstone, pp. 570–84.

Boulanger, C. and Luscher, T. F. (1990). Release of endothelin from the porcine aorta: inhibition by endothelium-derived nitric oxide. *J. Clin. Invest.*, **85**, 587–90.

Bower, S., Bewley, S. and Campbell, S. (1993). Improved prediction of preeclampsia by two-stage screening of uterine arteries using the early diastolic notch and color Doppler imaging. *Obstet. Gynecol.*, **82**, 78–83.

Bremme, K., Ostlund, E., Almquist, I., *et al.* (1992). Enhanced thrombin generation and fibrinolytic activity in normal pregnancy and the puerperium. *Obstet. Gynecol.*, **80**, 132–7.

Brockelsby, J., Hayman, R., Ahmed, A., *et al.* (1999). VEGF via VEGF receptor-1 (Flt-1) mimics pre-eclamptic plasma in inhibiting uterine blood vessel relaxation in pregnancy: implications in the pathogenesis of pre-eclampsia. *Lab. Invest.*, **79**, 1101–11.

Brown, M. A. and Gallery, E. D. M. (1994). Volume homeostasis in normal pregnancy and pre-eclampsia: physiology and clinical implications. *Baillieres Clin. Obst. Gynaecol.*, **8**, 287–310.

Calver, A., Collier, J., Leone, A., Moncada, S. and Vallance, P. (1993). Effect of local intra-arterial asymmetric dimethylarginine (ADMA) on the forearm arteriolar bed of healthy volunteers. *J. Hum. Hypertens.*, **7**, 193–4.

Cameron, I., van Papendorp, C. L., Palmer, R. M. J., *et al.* (1993). Relationship between nitric oxide synthesis and increase in systolic blood pressure in women with hypertension in pregnancy. *Hypertens. Preg.*, **12**, 85–92.

Castro, L. C., Hobel, C. J. and Gornbein, J. (1994). Plasma levels of atrial natriuretic peptide in normal and hypertensive pregnancies: a meta-analysis. *Am. J. Obstet. Gynecol.*, **171**, 1642–51.

Celermajer, D. S., Sorensen, K. E., Gooch, V. M., *et al.* (1992). Non-invasive detection of endothelial dysfunction in children and adults at risk of atherosclerosis. *Lancet*, **340**, 1111–15.

Chapman, A. B., Abraham, W. T., Zamudio, S., *et al.* (1998). Temporal relationships between hormonal and hemodynamic changes in early human pregnancy. *Kidney Int.*, **54**, 2056–63.

Chavarria, M. E., Lara-Gonzalez, L., Gonzalez-Gleason, A., *et al.* (2002). Maternal plasma cellular fibronectin concentrations in normal and pre-eclamptic pregnancies: a longitudinal study for early prediction of pre-eclampsia. *Am. J. Obstet. Gynecol.*, **187**, 595–601.

Chavarria, M. E., Lara-Gonzalez, L., Gonzalez-Gleason, A., *et al.* (2003). Prostacyclin/thromboxane early changes in pregnancies that are complicated by pre-eclampsia. *Am. J. Obstet. Gynecol.*, **188**, 986–92.

Chen, D. B., Bird, I. M., Zheng, J. and Magness, R. R. (2004). Membrane estrogen receptor-dependent extracellular signal-regulated kinase pathway mediates acute activation of endothelial nitric oxide synthase by estrogen in uterine artery endothelial cells. *Endocrinology*, **145**, 113–25.

Chen, G., Suzuki, H. and Weston, A. H. (1988). Acetylcholine releases endothelium-derived hyperpolarising factor and EDRF from rat blood vessels. *Br. J. Pharmacol.*, **95**, 1165–74.

Chen, G., Wilson, R., Wang, S. H., *et al.* (1996). Tumour necrosis factor alpha (TNF-α) gene polymorphism and expression in pre-eclampsia. *Clin. Exp. Immunol.*, **104**, 154–9.

Chirico, S., Smith, C., Merchant, C., *et al.* (1993). Lipid peroxidation in hyperlipidaemic patients: a study of plasma using an HPLC-based thiobarbituric acid test. *Free Rad. Res. Commun.*, **19**, 51–7.

Clark, B. A., Ludmire, J., Epstein, F. H., *et al.* (1997). Urinary cGMP, endothelin, and prostaglandin E_2 in normal pregnancy and preeclampsia. *Am. J. Perinatol.*, **14**, 559–62.

CLASP (Collaborative Low Dose Aspirin Study in Pregnancy) Collaborative group. (1994). CLASP: a randomised trial of low-dose aspirin for the prevention and treatment of preeclampsia among 9364 pregnant women. *Lancet*, **343**, 619–29.

Cockell, A. P. and Poston, L. (1997a). Flow mediated vasodilatation is enhanced in normal pregnancy but reduced in preeclampsia. *Hypertension*, **30**, 247–51.

Cockell, A. P. and Poston, L. (1997b). 17β estradiol stimulates flow-induced vasodilatation in isolated small mesenteric arteries from prepubertal female rats. *Am. J. Obstet. Gynaecol.*, **177**, 1432–8.

Cockell, A. P., Learmont, J. G., Smarason, A. L., *et al.* (1997). Human placental syncytiotrophoblast microvillous membranes impair maternal vascular endothelial cell function. *Br. J. Obstet. Gynaecol.*, **104**, 235–40.

Coleman, H. A., Tare, M. and Parkington, H. C. (2001). K^+ currents underlying the action of endothelium-derived hyperpolarizing factor in guinea-pig, rat and human blood vessels. *J. Physiol.*, **531**, 359–73.

Conrad, K. P. and Vernier, V. A. (1989). Plasma levels, urinary excretion and metabolic production of cGMP during gestation in rats. *Am. J. Physiol.*, **257**, R847–53.

Conrad, K. P. and Benyo, D. F. (1997). Placental cytokines and the pathogenesis of pre-eclampsia. *Am. J. Reprod. Immunol.*, **37**, 240–9.

Conrad, K. P., Joffe, G. M., Kruszyna, H., *et al.* (1993). Identification of increased nitric oxide biosynthesis during pregnancy in rats. *FASEB J.*, **7**, 566–71.

Coomerasamy, A., Honest, H., Papaionnou, S., *et al.* (2003). Aspirin for prevention of pre-eclampsia in women with historical risk factors: a systematic review. *Obstet. Gynecol.*, **101**, 1318–32.

Curtis, N. E., Gude, N. M., King, R. G., *et al.* (1995). Nitric oxide metabolites in normal human pregnancy and preeclampsia. *Hypertens. Preg.*, **23**, 1096–105.

Danielson, L. A. and Conrad, K. P. (1995). Acute blockade of nitric oxide synthase inhibits renal vasodilation and hyperfiltration during pregnancy in chronically instrumented conscious rats. *J. Clin. Investig.*, **96**, 482–90.

Davenport, A. P., Ashley, M. J., Easton, P., *et al.* (1990). A sensitive radioimmunoassay measuring endothelin-like immunoreactivity in human plasma: comparison of levels in patients with essential hypertension and normotensive control subjects. *Clin. Sci.*, **78**, 261–4.

Davidge, S. T. (2001). Prostaglandin H synthase and vascular function. *Circ. Res.*, **89**, 650–60.

Davidge, S. T., Signorella, A. P., Lykins, D. L., *et al.* (1996). Evidence of endothelial activation and endothelial activators in cord blood of infants of pre-eclamptic women. *Am. J. Obstet. Gynecol.*, **175**, 1301–6.

Davison, J. M. (1984). Renal haemodynamics and volume homeostasis in pregnancy. *Scand. J. Clin. Lab. Invest.*, **169**(Suppl.), 15–27.

Dayoub, H., Achan, V., Adimoolam, S., *et al.* (2003). Dimethylarginine dimethylaminohydrolase regulates nitric oxide synthesis. Genetic and physiological evidence. *Circulation*, **108**, 3042–7.

de Boer, K., ten-Cate, J. W., Sturk, A., *et al.* (1989). Enhanced thrombin generation in normal and hypertensive pregnancy. *Am. J. Obstet. Gynecol.*, **160**, 95–100.

Dunk, C. and Ahmed, A. (2001). Expression of VEGF-c and activation of its receptors VEGFR-2 and VEGFR-3 in trophoblast. *Histol. Histopathol.*, **16**, 359–75.

Dunlop, W. (1981). Serial changes in renal haemodynamics during normal human pregnancy. *Br. J. Obstet. Gynecol.*, **88**, 1–9.

Easterling, T. R., Watts, H., Schumucker, B. C. and Benedettie, T. J. (1987). Measurement of cardiac output during pregnancy: validation of Doppler technique and clinical observations in pre-eclampsia. *Obstet. Gynecol.*, **69**, 845–50.

Edwards, G., Dora, K. A., Gardener, M. J., *et al.* (1998). K$^+$ is an endothelium-derived hyperpolarizing factor in rat arteries. *Nature*, **396**, 269–72.

Edwards, G., Thollon, C., Gardener, M. J., *et al.* (2000). Role of gap junctions and EETs in endothelium-dependent hyperpolarisation of porcine artery. *Br. J. Pharmacol.*, **129**, 1145–54.

Endresen, M. J., Tosti, E., Lorentzen, B. and Henriksen, T. (1995). Sera of preeclamptic women is not cytotoxic to endothelial cells in culture. *Am. J. Obstet. Gynecol.*, **172**, 196–201.

Farhat, M. Y., Lavigne, M. C. and Ramwell, P. W. (1996). The vascular protective effects of estrogen. *FASEB J.*, **10**, 615–24.

Feletou, M. and Vanhoutte, P. M. (1988). Endothelium-dependent hyperpolarisation of canine coronary smooth muscle. *Br. J. Pharmacol.*, **93**, 515–24.

Fickling, S. A., Williams, D., Vallance, P., *et al.* (1993). Plasma concentrations of endogenous inhibitor of nitric oxide synthesis in normal pregnancy and pre-eclampsia. *Lancet*, **342**, 242–3.

Fitzgerald, D. J., Rocki, W., Murray, R., *et al.* (1990). Thromboxane A$_2$ synthesis in pregnancy-induced hypertension. *Lancet*, **335**, 751–4.

Flavahan, N. A. and Vanhoutte, P. M. (1995). Endothelial cell signalling and endothelial cell dysfunction. *Am. J. Hypertens.*, **8**, 28S–41S.

Ford, G. A., Robson, S. C. and Mahdy, Z. A. (1996). Superficial hand vein responses to N^G-monomethyl-L-arginine in post-partum and non-pregnant women. *Clin. Sci.*, **90**, 493–7.

Fostermann, U., Closs, E. I., Pollock, J. S., *et al.* (1994). Nitric oxide synthase isoenzymes. Characterization, purification, molecular cloning, and functions. *Hypertension*, **23**, 1211–31.

Freeman, B. A., Gutierrez, H. and Rubbo, H. (1995). Nitric oxide: a central regulatory species in pulmonary oxidant reactions. *Am. J. Physiol.*, **268**, L697–8.

Fried, G. and Samuelson, U. (1991). Endothelin and neuropeptide Y are vasoconstrictors in human uterine blood vessels. *Am. J. Obstet. Gynecol.*, **164**, 1330–6.

Furchgott, R. F. (1988). Studies on relaxation of rabbit aorta by sodium nitrite: the basis for the proposal that the acid-activatable inhibitory factor from retractor penis in inorganic nitrite and the endothelium-derived relaxing factor in nitric oxide. In *Vasodilatation: Vascular Smooth Muscle, Peptides, Autonomic Nerves and Endothelium*, ed. P. M. Vanhoutte. New York: Raven, pp. 401–14.

Furchgott, R. F. and Vanhoutte, P. M. (1989). Endothelium-derived relaxing and contracting factors. *FASEB J.*, **3**, 2007–18.

Furchgott, R. and Zawadzki, D. (1980). The obligatory role of endothelial cells in the relaxation of arterial smooth muscle by acetylcholine. *Nature*, **288**, 373–6.

Gargett, C. E., Bucak, K., Zaitseva, M., *et al.* (2002). Estrogen receptor-alpha and -beta expression in microvascular endothelial cells and smooth muscle cells of myometrium and leiomyoma. *Mol. Hum. Reprod.*, **8**, 770–5.

Garland, C. J., Plane, F., Kemp, B. K. and Cox, T. M. (1995). Endothelium-dependent hyperpolarisation: a role in the control of vascular tone. *Trends Pharmacol. Sci.*, **16**, 23–30.

Gerber, R. T., Anwar, M. A. and Poston, L. (1998). Enhanced acetylcholine induced relaxation in small mesenteric arteries from pregnant rats: an important role for endothelium-derived hyperpolarizing factor (EDHF). *Br. J. Pharmacol.*, **125**(3), 455–60.

Goodrum, L., Saade, G., Jahoor, F., *et al.* (1996). Nitric oxide production in normal human pregnancy. *J. Soc. Gynecol. Investig.*, **3**, 97A.

Goonasekera, C. D., Rees, D. D., Woolard, P., *et al.* (1997). Nitric oxide synthase inhibitors and hypertension in children and adolescents. *J. Hypertens.*, **15**, 901–9.

Granger, J. P., Alexander, B. T., Llinas, M. T., *et al.* (2001). Pathophysiology of hypertension during pre-eclampsia. Linking placental ischaemia with endothelial dysfunction. *Hypertension*, **38**(Suppl.), 718–22.

Greer, I. A., Haddad, N. G., Dawes, J., *et al.* (1989). Neutrophil activation in pregnancy-induced hypertension. *Br. J. Obstet. Gynaecol.*, **96**, 978–82.

Halligan, A., O'Brien, E., O'Malley, K., *et al.* (1993). 24 hour ambulatory blood pressure measurement in the primigravid population. *J. Hypertens.*, **11**, 869–73.

Hashimoto, M., Akishita, M., Eto, M., *et al.* (1995). Modulation of endothelium-dependent flow-mediated dilatation of the brachial artery by sex and menstrual cycle. *Circulation*, **92**, 3431–5.

Hecker, M., Bara, A. T., Bauersachs, J. and Busse, R. (1994). Characterization of endothelium-derived hyperpolarizing factor as a cytochrome P450-derived arachidonic acid metabolite in mammals. *J. Physiol. (Lond.)*, **481**, 407–14.

Hill, C. E., Phillips, J. K. and Sandow, S. L. (2001). Heterogeneous control of blood flow amongst different vascular beds. *Medic. Res. Rev.*, **21**, 1–60.

Holden, D. P., Fickling, S. A., StJ. Whitley, G. and Nussey, S. S. (1998). Plasma concentrations of asymmetric dimethylarginine, a natural inhibitor of nitric oxide synthase, in normal pregnancy and pre-eclampsia. *Am. J. Obstet. Gynecol.*, **178**, 551–6.

Hubel, C. A., McLaughlin, M. K., Evans, R. W., *et al.* (1996). Fasting serum triglycerides, free fatty acids and malondialdehyde are increased in pre-eclampsia, are positively correlated, and decrease within 48 hours post partum. *Am. J. Obstet. Gynecol.*, **174**, 975–82.

Ignarro, L. J., Byrns, R. E. and Wood, K. S. (1988). Biochemical and pharmacological properties of endothelium-derived relaxing factor and its similarity to nitric oxide radical. In *Vasodilatation: Vascular Smooth Muscle, Peptides, Autonomic Nerves and Endothelium*, ed. P. M. Vanhoutte. New York: Raven, pp. 401–14.

Kabbinavar, F., Hurwitz, H. I., Fehrenbacher, L., *et al.* (2003). Phase II, randomised trial comparing bevacizumab plus fluorouracil (FU)/leucovorin (LV) and FU/LV alone in patients with metastatic colorectal cancer. *J. Clin. Oncol.*, **21**, 60–5.

Kakimoto, Y. and Akazawa, S. (1970). Isolation and identification of N^G,N^G- and N^G,N'^G-dimethylarginine, N-epsilon-mono, di-, and trimethyllysine, and glucosylgalactosyl- and galactosyl-delta-hydroxylysine from human urine. *J. Biol. Chem.*, **245**, 5751–8.

Kenny, L. C., Baker, P. N., Kendall, D. A., *et al.* (2002a). Differential mechanisms of endothelium-dependent vasodilator responses in human myometrial small arteries in normal pregnancy and pre-eclampsia. *Clin. Sci.*, **103**, 67–73.

Kenny, L. C., Baker, P. N., Kendall, D. A., *et al.* (2002b). The role of gap junctions in mediating endothelium-dependent responses to bradykinin in myometrial small arteries isolated from pregnant women. *Br. J. Pharmacol.*, **136**, 1085–8.

Killam, A. P., Rosenfeld, C. R., Battaglia, F. C., *et al.* (1973). Effect of estrogens on the uterine blood flow of oophorectomised ewes. *Am. J. Obstet. Gynecol.*, **115**, 1045–52.

Kitching, A. R., Kong, Y. Z., Huang, X. R., *et al.* (2003). Plasminogen activator inhibitor-1 is a significant determinant of renal injury in experimental crescentic glomerulonephritis. *J. Am. Soc. Nephrol.*, **14**, 1487–95.

Knock, G. A. and Poston, L. (1996). Bradykinin-mediated relaxation of isolated maternal resistance arteries in normal pregnancy and preeclampsia. *Am. J. Obstet. Gynecol.*, **175**, 1668–74.

Koga, K., Osuga, Y., Yoshino, O., *et al.* (2003). Elevated serum soluble vascular endothelial growth factor receptor 1 (sVEGFR-1) levels in women with pre-eclampsia. *J. Clin. Endocrinol. Metab.*, **88**, 2348–51.

Kopp, L., Paradiz, G. and Tucci, J. R. (1977). Urinary excretion of cyclic 3′,5′-adenosine monophosphate and cyclic 3′,5′-guanosine monophosphate during and after pregnancy. *J. Clin. Endocrinol. Metabol.*, **44**, 590–4.

Kruithof, E. K., Tran-Thang, C., Gudinchet, A., *et al.* (1987). Fibrinolysis in pregnancy: a study of plasminogen activator inhibitors. *Blood*, **69**, 460–6.

Kublickiene, K. R., Kublickas, M., Lindblom, B., Lunell, N.-O. and Nisell, H. (1997a). A comparsion of myogenic and endothelial properties of myometrial and resistance vessels in late pregnancy. *Am. J. Obstet. Gynecol.*, **176**, 560–6.

Kublickiene, K. R., Cockell, A. P., Nisell, H. and Poston, L. (1997b). Role of nitric oxide in the regulation of vascular tone in pressurised and perfused resistance myometrial arteries from term pregnant women. *Am. J. Obstet. Gynecol.*, **177**, 1263–9.

Kublickiene, K. R., Gruenwald, C., Lindblom, B. and Nisell, H. (1998). Myogenic and endothelial properties of myometrial resistance arteries from women with pre-eclampsia. *Hypertens. Preg.*, **17**, 271–82.

Kuchan, M. J. and Frangos, J. A. (1994). Role of calcium and calmodulin in flow-induced nitric oxide production in endothelial cells. *Am. J. Physiol.*, **266**, C628–36.

Kupfermine, M., Peaceman, A. M., Wigton, T. R., *et al.* (1994). Tumour necrosis factor α is elevated in plasma and amniotic fluid of patients with severe preeclampsia. *Am. J. Obstet. Gynecol.*, **170**, 1752–9.

Learmont, J. G., Cockell, A. P., Knock, G. A. and Poston, L. (1996). Myogenic and flow mediated responses in isolated mesenteric small arteries from pregnant and non-pregnant rats. *Am. J. Obstet. Gynecol.*, **174**, 1631–6.

Leiper, J. and Vallance, P. (1999). Biological significance of endogenous methylarginines that inhibit nitric oxide synthases. *Cardiovasc. Res.*, **43**, 542–8.

Leiper, J. M., Santa Maria, J., Chubb, A., *et al.* (1999). Identification of two human dimethylarginine di-methyl-aminohydrolases with distinct tissue distributions and homology with microbial arginine deiminases. *Biochem. J.*, **343**, 209–14.

Letsky, E. A. (1995). Coagulation defects. In *Medical Disorders in Obstetric Practice*, ed. M. de Swiet. Oxford: Blackwell Scientific, pp. 71–115.

Levine, R. J., Maynard, S. E., Cong, Qian, *et al.* (2004). Circulating angiogenic factors and the risk of pre-eclampsia. *N. Engl. J. Med.*, **350**, 672–83.

Levine, R. J., Chun, Lam, Cong, Qian, *et al.* (2006). Soluble endoglin and other circulating antiangiogenic factors in pre-eclampsia. *N. Engl. J. Med.*, **355**, 992–1005.

Lincoln, J. and Burnstock, G. (1990). Neural–endothelial interactions in control of local blood flow. In *The Endothelium: An Introduction to Current Research*, ed. J. D. Warren. New York: Wiley-Liss, Inc., pp. 21–32.

Luscher, T. F. and Barton, M. (1997). Biology of the endothelium. *Clin. Cardiol.*, **20**, 3–10.

Luscher, T. F. and Vanhoutte, P. M. (1990). *The Endothelium: Modulator of Cardiovascular Function*. Boca Raton, FL: CRC Press.

Lyall, F. and Greer, I. A. (1996). The vascular endothelium in normal pregnancy and pre-eclampsia. *Rev. Reprod.*, **1**, 107–16.

Lyall, F., Greer, I. A., Boswell, F., *et al.* (1994). The cell adhesion molecule VCAM-1, is selectively elevated in serum in pre-eclampsia: does this indicate the mechanism of leucocyte activation? *Br. J. Obstet. Gynaecol.*, **101**, 485–7.

Lyall, F., Greer, I. A., Boswell, F. and Fleming, R. (1997). Suppression of serum vascular endothelial growth factor immunoreactivity in normal pregnancy and in pre-eclampsia. *Br. J. Obstet. Gynaecol.*, **104**, 223–8.

MacRitchie, A. N., Jun, S. S., Chen, Z., *et al.* (1997). Estrogen upregulates endothelial nitric oxide synthase gene expression in fetal pulmonary artery endothelium. *Circ. Res.*, **81**, 355–62.

Magness, R. R., Shaw, C. E., Phernetton, T. M., *et al.* (1997). Endothelial vasodilator production by uterine and systemic arteries. II Pregnancy effects on NO synthase expression. *Am. J. Physiol.*, **272**, H1730–40.

Mahdy, Z., Otun, H. A., Dunlop, W. and Gillespie, J. I. (1998). The responsiveness of isolated human hand vein endothelial cells in normal pregnancy and in pre-eclampsia. *J. Physiol.*, **508**, 609–17.

Mantovani, A. (1997). The interplay between primary and secondary cytokines. Cytokines involved in the regulation of monocyte recruitment. *Drugs*, **54**, 15–23.

Manyonda, I. T., Slater, D. M., Fenske, C., *et al.* (1988). A role for noradrenaline in pre-eclampsia: towards a unifying hypothesis for the pathophysiology. *Br. J. Obstet. Gynaecol.*, **105**, 641–8.

Marx, N., Imhof, A., Froehlich, J., *et al.* (2003). Effect of rosiglitazone treatment on soluble CD40L in patients with type II diabetes and coronary artery disease. *Circulation*, **107**, 1954–7.

Masaki, T. (1989). The discovery, the present state, and future prospects of endothelin. *J. Cardiovasc. Pharmacol.*, **13** (Suppl. 5), S1–4.

Maynard, S. E., Min, J. Y., Merchan, J., *et al.* (2003). Excess placental soluble fms-like tyrosine kinase 1 (sFlt-1) may contribute to endothelial dysfunction, hypertension, and proteinuria in pre-eclampsia. *J. Clin. Investig.*, **111**, 649–58.

McCarthy, A. L., Taylor, P., Graves, J., *et al.* (1994). Endothelium dependent relaxation of human resistance arteries in pregnancy. *Am. J. Obstet. Gynecol.*, **171**, 1309–15.

McDermott, J. R. (1976). Studies on the catabolism of NG-methylarginine, N^G,N^G-dimethylarginine and N^G,N^G-dimethylarginine in the rabbit. *Biochem. J.*, **154**, 179–84.

Mendelsohn, M. E. and Karas, R. H. (1994). Estrogen and the blood vessel wall. *Curr. Opin. Cardiol.*, **9**, 619–26.

Mills, J. L., DerSimonian, R., Raymond, E., *et al.* (1999). Prostacyclin and thromboxane changes predating clinical onset of pre-eclampsia. A multicenter prospective study. *J. Am. Med. Ass.*, **282**, 356–62.

Miyazaki, H., Matsuoka, H., Cooke, J. P., *et al.* (1999). Endogenous nitric oxide synthase inhibitor: a novel marker of atherosclerosis. *Circulation*, **99**, 1141–6.

Molnar, M. and Hertelendy, F. (1995). Signal transduction in rat myometrial cells: comparison of the actions of endothelin-1, oxytocin and prostaglandin F_2 alpha. *Eur. J. Endocrinol.*, **133**, 467–74.

Molnar, M., Suto, T., Toth, T., *et al.* (1994). Prolonged blockade of nitric oxide synthesis in gravid rats produces sustained hypertension, proteinuria, thrombocytopaenia and intrauterine growth retardation. *Am. J. Obstet. Gynecol.*, **170**, 1458–66.

Mombouli, J. V. and Vanhoutte, P. M. (1999). Endothelial dysfunction: from physiology to therapy. *J. Mol. Cell. Cardiol.*, **31**, 61–74.

Moncada, S. (1982). Biological importance of prostacyclin. *Br. J. Pharmacol.*, **76**, 3–31.

Moncada, S. (1992). The L-arginine-nitric oxide pathway. *Acta Physiol. Scand.*, **145**, 201–27.

Moncada, S. and Higgs, E. A. (1993). The L-arginine-nitric oxide pathway. *NJEM*, **329**, 2002–12.

Moncada, S., Gryglewski, R., Bunting, S. and Vane, J. R. (1976). An enzyme isolated from arteries transforms prostaglandin endoperoxides to an unstable substance that inhibits platelet aggregation. *Nature*, **263**, 663–5.

Moncada, S., Herman, A. G., Higgs, E. A. and Vane, J. R. (1977). Differential formation of prostacyclin (PGX or PGI$_2$) by layers of the arterial wall: an explanation for the anti-thrombotic properties of vascular endothelium. *Thromb. Res.*, **11**, 323–44.

Nobunaga, T., Tokugawa, Y., Hashimoto, K., *et al.* (1996). Plasma nitric oxide levels in pregnant patients with preeclampsia and essential hypertension. *Gynecol. Obstet. Investig.*, **41**, 189–93.

Palmer, R. M., Ferrige, A. G. and Moncada, S. (1987). Nitric oxide release accounts for the biological activity of endothelium-derived relaxing factor. *Nature*, **327**, 524–6.

Palmer, R. M., Ashton, D. S. and Moncada, S. (1988). Vascular endothelial cells synthesize nitric oxide from L-arginine. *Nature*, **333**, 664–6.

Pascoal, I. F. and Umans, J. G. (1996). Effect of pregnancy on mechanisms of relaxation in human omental microvessels. *Hypertension*, **28**, 183–7.

Pascoal, I. F., Lindheimer, M. D., Nalbantian-Brandt, C. and Umans, J. G. (1998). Preeclampsia selectively impairs endothelium-dependent relaxation and leads to oscillatory activity in small omental arteries. *J. Clin. Investig.*, **101**, 464–70.

Patrignani, P., Filabozzi, P. and Patrono, C. (1982). Selective cumulative inhibition of platelet thromboxane production by low-dose aspirin in healthy subjects. *J. Clin. Investig.*, **69**, 366–72.

Pedersen, A. K. and FitzGerald, G. A. (1984). Dose related kinetics of aspirin. *N. Engl. J. Med.*, **311**, 1206–11.

Penney, L. L., Frederick, R. J. and Parker, G. W. (1981). 17β-estradiol stimulation of uterine blood flow in oophorectomized rabbits with complete inhibition of uterine ribonucleic acid synthesis. *Endocrinology*, **109**, 1672–6.

Petty, R. G. and Pearson, J. D. (1989). Endothelium – the axis of vascular health and disease. *J. R. Coll. Physicians*, **23**, 92–101.

Phippard, A. F., Horvath, J. S., Glynn, E. M., *et al.* (1986). Circulatory adaptation to pregnancy: serial studies of haemodynamics, blood volume, renin and aldosterone in the baboon. *J. Hypertens.*, **4**, 773–9.

Pober, J. S. and Cotran, R. S. (1990). Cytokines and endothelial cell biology. *Physiol. Rev.*, **70**, 427–51.

Polliotti, B. M., Fry, A. G., Saller, D. N., *et al.* (2003). Second-trimester maternal serum placental growth factor and vascular endothelial growth factor for predicting severe, early-onset pre-eclampsia. *Obstet. Gynecol.*, **101**, 1266–74.

Poston, L., McCarthy, A. L. and Ritter, J. M. (1995). Control of vascular resistance in the maternal and feto-placental arterial beds. *Pharmacol. Ther.*, **65**, 215–39.

Poston, L. and Williams, D. J. (2000). The endothelium in human pregnancy. In *Vascular Endothelium in Human Physiology and Pathophysiology*, eds. P. J. T. Vallance and D. J. Webb. Harwood Academic Publishers, pp. 247–81.

Potter, J. M. and Nestel, P. J. (1979). The hyperlipidaemia of pregnancy in normal and complicated pregnancies. *Am. J. Obstet. Gynecol.*, **133**, 165–70.

Randall, M. D., Alexander, S. P. H., Bennett, T., *et al.* (1996). An endogenous cannabinoid as an endothelium-derived vasorelaxant. *Biochem. Biophys. Res. Commun.*, **229**, 114–20.

Redman, C. W., Sacks, G. P. and Sargent, I. L. (1999). Pre-eclampsia: an excessive maternal inflammatory response to pregnancy. *Am. J. Obstet. Gynecol.*, **180**, 499–506.

Rees, D. D., Palmer, R. M. and Moncada, S. (1989). Role of endothelium-derived nitric oxide in the regulation of blood pressure. *Proc. Natl Acad. Sci. USA*, **86**, 3375–8.

Resnick, N., Yahav, H., Schubert, S., *et al.* (2000). Signalling pathways in vascular endothelium activated by shear stress: relevance to atherosclerosis. *Curr. Opin. Lipidol.*, **11**, 167–77.

Ritter, J. M., Cockcroft, J. R., Doktor, H., *et al.* (1989). Differential effect of aspirin on thromboxane and prostaglandin biosynthesis in man. *Br. J. Clin. Pharm.*, **28**, 573–9.

Roberts, J. M. and Redman, C. W. G. (1993). Pre-eclampsia: more than pregnancy-induced hypertension. *Lancet*, **341**, 1447–51.

Roberts, J. M., Taylor, R. N., Musci, T. J., *et al.* (1989). Preeclampsia: an endothelial cell disorder. *Am. J. Obstet. Gynecol.*, **161**, 1200–4.

Roberts, M., Lindheimer, M. D. and Davison, J. M. (1996). Altered glomerular permselectivity to neutral dextrans and heteroporous membrane modeling in human pregnancy. *Am. J. Physiol.*, **270**, F338–43.

Robinson, L. J., Weremowicz, S., Morton, C. C. and Michel, T. (1994). Isolation and chromosomal localization of the human eNOS gene. *Genomics*, **19**, 350–7.

Robson, S. C., Hunter, S., Boys, R. J. and Dunlop, W. (1989). Serial study of factors influencing changes in cardiac output during human pregnancy. *Am. J. Physiol.*, **256**, H1060–5.

Rogers, G. M., Taylor, R. N. and Roberts, J. M. (1988). Pre-eclampsia is associated with a serum factor cytotoxic to human endothelial cells. *Am. J. Obstet. Gynecol.*, **159**, 908–14.

Russell, K. R., Haynes, M. P., Sinha, D., *et al.* (2000a). Human vascular endothelial cells contain membrane binding sites for estradiol, which mediate rapid intracellular signalling. *Proc. Natl Acad. Sci. USA*, **97**, 5930–5.

Russell, K. S., Haynes, M. P., Caulin-Glaser, T., *et al.* (2000b). Estrogen stimulates heat shock protein 90 binding to endothelial nitric oxide synthase in human vascular endothelial cells. Effects on calcium sensitivity and NO release. *J. Biol. Chem.*, **275**, 5026–30.

Sacks, G. P., Studena, K., Sargent, K., *et al.* (1998). Normal pregnancy and pre-eclampsia both produce inflammatory changes in peripheral blood leukocytes akin to those of sepsis. *Am. J. Obstet. Gynecol.*, **179**, 80–6.

Savvidou, M. D., Hingorani, A. D., Tsikas, D., *et al.* (2003). Endothelial dysfunction and raised plasma concentrations of asymmetric dimethylarginine in pregnant women who subsequently develop pre-eclampsia. *Lancet*, **361**, 1511–17.

Savvidou, M. D., Kametas, N. A., Donald, A. E. and Nicolaides, K. H. (2000). Non-invasive assessment of endothelial function in normal pregnancy. *Ultrasound Obstet. Gynecol.*, **15**, 502–7.

Schafer, K., Muller, K., Hecke, A., *et al.* (2003). Enhanced thrombosis in atherosclerosis-prone mice is associated with increased arterial expression of plasminogen activator inhibitor-1. *Arterioscler. Thromb. Vasc. Biol.*, **23**, 2097–103.

Schneider, F., Lutun, P., Balduf, J. J., *et al.* (1996). Plasma cyclic GMP concentrations and their relationship with changes of blood pressure levels in pre-eclampsia. *Acta Obstet. Gynecol. Scand.*, **75**, 40–4.

Schobel, H. P., Fischer, T., Heuszer, K., Geiger, H. and Schmieder, R. E. (1996). Pre-eclampsia – a state of sympathetic overactivity. *N. Engl. J. Med.*, **335**, 1480–5.

Seligman, S. P., Buyon, J. P., Clancy, R. M., *et al.* (1994). The role of nitric oxide in the pathogenesis of preeclampsia. *Am. J. Obstet. Gynecol.*, **171**, 944–8.

Sladek, S. M., Magness, R. R. and Conrad, K. P. (1997). Nitric oxide and pregnancy. *Am. J. Physiol.*, **272**, R441–63.

Smarason, A. K., Allman, K. G., Young, D. and Redman, C. W. G. (1997). Elevated levels of serum nitrate, a stable end product of nitric oxide, in women with pre-eclampsia. *Br. J. Obstet. Gynaecol.*, **104**, 538–43.

Sorensen, J., Secher, N. J. and Jespersen, J. (1995). Perturbed (procoagulant) endothelium and deviations within the fibrinolytic system during the third trimester of normal pregnancy. *Acta Obstet. Gynecol. Scand.*, **74**, 257–61.

Sudd, S. S., Gupta, I., Dhaliwal, L. K., *et al.* (1999). Serial plasma fibronectin levels in pre-eclamptic and normotensive women. *Int. J. Gynecol. Obstet.*, **66**, 123–8.

Taylor, R. N., Crombleholme, W. R., Friedman, S. A., *et al.* (1991). High plasma cellular fibronectin levels correlate with biochemical and clinical features of pre-eclampsia but cannot be attributed to hypertension alone. *Am. J. Obstet. Gynecol.*, **165**, 895–901.

Taylor, R. N., Grimwood, J., Taylor, R. S., *et al.* (2003). Longitudinal serum concentrations of placental growth factor: evidence for abnormal placental angiogenesis in pathologic pregnancies. *Am. J. Obstet. Gynecol.*, **188**, 177–82.

Tran, C. T., Fox, M. F., Vallance, P., *et al.* (2000). Chromosomal localization, gene structure, and expression pattern of DDAH I: comparison with DDAH II and implications for evolutionary origins. *Genomics*, **68**, 101–5.

Tsatsaris, V., Goffin, F., Munaut, C., *et al.* (2003). Overexpression of the soluble vascular endothelial growth factor in pre-eclamptic patients: pathophysiological consequences. *J. Clin. Endocrinol. Metab.*, **88**, 5555–63.

Vallance, P., Collier, J. and Moncada, S. (1989). Effects of endothelium-derived nitric oxide on peripheral arteriolar tone in man. *Lancet*, **2**, 997–1000.

Vallance, P., Leone, A., Calver, A., Collier, J. and Moncada, S. (1992). Accumulation of an endogenous inhibitor of nitric oxide synthesis in chronic renal failure. *Lancet*, **339**, 572–5.

Vane, J. R. (1983). Clinical potential of prostacyclin. *Adv. Prostaglandin Thromboxane Leukot. Res.*, **11**, 457–61.

Vangoni, K. E., Shaw, C. E., Phernetton, T. M., *et al.* (1998). Endothelial vasodilator production by uterine and systemic arteries. III. Ovarian and estrogen effects on NO synthase. *Am. J. Physiol.*, **275**, H1845–55.

Vaughan, D. E., Lazos, S. A. and Tong, K. (1995). Angiotensin II regulates the expression of plasminogen activator inhibitor-1 in cultured endothelial cells. A potential link between the renin–angiotensin system and thrombosis. *J. Clin. Invest.*, **95**, 995–1001.

Vanhoutte, P. M. and Rimele, T. J. (1983). Role of endothelium in the control of vascular smooth muscle function. *J. Physiol.*, **78**, 681–6.

Vedernikov, Y. P., Belfort, M. A., Saade, G. R. and Mosie, K. J. (1995). Preeclampsia does not alter the response to endothelin-1 in human omental artery. *J. Cardiovasc. Pharmacol.*, **3**, S233–5.

Wang, Z. Q., Millatt, L. J., Heiderstadt, N. T., *et al.* (1999). Differential regulation of renal angiotensin subtype AT_{1A} and A_{T2} receptor protein in rats with angiotensin-dependent hypertension. *Hypertension*, **33**, 96–101.

Weiner, C., Lizasoain, I., Baylis, S. A., *et al.* (1994a). Induction of calcium dependent nitric oxide synthases by sex hormones. *Proc. Natl Acad. Sci. USA*, **91**, 5212–16.

Weiner, C. P., Knowles, R. G. and Moncada, S. (1994b). Induction of nitric oxide synthases early in pregnancy. *Am. J. Obstet. Gynecol.*, **171**, 838–43.

Williams, D. J. (2003). Physiological changes of normal pregnancy. In *Oxford Textbook of Medicine* (fourth edition), eds. D. A. Warrell, T. M. Cox, J. D. Firth and E. J. Benz. Oxford: Oxford University Press, chapter, 13.1, pp. 383–5.

Williams, D. J., Vallance, P. J., Neild, G. H., *et al.* (1997). Nitric oxide mediated vasodilatation in human pregnancy. *Am. J. Physiol.*, **272**, H748–52.

Williams, M. A., Farrand, A., Mittendorf, R., *et al.* (1999). Maternal second trimester serum tumour necrosis factor-alpha-soluble receptor p55 (sTNFp55) and subsequent risk of pre-eclampsia. *Am. J. Epidemiol.*, **149**, 323–9.

Wolff, K., Nisell, H., Modin, A., *et al.* (1993). Contractile effects of endothelin 1 and endothelin 3 on myometrium and small intramyometrial arteries of pregnant women at term. *Gynecol. Obstet. Investig.*, **36**, 166–71.

Wolff, K., Kublickiene, K. R., Kublickas, M., *et al.* (1996a). Effects of endothelin-1 and the ET_A receptor antagonist BQ-123 on resistance arteries from normal pregnant and pre-eclamptic women. *Acta Obstet. Gynecol. Scand.*, **75**, 432–8.

Wolff, K., Nisell, H., Carlstom, K., *et al.* (1996b). Endothelin-1 and big endothelin-1 levels in normal term pregnancy and in preeclampsia. *Regul. Peptides*, **67**, 211–16.

Wolff, K., Carlstom, K., Fyhrquist, F., *et al.* (1997). Plasma endothelin in normal and diabetic pregnancy. *Diabetes Care*, **20**, 653–6.

Xu, D., Martin, P., St John, J., *et al.* (1996). Upregulation of endothelial and constitutive nitric oxide synthase in pregnant rats. *Am. J. Physiol.*, **271**, R1739–45.

Xu, H., Gonzalo, J. A., St Pierre, Y., *et al.* (1994). Leukocytosis and resistance to septic shock in intercellular adhesion molecule-1 deficient mice. *J. Exp. Med.*, **180**, 95–109.

Yallampalli, C. and Garfield, R. E. (1993). Inhibition of nitric oxide synthesis in rats during pregnancy produces signs similar to those of pre-eclampsia. *Am. J. Obstet. Gynecol.*, **169**, 1316–20.

Yang, J. C., Haworth, L., Sherry, R. M., *et al.* (2003). A randomised trial of bevacizumab, an antivascular endothelial growth factor antibody, for metastatic renal cancer. *N. Engl. J. Med.*, **349**, 427–34.

Yang, S., Bae, L. and Zhang, L. (2000). Estrogen increases eNOS and Nox release in human coronary artery endothelium. *J. Cardiovasc. Pharmacol.*, **36**, 242–7.

Yoshimura, T., Yoshimura, M., Tabata, A., *et al.* (2000). Association of the missense Glu298Asp variant of the endothelial nitric oxide synthase gene with severe preeclampsia. *J. Soc. Gynecol. Investig.*, **7**, 238–41.

Zemel, M. B., Zemel, P. C., Berry, S., *et al.* (1990). Altered platelet calcium metabolism as an early predictor of increased peripheral vascular resistance and pre-eclampsia in urban black women. *N. Engl. J. Med.*, **323**, 434–8.

Zhou, Y., McMater, M., Woo, K., *et al.* (2002). Vascular endothelial growth factor ligands and receptors that regulate human cytotrophoblast survival are dysregulated in severe pre-eclampsia and haemolysis, elevated liver enzymes, and low platelet syndrome. *Am. J. Path.*, **160**, 1405–23.

5

The renin–angiotensin system in pre-eclampsia

Fiona Broughton Pipkin

Angiotensin II (AngII) has suffered from being a hormone with a long history. Like an aging film star, it has tended to be overlooked. The renin–angiotensin system (RAS) was among the first hormone systems to be studied when Tigerstedt and Bergman described how intravenously injected saline extracts of kidney caused pronounced hypertension in rabbits (Tigerstedt and Bergman, 1898), and it is as a vasoconstrictor system that the RAS has largely been regarded ever since. This is, however, only one aspect of the chameleon-like RAS. AngII has autocrine and paracrine effects, as well as effects as a classic circulating hormone. Furthermore, fragments of angiotensin can have widely differing actions, and can work through receptors other than the well-described types 1 and 2. This chapter will consider the circulating RAS in pre-eclampsia as well as its effects as a paracrine system in relation to cell proliferation, differentiation and apoptosis, interaction with other cytokines, vascular media hypertrophy, endothelial dysfunction and athero-thrombosis. Many of these have not yet been studied in relation to pre-eclampsia, but the parallels with non-pregnant hypertension suggest strongly that they should be.

Synthesis

The enzyme renin, an aspartyl protease, has only one substrate, the α_2-globulin angiotensinogen (Aogen) (Poulsen and Jacobsen, 1993). The converse, however, is not true. Aogen acts as a substrate for a number of other enzymes, among them cathepsins D and G, tonin and tissue plasminogen activator (Dzau *et al.*, 1988; Klickstein *et al.*, 1982), all of which can cleave it, some apparently resulting in the direct synthesis of AngII without the intervening production of angiotensin I (AngI). AngI is acted upon by tissue- and plasma-converting enzymes to produce AngII, which in turn acts as a precursor for a number of biologically active angiotensin fragments (Figure 5.1). Angiotensin 2–8 (AngIII) is nearly as biologically active as AngII. Angiotensin 1–7 can also be synthesized directly from AngI (Figure 5.1). Aogen is known to be rate-limiting in normal pregnancy (Skinner *et al.*, 1972), although it is not usually so outside pregnancy.

Classically, these reactions are thought of as occurring in the plasma. However, it has been known for at least 20 years that there is a number of autonomous tissue RAS, within which all or most of the components of the cascade are synthesized. Since there is increasing evidence that inadequate placentation is a primary pathogenic factor in pre-eclampsia, this chapter will consider the utero-placental RAS in some detail.

Receptors

One of the fascinating features of AngII is that its function depends on which of its two receptors it is acting on. In most adult tissues, the type 1 receptor (AT1R) predominates. When AngII binds to the AT1Rs, it is a vasoconstrictor, but when either

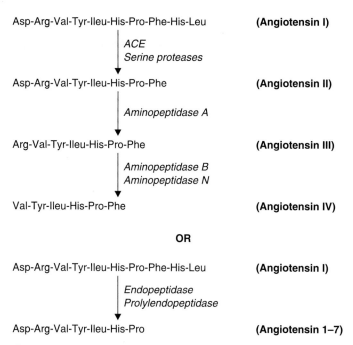

Asp-Arg-Val-Tyr-Ileu-His-Pro-Phe-His-Leu   **(Angiotensin I)**

| *ACE*
| *Serine proteases*
▼

Asp-Arg-Val-Tyr-Ileu-His-Pro-Phe   **(Angiotensin II)**

| *Aminopeptidase A*
▼

Arg-Val-Tyr-Ileu-His-Pro-Phe   **(Angiotensin III)**

| *Aminopeptidase B*
| *Aminopeptidase N*
▼

Val-Tyr-Ileu-His-Pro-Phe   **(Angiotensin IV)**

OR

Asp-Arg-Val-Tyr-Ileu-His-Pro-Phe-His-Leu   **(Angiotensin I)**

| *Endopeptidase*
| *Prolylendopeptidase*
▼

Asp-Arg-Val-Tyr-Ileu-His-Pro   **(Angiotensin 1–7)**

Figure 5.1 Pathways for the synthesis of the physiologically active angiotensins.

the AT1Rs are down-regulated either physiologically (pregnancy) or pharmacologically (AT1R blockers such as losartan), or the type 2 receptors (AT2Rs) are up-regulated (fetal life) then it can be a vasodilator. This capacity to exert opposing actions depending on the predominant receptor, as well as whether endogenous concentrations are low or high, is true for a number of AngII's actions (see below). The AT1R and AT2R are the best-characterized angiotensin receptors (de Gasparo *et al.*, 2000). These are 7-transmembrane receptors, with only a 30% sequence homology, specified on different chromosomes (3q21–q25 and Xq24–q25). The AT1Rs are G-protein coupled receptors; the third intracellular loop and the C-tail are important in regulating binding specificity. Their second messenger system involves G_q-mediated activation of phospholipase C followed by phosphoinositide hydrolysis and Ca^{2+} signaling. They also induce tyrosine phosphorylation of such effectors as JAK2, STATs, paxillin and MAPK and early response genes such

as c-*fos*, c-*jun*, and c-*myc*, effects also associated with growth factors (de Gasparo *et al.*, 2000). The AT1Rs mediate most of the "classic" effects of the RAS, for both AngII and AngIII.

It has been suggested that the AT2R is not a single entity, since its characteristics seem to vary depending on its cell type of origin. This, however, remains speculation. Activation of the AT2R blocks the MAPKs ERK1 and ERK2 by the activation of phosphotyrosine phosphatases via a G_1 or G_0 protein (de Gasparo *et al.*, 2000).

Angiotensin 1–7 and angiotensin 3–8 (AngIV) only bind weakly to the AT1 receptors. The *Mas* proto-oncogene encodes a protein with seven hydrophobic transmembrane domains, considered to be an "orphan" G protein-coupled receptor. It has recently been shown to bind angiotensin 1–7, and may be the receptor for this fragment (Santos *et al.*, 2003).

The receptor for AngIV is now known to be insulin-regulated aminopeptidase (IRAP), synthesized from a single gene on chromosome 5q14.2–q15 (Horio *et al.*, 1999). The human placenta expresses a high density of IRAP on the syncytiotrophoblast (Yamahara *et al.*, 2000). The extracellular domain of the receptor can be shed, and this occurs particularly in the second half of human pregnancy (Yamahara *et al.*, 2000). The second messenger systems for this receptor are still being investigated, but since binding of AngIV is insensitive to guanine nucleotides, the ATR4 may not be G-protein-linked.

Angiotensinases in normal and pre-eclamptic pregnancy

Angiotensin-converting enzyme (ACE) is a specialized angiotensinase. Concentrations of circulating ACE fall in the first half of normotensive human pregnancy, and then rise significantly over the third trimester towards non-pregnant levels (Oats *et al.*, 1981). In pre-eclamptic pregnancy, levels remain low in the third trimester (Rasmussen *et al.*, 1983). Plasma ACE is of endothelial origin, and these depressed concentrations may relate to the generalized endothelial dysfunction of pre-eclampsia. It is, however, usually assumed that [ACE] is not rate-limiting in the generation of AngII. There is a functional polymorphism in the ACE gene, the Insertion/Deletion (I/D) polymorphism, DD homozygotes having circulating [ACE] some 40% higher than the II homozygotes (Rigat *et al.*, 1990). Although this has been strongly associated with non-pregnant heart disease in a number of studies, studies in relation to pre-eclampsia have failed to show any association (Heiskanen *et al.*, 2001; Morgan *et al.*, 1999b).

Syncytial microvilli from human pregnancies have high concentrations of aminopeptidase A (angiotensinase A), which converts AngII to AngIII (Figure 5.1; Ino *et al.*, 2003; Johnson *et al.*, 1984). This is present from the first trimester. A series of papers from Mizutani's group suggests that the increased angiotensinase activity in normal pregnancy may contribute to the decreased pressor response to AngII (see Mizutani and Tomoda, 1996). In a prospective study, it was reported that aminopeptidase A was significantly raised prior to the onset of pre-eclampsia, but fell thereafter (Mizutani and Tomoda, 1996). Increasing villous trophoblastic aminopeptidase A has also been reported with increasing severity of pregnancy hypertension and pre-eclampsia (Mizutani and Tomoda, 1996; Neudeck *et al.*, 1996). Raised trophoblastic [aminopeptidase A] may be an initial homeostatic response protecting the placenta from the potentially deleterious effects of high concentrations of locally generated AngII. AngII is known to be a very potent vasoconstrictor in human villous stem arterioles (Tulenko, 1979), with a lower EC_{50} than 5-HT, prostaglandin $F_{2\alpha}$ or prostaglandin E_2 (Allen *et al.*, 1989). The sensitivity of villous stem arterioles in vitro to AngII does not differ between normotensive and pre-eclampsia pregnancy (Allen *et al.*, 1989). Interestingly, maternal omental (systemic) resistance arteries from women with pre-eclampsia do show significantly greater responsiveness to AngII (Aalkjaer *et al.*, 1984), paralleling the pressor responsiveness (see below). Further indirect support for the suggestion of an initially protective role for aminopeptidase A comes from the observation that while uterine venous [AngII] is lower than simultaneously measured peripheral venous AngII at elective Cesarean section in normal pregnancy, the converse is found in hypertensive pregnancy (Broughton Pipkin *et al.*, 1981).

The neutral endopeptidase 24.11 (neprilysin) is one of the enzymes capable of converting AngI and AngII to angiotensin (1–7). It is highly expressed on the cell surface of trophoblasts, particularly in the first trimester (Kikkawa *et al.*, 2002). Immunohistochemically, there is intense staining for the metallo-endopeptidase on extra-villous trophoblast, which is further enhanced in pre-eclampsia, when it is also present in the cytoplasm of the villous-associated trophoblast (Li *et al.*, 1995).

Angiotensin fragments

On a molecule-for-molecule basis, AngII is the most potent circulating vasoconstrictor yet described. The circulating concentrations of the angiotensins are normally very low ($\sim$8 pmol l^{-1} for AngII), and yet so potent is AngII as a vasoconstrictor that this concentration is only just below levels capable of increasing the blood pressure. High-performance liquid chromatography shows that in the venous plasma of normal male subjects, AngI is present at about twice the concentration of AngII, while AngIII is present at about one-tenth, and AngIV at about 7% of the concentration of AngII (Campbell and Kladis, 1990). In normal third-trimester pregnancy, circulating concentrations of AngII double but concentrations of AngIII and AngIV appear not to increase pro rata (Hanssens et al., 1991b). However, tissue concentrations of the peptides have not been measured in pregnancy, and local generation could result in differential increases in angiotensin fragments. This seems particularly likely in pregnancy, given the high capacity of human chorio-decidua and placenta to synthesize and release AngI into culture medium (Craven et al., 1983).

Angiotensin (1–7)

Both the cardiovascular and renal effects of angiotensin (1–7) oppose those of AngII (Cesari et al., 2002). It seems likely that it is locally generated, and acts locally, with a half-life as short as that of nitric oxide (NO). In animal experiments it is vasodilator, natriuretic and diuretic, these effects being particularly pronounced when the RAS is activated (Ferrario, 2002). Pregnancy is, of course, such a state. Angiotensin (1–7) acts at least in part by stimulating the release of NO (Li et al., 1997) prostacyclin (PGI2) and endothelium-derived hyperpolarizing factor (EDMF) (Ferrario et al., 1997).

Since the placenta is a rich source of the endopeptidase which converts AngI and AngII to angiotensin (1–7) (see above), one might expect concentrations to rise in pregnancy. Both plasma (Merrill et al., 2002) and urinary angiotensin (1–7) (Valdes et al., 2001) indeed do show similar patterns of increase to that of AngII in normal pregnancy. Maternal plasma concentrations have been reported to be lower in women with pre-eclampsia (Merrill et al., 2002). However, the further increased expression of neutral endopeptidase in placentae in pre-eclampsia (Li et al., 1995) suggests the possibility of greater local generation, perhaps counterbalancing the effects of endothelial damage. Several studies have suggested a similar possible role for NO in pre-eclampsia.

Angiotensin III (AIII)

Like AngII, AngIII is a pressor agent which can also stimulate vasopressin release and drinking (Ardaillou and Chansel, 1997). However, it is thought mainly to exert these effects in the central nervous system, and will not be further discussed here.

Angiotensin IV (AngIV)

Much of the current research on the role of AngIV centers on its capacity to promote learning in rodents. However, the recent identification of its receptor as being insulin-regulated aminopeptidase (IRAP; Albiston et al., 2001), which is widespread in the placenta, raises intriguing hypotheses. For example, AngIV functions as an endogenous inhibitor of ACE (Fruitier-Arnaudin et al., 2002). In vitro, it stimulates both DNA and RNA synthesis and cellular proliferation in endothelial cells. The expression of the AT4R more than doubles in rabbit carotid artery following balloon injury, and its mitogenic properties suggest that it could be involved in vascular remodeling after injury (Moeller et al., 1999). Another property of AngIV is that it can increase the expression of plasminogen activator inhibitor-1 (PAI-1) mRNA and protein expression in endothelial cells (Kerins et al., 1995).

It is also a vasodilator, at least in the cerebral vessels. These properties suggest that the local generation of AngIV in the placenta via aminopeptidase N could be involved in the local control of apoptosis and remodeling.

The circulating RAS in pre-eclampsia – early and late roles?

Normal pregnancy is a state of activation of the RAS, which is one of the earliest systems to recognize pregnancy. There is activation of the circulating system in the luteal phase of every ovulatory menstrual cycle and, should conception occur, this activation is maintained and rapidly amplified. It is thought that the activation is initially a response to the increased [progesterone], which is natriuretic, but it may also be a response to the perceived "underfilling" of the circulation in very early pregnancy (Chapman et al., 1998). This is sensed at the macula densa and renin synthesis and release from the juxtaglomerular apparatus is stimulated. At the same time, increasing [estrogen], acting at the promoter region of the Aogen gene, stimulates the synthesis of angiotensinogen. Plasma [AngII] rises, and in turn stimulates aldosterone synthesis and release from the zona glomerulosa (Chapman et al., 1998). The pregnant woman is protected from the potential pressor effects of the raised circulating concentrations of AngII by a specific diminution in pressor response to AngII, via down-regulation of the AT1Rs (Baker et al., 1992), while adrenal cortical responsiveness is maintained (both AT1Rs and AT2Rs are present). This general picture has been known for more than a generation. For reviews of early studies, see Broughton Pipkin (1993) and Skinner (1993).

There is good evidence that in established pre-eclampsia, the circulating RAS is suppressed. A lower plasma total renin concentration was first noted almost 40 years ago (Brown et al., 1964b), an observation which has since been confirmed repeatedly, and extended to plasma active renin

and plasma renin activity (PRA). Interestingly, a recent report including further confirmation of suppressed PRA in established pre-eclampsia found no such suppression in women with HELLP (hemolysis, elevated liver enzymes and low platelets) (Bussen et al., 1998). Aogen is usually only measured in research laboratories. It exists in two forms in pregnancy, one being a high-molecular weight (HMW Aogen) form. This HMW Aogen can be detected early in the first trimester and about half of the women who develop pre-eclampsia have significantly raised HMW Aogen (Tewksbury et al., 2001). The pattern of increase is, however, very variable.

We have previously reported, in a series of just under 200 patients, that maternal plasma [Aogen] at the time of the booking visit (~18 weeks gestation) is significantly inversely associated with the subsequent birthweight of the baby, both raw and corrected for gestation age at delivery and maternal build and parity (Broughton Pipkin et al., 1995) and with the baby's head circumference at birth ($p < 0.05$). When one considers the number of parameters which might have impinged on the birthweight some 20 weeks later, the implication has to be that Aogen is an early determinant of fetal growth. The number of women who developed pre-eclampsia in this prospective study is too small to allow subgroup analysis.

However, a number of papers have reported that when patients who had developed de novo pregnancy-induced hypertension without significant proteinuria were studied, no significant depression in PRA was found (Gallery et al., 1980; Kaaja et al., 1999; Symonds and Andersen, 1974). Indeed, there is some evidence from small-scale prospective studies that PRA may be increased in the second trimester in women who go on to develop pre-eclampsia, only later being suppressed (Gordon et al., 1969, 1973). Furthermore, a group of women who developed pregnancy-induced hypertension very early (~24 weeks gestation) had significantly raised PRA at this time (Ruilope et al., 1984). The measurement of AngII is less often undertaken, but the same picture emerges, of a normal or even raised plasma [AngII] in women with non-proteinuric pregnancy hypertension (Hayashi *et al.*, 1977; Symonds *et al.*, 1975), but indubitably suppressed levels in pre-eclampsia (Hanssens *et al.*, 1991a). This suggests the possibility that the fall in [renin] is a late homeostatic response to hypertension evoked through other mechanisms.

The pressor response to AngII is well known to be enhanced before pre-eclampsia is clinically detectable and is associated with an increased density of AngII binding sites having the characteristics of AT1Rs (Morgan *et al.*, 1997a). Similar increases in AT1R expression have also been found on syncytiotrophoblasts from pre-eclamptic placentae.

Given the very early activation of the RAS in pregnancy, and the known long-term effects of subpressor infusion of AngII on vascular structure (Lever, 1993), it is tempting to propose an hypothesis. If, for some reason, perhaps genetically determined or related to a relatively hypoxic implantation site, there is early increased activation of the RAS in pregnancy, either locally in the placenta or in the maternal systemic circulation, then subtle structural changes in the vasculature could occur, with an increased tendency to hypertension later in gestation when absolute fetal demands increase. The RAS could then be suppressed by the normal baroreflex reduction in renal renin release.

The utero-placental RAS

This was the first extra-renal RAS to be characterized. The existence of "big" renin (prorenin) was identified by serendipity, in human amniotic fluid, nearly 40 years ago (Brown *et al.*, 1964a) and the ability of cultured human chorion to synthesize renin was described soon after (Symonds *et al.*, 1968). A particular curiosity of the utero-placental RAS is the very considerable between-species variability, which means that it is particularly unsafe to extrapolate across species.

All components of the RAS are present in human endometrium and decidua (Hagemann, 1994) and endometrial renin. Aogen and ATRs vary cyclically in the non-pregnant woman (Johnson, 1980; Li and Ahmed, 1996). AT2Rs predominate in the non-pregnant endometrium (Ahmed *et al.*, 1995). mRNA for renin, Aogen, ACE and AT1R has been identified in human decidua from as early as 5 weeks gestation (Morgan *et al.*, 1997b, 1998). Renin and Aogen have been localized histochemically round the unremodeled spiral arteries, while AT1R is mainly found in decidual perivascular stromal cells, with only a faint signal from spiral artery smooth muscle cells. This suggests strongly that locally generated AngII may be involved in the spiral artery remodeling central to successful placentation. AT2Rs have not been reported in pregnant human endometrium or decidua, but are known to be markedly down-regulated in pregnant human myometrium (Bing *et al.*, 1996; de Gasparo *et al.*, 2000).

In the placenta itself, conflicting results have been reported for the expression of mRNA and protein for the components of the RAS in pre-eclampsia. A study of nulliparous African-American women with pre-eclampsia (Sowers *et al.*, 1993) reported somewhat higher active and inactive renin concentration and renin mRNA (blot hybridization) in placental homogenates than in controls, while Aogen mRNA and tissue concentration did not differ. However, more recently, using the more sensitive RT-PCR, mRNA and protein expression of AT1Rs and mRNA for Aogen were shown to be more than doubled in established pre-eclampsia in Chinese women (Leung *et al.*, 2001). Another study, using micro-dissection to identify the specific tissue source of placental renin expression, reported the level of renin gene expression in the basal decidua and chorionic villi of PE and control placentae to be the same, although, curiously, expression in the decidua vera was some threefold higher in pre-eclamptic placentae (Shah *et al.*, 2000). Studies using in vitro autoradiography identified a lower capacity and affinity of AngII binding sites identified as

AT1Rs in placental villous blood vessels in PE (Knock *et al.*, 1994). However, using RT-PCR and Western blotting, mRNA and protein expression of AT1Rs were shown to be more than doubled in established pre-eclampsia in Chinese women (Leung *et al.*, 2001). These authors noted that enhanced immunoreactivity for AT1Rs was localized in the syncytiotrophoblast of the placental villi from pre-eclamptic placentae. The differences in approach may account for the reported differences.

The macrophage RAS

Macrophages are mobile RAS factories. They are known to contain mRNA for prorenin, ACE and the AT1R (Jikihara *et al.*, 1995; Keidar *et al.*, 2002; Viinikainen, 2002). The possible implications in relation to pathogenesis of pre-eclampsia are discussed below.

Some less well-known local functions of AngII

AngII, vascular permeability and angiogenesis

One of the prerequisites for successful placentation involves an increase in vascular permeability, allowing tissue growth and remodeling and angiogenesis. Vascular endothelial growth factor (VEGF-A; originally known as vascular permeability factor) is an endothelial cell mitogen which promotes localized vascular permeability and angiogenesis and is believed to be integral in placentation. VEGF synthesis can be induced in vascular smooth muscle cells by either hypoxic or hormonal stimuli such as AngII (Richard *et al.*, 2000; Williams *et al.*, 1995). AngII can induce up to fourfold increases in vascular endothelial cell VEGF mRNA via the AT1Rs (Williams *et al.*, 1995). It can also induce angiogenic activity through a several-fold increase of the VEGF receptor KDR/Flk-1. Hypoxia-inducible factor (HIF-1)

induces transcriptional upregulation of the VEGF gene. The HIF-1α subunit can also be induced by non-hypoxic stimuli, including AngII (Otani *et al.*, 1998; Page *et al.*, 2002). AngII in this context acts via two mechanisms: a protein kinase C (PKC)-mediated effect on transcription and a reactive oxygen species (ROS)-dependent increase in HIF-1 α protein expression.

VEGF stimulates endothelial cell migration and tube formation, both of which play an important role in the process of angiogenesis. As noted above, stimulation of the AT2Rs is antiangiogenic. AngII has been variously reported to stimulate or inhibit human vascular endothelial cell migration. The reported differences may well relate to whether the tissue from which the test cells were isolated expresses predominantly AT1R or AT2Rs. For example, in retinal microvascular pericytes, AngII stimulated migration via AT1Rs (Nadal *et al.*, 2002). However, in human coronary artery endothelial cells, AngII was associated with inhibition of migration, mediated via the AT2Rs (Benndorf *et al.*, 2003). This was related to inhibition of the VEGF-mediated phosphorylation of endothelial NO synthase (eNOS).

AngII also stimulates expression of angiopoietin 2 (Ang-2) mRNA, through the protein kinase C and mitogen-activated protein kinase pathways (Otani *et al.*, 2001). Ang-2 is the ligand for the Tie-2 receptor. It has been suggested that Ang-2 may be either pro- or antiangiogenic depending on whether endogenous VEGF-A is present. When it is, Ang-2 promotes a rapid increase in capillary diameter, remodeling of the basal lamina, proliferation and migration of endothelial cells, and stimulates sprouting of new blood vessels in an angiogenic model in the eye. However, if the activity of endogenous VEGF is inhibited, Ang-2 promotes endothelial cell death and vessel regression (Lobov *et al.*, 2002).

Some 97% of the Aogen molecule gives the impression of simply acting as a "carrier" for the decapeptide angiotensin I. However, both the native Aogen and the [des Asp[1]] Aogen have recently been shown to inhibit angiogenesis both in vivo and in vitro (Celerier et al., 2002), as do other serpins. The effects of the RAS on angiogenesis might therefore depend not only on the ratio of expression of AT1R/AT2Rs, but also on whether Aogen is locally synthesized. The presence of mRNA for Aogen in human placenta from the first trimester has been shown by several groups (Cooper et al., 1999; Morgan et al., 1998). In decidua, Aogen expression and transcription is localized to the spiral arteries (Morgan et al., 1998), suggesting that a local generation of AngII is indeed involved in angiogenesis.

The genetics of the RAS in pre-eclampsia

The M235T polymorphism is a common polymorphism of the Aogen gene. Although there are considerable population differences in allele frequency, a recent meta-analysis of 45,267 non-pregnant patients showed a stepwise increase in both plasma [Aogen] and in the odds ratio for hypertension with increasing dosage of the T allele (Sethi et al., 2003). In the first published study of pre-eclamptic patients (Ward et al., 1993), the variant M235T was found in significantly increased frequency in 45 pre-eclamptic women, in association with a raised plasma angiotensinogen concentration. However, later studies in different populations have shown discrepant results. For example, while a similar association between the 235T allele and pre-eclampsia was reported in one Japanese population (Kobashi et al., 2001), it was not in another (Suzuki et al., 1999). Nor has it been confirmed in a different population in the USA (Bashford et al., 2001) or in Australian, Chinese or UK populations (Guo et al., 1997; Morgan et al., 1999a; Suzuki et al., 1999). Published T allele frequencies range between 0.36 and 0.91 in non-pregnant populations so that the possibility of differing interactions with other genes or the environment must exist.

However, in pre-eclamptic pregnancies, 11/14 mothers heterozygous for the dinucleotide repeat allele designated A9 in the Aogen gene transmitted this allele to the fetus, more frequently than would be expected by chance ($p = 0.02$; Morgan et al., 1999a). In our normal pregnant population, the A9 allele is associated with significantly low [Aogen] and high [renin].

The T allele is in tight linkage disequilibrium with a functional mutation in the promoter region (Inoue et al., 1997), promoting increased protein synthesis. Studies of first trimester decidua suggest that tissues from TT women have less effective remodeling of the spiral arteries (Morgan et al., 1999c) and that 235T expression is increased in the vessel wall (Morgan et al., 1997b).

We have subsequently reported that in our population, plasma angiotensinogen concentrations are actually lower in pregnant normotensive TT homozygotes (Morgan et al., 1999a). There is evidence of variation in the frequency of several diallelic mutations of the angiotensinogen gene even between populations described as "Caucasian" (Morgan et al., 1996), suggesting the possibility of cryptic ethnic differences, and marked variability between Asian, African and Caucasian populations.

The substitution of threonine for methionine is not known to have any functional effects, although there might be an effect on three-dimensional structure. However, another mutation has been reported in one pre-eclamptic patient, which results in the replacement of leucine by phenylalanine at position 10 of angiotensinogen (the LF10 mutation). Since this is the cleavage site for renin, it might be expected that some alterations in kinetics would occur, and a tenfold decrease in Km and a doubling in catalytic efficiency was reported (Inoue et al., 1997). However, a more recent study of 32 women of various ethnic groups with well-defined pre-eclampsia reported no instance of the LF10 mutation (Curnow et al., 2000).

The renin gene has been much studied with respect to non-pregnant essential hypertension in co-segregation studies. However, so far no mutation has been associated with a functionally significant phenotypic alteration. A small linkage analysis study of nine families in Iceland, presenting with pre-eclampsia in two or three generations, provided no evidence for any involvement of the renin gene in this disease either (Arngrimsson et al., 1994).

The impact of the angiotensin converting enzyme (ACE) insertion : deletion polymorphism on circulating [ACE] was mentioned above. However, a small-scale study of this polymorphism in pregnant African-American women failed to reveal any association with the development of pregnancy-induced hypertension (Tamura et al., 1996). More recent association studies of 66 British (Morgan et al., 1999b) and 133 Finnish women (Heiskanen et al., 2001) with carefully defined pre-eclampsia have also failed to demonstrate any association.

A study investigating possible linkage between AT1R genotype and the development of PE found no evidence that the three best-known polymorphisms in the gene were associated with pre-eclampsia (Morgan et al., 1997a). However, there is a dinucleotide repeat polymorphism in the 3′ flanking region of the AT_1 receptor gene, and a marked distortion of maternal–fetal transmission of one of these alleles was shown in pre-eclampsia (Morgan et al., 1997a). Mothers heterozygous for the dinucleotide repeat allele designated A4 transmitted this allele to the fetus in 15/18 informative pre-eclamptic pregnancies, but only 8/26 normotensive pregnancies. This allele is in partial linkage disequilibrium with the C573T variant, which in normotensive pregnancy is associated with higher levels of platelet AT_1 receptors (Morgan et al., 1997a). Polymorphisms in the AT2R seem not to have been studied yet in relation to pre-eclampsia.

Conclusion

One of the most fascinating series of papers linking the RAS to pre-eclampsia has recently come from Luft's group in Berlin. In 1999 they demonstrated the existence of circulating stimulatory autoantibodies to the second extracellular loop of the AT1R in all pre-eclamptic patients studied (Wallukat et al., 1999) an observation subsequently confirmed by others (Xia et al., 2003). Such autoantibodies have also been found in a proportion of patients with non-pregnant hypertension (Fu et al., 2000). These autoantibodies can stimulate the AT1Rs on vascular smooth muscle to activate tissue factor (Dechend et al., 2000). This could contribute to the activation of the coagulation cascade. Furthermore, activation of the AT1Rs by purified autoantibodies resulted in increased PAI-1 expression, but lesser trophoblast invasiveness (Matrigel invasion assay) (Xia et al., 2003), in agreement with data obtained after activation of AT1Rs by AngII (Xia et al., 2002). We have preliminary data to suggest that AngII does stimulate invasiveness of human trophoblast cells in vitro (Lash and Broughton Pipkin, unpublished data). Since expression of both mRNA and protein for AT1Rs are approximately doubled in syncytiotrophoblasts from pre-eclamptic placentae (Leung et al., 2001), the possibility that invasiveness has been impaired by such a mechanism can at least be considered. However, tissues from third trimester pregnancies are many weeks removed from those involved in early placentation, and could be showing adaptive or secondary, rather than causal, changes.

The AT1R autoantibodies from pre-eclamptic women have also been shown to stimulate reactive oxygen species (ROS) and NADPH oxidase (Dechend et al., 2003). AngII is known to stimulate an increase in several membrane components of NADPH oxidase, leading to increased activity of the oxidase (Hanna et al., 2002). Reactive oxygen species act as intracellular second messengers in the activation of such downstream signaling molecules as mitogen-activated protein kinase, protein tyrosine phosphatases, protein tyrosine kinases and transcription factors. This can lead to growth, proliferation and migration of vascular smooth muscle cells, expression of pro-inflammatory mediators and modification of extracellular matrix. The inactivation of NO could then lead to decreased endothelium-dependent vasodilatation, a clotting tendency, cellular infiltration and inflammatory reaction. It has been suggested that the now well-documented interactions between AngII and NO particularly affect the capacity of the vascular endothelium to adapt to dyslipidemia, and may exacerbate atherogenesis. AngII can stimulate macrophages, platelet aggregation and plasminogen activator inhibitor 1 synthesis, as well as its other actions noted above. These aspects of AngII's less well-known functions have been reviewed recently (de Gasparo, 2002; Strawn and Ferrario, 2002).

Put all these features together, and a picture emerges of a pluripotent molecule, capable of acting from the very earliest pregnancy as an autocrine or paracrine agent, capable of affecting implantation and placentation and moving through to its classical actions in late pregnancy as a circulating hormone. If the analogy with the ''slow pressor response'' to AngII is valid, then its role in pre-eclampsia may well lie in very early pregnancy, long before pre-eclampsia can be diagnosed.

REFERENCES

Aalkjaer, C., Johannesen, P., Pedersen, E. B., Rasmussen, A. and Mulvany, M. J. (1984). Morphology and angiotensin II responsiveness of isolated resistance vessels from patients with pre-eclampsia. *Scand. J. Clin. Lab. Invest.*, **169**(Suppl.), 57–60.

Ahmed, A., Li, X. F., Shams, M., *et al.* (1995). Localization of the angiotensin II and its receptor subtype expression in human endometrium and identification of a novel high-affinity angiotensin II binding site. *J. Clin. Invest.*, **96**, 848–57.

Albiston, A. L., McDowall, S. G., Matsacos, D., *et al.* (2001). Evidence that the angiotensin IV (AT4) receptor is the enzyme insulin-regulated aminopeptidase. *J. Biol. Chem.*, **276**, 48,623–6.

Allen, J., Forman, A., Maigaard, S., Jespersen, L. T. and Andersson, K. E. (1989). Effect of endogenous vasoconstrictors on maternal intramyometrial and fetal stem villous arteries in pre-eclampsia. *J. Hypertens.*, **7**, 529–36.

Ardaillou, R. and Chansel, D. (1997). Synthesis and effects of active fragments of angiotensin II. *Kidney Int.*, **52**, 1458–68.

Arngrimsson, R., Geirsson, R. T., Cooke, A., Connor, M., Bjornsson, S. and Walker, J. J. (1994). Renin gene restriction fragment length polymorphisms do not show linkage with preeclampsia and eclampsia. *Acta Obstet. Gynecol. Scand.*, **73**, 10–13.

Baker, P. N., Broughton Pipkin, F. and Symonds, E. M. (1992). Longitudinal study of platelet angiotensin II binding in human pregnancy. *Clin. Sci. (Lond.)*, **82**, 377–81.

Bashford, M. T., Hefler, L. A., Vertrees, T. W., Roa, B. B. and Gregg, A. R. (2001). Angiotensinogen and endothelial nitric oxide synthase gene polymorphisms among Hispanic patients with preeclampsia. *Am. J. Obstet. and Gynecol.*, **184**, 1345–50.

Benndorf, R., Boge, R. H., Ergun, S., Steenpass, A. and Wieland, T. (2003). Angiotensin II type 2 receptor inhibits vascular endothelial growth factor-induced migration and in vitro tube formation of human endothelial cells. *Circ. Res.*, **93**, 438–47.

Bing, C., Johnson, I. R. and Broughton Pipkin, F. (1996). Angiotensin receptors in myometrium and myometrial vessels from uteri of women during the follicular and luteal phases of the menstrual cycle and in late pregnancy. *Clin. Sci. (Lond.)*, **90**, 499–505.

Broughton Pipkin, F. (1993). The renin system and reproduction in animals. In *The Renin–Angiotensin System*, vol. **1**. ed. J. I. S. N. Robertson and M. G. Nicholls. London: Gower Medical Publishing. pp. 49.41–49.49.

Broughton Pipkin, F., Craven, D. J. and Symonds, E. M. (1981). The utero-placental renin–angiotensin system in normal and hypertensive pregnancy. *Contrib. Nephrol.*, **25**, 49–52.

Broughton Pipkin, F., Sharif, J. and Lal, S. (1995). Angiotensin and asymmetric fetal growth. *Lancet*, **346**, 844–5.

Brown, J. J., Davies, D. L., Doak, P. B., Lever, A. F., Robertson, J. I. and Tree, M. (1964a). The presence of renin in human amniotic fluid. *Lancet*, **ii**, 64–6.

Brown, J. J., Davies, D. L., Doak, P. B., Lever, A. F., Robertson, J. I. and Trust, P. (1964b). Plasma renin concentration in the hypertensive diseases of pregnancy. *J. Obst. Gynaecol. Br. Commonwlth*, **73**, 410–17.

Bussen, S. S., Sutterlin, M. W. and Steck, T. (1998). Plasma renin activity and aldosterone serum concentration are decreased in severe preeclampsia but not in the HELLP-syndrome. *Acta Obstet. Gynecol. Scand.*, **77**, 609–13.

Campbell, D.C. and Kladis, A. (1990). Simultaneous radioimmunoassay of six angiotensin peptides in arterial and venous plasma of man. *J. Hypertens.*, **8**, 165–72.

Celerier, J., Cruz, A., Lamande, N., Gasc, J.M. and Corvol, P. (2002). Angiotensinogen and its cleaved derivatives inhibit angiogenesis. *Hypertension*, **39**, 224–8.

Cesari, M., Rossi, G.P. and Pessina, A.C. (2002). Biological properties of the angiotensin peptides other than angiotensin II: implications for hypertension and cardiovascular diseases. *J. Hypertens.*, **20**, 793–9.

Chapman, A.B., Abraham, W.T., Zamudio, S., et al. (1998). Temporal relationships between hormonal and hemodynamic changes in early human pregnancy. *Kidney Int.*, **54**, 2056–63.

Cooper, A.C., Robinson, G., Vinson, G.P., Cheung, W.T. and Broughton Pipkin, F. (1999). The localization and expression of the renin–angiotensin system in the human placenta throughout pregnancy. *Placenta*, **20**, 467–74.

Craven, D.J., Warren, A.Y. and Symonds, E.M. (1983). Generation of angiotensin I by tissues of the human female genital tract. *Am. J. Obstet. Gynecol.*, **145**, 749–51.

Curnow, K.M., Pham, T. and August, P. (2000). The L10F mutation of angiotensinogen is rare in pre-eclampsia. *J. Hypertens.*, **18**, 173–8.

de Gasparo, M. (2002). Angiotensin II and nitric oxide interaction. *Heart Fail. Rev.*, **7**, 347–58.

de Gasparo, M., Catt, K.J., Inagami, T., Wright, J.W. and Unger, T. (2000). The angiotensin II receptors. *Pharmacol. Rev.*, **52**, 415–72.

Dechend, R., Homuth, V., Wallukat, G., et al. (2000). AT1 receptor agonistic antibodies from preeclamptic patients cause vascular cells to express tissue factor. *Circulation*, **101**, 2382–7.

Dechend, R., Viedt, C., Muller, D.N., et al. (2003). AT1 receptor agonistic antibodies from preeclamptic patients stimulate NADPH oxidase. *Circulation*, **107**, 1632–9.

Dzau, V.J., Burt, D.W. and Pratt, R.E. (1988). Molecular biology of the renin–angiotensin system. *Am. J. Physiol. Renal, Fluid Electro. Physiol.*, **255**, F563–73.

Ferrario, C. (2002). Angiotensin I, angiotensin II and their biologically active peptides. *J. Hypertens.*, **20**, 805–7.

Ferrario, C.M., Chappell, M.C., Tallant, E.A., Brosnihan, K.B. and Diz, D.I. (1997). Counterregulatory actions of angiotensin-(1–7). *Hypertension*, **30**, 535–41.

Fruitier-Arnaudin, I., Cohen, M., Bordenave, S., Sannier, F. and Piot, J.M. (2002). Comparative effects of angiotensin IV and two hemorphins on angiotensin-converting enzyme activity. *Peptides*, **23**, 1465–70.

Fu, M.L., Herlitz, H., Schulze, W., et al. (2000). Autoantibodies against the angiotensin receptor (AT1) in patients with hypertension. *J. Hypertens.*, **18**, 945–53.

Gallery, E.D., Stokes, G.S., Gyory, A.Z., Rowe, J. and Williams, J. (1980). Plasma renin activity in normal human pregnancy and in pregnancy-associated hypertension, with reference to cryoactivation. *Clin. Sci.*, **59**, 49–53.

Gordon, R.D., Parsons, S. and Symonds, E.M. (1969). A prospective study of plasma-renin activity in normal and toxaemic pregnancy. *Lancet*, **i**(7590), 347–9.

Gordon, R.D., Symonds, E.M., Wilmshurst, E.G. and Pawsey, C.G. (1973). Plasma renin activity, plasma angiotensin and plasma and urinary electrolytes in normal and toxaemic pregnancy, including a prospective study. *Clin. Sci.*, **45**, 115–27.

Guo, G., Wilton, A.N., Fu, Y., Qiu, H., Brennecke, S.P. and Cooper, D.W. (1997). Angiotensinogen gene variation in a population case-control study of preeclampsia/eclampsia in Australians and Chinese. *Electrophoresis*, **18**, 1646–9.

Hagemann, A., Nielsen, A.H. and Poulsen, K. (1994). The uteroplacental renin–angiotensin system: a review. *Exp. Clin. Endocrinol.*, **102**(3), 252–61.

Hanna, I.R., Taniyama, Y., Szocs, K., Rocic, P. and Griendling, K.K. (2002). NAD(P)H oxidase-derived reactive oxygen species as mediators of angiotensin II signaling. *Antioxid. Redox. Signal.*, **4**, 899–914.

Hanssens, M., Keirse, M.J., Spitz, B. and van Assche, F.A. (1991a). Angiotensin II levels in hypertensive and normotensive pregnancies. *Br. J. Obstet. Gynaecol.*, **98**, 155–61.

Hanssens, M., Keirse, M.J.N.C., Spitz, B. and van Assche, F.A. (1991b). Measurement of individual plasma angiotensins in normal pregnancy and pregnancy-induced hypertension. *J. Clin. Endocrinol. Metab.*, **73**, 489–94.

Hayashi, R.H., Becker, R.A., Evans, G.T., Morris, K. and Franks, R.C. (1977). Prospective study of angiotensin II response to positional change in pregnancy-induced hypertension. *Am. J. Obstet. Gynecol.*, **128**, 872–8.

Heiskanen, J. T., Pirskanen, M. M., Hiltunen, M. J., Mannermaa, A. J., Punnonen, K. R. and Heinonen, S. T. (2001). Insertion–deletion polymorphism in the gene for angiotensin-converting enzyme is associated with obstetric cholestasis but not with preeclampsia. *Am. J. Obstet. Gynecol.*, **185**, 600–3.

Horio, J., Nomura, S., Okada, M., *et al.* (1999). Structural organization of the 5'-end and chromosomal assignment of human placental leucine aminopeptidase/insulin-regulated membrane amino-peptidase gene. *Biochem. Biophys. Res. Commun.*, **262**, 269–74.

Ino, K., Uehara, C., Kikkawa, F., *et al.* (2003). Enhancement of aminopeptidase A expression during angiotensin II-induced choriocarcinoma cell proliferation through AT1 receptor involving protein kinase C- and mitogen-activated protein kinase-dependent signaling pathway. *J. Clin. Endocrinol. Metab.*, **88**, 3973–82.

Inoue, I., Nakajima, T., Williams, C. S., *et al.* (1997). A nucleotide substitution in the promoter of human angiotensinogen is associated with essential hypertension and affects basal transcription in vitro. *J. Clin. Invest.*, **99**, 1786–97.

Jikihara, H., Poisner, A. M., Hirsch, R. and Handwerger, S. (1995). Human uterine decidual macrophages express renin. *J. Clin. Endocrinol. Metab.*, **80**, 1273–7.

Johnson, A. R., Skidgel, R. A., Gafford, J. T. and Erdos, E. G. (1984). Enzymes in placental microvilli: angiotensin I converting enzyme, angiotensinase A, carboxypeptidase, and neutral endopeptidase ("enkephalinase"). *Peptides*, **5**, 789–96.

Johnson, I. R. (1980). Renin substrate, active and acid-activatable renin concentrations in human plasma and endometrium during the normal menstrual cycle. *Br. J. Obstet. Gynaecol.*, **87**, 875–82.

Kaaja, R. J., Moore, M. P., Yandle, T. G., Ylikorkala, O., Frampton, C. M. and Nicholls, M. G. (1999). Blood pressure and vasoactive hormones in mild preeclampsia and normal pregnancy. *Hypertens. Pregn.*, **18**, 173–87.

Keidar, S., Heinrich, R., Kaplan, M. and Aviram, M. (2002). Oxidative stress increases the expression of the angiotensin-II receptor type 1 in mouse peritoneal macrophages. *J. Renin Angiotensin Aldosterone Syst.*, **3**, 24–30.

Kerins, D. M., Hao, Q. and Vaughan, D. E. (1995). Angiotensin induction of PAI-1 expression in endothelial cells is mediated by the hexapeptide angiotensin IV. *J. Clin. Invest.*, **96**, 2515–20.

Kikkawa, F., Kajiyama, H., Ino, K., *et al.* (2002). Possible involvement of placental peptidases that degrade gonadotropin-releasing hormone (GnRH) in the dynamic pattern of placental hCG secretion via GnRH degradation. *Placenta*, **23**, 483–9.

Klickstein, L. B., Kaempfer, C. E. and Wintroub, B. U. (1982). The granulocyte–angiotensin system. Angiotensin I-converting activity of cathepsin G. *J. Biol. Chem.*, **257**, 15,042–6.

Knock, G. A., Sullivan, M. H., McCarthy, A., Elder, M. G., Polak, J. M. and Wharton, J. (1994). Angiotensin II (AT1) vascular binding sites in human placentae from normal-term, preeclamptic and growth retarded pregnancies. *J. Pharmacol. Exp. Therap.*, **271**, 1007–15.

Kobashi, G., Shido, K., Hata, A., *et al.* (2001). Multivariate analysis of genetic and acquired factors; T235 variant of the angiotensinogen gene is a potent independent risk factor for preeclampsia. *Semin. Thromb. Hemost.*, **27**, 143–7.

Leung, P. S., Tsai, S. J., Wallukat, G., Leung, T. N. and Lau, T. K. (2001). The upregulation of angiotensin II receptor AT1 in human preeclamptic placenta. *Molec. Cell. Endocrinol.*, **184**, 95–102.

Lever, A. F. (1993). Slow developing pressor effect of angiotensin II and vascular structure. *J. Hypertens.*, **11**(Suppl.), S27–8.

Li, P., Chappell, M. C., Ferrario, C. M. and Brosnihan, K. B. (1997). Angiotensin-(1–7) augments bradykinin-induced vasodilation by competing with ACE and releasing nitric oxide. *Hypertension*, **29**, 394–400.

Li, X. F. and Ahmed, A. (1996). Dual role of angiotensin II in the human endometrium. *Hum. Reprod.*, **11**, 95–108.

Li, X. M., Moutquin, J. M., Deschenes, J., Bourque, L., Marois, M. and Forest, J. C. (1995). Increased immuno-histochemical expression of neutral metalloendo-peptidase (enkephalinase; EC 3.4.24.11) in villi of the human placenta with pre-eclampsia. *Placenta*, **16**, 435–45.

Lobov, I. B., Brooks, P. C. and Lang, R. A. (2002). Angiopoietin-2 displays VEGF-dependent modulation of capillary structure and endothelial cell survival in vivo. *Proc. Natl Acad. Sci. USA*, **99**, 11,205–10.

Merrill, D. C., Karoly, M., Chen, K., Ferrario, C. M. and Brosnihan, K. B. (2002). Angiotensin-(1–7) in normal and preeclamptic pregnancy. *Endocrine J.*, **18**, 239–45.

Mizutani, S. and Tomoda, Y. (1996). Effects of placental proteases on maternal and fetal blood pressure in normal pregnancy and preeclampsia. *Am. J. Hypertens.*, **9**, 591–7.

Moeller, I., Clune, E. F., Fennessy, P. A., *et al.* (1999). Up regulation of AT4 receptor levels in carotid arteries following balloon injury. *Regul. Peptides*, **83**, 25–30.

Morgan, L., Crawshaw, S., Baker, P. N., Edwards, R., Broughton Pipkin, F. and Kalsheker, N. (1997a). Functional and genetic studies of the angiotensin II type 1 receptor in pre-eclamptic and normotensive pregnant women. *J. Hypertens.*, **15**, 1389–96.

Morgan, T., Craven, C., Nelson, L., Lalouel, J. M. and Ward, K. (1997b). Angiotensinogen T235 expression is elevated in decidual spiral arteries. *J. Clin. Invest.*, **100**, 1406–15.

Morgan, T., Craven, C. and Ward, K. (1998). Human spiral artery renin–angiotensin system. *Hypertension*, **32**, 683–7.

Morgan, L., Crawshaw, S., Baker, P. N., Broughton Pipkin, F. and Kalsheker, N. (1999a). Maternal and fetal angiotensinogen gene allele sharing in pre-eclampsia. *Br. J. Obstet. Gynaecol.*, **106**, 244–51.

Morgan, L., Foster, F., Hayman, R., *et al.* (1999b). Angiotensin-converting enzyme insertion–deletion polymorphism in normotensive and pre-eclamptic pregnancies. *J. Hypertens.*, **17**, 765–8.

Morgan, T., Craven, C., Lalouel, J. M. and Ward, K. (1999c). Angiotensinogen Thr235 variant is associated with abnormal physiologic change of the uterine spiral arteries in first-trimester decidua. *Am. J. Obstet. Gynecol.*, **180**, 95–102.

Nadal, J. A., Scicli, G. M., Carbini, L. A. and Scicli, A. G. (2002). Angiotensin II stimulates migration of retinal microvascular pericytes: involvement of TGF-beta and PDGF-BB. *Am. J. Physiol. Heart Circ. Physiol.*, **282**, H739–48.

Neudeck, H., Schuster, C., Hildebrandt, R., *et al.* (1996). Histochemical evaluation of placental angiotensinase A in pre-eclampsia: enzyme activity in villous trophoblast indicates an enhanced likelihood of gestational proteinuric hypertension. *Placenta*, **17**, 155–63.

Oats, J. N., Broughton Pipkin, F., Symonds, E. M. and Craven, D. J. (1981). A prospective study of plasma angiotensin-converting enzyme in normotensive primigravidae and their infants. *Br. J. Obstet. Gynaecol.*, **88**, 1204–10.

Otani, A., Takagi, H., Suzuma, K. and Honda, Y. (1998). Angiotensin II potentiates vascular endothelial growth factor-induced angiogenic activity in retinal microcapillary endothelial cells. *Circ. Res.*, **82**, 619–28.

Otani, A., Takagi, H., Oh, H., Koyama, S. and Honda, Y. (2001). Angiotensin II induces expression of the Tie2 receptor ligand, angiopoietin-2, in bovine retinal endothelial cells. *Diabetes*, **50**, 867–75.

Page, E. L., Robitaille, G. A., Pouyssegur, J. and Richard, D. (2002). Induction of hypoxia-inducible factor-1alpha by transcriptional and translational mechanisms. *J. Biol. Chem.*, **277**, 48,403–9.

Poulsen, K. and Jacobsen, J. (1993). Enzymic reactions of the renin–angiotensin system. In *The Renin–Angiotensin System*, vol. **1**. ed. J. I. S. Robertson and M. G. Nicholls, London: Gower Medical Publishing, pp. 5.1–5.12.

Rasmussen, A. B., Pedersen, E. B., Romer, F. K., *et al.* (1983). The influence of normotensive pregnancy and pre-eclampsia on angiotensin-converting enzyme. *Acta Obstet. Gynecol. Scand.*, **62**, 341–4.

Richard, D. E., Berra, E. and Pouyssegur, J. (2000). Nonhypoxic pathway mediates the induction of hypoxia-inducible factor 1alpha in vascular smooth muscle cells. *J. Biol. Chem.*, **275**, 26,765–71.

Rigat, B., Hubert, C., Alhenc-Gelas, F., Cambien, F., Corvol, P. and Soubrier, F. (1990). An insertion/deletion polymorphism in the angiotensin I-converting enzyme gene accounting for half the variance of serum enzyme levels. *J. Clin. Invest.*, **86**, 1343–6.

Ruilope, L., Paya, C., Alcazar, J. M., *et al.* (1984). Failure of angiotensin II to reduce plasma renin activity in hypertensive pregnant women. *J. Hypertens.*, **2**, S251–4.

Santos, R. A., Simoes e Silva, A. C., Maric, C., *et al.* (2003). Angiotensin-(1–7) is an endogenous ligand for the G protein-coupled receptor Mas. *Proc. Natl Acad. Sci. USA*, **100**, 8258–63.

Sethi, A. A., Nordestgaard, B. G. and Tybjaerg-Hansen, A. (2003). Angiotensinogen gene polymorphism, plasma angiotensinogen, and risk of hypertension and ischemic heart disease: a meta-analysis. *Arterioscl. Thromb. Vasc. Biol.*, **23**, 1269–75.

Shah, D. M., Banu, J. M., Chirgwin, J. M. and Tekmal, R. R. (2000). Reproductive tissue renin gene expression in preeclampsia. *Hypertens. Pregn.*, **19**, 341–51.

Skinner, S. L. (1993). The renin system in fertility and normal human pregnancy. In *The Renin–Angiotensin System*, vol. **1**. ed. J. I. S. N. Robertson and M. G. Nicholls, London: Gower Medical Publishing, pp. 50.1–50.16.

Skinner, S. L., Lumbers, E. R. and Symonds, E. M. (1972). Analysis of changes in the renin–angiotensin system during pregnancy. *Clin. Sci.*, **42**, 479–88.

Sowers, J. R., Eggena, P., Kowal, D. K., Simpson, L., Zhu, J.-H. and Barrett, J. D. (1993). Expression of renin and angiotensinogen genes in preeclamptic and normal human placental tissue. *Hypertens. Pregn.*, **12**, 163–71.

Strawn, W. B. and Ferrario, C. M. (2002). Mechanisms linking angiotensin II and atherogenesis. *Curr. Opin. Lipidol.*, **13**, 505–12.

Suzuki, Y., Tanemura, M., Suzuki, Y., Murakami, I. and Suzumori, K. (1999). Is angiotensinogen gene polymorphism associated with hypertension in pregnancy? *Hypertens. Pregn.*, **18**, 261–71.

Symonds, E. M. and Andersen, G. J. (1974). The effect of bed rest on plasma renin in hypertensive disease of pregnancy. *J. Obstet. Gynaecol. Br. Commonwlth*, **81**, 676–81.

Symonds, E. M., Stanley, M. A. and Skinner, S. L. (1968). Production of renin by in vitro cultures of human chorion and uterine muscle. *Nature*, **217**, 1152–3.

Symonds, E. M., Broughton Pipkin, F. and Craven, D. J. (1975). Changes in the renin-angiotensin system in primigravidae with hypertensive disease of pregnancy. *Br. J. Obstet. Gynaecol.*, **82**, 643–50.

Tamura, T., Johanning, G. L., Goldenberg, R. L., Johnston, K. E. and DuBard, M. B. (1996). Effect of angiotensin-converting enzyme gene polymorphism on pregnancy outcome, enzyme activity, and zinc concentration. *Obstet. Gynecol.*, **88**, 497–502.

Tewksbury, D. A., Kaiser, S. J. and Burrill, R. E. (2001). A study of the temporal relationship between plasma high molecular weight angiotensinogen and the development of pregnancy-induced hypertension. *Am. J. Hypertens.*, **14**, 794–7.

Tigerstedt, R. and Bergman, P. (1898). Niere und Kreislauf. *Skandi. Archiv Physiol.*, **8**, 223–71.

Tulenko, T. N. (1979). Regional sensitivity to vasoactive polypeptides in the human umbilicoplacental vasculature. *Am. J. Obstet. Gynecol.*, **135**, 629–36.

Valdes, G., Germain, A. M., Corthorn, J., *et al.* (2001). Urinary vasodilator and vasoconstrictor angiotensins during menstrual cycle, pregnancy, and lactation. *Endocrine J.*, **16**, 117–22.

Viinikainen, A., Nyman, T., Fyhrquist, F. and Saijonmaa, O. (2002). Downregulation of angiotensin converting enzyme by TNF-alpha in differentiating human macrophages. *Cytokine*, **18**(6), 304–10.

Wallukat, G., Homuth, V., Fischer, T., *et al.* (1999). Patients with preeclampsia develop agonistic autoantibodies against the angiotensin AT1 receptor. *J. Clin. Invest.*, **103**, 945–52.

Ward, K., Hata, A., Jeunemaitre, X., *et al.* (1993). A molecular variant of angiotensinogen associated with preeclampsia. *Nature Genet.*, **4**, 59–61.

Williams, B., Baker, A. Q., Gallacher, B. and Lodwick, D. (1995). Angiotensin II increases vascular permeability factor gene expression by human vascular smooth muscle cells. *Hypertension*, **25**, 913–17.

Xia, Y., Wen, H., Bobst, S., Day, M. C. and Kellems, R. E. (2003). Maternal autoantibodies from preeclamptic patients activate angiotensin receptors on human trophoblast cells. *J. Soc. Gynecol. Invest.*, **10**, 82–93.

Xia, Y., Wen, H. Y. and Kellems, R. E. (2002). Angiotensin II inhibits human trophoblast invasion through AT1 receptor activation. *J. Biol. Chem.*, **277**, 24,601–8.

Yamahara, N., Nomura, S., Suzuki, T., *et al.* (2000). Placental leucine aminopeptidase/oxytocinase in maternal serum and placenta during normal pregnancy. *Life Sci.*, **66**, 1401–10.

Immunological factors and placentation: implications for pre-eclampsia

Ashley Moffett and Susan E. Hiby

Introduction

Pre-eclampsia only occurs during pregnancy, a physiological situation where allogeneic cells from two different individuals come into close contact. Furthermore, the development of the disease is dependent only on the presence of the placenta and not the fetus as the disease is frequently seen in complete hydatidiform mole where no fetus is present. Numerous epidemiological studies have given rise to the widely held view that immunological mechanisms probably contribute to the pathogenesis of this disease (and indeed other pregnancy disorders) (Dekker, 2002; Redman, 1991; Roberts and Lain, 2002; Walker, 2000). However, the molecular and biological mechanisms underlying this presumed maternal immune maladaptation remain unknown.

During pregnancy both the maternal and fetal immune systems would be expected to recognize the presence of each other's allogeneic cells. However, the acceptance of the fetal allograft by the mother is at variance with the rejection typically seen with organ grafts. If the transplant analogy is extended further it would be expected that the maternal immune reaction would exhibit both specificity and memory for particular paternal genes expressed by the placenta. In other words, is there a partner-specific effect which contributes to pregnancy success or failure? Therefore, in considering possible immunological factors in pre-eclampsia two broad questions arise: first, how does the maternal immune system normally allow a symbiotic relationship with the feto-placental unit and, second, can this symbiosis be altered in a partner-specific way in pre-eclampsia?

Epidemiology

The strongest risk factor for pre-eclampsia is primiparity with 75% of cases occurring in primips, indicating that a previous pregnancy is protective in the development of the disease (Eskenazi et al., 1991; MacGillivray, 1958; Roberts and Redman, 1993). One interpretation is that the mother has immunological memory for her first pregnancy. However, in contrast to the memory characteristic of a transplanted organ where the rejection reaction to a second graft from the same individual is accelerated and more vigorous, the second pregnancy is more successful. Viewed in conventional immunological terms, pregnancy appears to induce tolerance rather than sensitization. There is still no satisfactory explanation why first pregnancies are so at risk from pre-eclampsia and why subsequent pregnancies generally proceed normally.

Intriguingly, a partner-specific effect may also be important. If subsequent pregnancy occurs with a different father, then the protective effect of primiparity will be lost. This "change of partner" effect has been found in many studies (Feeney and Scott, 1980; Li and Wi, 2000; Lie et al., 1998; Trupin et al., 1996; Tubbergen et al., 1999). Furthermore, after change of partner, it seems that the risk of developing pre-eclampsia increases if the woman has no previous history of pre-eclampsia but may conversely actually decrease if she has experienced pre-eclampsia in her first pregnancy. Recently, other reports have challenged these findings and concluded it is the longer birth interval – more likely to occur when a new partner intervenes between pregnancies – rather than the new partner himself which is important (Basso *et al.*, 2001; Skjaerven *et al.*, 2002; Trogstad *et al.*, 2001). Disentangling the effect of paternal change from this time aspect (which will involve other factors such as infertility, length of cohabitation and age) would be difficult.

At present, therefore, it is unclear whether the first pregnancy and change of partner effects do indicate immune mechanisms in pre-eclampsia. More prosaic explanations are possible. For example, the structural modifications of the uterine arteries may be more difficult to achieve optimally the first time the placenta is established (Redman, 1991). It might be easier to re-modify the uterine arteries in a subsequent pregnancy after a short birth interval than after a longer interval when the arteries may have returned more closely to their "virgin" untransformed state.

Despite these caveats other reports do suggest immunological factors may be operative. For example, a protective effect of sperm/seminal fluid from the father in a subsequent pregnancy is suggested from several studies. Barrier contraception seems to increase the risk (Klonoff-Cohen *et al.*, 1989) and, conversely, a prolonged period of sexual contact reduces the risk (Marti and Herrmann, 1977; Robillard *et al.*, 1994, 1998). Similarly, an increased incidence of pre-eclampsia has been seen in IVF pregnancies when donated sperm rather than sperm from the cohabiting partner are used (Dekker *et al.*, 1998; Hoy *et al.*, 1999; Need *et al.*, 1983). The effect seems to be due to the father's sperm rather than other soluble or cellular components of seminal fluid because the risk of pre-eclampsia is also increased in women who were treated by intracytoplasmic sperm injection (ICSI) performed with surgically obtained sperm (Wang *et al.*, 2002).

The most compelling evidence that there is an immunological basis to pre-eclampsia comes from studies comparing the incidence of pre-eclampsia in women undergoing IVF with donated oocytes with those who have used their own oocytes (Abdalla *et al.*, 1998; Boks and Braat, 1997; Salha *et al.*, 1999; Serhal and Craft, 1989; Soderstrom-Anttila *et al.*, 1998). The incidence of pre-eclampsia rises to ∼30% with donated oocytes. In these pregnancies the fetus and placenta will have no genetic contribution from the mother and the conceptus is completely non-self or foreign to her.

A maternally inherited predisposition has long been noted with a fourfold increased risk of a woman developing severe pre-eclampsia if she has a family history (Adams and Finlayson, 1961; Cincotta and Brennecke, 1998; Sutherland *et al.*, 1981). Recently, large population-based studies have indicated that paternal genes also contribute to a woman's risk of developing pre-eclampsia. Indeed, the role of the fetus is as important as that of the mother (Esplin *et al.*, 2001; Lie *et al.*, 1998). Twin studies also do not support sole maternal genetic influences as no concordant twin pairs have been found in pre-eclampsia (Treloar *et al.*, 2001). The genetics of the disease cannot be explained by any simple model (Cross, 2003). Instead a combined genetic contribution from both the mother and the fetus is likely to be important. Could these genes belong to the immune system? If so, what genes might be involved?

Pathogenesis of pre-eclampsia

The pathogenesis of the disease is generally considered in several stages (Redman, 1991). In the first stage the placental trophoblast cells fail to invade adequately into the decidua and the spiral arteries to achieve the transformation necessary for the increase in the feto-placental blood flow. The second stage results from the poor placental perfusion through the inadequately transformed arteries. The placenta fails to grow and develop normally so that an abnormal placental structure with defective branching morphogenesis of the villous tree results. Finally, in the third stage a systemic leukocytic–endothelial inflammatory syndrome is triggered by factors released by the ischemic placenta. At what stage might immunological effects be operating?

The main area of tissue contact between the immune cells of the mother and her fetus is at the implantation site where the vascular modification of the arteries takes place. We have proposed that the control of trophoblast invasion into the decidua and arteries has an immunological basis (Moffett-King, 2002). The immunological changes occurring in decidua during placentation must be separated clearly from the systemic immune and inflammatory changes seen in the periphery once that disease is established. When considering the maternal immune response there are still many questions that need to be addressed. How does the maternal local immune system operating in the decidua recognize and respond to the invading placenta? How is the balance between under and over invasion achieved and how could partner-specific effects be explained in terms of this putative immunological control mechanism?

Maternal immune system and trophoblast invasion

The trophoblast cells which invade are derived from the anchoring villi and are known as extravillous trophoblast (EVT) (Loke and King, 1995). These invade into maternal decidua which is infiltrated by abundant NK cells, together with macrophages and a few $CD3^+$ T cells. As trophoblasts are allogeneic cells the MHC status is important in considering how the uterine immune cells perceive their presence. EVT expresses no HLA class II but do express three class I molecules, HLA-G, HLA-E and HLA-C. It is important to note that the classical MHC molecules, HLA-A and B, which are the dominant ligands used by T cells, are never expressed by trophoblast. Of the three which are expressed, HLA-G and HLA-E show very limited polymorphism and it can be assumed that trophoblast cells derived from all individuals will be recognized by maternal leukocytes in a similar manner. This has been demonstrated experimentally for HLA-E, where tetramers bind to the inhibitory CD94/NKG2A receptors found on all uterine NK cells (King et al., 2000a; Moffett-King, 2002). HLA-E, therefore, may function as an inhibitory ligand. The function of the trophoblast-specific HLA class I molecule, HLA-G, is still unknown. It may bind to receptors on uterine NK cells and/or macrophages signaling the presence of an implanting placenta. Neither polymorphisms of HLA-G or its putative receptor KIR2DL4 have been shown to be correlated with pre-eclampsia (Aldrich et al., 2000; Bermingham et al., 2000; Humphrey et al., 1995; Witt et al., 2002).

HLA-C is expressed at the trophoblast cell surface and is up-regulated by IFN-γ (King et al., 1996, 2000b). Importantly, it is highly polymorphic (74 alleles are known) and the paternal allele is expressed in trophoblast (Hiby et al., 1999). Therefore, in terms of allorecognition in reproduction, trophoblast non-self HLA-C is the most important MHC molecule to consider. Although there are receptors for HLA-C on T cells and macrophages, the dominant influence of HLA-C is on NK cells (Colonna et al., 1992; Valiante et al., 1997). The profusion of NK cells at the implantation site indicate that maternal NK cell/trophoblast HLA-C interaction deserves particular attention when considering regulation of trophoblast invasion and arterial transformation.

NK cells and killer immunoglobulin-like receptors (KIR)

NK cells are effector lymphocytes that act by production of cytokines and chemokines. Regulation of NK cell function is accomplished through a diverse repertoire of receptors mediating

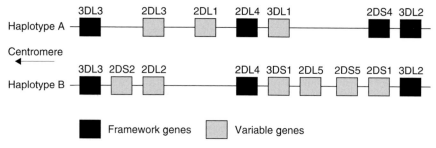

Figure 6.1 Two representative KIR haplotypes of the A and B type.

both activating and inhibitory signals (Lanier, 1998). Of the NK receptors identified it is the Killer Immunoglobulin-like Receptors (KIR) family that have members that will bind to HLA-C (Vilches and Parham, 2002). The KIR multigene family is located on chromosome 19q13.4 within the leukocyte receptor complex (Trowsdale, 2001). This KIR region exhibits an extensive degree of diversity achieved by a combination of presence/absence of genes and allelic polymorphism. It is estimated that such is the diversity that only 0.24% of unrelated individuals can expect an identical genotype. Underlying this diversity are conserved patterns with three framework genes, present in all individuals, defining the borders of the region (3DL3 and 3DL2) with 2DL4 in the middle. The regions between these framework genes contain a variable number of genes and the combination of genes on one chromosome is known as the KIR haplotype (Carrington and Norman, 2003; Vilches and Parham, 2002; Yawata et al., 2002). There are two main types of haplotype, A and B (Figure 6.1). The A haplotypes (present at a frequency of ~50% in Caucasians) have the least number of genes and most encode inhibitory receptors which have a long (L) cytoplasmic tail. The B haplotypes exhibit much greater variability and the extra genes present encode activating receptors with a short (S) cytoplasmic tail.

The KIR family includes inhibitory receptors (KIR2DL1, 2DL2 and 2DL3), for polymorphic determinants of all HLA-C allotypes, the latter are

HLA-C group 1 (C1 epitope) Ser 77 Asn 80	HLA-C group 2 (C2 epitope) Asn 77 Lys 80
Cw 01	Cw 02
03 – now 09 and 10)	04
	05
	06
07 (01–06, 08, 10–14)	07 (07, 09)
08	
12 (02, 03, 06, 07)	12 (04, 05)
13	
14	
15 (07)	15 (02 – 06, 08, 09)
16 (01, 04)	16 (02)
	17
	18
KIR receptors: **2DL2** **2DL3** **(2DS2)** **(2DS4)**	**KIR receptors:** **2DL1** **2DS1** **(2DS3)** **(2DS5)**

The ligand specificity of the 2DS activating receptors (in brackets) is predicted on the basis of sequence similarity but is not proven.

Figure 6.2 HLA-C alleles and their KIR receptors.

known as the KIR epitopes of HLA-C. All HLA-C alleles have either asparagine or lysine at position 80 of the $\alpha 1$ domain and this dimorphism distinguishes the two KIR epitopes and divides HLA-C allotypes into two groups known as group 1 (HLA-C^{asn80}) and group 2 (HLA-C ^{lys80}) (Figure 6.2). An activating receptor for HLA-C^{lys80} (KIR2DS1) will also bind group 2 HLA-C allotypes and KIR2DS2 has been reported to bind group 1 HLA-C. These activating receptors are present on some B haplotypes but absent from all A haplotypes. The other KIR2DS receptors (2DS3, 2DS4 and 2DS5) may also bind HLA-C molecules although the ligand specificity of all activating receptors is still not well defined (Vilches and Parham, 2002).

HLA and KIR genes are on different chromosomes and segregate independently meaning that in an individual KIR may be expressed for which there is no HLA ligand. Alternatively, activating KIR for non-self and self HLA molecules may be present in an individual although, as all NK cells acquire an inhibitory receptor for self HLA during development, NK cells will not kill self cells under normal circumstances. However, NK cells can lack inhibitory receptors for non-self HLA and in this case the activating KIR for non-self may stimulate the NK cell. As there is the potential for interaction between particular KIR receptors and HLA molecules in an individual, epistatic effects of KIR and HLA genes might be expected and indeed have now been reported. Subjects with psoriasis with activating KIR2DS1 and/or 2DS2/3 are susceptible to the development of the disease only if the HLA-C ligands for the corresponding inhibitory KIR, 2DL1 and 2DL2/3 are missing (Martin *et al.*, 2002a). Progression to AIDS is influenced by the combination of expressing both KIR3DS1 and the ligands for this activating KIR which are certain Bw4 alleles (Martin *et al.*, 2002b). In defining the role for KIR in the predisposition to particular diseases, both these studies highlight the importance of the presence/absence of the activating KIR which are found on the B haplotypes.

NK allorecognition and pregnancy

HLA-C plays a key role in allorecognition by NK cells. Indeed, allospecificities were originally mapped by family studies in the MHC in close linkage to HLA-C (Colonna *et al.*, 1992, 1993).

Recently, KIR ligand incompatibility or mismatch in HLA-C groups between host and donor has been shown to influence the outcome of bone marrow transplantation (Giebel *et al.*, 2003; Parham and McQueen, 2003). A beneficial graft versus leukemia effect was seen when the donor NK cells express an inhibitory KIR for a ligand lacking in the recipient resulting in killing of the recipient's leukemic cells. In this situation NK cell alloreactivity was associated with a better outcome. NK cells when confronted by allogeneic targets lacking their own inhibiting class I alleles may react. Although these studies need confirmation this has given rise to the concept of the ''perfectly mismatched'' donor (Karre, 2002). The analogy with pregnancy is obvious and raises the question whether there could be ''perfectly mismatched'' couples.

Pregnancy is a natural allograft and the mother could possess KIR genes for paternal HLA-C that belong to a different group than her own (non-self). Alternatively, if the mother has two HLA-C allotypes belonging to both Group 1 and Group 2 and the father is homozygous for either Group 1 or Group 2, then the trophoblast might lack one of the HLA-C groups belonging to the mother. In other words, the trophoblast would be ''Missing Self'' (Figure 6.3). Of interest also is the observation that the phenotypic expression of KIR is skewed in decidual NK cells with a higher proportion of decidual NK cells expressing KIR 2D receptors with specificities for HLA-C allotypes than is found in peripheral blood from the same individual (Verma *et al.*, 1997).

The particular combinations of maternal KIR2D and paternal HLA-C may have a profound influence on NK cell function in terms of cytokine/chemokine production and hence the depth of trophoblast infiltration. In this way chance events could determine which HLA-C alleles the child possesses and which KIR genes the mother possesses and pre-eclampsia would arise as a consequence of unfavorable combinations of maternal KIR and paternal HLA-C. This is one mechanism whereby a particular genotype in the mother might interact detrimentally with a

HLA-C combinations in mother and fetus

Mother may have KIR for a ligand she does not have but which is present in fetus.

Mother	Fetus
Gp1 + Gp1	Gp1 + **Gp2**
Gp2 + Gp2	**Gp1** + Gp2

Fetus is **Non-Self** for HLA-C group.

Mother may have KIR for ligands which she possesses but is lacking in fetus.

Mother	Fetus
Gp1 + **Gp2**	Gp1 + Gp1
Gp1 + Gp2	Gp2 + Gp2

Fetus is **Missing Self** for one of the Maternal HLA-C groups

Figure 6.3 HLA-C combinations in mother and fetus.

particular genotype in the father to give rise to inadequate placentation and pre-eclampsia. Recent work shows that this is indeed the case (Hiby *et al.*, 2004).

NK, KIR and HLA-C

This hypothesis would explain the high incidence of pre-eclampsia in oocyte donation where the conceptus may possess HLA-C allotypes which are both in a different group from the mother. It could also theoretically explain the lack of concordance in twins as development of the disease would depend on the HLA-C of the fathers. There are striking differences in the frequency of both KIR haplotypes and HLA-C allotypes in different ethnic groups (Cook *et al.*, 2003; Vilches and Parham, 2002). Racial dissimilarity has been found to be associated with an increased risk of pre-eclampsia (Alderman *et al.*, 1986). More difficult to envisage is how the previous pregnancy is protective and, if true, how a change of partner may increase (or decrease) the risk in a subsequent pregnancy. How the expressed repertoire of KIR genes is acquired in decidua, why this repertoire is

different from that in circulating blood NK cells, and whether there could be any learning or memory for KIR are all questions to be addressed in the future.

T cell responses in pregnancy and pre-eclampsia

Viewing the fetus as an allograft drove reproductive immunologists to think like transplantation immunologists, who are mainly pre-occupied with suppression of recipient T cell responses to prevent rejection (Moffett and Loke, 2006). The idea that maternal T cells need to be suppressed during pregnancy has dominated research in reproduction. Is there any evidence for aberrations in maternal T cell responses in pre-eclampsia?

The main points of contact between the maternal immune system and the fetus are at two anatomical sites: the systemic immune response between maternal blood and syncytiotrophoblast, or the local immune response between maternal decidua and extravillous trophoblast (Loke and King, 1995). The syncytiotrophoblast is entirely devoid of expression of Major Histocompatibility Complex (MHC) antigens, the main polymorphic antigen system used by the immune system to recognize allogeneic cells. It is unlikely, therefore, that this tissue can provide a sufficient antigenic stimulus to the maternal systemic immune system. Indeed no antibodies or T cell responses directed at syncytiotrophoblast have ever been demonstrated.

When considering maternal systemic T cell responses during pregnancy, there are two potential sources of confusion. First, antibodies (and even occasionally cytotoxic T cells) to paternal HLA antigens are present in pregnancy. These are mainly directed at the classical HLA class I antigens, HLA-A and HLA-B, and, since these molecules are never expressed by trophoblast, these placental cells at the maternal–fetal interface cannot be the immunogenic source. These antibodies are found mainly in multips and are likely to be the result of sensitization by fetal cells crossing the placenta which occurs at delivery. Importantly, the presence or absence of these anti-paternal HLA antibodies has no correlation with pregnancy success and they have no role in pre-eclampsia.

The second source of confusion is the nature of T cell responses during pregnancy. CD4$^+$ Th cells differentiate into two subsets of effector cells (Th1 and Th2) which produce distinct sets of cytokines with different effector functions. The main cytokine produced by Th1 cells is IFN-γ whilst IL-4 and IL-5 define the Th2 subset (O'Garra, 1998). Th1 and Th2 cells develop from the same precursors, naïve Th0 CD4$^+$ cells, and the pattern of differentiation is determined by stimuli present locally during the early initiation of the immune response. These stimuli include IL-12 (Th1) and IL-4 (Th2) itself but other cytokines and hormones, particularly estrogen, progesterone and steroids also influence the pattern of T cell differentiation (Miyaura and Iwata, 2002; Piccini et al., 1995). Murine studies have demonstrated a shift in T cell responses during pregnancy toward Th2 (Krishnan et al., 1996a,b). In humans, the evidence is less convincing, although there are reports that where elimination of a pathogen requires a vigorous Th1-type response (e.g. chicken pox), the disease is far more severe in pregnancy. In addition, the severity of auto-immune diseases (e.g. SLE, multiple sclerosis and rheumatoid arthritis) can vary in pregnancy with either an improvement or exacerbation of symptoms. These clinical observations indicate that the nature of maternal T cell responses to all antigens (infections, self or fetal) may deviate toward Th2 differentiation probably due to the dramatic changes in hormonal stimuli during pregnancy (Kim et al., 1999; Ostensen, 1999). It is important to note that this Th2 deviation is not essential for pregnancy as mice deficient in all Th2 cytokines reproduce successfully (Fallon et al., 2002; Svensson et al., 2001).

Some experimental studies on circulating T cells during normal pregnancy have suggested that a shift toward Th2 cell differentiation does occur (Holmes et al., 2003; Suzuki et al., 2002), although not all aspects of Th2/Th1 responses are affected, for example IL-12 production by monocytes was found to be unaltered (Sacks et al., 2003). In pre-eclampsia an imbalance in the Th1/Th2 ratio has been proposed with deviation toward Th1 responses rather than the normal pregnancy Th2 differentiation (Darmochwal-Kolarz et al., 2002; Rein et al., 2002; Saito et al., 1999; Yoneyama et al., 2002). However, this seems more likely to be a component of the excessive inflammatory response seen in pre-eclamptic pregnancy (Redman and Sargent, 2003). These systemic inflammatory changes are part of the tertiary systemic stage of the disease and are not related to placentation. It is clear that it is premature to conclude that failure to deviate toward Th2 responses plays any part in the primary pathogenesis of pre-eclampsia.

The other main point of contact is between the maternal decidua and EVT. T cells are also present in the early decidua in close proximity to trophoblast cells which express one polymorphic HLA class I molecule, HLA-C. Other polymorphic genes may also be expressed by trophoblast and could, in the context of transplantation, be considered as minor histocompatibility antigens. In the transplant situation the responding T cells can respond *directly* or *indirectly* to the polymorphic antigens of the donor. In *direct* presentation, the donor cells express HLA molecules and are thus Antigen Presenting Cells (APC) (Gould and Auchincloss, 1999). The recipient T cell recognizes unprocessed allogeneic MHC molecules on the donor APC. As extravillous trophoblast cells only express one polymorphic HLA class I molecule and never express HLA class II molecules, this mechanism is unlikely to be very important. In *indirect* presentation allogeneic MHC molecules are taken up and processed by recipient APC so the processed peptides are presented to recipient T cells in the context of self MHC. In the decidua, maternal dendritic cells and HLA-DR$^+$ macrophages would fulfill this role. To generate an immune response they would mature and migrate to regional lymph modes where trophoblast-specific CTL and antibody-producing B cells would be generated, and subsequently migrate back to the site of the antigenic stimulus. The observation that there is a paucity of T cells at the implantation site and an almost complete absence of B cells would suggest that the local decidual T cells and B cells have not been activated by extravillous trophoblast.

The reasons for this are, as yet, unknown, but there are likely to be several overlapping mechanisms to prevent decidual T cell activation. For example, the type of dendritic cells present in decidua and the microenvironment are likely to induce a tolerogenic rather than an immunogenic signal to the T cells (Gardner and Moffett, 2003). Local tryptophan concentrations in the decidua may be low due to catabolism by indoleamine 2,3-dioxygenase (IDO) and tryptophan is an essential amino acid for T cell proliferation (Mellor and Munn, 2003). As yet there is no evidence that any derangement of decidual T cell function occurs in pre-eclampsia.

Conclusion

The original self/non-self paradigm has always provided the framework with which to view the problem of the fetal allograft. Since then, other models have been proposed to explain how the immune system operates to maintain the integrity of the host. These include: self/infectious non-self model where germ-line encoded receptors recognize pathogen-associated molecular patterns (PAMPs) (Janeway, 1992); the Missing Self hypothesis where leukocyte activation is prevented by inhibitory receptors for ligands on normal healthy cells (Karre et al., 1986); and the Danger Hypothesis where immune cells discern tissue damage (Matzinger, 1994). Although some insights can be gained in examining these models in the context of the uterine–placental interaction, none of them are really appropriate because the interface

between trophoblast cells and decidual leukocytes is unique (Moffett and Loke, 2004). Any immunological mechanisms which might be responsible for the inadequate trophoblast-mediated transformation of vessels must explain how decidual leukocytes recognize and respond to the trophoblast with memory and partner-specificity. The effector mechanisms must result in neither rejection nor parasitism, but provide a balanced co-existence of the two different individuals.

There are only two types of leukocytes which are known to be capable of allorecognition – T cells and NK cells. As discussed in this chapter, there is no evidence that decidual T cells can recognize EVT and are activated in either normal or abnormal pregnancy. However, the dominant population of decidual NK cells do express receptors (KIR) which can distinguish between two groups of HLA-C allotypes and are potentially capable of NK allorecognition during pregnancy. As both KIR and HLA-C are polymorphic, it is possible that certain combinations will prove unfavorable to successful placentation. In this way two polymorphic gene systems which segregate independently may influence reproductive success. The cumulative evidence would seem to indicate that the NK cell system is more important than the T cell system in reproductive immunology and by extension may influence the pathogenesis of pre-eclampsia.

REFERENCES

Abdalla, H. I., Billett, A., Kan, A. K., et al. (1998). Obstetric outcome in 232 ovum donation pregnancies. Br. J. Obstet. Gynaecol., **105**, 332–7.

Adams, E. M. and Finlayson, A. (1961). Familial aspects of preeclampsia and hypertension in pregnancy. Lancet, **2**, 1357.

Alderman, B. W., Sperling, R. S. and Daling, J. R. (1986). An epidemiological study of the immunogenetic aetiology of pre-eclampsia. Br. Med. J., **292**, 372–4.

Aldrich, C., Verp, M. S., Walker, M. A. and Ober, C. (2000). A null mutation in HLA-G is not associated with preeclampsia or intrauterine growth retardation. J. Reprod. Immunol., **47**, 41–8.

Basso, O., Christiansen, K. and Olsen, J. (2001). Higher risk of pre-eclampsia after change of partner. An effect of longer interpregnancy intervals? *Epidemiology*, **12**, 624–9.

Bermingham, J., Jenkins, D., McCarthy, T. and O'Brien, M. (2000). Genetic analysis of insulin-like growth factor II and HLA-G in pre-eclampsia. *Biochem. Soc. Trans.*, **28**, 215–19.

Boks, D. E. and Braat, D. D. (1997). Pregnancy following oocyte donation. *Ned. Tijdschr. Geneeskd.*, **141**, 1641–3.

Carrington, M. and Norman, P. J. (2003). *The KIR Gene Cluster*, Vol. 2003, National Library of Medicine (US), National Center for Biotechnology Information, Bethesda, MD.

Cincotta, R. B. and Brennecke, S. P. (1998). Family history of pre-eclampsia as a predictor for pre-eclampsia in primigravidas. *Int. J. Gynaecol. Obstet.*, **60**, 23–7.

Colonna, M., Spies, T., Strominger, J. L., *et al.* (1992). Alloantigen recognition by two human natural killer cell clones is associated with HLA-C or a closely linked gene. *Proc. Natl Acad. Sci. USA*, **89**, 7983–5.

Colonna, M., Brooks, E. G., Falco, M., Ferrara, G. B. and Strominger, J. L. (1993). Generation of allospecific natural killer cells by stimulation across a polymorphism of HLA-C. *Science*, **260**, 1121–4.

Cook, M. A., Moss, P. A. and Briggs, D. C. (2003). The distribution of 13 killer-cell immunoglobulin-like receptor loci in UK blood donors from three ethnic groups. *Eur. J. Immunogen.*, **30**, 213–21.

Cross, J. (2003). The genetics of pre-eclampsia: a feto-placental or maternal problem? *Clin. Genet.*, **64**, 96–103.

Darmochwal-Kolarz, D., Rolinski, J., Leszczynska-Goarzelak, B. and Oleszczuk, J. (2002). The expressions of intracellular cytokines in the lymphocytes of preeclamptic patients. *Am. J. Reprod. Immunol.*, **48**, 381–6.

Dekker, G. (2002). The partner's role in the etiology of preeclampsia. *J. Reprod. Immunol.*, **57**, 203–15.

Dekker, G. A., Robillard, P. Y. and Hulsey, T. C. (1998). Immune maladaptation in the etiology of preeclampsia: a review of corroborative epidemiologic studies. *Obstet. Gynecol. Surv.*, **53**, 377–82.

Eskenazi, B., Fenster, L. and Sidney, S. (1991). A multivariate analysis of risk factors for preeclampsia. *J. Am. Med. Ass.*, **266**, 237–41.

Esplin, M. S., Fausett, M. B., Fraser, A., *et al.* (2001). Paternal and maternal components of the predisposition to preeclampsia. *N. Engl. J. Med.*, **344**, 867–72.

Fallon, P. G., Jolin, H. E., Smith, P., *et al.* (2002). IL-4 induces characteristic Th2 responses even in the combined absence of IL-5, IL-9 and IL-13. *Immunity*, **17**, 7–17.

Feeney, J. G. and Scott, J. S. (1980). Pre-eclampsia and changed paternity. *Eur. J. Obstet. Gynecol. Reprod. Biol.*, **11**, 35–8.

Gardner, L. and Moffett, A., (2003). Dendritic cells in the human decidua. *Biol. Reprod.*, **69**, 1438–46.

Giebel, S., Locatelli, F., Lamparelli, T., *et al.* (2003). Survival advantage with KIR ligand incompatibility in hematopoietic stem cell transplantation from unrelated donors. *Blood*, **102**, 814–19.

Gould, D. S. and Auchincloss, H. (1999). Direct and indirect recognition: the role of MHC antigens in graft rejection. *Immunol. Today*, **20**, 77–82.

Hiby, S. E., King, A., Sharkey, A. and Loke, Y. W. (1999). Molecular studies of trophoblast HLA-G: polymorphisms, isoforms, imprinting and expression in preimplantation embryo. *Tissue Antigens*, **53**, 1–13.

Hiby, S. E., Walker, J. J., O'Shaughnessy, K. M., Redman, C. W., Carrington, M., Trowsdale, J. and Moffett, A. (2004). Combination of maternal KIR and fetal HLA-C genes influence the risk of preeclampsia and reproductive success. *J. Exp. Med.*, **200**, 957–65.

Holmes, V. A., Wallace, J. M., Gilmore, W. S., McFaul, P. and Alexander, H. D. (2003). Plasma levels of the immunomodulatory cytokine interleukin-10 during normal human pregnancy: a longitudinal study. *Cytokine*, **21**, 265–9.

Hoy, J., Venn, A., Halliday, J., Kovacs, G. and Waalwyk, K. (1999). Perinatal and obstetric outcomes of donor insemination using cryopreserved semen in Victoria, Australia. *Hum. Reprod.*, **14**, 1760–4.

Humphrey, K. E., Harrison, G. A., Cooper, D. W., Wilton, A. N., Brennecke, S. P. and Trudinger, B. J. (1995). HLA-G deletion polymorphism and pre-eclampsia/eclampsia. *Br. J. Obstet. Gynaecol.*, **102**, 707–10.

Janeway, C. A. (1992). The immune system evolved to discriminate infectious nonself from non-infectious self. *Immunol. Today*, **13**, 11–16.

Karre, K. (2002). Immunology. A perfect mismatch. *Science*, **295**, 2029–31.

Karre, K., Ljunggren, H. G., Piontek, G. and Kiessling, R. (1986). Selective rejection of H-2 deficient lymphoma variants suggests alternative immune defence strategy. *Nature*, **319**, 675–8.

Kim, S., Liva, S. M., Dalal, M. A., Verity, M. A. and Voskuhl, R. R. (1999). Estriol ameliorates autoimmune demyelinating disease: implications for multiple sclerosis. *Neurology*, **52**, 1230–8.

King, A., Boocock, C., Sharkey, A. M., *et al.* (1996). Evidence for the expression of HLA-C class I mRNA and protein by human first trimester trophoblast. *J. Immunol.*, **156**, 2068–76.

King, A., Allan, D. S., Bowen, M., *et al.* (2000a). HLA-E is expressed on trophoblast and interacts with CD94/NKG2 receptors on decidual NK cells. *Eur. J. Immunol.*, **30**, 1623–31.

King, A., Burrows, T. D., Hiby, S. E., *et al.* (2000b). Surface expression of HLA-C antigen by human extravillous trophoblast. *Placenta*, **21**, 376–87.

Klonoff-Cohen, H. S., Savitz, D. A., Cefalo, R. C. and McCann, M. F. (1989). An epidemiologic study of contraception and preeclampsia. *J. Am. Med. Ass.*, **262**, 3143–7.

Krishnan, L., Guilbert, L. J., Wegmann, T. G., Belosevic, M. and Mosmann, T. R. (1996a). T helper 1 response against *Leishmania major* in pregnant C57BL/6 mice increases implantation failure and fetal resorptions. Correlation with increased IFN-gamma and TNF and reduced IL-10 production by placental cells. *J. Immunol.*, **156**, 653–62.

Krishnan, L., Guilbert, L. J., Russell, A. S., Wegmann, T. G., Mosmann, T. R. and Belosevic, M. (1996b). Pregnancy impairs resistance of C57BL/6 to *Leishmania major* infection and causes decreased antigen-specific IFN-gamma response and increased production of T helper 2 cytokines. *J. Immunol.*, **156**, 644–52.

Lanier, L. L. (1998). NK cell receptors. *Ann. Rev. Immunol.*, **16**, 359–93.

Li, D. K. and Wi, S. (2000). Changing paternity and the risk of preeclampsia/eclampsia in the subsequent pregnancy. *Am. J. Epidemiol.*, **151**, 57–62.

Lie, R. T., Rasmussen, S., Brunborg, H., Gjessing, H. K., Lie-Nielsen, E. and Irgens, L. M. (1998). Fetal and maternal contributions to risk of pre-eclampsia: population based study. *Br. Med. J.*, **316**, 1343–7.

Loke, Y. W. and King, A. (1995). *Human Implantation: Cell Biology and Immunology*. Cambridge: Cambridge University Press.

MacGillivray, I. (1958). Some observations on the incidence of preeclampsia. *Obstet. Gynaecol. Br. Emp.*, **65**, 536–9.

Marti, J. J. and Herrmann, U. (1977). Immunogestosis: a new etiologic concept of 'essential' EPH gestosis, with special consideration of the primigravid patient. *Am. J. Obstet. Gynecol.*, **128**, 489–93.

Martin, M. P., Nelson, G., Lee, J.-H., *et al.* (2002a). Susceptibility to psoriatic arthritis: influence of activating killer Ig-like receptor genes in the absence of specific HLA-C alleles. *J. Immunol.*, **169**, 2818–22.

Martin, M. P., Gao, X., Lee, J.-H., *et al.* (2002b). Epistatic interaction between KIR3DS1 and HLA-B delays the progression to AIDS. *Nature Genet.*, **31**, 429–34.

Matzinger, P. (1994). Tolerance, danger, and the extended family. *Ann. Rev. Immunol.*, **12**, 991–1045.

Mellor, A. L. and Munn, D. H. (2003). Tryptophan catabolism and regulation of adaptive immunity. *J. Immunol.*, **170**, 5809–13.

Miyaura, H. and Iwata, M. (2002). Direct and indirect inhibition of Th1 development by progesterone and glucocorticoids. *J. Immunol.*, **168**, 1087–94.

Moffett, A. and Loke, Y. W. (2004). The immunological paradox of pregnancy: a reappraisal. *Placenta*, **24**, 1–8.

Moffett, A. and Loke, Y. W. (2006). Immunology of placentation in eutherian mammals. *Nat. Rev. Immunol.*, **6**, 584–94.

Moffett-King, A. (2002). Natural killer cells and pregnancy. *Nature Rev. Immunol.*, **2**, 656–63.

Need, J. A., Bell, B., Meffin, E. and Jones, W. R. (1983). Pre-eclampsia in pregnancies from donor inseminations. *J. Reprod. Immunol.*, **5**, 329–38.

O'Garra, A. (1998). Cytokines induce the development of functionally heterogeneous T helper cell subsets. *Immunity*, **8**, 275–83.

Ostensen, M. (1999). Sex hormones and pregnancy in rheumatoid arthritis and systemic lupus erythematosus. *Annals N.Y. Acad. Sci.*, **876**, 131–43.

Parham, P. and McQueen, K. L. (2003). Alloreactive killer cells: hindrance and help for haematopoietic transplants. *Nature Rev. Immunol.*, **3**, 108–22.

Piccinni, M. P., Giudizi, M. G., Biagiotti, R., *et al.* (1995). Progesterone favors the development of human T helper cells producing Th2-type cytokines and promotes both IL-4 production and membrane CD30 expression in established Th1 cell clones. *J. Immunol.*, **155**, 128–33.

Redman, C. W. (1991). Current topic: pre-eclampsia and the placenta. *Placenta*, **12**, 301–8.

Redman, C. W. and Sargent, I. L. (2003). Pre-eclampsia, the placenta and the maternal systemic inflammatory response – a review. *Placenta*, **24**, S21–7.

Rein, D. T., Schondorf, T., Gohring, U. J., *et al.* (2002). Cytokine expression in peripheral blood lymphocytes indicates a switch to T(HELPER) cells in patients with preeclampsia. *J. Reprod. Immunol.*, **54**, 133–42.

Roberts, J. M. and Redman, C. W. (1993). Pre-eclampsia: more than pregnancy-induced hypertension. *Lancet*, **341**, 1447–51.

Roberts, J. M. and Lain, K. Y. (2002). Recent insights into the pathogenesis of pre-eclampsia. *Placenta*, **23**, 359–72.

Robillard, P.-Y., Hulsey, T. C., Perianin, J., Janky, E., Miri, E. H. and Papiernik, E. (1994). Association of pregnancy-induced hypertension with duration of sexual cohabitation before conception. *Lancet*, **344**, 973–5.

Robillard, P.-Y., Dekker, G. A. and Hulsey, T. C. (1998). Primipaternities in families: is the incidence of pregnancy-induced hypertensive disorders in multigravidas an anthropological marker of reproduction. *Austr. N. Zeal. J. Obstet. Gynecol.*, **38**, 284–7.

Sacks, G. P., Redman, C. W. and Sargent, I. L. (2003). Monocytes are primed to produce the Th1 type cytokine IL-12 in normal human pregnancy: an intracellular flow cytometric analysis of peripheral blood mononuclear cells. *Clin. Exp. Immunol.*, **131**, 490–7.

Saito, S., Umekage, H., Sakamoto, Y., *et al.* (1999). Increased T-helper-1-type immunity and decreased T-helper-2-type immunity in patients with preeclampsia. *Am. J. Reprod. Immunol.*, **41**, 297–306.

Salha, O., Sharma, V., Dada, T., *et al.* (1999). The influence of donated gametes on the incidence of hypertensive disorders of pregnancy. *Hum. Reprod.*, **14**, 2268–73.

Serhal, P. F. and Craft, I. L. (1989). Oocyte donation in 61 patients. *Lancet*, **1**, 1185–7.

Skjaerven, R., Wilcox, A. J. and Lie, R. T. (2002). The interval between pregnancies and the risk of preeclampsia. *N. Engl. J. Med.*, **346**, 33–8.

Soderstrom-Anttila, V., Tiitinen, A., Foudila, T. and Hovatta, O. (1998). Obstetric and perinatal outcome after oocyte donation: comparison with *in vitro* fertilization pregnancies. *Hum. Reprod.*, **13**, 483–90.

Sutherland, A., Cooper, D. W., Howie, P. W., Liston, W. A. and MacGillivray, I. (1981). The incidence of severe pre-eclampsia amongst mothers and mothers-in-law of pre-eclamptics and controls. *Br. J. Obstet. Gynaecol.*, **88**, 785–91.

Suzuki, S., Kuwajima, T., Yoneyama, Y., Sawa, R. and Araki, T. (2002). Maternal peripheral T-helper 1-type and T-helper 2-type immunity in non preeclamptic twin pregnancies. *Gynecol. Obstet. Invest.*, **53**, 140–3.

Svensson, L., Arvola, M., Sallstrom, M. A., Holmdahl, R. and Mattsson, R. (2001). The Th2 cytokines IL-4 and IL-10 are not crucial for the completion of allogeneic pregnancy in mice. *J. Reprod. Immun.*, **51**, 3–7.

Treloar, S. A., Cooper, D. W., Brennecke, S. P., Grehan, M. M. and Martin, N. G. (2001). An Australian twin study of the genetic basis of preeclampsia and eclampsia. *Am. J. Obstet. Gynecol.*, **184**, 374–81.

Trogstad, L. I., Eskild, A., Magnus, P., Samuelsen, S. O. and Nesheim, B. I. (2001). Changing paternity and time since last pregnancy; the impact on pre-eclampsia risk. A study of 547 238 women with and without previous pre-eclampsia. *Int. J. Epidemiol.*, **30**, 1317–22.

Trowsdale, J. (2001). Genetic and functional relationships between MHC and NK receptor genes. *Immunity*, **15**, 363–74.

Trupin, L. S., Simon, L. P. and Eskenazi, B. (1996). Change in paternity: a risk factor for preeclampsia in multiparas. *Epidemiology*, **7**, 240–4.

Tubbergen, P., Lachmeijer, A. M., Althuisius, S. M., Vlak, M. E., van Geijn, H. P. and Dekker, G. A. (1999). Change in paternity: a risk factor for pre-eclampsia in multiparous women? *J. Reprod. Immunol.*, **45**, 81–8.

Valiante, N. M., Uhrberg, M., Shilling, H. G., *et al.* (1997). Functionally and structurally distinct NK cell receptor repertoires in the peripheral blood of two human donors. *Immunity*, **7**, 739–51.

Verma, S., King, A. and Loke, Y. W. (1997). Expression of killer-cell inhibitory receptors on human uterine NK cells. *Eur. J. Immunol.*, **27**, 979–83.

Vilches, C. and Parham, P. (2002). KIR: diverse, rapidly evolving receptors of innate and adaptive immunity. *Ann. Rev. Immunol.*, **20**, 217–51.

Walker, J. J. (2000). Pre-eclampsia. *Lancet*, **356**, 1260–5.

Wang, J. X., Knottnerus, A.-M., Schuit, G., Norman, R. J., Chan, A. and Dekker, G. A. (2002). Surgically obtained sperm, and risk of gestational hypertension and pre-eclampsia. *Lancet*, **359**, 673–4.

Witt, C. S., Whiteway, J. M., Warren, H. S., *et al.* (2002). Alleles of the KIR2DL4 receptor and their lack of association with pre-eclampsia. *Eur. J. Immunol.*, **32**, 18–29.

Yawata, M., Yawata, N., Abi-Rached, L. and Parham, P. (2002). Variation within the human killer cell immunoglobulin-like receptor (KIR) gene family. *Criti. Rev. Immunol.*, **22**, 463–82.

Yoneyama, Y., Suzuki, S., Sawa, R., Yoneyama, K., Power, G. G. and Araki, T. (2002). Relation between adenosine and T-helper 1/T-helper 2 imbalance in women with preeclampsia. *Obstet. Gynaecol.*, **99**, 641–6.

7

Immunological factors and placentation: implications for pre-eclampsia

C. W. G. Redman and I. L. Sargent

In this chapter what constitutes a systemic inflammatory response is described. Evidence is presented that normal pregnancy evokes such a response and that pre-eclampsia arises when the response becomes extreme and decompensates. The possible causes of systemic inflammation in pregnancy are reviewed, as is the relation between the inflammatory response and systemic oxidative stress. The interaction between systemic inflammation and changes in lipid and glucose metabolism are described and the relevance of long-term systemic inflammation as a predisposing risk factor is outlined. It is suggested that the metabolic results of systemic inflammation may endow a survival advantage for the fetus. Last, the systemic inflammation is related to other immune responses that are thought to be important for the success or failure of pregnancy.

Immune and inflammatory responses

In evolutionary terms, inflammatory responses are older than immune responses. The latter are superimposed on the former and cannot work without it. The primitive innate (inflammatory) system responds quickly and is relatively non-specific. The more sophisticated adaptive immune system is slow but precise, delivering antigen-specific responses with astonishing versatility and accuracy. The innate and adaptive systems are asymmetrically interdependent. The innate system does not need the adaptive system to function, whereas the adaptive system cannot function

without signals from the innate system, nor need it provoke antibodies of antigen-specific cytotoxicity. This is a crucial consideration in relation to this chapter. A systemic inflammatory response is not necessarily generated by antigenic stimulation. In relation to normal and abnormal pregnancy it may not result, indeed almost certainly does not result, from antigenic stimulation by the genetically foreign fetus.

The adaptive immune system distinguishes self from non-self antigens and responds to the latter. The innate immune system responds, more widely, to "danger" signals (Matzinger, 2002) using a range of "pattern recognition receptors" that have evolved to respond in a wide but essentially stereotyped way. The danger signal may be external (from pathogens) or internal (from products of trauma, ischemia, necrosis or oxidative stress). When external stimuli activate inflammatory cells they release signals such as cytokines or chemokines that, in turn, attract and "instruct" adaptive immune cells (T or B lymphocytes) to generate antigen-specific responses from antibodies or cytotoxic cells. Hence the two systems, innate and adaptive, operate together and in sequence.

The inflammatory network

Inflammatory responses involve more than inflammatory leukocytes (granulocytes, macrophages and natural killer lymphocytes). Endothelial cells are major players. They have many of the receptors that activate innate immune responses, can present antigen to T cells after appropriate stimulation,

Table 7.1. Components of the inflammatory or innate immune system

Inflammatory leukocytes:
  Granulocytes
  Monocytes
  Natural killer lymphocytes
  Certain B cells producing "natural antibodies"
Endothelium
Platelets
Coagulation cascade
Complement system
Cytokines and chemokines
Adipocytes
Hepatocytes

Table 7.2. Danger signals that activate the innate (inflammatory) immune system

Stimulants of inflammation	Corresponding receptors
Bacterial products	Toll-like receptors
Products of oxidative stress	Scavenger receptors
Products of cell trauma	Toll-like and scavenger receptors
Thrombin	Protease-activated receptors
Heat shock proteins	Various
Soluble DNA	Toll-like receptor 9

produce pro-inflammatory cytokines and can stimulate, as well as be stimulated by, inflammatory leukocytes. Platelets and a variety of humoral components are also part of the process (Table 7.1). Other cells, such as hepatocytes and adipocytes that are not normally considered to be inflammatory, have key or central roles (see below). The innate immune response is therefore not simple. It contains many cross-regulating and synergistic pathways, which are not yet understood fully. The range of the inflammatory network may not be appreciated, nor the two-way interactions between its components. For example, blood coagulation is not only activated by inflammatory processes but thrombin, the final trigger to coagulation, also stimulates inflammation via specific receptors.

Receptors that activate inflammation are listed in Table 7.2. They include pattern recognition receptors that recognize conserved molecular structures, which comprise danger signals and scavenger receptors. The former include an important family of conserved structures called Toll-like receptors (TLRs) (Rock et al., 1998). As well as binding products largely derived from pathogenic bacteria they also recognize endogenous products of stress, trauma, oxidative stress or other responses to danger. These proteins signal danger through various receptors including scavenger and TLRs (Gallucci and Matzinger, 2001).

Systemic inflammation and the acute phase response

Inflammation may be local or systemic (generalized). The complete range of events stimulated by systemic inflammation is termed the acute phase response. The term is a misnomer because it includes acute and chronic changes. The response is not identical under all situations. It comprises alterations in circulating plasma protein concentrations as well as other phenomena such as fever, anemia, leukocytosis, and metabolic adaptations especially involving the liver and adipose tissue (Gabay and Kushner, 1999). Proteins linked to the acute phase response (acute phase proteins) are typically synthesized in the liver. They are classified as positive, that is increase with systemic inflammation, of which C-reactive protein is the best known, or negative which means that they decrease. Albumin is an example of the latter.

C-reactive protein (CRP) is the classical acute phase reactant. Circulating concentrations can increase within hours by several orders of magnitude in response to inflammatory stimuli. Human CRP binds with highest affinity to phosphocholine residues, but also to a variety of other intrinsic and extrinsic ligands, including native and modified plasma lipoproteins, damaged cell membranes, a number of different phospholipids and related compounds and small nuclear ribonucleoprotein

Table 7.3. Changes in concentrations of plasma proteins in the acute phase response

Proteins whose plasma concentrations increase

Proteinase inhibitors
  α_1-Antitrypsin, α_1-antichymotrypsin

Coagulation proteins
  Fibrinogen, prothrombin, factor VIII, plasminogen, plasminogen-activator inhibitor 1

Complement proteins
  C1s, C2, Factor B, C3, C4, C5, C1 inhibitor, mannose-binding lectin

Transport proteins
  Haptoglobin, hemopexin, caeruloplasmin

Participants in inflammatory responses
  Soluble phospholipase A2, interleukin-1-receptor antagonist, lipopolysaccharide binding protein

Miscellaneous
  CRP, serum amyloid A, fibronectin, ferritin, α_1-acid glycoprotein, Gc globulin, proteins whose plasma concentrations decrease

Miscellaneous
  Albumin, transferrin, insulin-like growth factor 1, transthyretin, HDL, LDL

particles. Extrinsic factors that bind to CRP include many constituents of microorganisms and plant products. Human CRP potently activates the classical complement pathway. It functions as a typical component of the innate immune system acting as a scavenger protein and responding to a range of "dangerous" molecules (Pepys and Hirschfield, 2003). Some acute phase proteins are listed in Table 7.3. In the mouse liver the acute phase response involves nearly 10% of the genome (Yoo and Desiderio, 2003), which indicates the enormous complexity and broad range of the response.

Systemic inflammation and oxidative stress

Oxidative stress is a disequilibrium between anti-oxidant defenses and production of reactive oxygen species in favor of the latter. Reactive oxygen species are toxic. Natural antioxidant mechanisms

have evolved to stop and so limit oxidative damage. The process is discussed in extended detail in the chapter by Raijmakers and Poston. The key feature which is central to this chapter is that oxidative stress and chronic inflammation are related, perhaps inseparable phenomena (Hensley et al., 2000). An inflammatory response generates oxidative stress. In a converse fashion, oxidative stress from other causes stimulates an inflammatory response. You cannot have one without the other. There are multiple reasons for this, including the fact that reactive oxygen species are used as second messengers in the inflammatory response.

Metabolism and the systemic inflammatory response

Systemic inflammation has complex effects on metabolism, of which many are stimulated by components of the acute phase response. Inflammatory responses, stimulated by endotoxin, TNF-α or other pro-inflammatory factors cause insulin resistance and hyperlipidemia. The hyperlipidemia of sepsis has been known for many years (Harris et al., 2001). TNF-α is an important mediator of these changes because it induces insulin resistance and inhibits lipogenesis while increasing lipolysis (Sethi and Hotamisligil, 1999). It inhibits proximal steps of insulin signaling in varying ways depending on cell type. Increased release of free fatty acids (FFAs) contributes also to the insulin resistance peripherally (Hirosumi et al., 2002). The catabolic state induced by TNF-α led to its early designation as cachectin (Beutler et al., 1985).

It is an apparent paradox that obesity is associated with a systemic inflammatory response involving TNF-α, a cytokine that induces cachexia among its other actions. A cluster of clinical features including obesity is variously called the metabolic syndrome, syndrome X or the insulin resistance syndrome (Isomaa, 2003). Components of the syndrome include insulin resistance, impaired glucose tolerance or overt diabetes, dyslipidemia and hypertension. The syndrome results from the fact that adipose tissue is not merely an energy store but a source of pro-inflammatory cytokines and other metabolic mediators. It is a major source of TNF-α, interleukin-6 (IL-6), leptin, a hormone that regulates appetite and energy expenditure, and plasminogen activator-1 (PAI-1). Thus there is a significant correlation between body mass index, circulating leptin and TNF-α and IL-6 in humans (Mantzoros et al., 1997). Leptin has pro-inflammatory actions as does TNF-α (Zarkesh-Esfahani et al., 2001). The net effect is that obesity is a state of chronic systemic inflammation. IL-6 induces the acute phase response, of which circulating C-reactive protein (CRP) is the classical example (Bastard et al., 2000; Yudkin et al., 1999). The importance of obesity in generating the inflammatory response is demonstrated by its reversal after weight loss (Ziccardi et al., 2002).

Systemic inflammation is accompanied by an increase in triglyceride-rich lipoproteins, a reduction in high-density lipoprotein cholesterol, and impairment of cholesterol transport. These metabolic alterations, which promote atherosclerosis, may explain an epidemiological link between chronic inflammation and cardiovascular disease (Hansson et al., 2002).

A master regulator of inflammation

Many aspects of the inflammatory response are coordinated by a single transcription factor, nuclear factor kappa-B (NF-κB). Genes that contain NF-κB binding elements include those for inflammatory cytokines, acute phase proteins and adhesion molecules (Haddad, 2002). There is uncertainty about the relationship between NF-κB and oxidative stress (Hayakawa et al., 2003; Li and Karin, 1999). Indirect activation by way of the inflammatory responses to lipid peroxides or other products of cell damage undoubtedly occurs (Hensley et al., 2000).

Normal pregnancy evokes a systemic inflammatory response

Normal pregnancy is associated with systemic inflammation. The changes are mild and do not imply that pregnant women are, in any sense, ill. Many features of pregnancy that are considered to be physiological are components of the acute phase response. They include increases in plasma fibrinogen (Gatti et al., 1994), plasminogen activator inhibitor 1 (Halligan et al., 1994) and complement component C3 (Schena et al., 1982). The intensity increases modestly as normal gestation advances. The classical acute phase reactant CRP has not been studied in detail during pregnancy. What little evidence there is points to a small significant increase in the circulation, which begins in the first trimester (Sacks et al., 2004). Leukocytosis is also already evident in the first trimester (Pitkin and Witte, 1979; Smarason et al., 1986).

The numbers of circulating neutrophils increase during normal pregnancy and the cells are activated (Rebelo et al., 1995). Phagocytosis (Barriga et al., 1994) and the chemiluminescent responses of polymorphonuclear leukocytes (PMN) after stimulation are increased (Shibuya et al., 1987). Circulating neutrophil elastase concentrations are significantly higher in normal pregnancy than in non-pregnant women (Greer et al., 1989). However, not all investigators agree that granulocytes are activated, with contrary findings in normal pregnancy (Crouch et al., 1995). Monocytes are also primed or activated (Sacks et al., 2003). The weight of evidence is overwhelmingly in favor of activation.

As pregnancy advances the systemic inflammatory response strengthens and peaks during the third trimester. It was not until the late 1990s that this concept was formally consolidated (Redman et al., 1999; Sacks et al., 1998).

Activation during pregnancy extends to lymphocytes and monocytes (Sacks et al., 1998). Other evidence comes from measures of circulating inflammatory cytokines. Because TNF-α has a short half-life, levels of its circulating soluble receptors are used as surrogate markers. By this indirect measure (Arntzen et al., 1995) or by direct assay, circulating TNF-α is increased in normal pregnancy (Melczer et al., 2003). Interleukin-6 is similarly increased (Austgulen et al., 1994). In summary, normal pregnancy can be viewed as a state of mild systemic inflammation complete with evidence for an acute phase reaction and activation of multiple components of the inflammatory network.

Given these findings it would be predicted that circulating inflammatory cells would display upregulation of the NF-κB system. Paradoxically, the opposite is found (McCracken et al., 2004).

Metabolic changes and the inflammatory response in normal pregnancy

The metabolic adaptations of systemic inflammation, namely an acute phase response (as discussed above), oxidative stress, hyperlipidemia and insulin resistance, also occur during normal pregnancy. Markers of oxidative stress (Morris et al., 1998; Zusterzeel et al., 2000) are increased at least in the third trimester. In normal pregnancy insulin resistance develops early and persists until delivery (Stanley et al., 1998). To some extent this parallels the development of systemic inflammation during pregnancy outlined above. Hypertriglyceridemia, as occurs in systemic inflammation, also becomes detectable in the second trimester (Martin et al., 1999). The cause of the insulin resistance is undecided (Hornnes, 1985). Recently the list of potential placental factors has been enlarged by the inclusion of human placental growth hormone (Barbour et al., 2002) and the discovery that the adipokine resistin, which causes insulin resistance, is also expressed in the human placenta, particularly by trophoblast (Yura et al., 2003). The fact that inflammatory responses themselves can engender insulin resistance raises the possibility that they contribute to the insulin resistance and ensuing metabolic changes of pregnancy.

The metabolic changes of the systemic inflammatory response may have survival advantages. It has been proposed (Haig, 1993) that the insulin resistance of normal pregnancy could divert maternal glucose to meet the needs of the fetus and that this may represent fetal–maternal genetic conflict. Indeed there is evidence that this diversion does occur (Arkwright et al., 1993).

The systemic inflammatory response in normal pregnancy is not a form of immune rejection

It is important to appreciate, especially in the context of the remarks above about the relation between innate and adaptive immunity, that these responses do not imply that there is some form of alloimmune recognition of the fetus with either antigen-specific tolerance or conversely immune rejection. The key issue is that the major interface between mother and fetus, the syncytiotrophoblast, expresses no known polymorphic major histocompatibility (HLA) antigens. It is possible that it secretes a soluble isotype of the HLA-G, the non-classical histocompatibility molecule that is specifically confined to trophoblast (Blaschitz et al., 2001). However, there are no important allelic variants of HLA-G. Histocompatibility antigens are the targets for immune rejection which is executed by cytotoxic T cells. Since the placental hemochorial surface is a syncytium, it is problematic to envisage how it could be susceptible to cytolytic attack from single T cells, since this huge unicellular layer would be too large. However, the concept of maternal immune rejection of the "foreign" fetus continues to be developed. In mouse pregnancy this may be appropriate. In human pregnancy there is, so far, remarkably little direct evidence that such a process can occur. Current concepts are focused on the phenomenon of T cell differentiation into two sorts of helper cells: type 1 (Th1) and type 2 (Th2). Th1 cells characteristically secrete interferon gamma (IFNγ) and promote antigen-specific cell-mediated immunity (cytotoxicity), whereas Th2 cells are distinguished by interleukin-4 (IL-4) production and can stimulate the development of humoral immunity (antibodies). Graft rejection is a type 1 phenomenon. The hypothesis, first proposed by Wegmann and colleagues (1993), has been that Th1 responses are suppressed in normal pregnancy to avoid immune rejection of the fetus. There is some evidence of such regulation in human pregnancy in that Th1 activity is partially suppressed (Marzi *et al.*, 1996; Sacks *et al.*, 2003), but that is as far as the concept goes. In the absence of a placental target for maternal T cells it is not possible at the moment to see the relevance of this mechanism. It is now believed that the Th1/Th2 paradigm has served its purpose and should be superseded to take account of rapidly expanding knowledge of the complexity of the interactions between the innate and adaptive immune systems (Chaouat, 2003).

The inflammatory (innate) immune system can be activated in several ways which do not depend on activated antigen-specific T cells. It is not known how normal pregnancy provokes a mild maternal systemic response. That it arises from the placenta is self-evident. As already mentioned, it appears to be heralded in the luteal phase of the menstrual cycle before the placenta exists. Systemic inflammatory changes can be detected in the luteal phase (Willis *et al.*, 2003). Furthermore, it has long been known that body temperature rises (an effect of systemic inflammation) at this time, and that after successful conception this is sustained until the uteroplacental circulation develops. This issue is elaborated in more detail below in relation to pre-eclampsia.

Pre-eclampsia is associated with a more extreme systemic inflammatory response than occurs in normal pregnancy

In other chapters the clinical nature of pre-eclampsia is described. It must be borne in mind that it has to be recognized as a syndrome, a cluster of features that together define the disorder. All current definitions arise from consensus, not an understanding of the pathogenesis of pre-eclampsia. In clinical terms the disease presents in an extraordinarily variable way: varying in time of onset, speed of progression, degree to which the mother or fetus or both are endangered and the pattern of maternal organ involvement. The diversity of the features of the maternal syndrome could not be explained until it was proposed that they arise from the sum of the circulatory disturbances caused by systemic maternal endothelial cell dysfunction or activation (Roberts *et al.*, 1989). Subsequent work from many investigators strengthened the hypothesis. Pathological alterations in the endothelium can be seen in the kidney as glomerular endotheliosis (Gaber *et al.*, 1994). Comparable endothelial pathology is evident in other organs (Barton *et al.*, 1991; Shanklin and Sibai, 1989).

As a result of the work described by Sacks *et al.* (1998) and its interpretation in the context of other findings, some of them relatively old (Redman *et al.*, 1999), the endothelial theory of pre-eclampsia can now be expanded by placing the endothelium in its larger context as part of the inflammatory network. Activated leukocytes will activate endothelium, and vice versa (Zimmerman *et al.*, 1992). Hence it is inevitable that, on average, all the markers of inflammation that are already changed in normal pregnancy (see above) are more severely affected in pre-eclampsia (Table 7.4). The inflammatory changes may progress to the point of decompensation, giving one or other of the well-known crises of the condition.

It is a new concept that the systemic inflammatory response of pre-eclampsia is not different from that of normal pregnancy, except that it is more severe. Hence we have proposed that pre-eclampsia develops when the systemic inflammatory process, common to all women in the second half of their pregnancies, causes one or other maternal system to decompensate (Redman *et al.*, 1999). In other words, the disorder is not a separate condition but simply the extreme end of a continuum of maternal systemic inflammatory responses engendered by pregnancy itself.

Table 7.4. The systemic inflammatory network is stimulated in pre-eclampsia relative to normal pregnancy

*Leukocytosis	Terrone *et al.*, 2000
*Increased leukocyte activation	Sacks *et al.*, 1998
*Complement activation	Haeger *et al.*, 1989
*Activation of the clotting system	Perry and Martin, 1992
*Activation of platelets	Konijnborg *et al.*, 1997
*Markers of endothelial activation	Taylor *et al.*, 1991
*Markers of oxidative stress	Gratacos *et al.*, 1998
*Hypertriglyceridemia	Hubel *et al.*, 1996
	Lorentzen *et al.*, 1995
*Increased circulating pro-inflammatory cytokines	
Tumor necrosis factor-α	Vince *et al.*, 1995
	Kupferminc *et al.*, 1994
	Teran *et al.*, 2001
⊥Interleukin-6	Vince *et al.*, 1995
	Conrad *et al.*, 1998
	Greer *et al.*, 1994
⊥Interleukin-8	Stallmach *et al.*, 1995
	Ellis *et al.*, 2001

*Significant change(s) relative to normal non-pregnant women.
⊥Not all authors agree, see text.
There are usually multiple references to justify each change.

This concept has profound implications for prediction, screening, studies of genetic susceptibility or treatment, and can explain why pre-eclampsia is impossible to distinguish clearly, in terms of any definition, diagnostic test or pathological lesion from normal pregnancy. Even the renal glomerular lesion of endotheliosis has now been found in an early form in biopsies from totally normal women (Strevens *et al.*, 2003). The old view that systemic inflammation equates with sepsis, and sepsis causes profound hypotension, seems contrary to the idea that systemic inflammation can be associated with hypertension. However, it is accepted that the endothelium (which is part of the inflammatory system) is the final controller of the microcirculation and is a potential source of potent vasoconstrictors such as endothelin-1 or thromboxane-A2. A number of more recent studies have shown how pro-inflammatory stimuli can impair endothelial dependent relaxation (Eiserich *et al.*, 2002). The hypotension of sepsis represents complete failure of vascular homeostasis. A rat model of pre-eclampsia depends on using a classical pro-inflammatory stimulus, a single administration of endotoxin to pregnant rats at 14 days. This causes hypertension and proteinuria, which persist until the end of pregnancy. The same dose has no effect on non-pregnant animals (Faas *et al.*, 1994). Infusion of the pro-inflammatory cytokine, TNF-α, provokes systemic hypertension but only in pregnant and not in non-pregnant rats (Alexander *et al.*, 2002). These are direct demonstrations of how systemic inflammation can cause hypertension and the features of pre-eclampsia. Sepsis is also associated with fever, which is not considered to be a feature of pre-eclampsia. However, fever occurs significantly more often in pre-eclamptic women during labor, even after adjustment for confounding factors (Impey *et al.*, 2001).

In terms of adaptive immunity, type 1 responses are not suppressed to the same degree in pre-eclampsia as they are in normal pregnancy (Saito *et al.*, 1999). Some interpret this observation, which has been confirmed by others (Rein *et al.*, 2002; Sakai *et al.*, 2002), to indicate activation of a partial maternal alloimmune rejection of the fetus, but there is little evidence to support this hypothesis and none for allospecific immune rejection mechanisms. Hence, the working model is that since pregnancy stimulates systemic inflammation, there are mechanisms (largely undefined) that regulate its expression (Sacks *et al.*, 1999), such that homeostasis is preserved, possibly by placental production of type 2 cytokines that induce a bias to type 2 innate immune activity. Our recent evidence is that it is peripheral blood NK cells (which are lymphocytes with primarily innate immune characteristics) and not T cells that are the main participants in the type 1/type 2 immune balance in pregnancy and pre-eclampsia, with reversion to a type 1 response in pre-eclampsia (Borzychowski *et al.*, 2005).

Pre-eclampsia, oxidative stress and other metabolic changes

Pre-eclampsia is associated with increased markers of oxidative stress in placental tissue, as described in the chapter by Raijmakers and Poston. As already mentioned, inflammation and oxidative stress are closely related. The oxidative stress of pre-eclampsia is not localized to the placenta but disseminated in the maternal circulation (Hubel, 1998) and is an expected part of the systemic inflammatory response. Just as normal pregnancy is associated with increased circulating markers of oxidative stress, the more intense systemic inflammatory response of pre-eclampsia is matched by evidence for greater systemic oxidative stress (Hubel, 1998; Wickens *et al.*, 1981). Of great clinical relevance is the fact that anti-oxidants, including the anti-oxidant vitamins that have a potential use in preventing pre-eclampsia, also have anti-inflammatory actions (Hensley *et al.*, 2000).

There is no agreement about the occurrence in pre-eclampsia of the other metabolic changes that have been associated with systemic inflammation. There is modest evidence for a more intense acute phase response which, with respect to some markers, for example caeruloplasmin (Vitoratos *et al.*, 1999), complement proteins C3 and Factor B (Johansen *et al.*, 1981; Tedder *et al.*, 1975) is more marked than in normal pregnancy. Serum CRP may be elevated (Teran *et al.*, 2001), but there is difficulty in separating the changes due to pre-eclampsia to the chronic changes associated with risk features such as obesity. Some can find evidence of insulin resistance in pre-eclampsia (Kaaja *et al.*, 1999), others cannot (Roberts *et al.*, 1998). As with measures of serum CRP, it is a concern whether the changes are specific to the woman or to the pregnancy. The fact that the insulin resistance may persist for long periods after

delivery (Nisell *et al.*, 1999) suggests the possibility that they may be constitutional attributes of the woman rather than a specific feature of pre-eclampsia.

The role of the placenta

It has been known for nearly 100 years that pre-eclampsia is a placental condition (Holland, 1909; Redman, 1991). Other workers have clarified that an important placental pathology is an insufficient uteroplacental circulation leading to placental hypoxia, oxidative stress and, in the most severe cases, infarction (described in the chapter by Pijnenborg).

The question of how the placental problem becomes a generalized maternal problem needs to be considered. One or several undefined placental factors, which we have previously denoted "factor X" (Redman, 1992), must circulate to cause the maternal disorder. There are two aspects to consider. What is the relevant placental function, and how does this translate into systemic dysfunction? The stimulus should originate in the placenta, must be released during all pregnancies to account for the systemic inflammatory response encountered in normal pregnant women, and be atypically large when the placenta is oxidatively stressed. There are three interrelated possibilities: dissemination of growth factors, their soluble regulators or inflammatory cytokines released by syncytiotrophoblast or, second, placental oxidative stress or, last, placental debris.

The strongest candidate so far is the soluble receptor for vascular endothelial growth factor (VEGFR-1), also known as sFlt-1, which inhibits the actions of VEGF (Kendall *et al.*, 1996). sFlt-1 is synthesized and released by endothelial cells and peripheral blood monocytes (Barleon *et al.*, 2001). VEGF is an important survival factor for endothelium so systemic inhibition would be expected to cause generalized endothelial dysfunction. This has been confirmed in human and animal studies. Clinical trials of a neutralizing monoclonal antibody to VEGF for the treatment of metastatic colorectal or renal cancer have shown that hypertension and proteinuria are the commonest side effects (Kabbinavar *et al.*, 2003; Yang *et al.*, 2003). Likewise, the infusion of sFlt-1 into rats (Maynard *et al.*, 2003) causes these signs to appear. In the latter study the associated glomerular lesions were the same as those seen specifically in preeclampsia (Pollak and Nettles, 1960). Serum-soluble flt-1 is increased in pre-eclampsia (Maynard *et al.*, 2003). Because it is complexed to VEGF, its high levels in pre-eclampsia can explain the variable reports of changes of plasma VEGF in this condition. If total VEGF is measured it is increased, whereas if only free VEGF is assayed it is reduced. The origin of the circulating sFlt-1 is presumed to be the placenta, although this has not yet been directly demonstrated (Clark *et al.*, 1998; Maynard *et al.*, 2003). The most compelling evidence is its rapid decline in concentration after delivery (Maynard *et al.*, 2003). If soluble Flt-1 were the main cause of pre-eclampsia this could explain the paradoxical protective effect of cigarette smoking on the occurrence of pre-eclampsia (Zabriskie, 1963). Non-pregnant cigarette smokers have lower levels of circulating sFlt-1 than controls who do not smoke (Belgore *et al.*, 2000). The fact that fetuses with trisomy 13 are particularly likely to provoke pre-eclampsia in their mothers (Boyd *et al.*, 1987) is consistent with the location of the gene for soluble flt-1 on chromosome 13 (Barr *et al.*, 1991).

How does this link to the model that is presented here? The most direct attempt to chart the sources of soluble Flt-1 in the human pregnancy showed that it is predominantly produced by extravillous trophoblast in the decidua and by endothelial and stromal cells in the chorionic villi, but not by the villous trophoblast (Clark *et al.*, 1998). Villous explants release sFlt-1 into the culture supernatant in significantly greater amounts when cultured under hypoxic conditions (Ahmed *et al.*, 2000), which is consistent with the view that placental hypoxia is an important part of the pathogenesis. The fact that it is also released by endothelium and monocytes (Barleon *et al.*, 2001) suggests an

alternative possible source of this factor. In non-pregnant individuals, chronic medical conditions that are associated with mild systemic inflammatory responses yield conflicting findings with sFlt-1 measured as increased (Belgore *et al.*, 2001) or decreased (Felmeden *et al.*, 2003). It is likely that sFlt-1 is a relevant placental factor in the direct causation of the features of pre-eclampsia.

It is possible that syncytiotrophoblast could synthesize and release excessive amounts of pro-inflammatory cytokines. However, an analysis of production from chorionic villous explants failed to show increases in TNF-α, IL-6, IL-α and IL-1β (Benyo *et al.*, 2001) when tissues from pre-eclamptic and normal pregnancies were compared. Thus, there is no convincing evidence that the pre-eclampsia placenta disseminates inflammatory cytokines into the maternal circulation.

Dissemination may also involve oxidative stress and the disseminators may be inflammatory leukocytes themselves exposed to oxidatively altered trophoblast in the intervillous space. Leukocytes in the uterine vein are significantly activated relative to those in the peripheral circulation in pre-eclampsia. Transient hypoxia in the intervillous space could account for at least some of the observed changes (Mellembakken *et al.*, 2002).

Cellular, subcellular and molecular debris from the syncytial surface of the placenta is shed into the maternal circulation. We have proposed that its clearance comprises the systemic inflammatory stimulus in normal and pre-eclamptic pregnancies. Such debris is detected in the plasma of normal pregnant women but in significantly increased amounts in pre-clampsia and is probably the product of syncytial apoptosis and necrosis (Redman and Sargent, 2000).

The placental villi of the pre-eclamptic woman are characterized by focal syncytial necrosis, with loss and distortion of microvilli (Jones and Fox, 1980). However, necrosis is not a marked feature of normal placentas and is therefore unlikely to cause the release of the circulating syncytial debris found in normal pregnancies

programmed cell death. Distinct from necrosis in which uncontrolled cell death leads to lysis of cells (inflammatory responses and potential serious health probs

near term. The debris includes syncytiotrophoblast microparticles (Knight et al., 1998), which are the hallmark of apoptosis (Aupeix et al., 1997). Apoptosis of normal human syncytiotrophoblast results in characteristic features including loss of microvilli and blebbing of the surface membrane (Nelson, 1996). It has been proposed that apoptosis plays a central role in turnover of cytotrophoblast and renewal of the syncytial surface of chorionic villi (Huppertz et al., 1998). Apoptosis rates are significantly increased in the syncytiotrophoblast in pre-eclampsia (Ishihara et al., 2002). It is also known that in vitro hypoxia induces apoptosis of cultured human cytotrophoblasts (Levy et al., 2000). Hence, if syncytiotrophoblast microparticles were derived from apoptotic processes, then the observation that more circulates in pre-eclampsia may be related to the degree of apoptosis in, and shedding from, the syncytiotrophoblast. The argument is strengthened by the increased concentrations, in pre-eclampsia, of other circulating markers of syncytial debris including cytokeratin (Schrocksnadel et al., 1993) and soluble fetal DNA (Lo et al., 1999). At the other end of the spectrum is the evidence for increased shedding of syncytial cells (Johansen et al., 1999), a process long known as trophoblast deportation.

Shedding of debris from the syncytial surface would be expected to increase in two situations. The first is with increased placental size. Pre-eclampsia is predominantly a disorder of the third trimester, when the placenta reaches its greatest size. The placenta grows larger with multiple pregnancies, which also increase the likelihood of pre-eclampsia. The second would be associated with placental oxidative stress, as with the most severe pre-eclampsia, typically of early onset and associated with intense fetal growth retardation. The placentas are usually abnormally small. Here, it must be presumed that there is an alteration in the quality of the inflammatory stimulus generated by the placenta, for example, by its content of peroxidized lipids (Cester et al., 1994).

The current evidence is that circulating placental debris is likely to be an important part of the systemic inflammatory stimulus associated with both normal and pre-eclamptic pregnancies. We have shown that they are directly damaging to endothelium (Smarason et al., 1993) which is stimulated to release pro-inflammatory substances (von Dadelszen et al., 1999). Our preliminary evidence is that they are directly pro-inflammatory (Sacks et al., unpublished observations; Branton et al., unpublished observations). It is possible that it is this circulating debris which is the danger signal of pregnancy to which the inflammatory system responds appropriately.

Maternal predisposing factors

Some medical conditions are well known to predispose to pre-eclampsia, including obesity (Ros et al., 1998), diabetes (Garner et al., 1990) and chronic hypertension (Sibai et al., 1995). Low grade systemic inflammation is a feature of all these conditions in men or non-pregnant women. It also is evident in chronic arterial disease such as ischemic heart disease (Hansson et al., 2002). For example, elevated circulating C-reactive protein is as important a risk factor for chronic arterial disease as circulating cholesterol (Ridker, 2001). Arterial disease and chronic hypertension are closely associated, and the latter is also associated with a systemic inflammatory response. Angiotensin II and endothelin-I, both potent vasoconstrictors, are pro-inflammatory (Luft, 2002), and chronic hypertension is also a state of systemic inflammation (Dalekos et al., 1996).

Hyperglycemia stimulates a systemic inflammatory response (Esposito et al., 2002) as does both type 1 (Lechleitner et al., 2000) and type 2 diabetes (Pickup et al., 2000). Type 2 diabetes is strongly associated with increased insulin resistance, chronic hypertension, disordered lipid regulation and obesity, which is Syndrome X (Ukkola and Bouchard, 2001), as described earlier in this chapter. Hence these various chronic conditions are strongly interrelated.

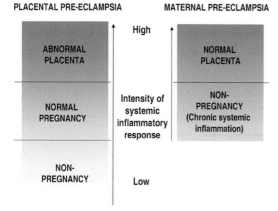

PLACENTAL PRE-ECLAMPSIA   MATERNAL PRE-ECLAMPSIA

Figure 7.1 Placental and maternal pre-eclampsia.
A hypothetical gray scale of increasing systemic
inflammation is shown. In a completely normal woman,
although normal pregnancy stimulates a systemic
inflammatory response, it is not intense enough to
generate the signs of pre-eclampsia. To do that requires
the abnormal stimulus from an oxidatively stressed
placenta (left – placental pre-eclampsia). In a woman
with a chronic systemic inflammatory response associated
with conditions such as chronic hypertension, diabetes
or obesity that predispose to pre-eclampsia, the
starting point is abnormal enough such that even a
normal placenta can stimulate a systemic response
of an intensity to give the signs of pre-eclampsia
(right – maternal pre-eclampsia). In clinical practice
there are many mixed presentations with both maternal
constitution and placental ischemia contributing to the
presentation.

The effect of such medical problems is to elevate
the baseline of systemic inflammation upon which
the changes of pregnancy are superimposed
(Figure 7.1). We propose that, in pregnancy, the
decompensation from excessive systemic inflammation will happen earlier and at a lower threshold, accounting for the predisposition of affected
women to pre-eclampsia.

Maternal and placental pre-eclampsia

This concept was first proposed to distinguish
between pre-eclampsia caused by an abnormal

placenta and that caused by an increased maternal
susceptibility, owing to the predisposing conditions discussed in the preceding section (Ness and
Roberts, 1996). They summarized the evidence
that the maternal and placental causes converge
downstream from the effects of reduced placental
perfusion, at the point of maternal endothelial
injury. This extremely useful concept is here
extended in four ways. First, we show that the
endothelial problems occur in a larger context of
systemic inflammation. Second, the inflammatory
response of pre-eclampsia is not a new event but
an intensification of what happens in all pregnancies. Third, the inflammatory response associated
with normal pregnancy added to that associated
with chronic predisposing conditions such as
obesity can account for maternal pre-eclampsia.
Fourth, the systemic inflammatory response is
consistent with many other metabolic features of
normal and pre-eclamptic pregnancies such as
changes in acute phase reactants.

The two-stage model of pre-eclampsia (Figure 7.2)

The two-stage model of pre-eclampsia, originally
proposed more than a decade ago (Redman, 1991)
and described elsewhere in this volume, envisages
that pre-eclampsia arises in various ways including
from placental ischemia secondary to deficient
placentation. Whereas some consider abnormal
placentation to be the start and invariable cause
of pre-eclampsia, it is much more likely that it is
a completely separate but predisposing condition
(Redman and Sargent, 2000). Placentation is
described elsewhere in this volume and may be
abnormally shallow in pre-eclampsia, such that the
spiral arteries are maladapted and unable to meet
the perfusion needs of the second and third
trimester fetoplacental unit. The mechanisms,
which involve invasion of the placental bed by
extravillous cytotrophoblasts and their close association with large granular lymphocytes in the
decidua, remain to be defined. It is a local process,
without evidence that systemic inflammatory

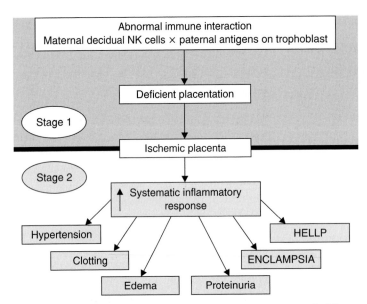

Figure 7.2 The two possible stages of evolution of pre-eclampsia with different contributions from the maternal immune system in each stage. Other types of pre-eclampsia that do not depend on poor placentation but excessively large placentas or increased maternal susceptibility to the inflammatory stresses of an otherwise normal pregnancy (Redman and Sargent, 2000) will not depend on the first stage as depicted here.

responses are involved. There are, however, important data, described in chapter 6, which suggest that maternal immune recognition of trophoblast in the decidua may control placentation and, if deficient, cause poor placentation. The proposal is for a novel form of immune recognition, of paternally expressed genes on trophoblast by decidual natural killer cells. If such immune mechanisms operate they could explain particular features of pre-eclampsia, such as its first pregnancy preponderance and apparent partner specificity (Li and Wi, 2000; Lie *et al.*, 1998).

Conclusions

Pregnancy imposes a substantial systemic inflammatory stress on all pregnant women in the second half of pregnancy. Part or all of the stimulus may arise from debris shed into the maternal circulation from the syncytiotrophoblast, which signals danger to the maternal innate immune system. Pre-eclampsia occurs when this response is increased to the point of decompensation. These features, which are clinically apparent, comprise the second stage of pre-eclampsia. Some, but not all, cases of pre-eclampsia are associated with poor placentation. This comprises the first stage, which would appear to have a different origin. First stage immune responses, localized in the decidua, involving maternal recognition of paternal antigens on trophoblast, could account for the first pregnancy and possible partner specificity of pre-eclampsia. Second stage responses, which we propose are all secondary to the systemic inflammatory response, could explain why women bearing pregnancies with unusually large placentas are susceptible to pre-eclampsia. Chronic systemic inflammation in women who are obese, chronically hypertensive or diabetic to pre-eclampsia combined with the added stimulus from that of even a normal pregnancy could explain the special susceptibility of these women to the pregnancy disorder.

Many of the metabolic features of normal and pre-eclamptic pregnancy such as insulin resistance, hyperlipidemia, increased blood coagulability or hypoalbuminemia, previously seen in isolation as hormonally induced, could instead be different consequences of the one process of a systemic inflammatory response. It is proposed that the maternal inflammatory response may represent maternal–fetal genetic conflict. The placenta signals danger to the mother but the ensuing inflammatory response generates these metabolic consequences, which are beneficial for the fetus.

REFERENCES

Ahmed, A., Dunk, C., Ahmad, S. and Khaliq, A. (2000). Regulation of placental vascular endothelial growth factor (VEGF) and placenta growth factor (PlGF) and soluble Flt-1 by oxygen – a review. *Placenta*, 21(Suppl. A), S16–24.

Alexander, B.T., Cockrell, K.L., Massey, M.B., Bennett, W.A. and Granger, J.P. (2002). Tumor necrosis factor-alpha-induced hypertension in pregnant rats results in decreased renal neuronal nitric oxide synthase expression. *Am. J. Hypertens.*, 15, 170–5.

Arkwright, P.D., Rademacher, T.W., Dwek, R.A. and Redman, C.W.G. (1993). Pre-eclampsia is associated with an increase in trophoblast glycogen content and glycogen synthase activity, similar to that found in hydatidiform moles. *J. Clin. Invest.*, 91, 2744–53.

Arntzen, K.J., Liabakk, N.B., Jacobsen, G., Espevik, T. and Austgulen, R. (1995). Soluble tumor necrosis factor receptor in serum and urine throughout normal pregnancy and at delivery. *Am. J. Reprod. Immunol.*, 34, 163–9.

Aupeix, K., Hugel, B., Martin, T., *et al.* (1997). The significance of shed membrane particles during programmed cell death in vitro, and in vivo, in HIV-1 infection. *J. Clin. Invest.*, 99, 1546–54.

Austgulen, R., Lien, E., Liabakk, N.B., Jacobsen, G. and Arntzen, K.J. (1994). Increased levels of cytokines and cytokine activity modifiers in normal pregnancy. *Eur. J. Obstet. Gynecol. Reprod. Biol.*, 57, 149–55.

Barbour, L.A., Shao, J., Qiao, L., *et al.* (2002). Human placental growth hormone causes severe insulin resistance in transgenic mice. *Am. J. Obstet. Gynecol.*, 186, 512–17.

Barleon, B., Reusch, P., Totzke, F., *et al.* (2001). Soluble VEGFR-1 secreted by endothelial cells and monocytes is present in human serum and plasma from healthy donors. *Angiogenesis*, 4, 143–54.

Barr, F.G., Biegel, J.A., Sellinger, B., Womer, R.B. and Emanuel, B.S. (1991). Molecular and cytogenetic analysis of chromosomal arms 2q and 13q in alveolar rhabdomyosarcoma. *Genes Chromosomes Cancer*, 3, 153–61.

Barriga, C., Rodriguez, A.B. and Ortega, E. (1994). Increased phagocytic activity of polymorphonuclear leukocytes during pregnancy. *Eur. J. Obstet. Gynecol. Reprod. Biol.*, 57, 43–6.

Barton, J.R., Hiett, A.K., O'Connor, W.N., Nissen, S.E. and Greene, J.-W.J. (1991). Endomyocardial ultrastructural findings in preeclampsia. *Am. J. Obstet. Gynecol.*, 165, 389–91.

Bastard, J.P., Jardel, C., Bruckert, E., *et al.* (2000). Elevated levels of interleukin 6 are reduced in serum and subcutaneous adipose tissue of obese women after weight loss. *J. Clin. Endocrinol. Metab.*, 85, 3338–42.

Belgore, F.M., Lip, G.Y. and Blann, A.D. (2000). Vascular endothelial growth factor and its receptor, Flt-1, in smokers and non-smokers. *Br. J. Biomed. Sci.*, 57, 207–13.

Belgore, F.M., Blann, A.D., Li, S.H., Beevers, D.G. and Lip, G.Y. (2001). Plasma levels of vascular endothelial growth factor and its soluble receptor (SFlt-1) in essential hypertension. *Am. J. Cardiol.*, 87, 805–7, A9.

Benyo, D.F., Smarason, A., Redman, C.W.G., Sims, C. and Conrad, K.P. (2001). Expression of inflammatory cytokines in placentas from women with preeclampsia. *J. Clin. Endocrinol. Metab.*, 86, 2505–12.

Beutler, B., Mahoney, J., Le-Trang, N., Pekala, P. and Cerami, A. (1985). Purification of cachectin, a lipoprotein lipase-suppressing hormone secreted by endotoxin-induced RAW 264.7 cells. *J. Exp. Med.*, 161, 984–95.

Blaschitz, A., Hutter, H. and Dohr, G. (2001). HLA Class I protein expression in the human placenta. *Early Pregnancy*, 5, 67–9.

Borzychowski, A.M., Croy, B.A., Chan, W.L., Redman, C.W.G. and Sargent, I.S. (2005). Changes in type 1 and type 2 immunity in normal pregnancy and pre-eclampsia may be mediated by NK cells. *Eur. J. Immunol.*, 35, 3054–63.

Boyd, P. A., Lindenbaum, R. H. and Redman, C. W. G. (1987). Pre-eclampsia and trisomy 13: a possible association. *Lancet*, **ii**, 425–7.

Cester, N., Staffolani, R., Rabini, R. A., *et al.* (1994). Pregnancy induced hypertension, a role for peroxidation in microvillus plasma membranes. *Mol. Cell. Biochem.*, **131**, 151–5.

Chaouat, G. (2003). Innately moving away from the Th1/Th2 paradigm in pregnancy. *Clin. Exp. Immunol.*, **131**, 393–5.

Clark, D. E., Smith, S. K., He, Y., *et al.* (1998). A vascular endothelial growth factor antagonist is produced by the human placenta and released into the maternal circulation. *Biol. Reprod.*, **59**, 1540–8.

Conrad, K. P., Miles, T. M. and Benyo, D. F. (1998). Circulating levels of immunoreactive cytokines in women with preeclampsia. *Am. J. Reprod. Immunol.*, **40**, 102–11.

Crouch, S. P., Crocker, I. P. and Fletcher, J. (1995). The effect of pregnancy on polymorphonuclear leukocyte function. *J. Immunol.*, **155**, 5436–43.

Dalekos, G. N., Elisaf, M. S., Papagalanis, N., Tzallas, C. and Siamopoulos, K. C. (1996). Elevated interleukin-1 beta in the circulation of patients with essential hypertension before any drug therapy: a pilot study. *Eur. J. Clin. Invest.*, **26**, 936–9.

Eiserich, J. P., Baldus, S., Brennan, M. L., *et al.* (2002). Myeloperoxidase, a leukocyte-derived vascular NO oxidase. *Science*, **296**, 2391–4.

Ellis, J., Wennerholm, U. B., Bengtsson, A., *et al.* (2001). Levels of dimethylarginines and cytokines in mild and severe preeclampsia. *Acta Obstet. Gynecol. Scand.*, **80**, 602–8.

Esposito, K., Nappo, F., Marfella, R., *et al.* (2002). Inflammatory cytokine concentrations are acutely increased by hyperglycemia in humans: role of oxidative stress. *Circulation*, **106**, 2067–72.

Faas, M. M., Schuiling, G. A., Baller, J. F., Visscher, C. A. and Bakker, W. W. (1994). A new animal model for human preeclampsia: ultra-low-dose endotoxin infusion in pregnant rats. *Am. J. Obstet. Gynecol.*, **171**, 158–64.

Felmeden, D. C., Spencer, C. G., Belgore, F. M., Blann, A. D., Beevers, D. G. and Lip, G. Y. (2003). Endothelial damage and angiogenesis in hypertensive patients: relationship to cardiovascular risk factors and risk factor management. *Am. J. Hypertens.*, **16**, 11–20.

Gabay, C. and Kushner, I. (1999). Acute-phase proteins and other systemic responses to inflammation. *N. Engl. J. Med.*, **340**, 448–54.

Gaber, L. W., Spargo, B. M. and Lindheimer, M. D. (1994). Renal pathology in pre-eclampsia. *Bailliere's Clin. Obstet. Gynaecol.*, **8**, 443–68.

Gallucci, S. and Matzinger P. (2001). Danger signals: SOS to the immune system. *Curr. Opin. Immunol.*, **13**, 114–19.

Garner, P. R., D'Alton, M. E., Dudley, D. K., Huard, P. and Hardie, M. (1990). Preeclampsia in diabetic pregnancies. *Am. J. Obstet. Gynecol.*, **163**, 505–8.

Gatti, L., Tenconi, P. M., Guarneri, D., *et al.* (1994). Hemostatic parameters and platelet activation by flow-cytometry in normal pregnancy: a longitudinal study. *Int. J. Clin. Lab. Res.*, **24**, 217–19.

Gratacos, E., Casals, E., Deulofeu, R., Cararach, V., Alonso, P. L. and Fortuny, A. (1998). Lipid peroxide and vitamin E patterns in pregnant women with different types of hypertension in pregnancy. *Am. J. Obstet. Gynecol.*, **178**, 1072–6.

Greer, I. A., Haddad, N. G., Dawes, J., Johnstone, F. D. and Calder, A. A. (1989). Neutrophil activation in pregnancy-induced hypertension. *Br. J. Obstet. Gynaecol.*, **96**, 978–82.

Greer, I. A., Lyall, F., Perera, T., Boswell, F. and Macara, L. M. (1994). Increased concentrations of cytokines interleukin-6 and interleukin-1 receptor antagonist in plasma of women with preeclampsia: a mechanism for endothelial dysfunction? *Obstet. Gynecol.*, **84**, 937–40.

Haddad, J. J. (2002). Antioxidant and prooxidant mechanisms in the regulation of redox(y)-sensitive transcription factors. *Cell Signal*, **14**, 879–97.

Haeger, M., Bengtson, A., Karlsson, K. and Heideman, M. (1989). Complement activation and anaphylatoxin (C3a and C5a) formation in preeclampsia and by amniotic fluid. *Obstet. Gynecol.*, **73**, 551–6.

Haig, D. (1993). Genetic conflicts in human pregnancy. *Q. Rev. Biol.*, **68**, 495–532.

Halligan, A., Bonnar, J., Sheppard, B., Darling, M. and Walshe, J. (1994). Haemostatic, fibrinolytic and endothelial variables in normal pregnancies and pre-eclampsia. *Br. J. Obstet. Gynaecol.*, **101**, 488–92.

Hansson, G. K., Libby, P., Schönbeck, U. and Yan, Z. Q. (2002). Innate and adaptive immunity in the pathogenesis of atherosclerosis. *Circ. Res.*, **91**, 281–91.

Harris, H. W., Gosnell, J. E. and Kumwenda, Z. L. (2001). The lipemia of sepsis: triglyceride-rich lipoproteins as agents of innate immunity. *J. Endotoxin Res.*, **6**, 421–30.

Hayakawa, M., Miyashita, H., Sakamoto, I., *et al.* (2003). Evidence that reactive oxygen species do not mediate NF-kappaB activation. *EMBO J.*, **22**, 3356–66.

Hensley, K., Robinson, K. A., Gabbita, S. P., Salsman, S. and Floyd, R. A. (2000). Reactive oxygen species, cell signaling, and cell injury. *Free Rad. Biol. Med.*, **28**, 1456–62.

Hirosumi, J., Tuncman, G., Chang, L., *et al.* (2002). A central role for JNK in obesity and insulin resistance. *Nature*, **420**, 333–6.

Holland, E. (1909). Recent work on the aetiology of eclampsia. *J. Obstet. Gynaecol. Br. Emp.*, **16**, 255–73.

Hornnes, P. J. (1985). On the decrease of glucose tolerance in pregnancy. A review. *Diabet. Metab.*, **11**, 310–15.

Hubel, C. A. (1998). Dyslipidemia, iron, and oxidative stress in preeclampsia, assessment of maternal and feto-placental interactions. *Semin. Reprod. Endocrinol.*, **16**, 75–92.

Hubel, C. A., McLaughlin, M. K., Evans, R. W., Hauth, B. A., Sims, C. J. and Roberts, J. M. (1996). Fasting serum triglycerides, free fatty acids, and malondialdehyde are increased in preeclampsia, are positively correlated, and decrease within 48 hours post partum. *Am. J. Obstet. Gynecol.*, **174**, 975–82.

Huppertz, B., Frank, H. G., Kingdom, J. C., Reister, F. and Kaufmann, P. (1998). Villous cytotrophoblast regulation of the syncytial apoptotic cascade in the human placenta. *Histochem. Cell Biol.*, **110**, 495–508.

Impey, L., Greenwood, C., Sheil, O., MacQuillan, K., Reynolds, M. and Redman, C. (2001). The relation between pre-eclampsia at term and neonatal encephalopathy. *Arch. Dis. Child. Fetal Neonatal Ed.*, **85**, F170–2.

Ishihara, N., Matsuo, H., Murakoshi, H., Laoag-Fernandez, J. B., Samoto, T. and Maruo, T. (2002). Increased apoptosis in the syncytiotrophoblast in human term placentas complicated by either preeclampsia or intrauterine growth retardation. *Am. J. Obstet. Gynecol.*, **186**, 158–66.

Isomaa, B. (2003). A major health hazard: the metabolic syndrome. *Life Sci.*, **73**, 2395–411.

Johansen, K. A., Williams, J. H. and Stark, J. M. (1981). Acute-phase C56-forming ability and concentrations of complement components in normotensive and hypertensive pregnancies. *Br. J. Obstet. Gynaecol.*, **88**, 504–12.

Johansen, M., Redman, C. W. G., Wilkins, T. and Sargent, I. L. (1999). Trophoblast deportation in human pregnancy – its relevance for pre-eclampsia. *Placenta*, **20**, 531–9.

Jones, C. J. and Fox, H. (1980). An ultrastructural and ultrahistochemical study of the human placenta in maternal pre-eclampsia. *Placenta*, **1**, 61–76.

Kaaja, R., Laivuori, H., Laakso, M., Tikkanen, M. J. and Ylikorkala, O. (1999). Evidence of a state of increased insulin resistance in preeclampsia. *Metabolism*, **48**, 892–6.

Kabbinavar, F., Hurwitz, H. I., Fehrenbacher, L., *et al.* (2003). Phase II, randomized trial comparing bevacizumab plus fluorouracil (FU)/leucovorin (LV) with FU/LV alone in patients with metastatic colorectal cancer. *J. Clin. Oncol.*, **21**, 60–5.

Kendall, R. L., Wang, G. and Thomas, K. A. (1996). Identification of a natural soluble form of the vascular endothelial growth factor receptor, FLT-1, and its heterodimerization with KDR. *Biochem. Biophys. Res. Commun.*, **226**, 324–8.

Knight, M., Redman, C. W., Linton, E. A. and Sargent, I. L. (1998). Shedding of syncytiotrophoblast microvilli into the maternal circulation in pre-eclamptic pregnancies. *Br. J. Obstet. Gynaecol.*, **105**, 632–40.

Konijnenberg, A., Stokkers, E. W., van der Post, J., *et al.* (1997). Extensive platelet activation in preeclampsia compared with normal pregnancy, enhanced expression of cell adhesion molecules. *Am. J. Obstet. Gynecol.*, **176**, 461–9.

Kupferminc, M. J., Peaceman, A. M., Wigton, T. R., Rehnberg, K. A. and Socol, M. L. (1994). Tumor necrosis factor-alpha is elevated in plasma and amniotic fluid of patients with severe preeclampsia. *Am. J. Obstet. Gynecol.*, **170**, 1752–7.

Lechleitner, M., Koch, T., Herold, M., Dzien, A. and Hoppichler, F. (2000). Tumour necrosis factor-alpha plasma level in patients with type 1 diabetes mellitus and its association with glycaemic control and cardiovascular risk factors. *J. Intern. Med.*, **248**, 67–76.

Levy, R., Smith, S. D., Chandler, K., Sadovsky, Y. and Nelson, D. M. (2000). Apoptosis in human cultured trophoblasts is enhanced by hypoxia and diminished by epidermal growth factor. *Am. J. Physiol. Cell Physiol.*, **278**, C982–8.

Li, D. K. and Wi, S. (2000). Changing paternity and the risk of preeclampsia/eclampsia in the subsequent pregnancy. *Am. J. Epidemiol.*, **151**, 57–62.

Li, N. and Karin, M. (1999). Is NF-kappaB the sensor of oxidative stress? *FASEB J.*, **13**, 1137–43.

Lie, R. T., Rasmussen, S., Brunborg, H., Gjessing, H. K., Lie, N. E. and Irgens, L. M. F. (1998). Fetal and maternal contributions to risk of pre-eclampsia: population based study. *Br. Med. J.*, **316**, 1343–7.

Lo, Y. M., Leung, T. N., Tein, M. S., *et al.* (1999). Quantitative abnormalities of fetal DNA in maternal serum in preeclampsia. *Clin. Chem.*, **45**, 184–8.

Lorentzen, B., Drevon, C. A., Endresen, M. J. and Henriksen, T. (1995). Fatty acid pattern of esterified and free fatty acids in sera of women with normal and pre-eclamptic pregnancy. *Br. J. Obstet. Gynaecol.*, **102**, 530–7.

Luft, F. C. (2002). Proinflammatory effects of angiotensin II and endothelin: targets for progression of cardiovascular and renal diseases. *Curr. Opin. Nephrol. Hypertens.*, **11**, 59–66.

McCracken, S. A., Gallery, E. D. M. and Morris, J. M. (2004). Pregnancy-specific down regulation of NF-kappaB expression in T cells is essential for the maintenance of cytokine profile required for pregnancy success. *J. Immunol.*, **172**, 4583–91.

Mantzoros, C. S., Moschos, S., Avramopoulos, I., *et al.* (1997). Leptin concentrations in relation to body mass index and the tumor necrosis factor-alpha system in humans. *J. Clin. Endocrinol. Metab.*, **82**, 3408–13.

Martin, U., Davies, C., Hayavi, S., Hartland, A. and Dunne, F. (1999). Is normal pregnancy atherogenic? *Clin. Sci. Colch.*, **96**, 421–5.

Marzi, M., Vigano, A., Trabattoni, D., *et al.* (1996). Characterization of type 1 and type 2 cytokine production profile in physiologic and pathologic human pregnancy. *Clin. Exp. Immunol.*, **106**, 127–33.

Matzinger, P. (2002). The danger model: a renewed sense of self. *Science*, **296**, 301–5.

Maynard, S. E., Min, J. Y., Merchan, J., *et al.* (2003). Excess placental soluble fms-like tyrosine kinase 1 (sFlt1) may contribute to endothelial dysfunction, hypertension, and proteinuria in preeclampsia. *J. Clin. Invest.*, **111**, 649–58.

Melczer, Z., Banhidy, F., Csomor, S., *et al.* (2003). Influence of leptin and the TNF system on insulin resistance in pregnancy and their effect on anthropometric parameters of newborns. *Acta Obstet. Gynecol. Scand.*, **82**, 432–8.

Mellembakken, J. R., Aukrust, P., Olafsen, M. K., Ueland, T., Hestdal, K. and Videm, V. (2002). Activation of leukocytes during the uteroplacental passage in preeclampsia. *Hypertension*, **39**, 155–60.

Morris, J. M., Gopaul, N. K., Endresen, M. J., *et al.* (1998). Circulating markers of oxidative stress are raised in normal pregnancy and pre-eclampsia. *Br. J. Obstet. Gynaecol.*, **105**, 1195–9.

Nelson, D. M. (1996). Apoptotic changes occur in syncytiotrophoblast of human placental villi where fibrin type fibrinoid is deposited at discontinuities in the villous trophoblast. *Placenta*, **17**, 387–91.

Ness, R. B. and Roberts, J. M. (1996). Heterogeneous causes constituting the single syndrome of preeclampsia: a hypothesis and its implications. *Am. J. Obstet. Gynecol.*, **175**, 1365–70.

Nisell, H., Erikssen, C., Persson, B. and Carlstrom, K. (1999). Is carbohydrate metabolism altered among women who have undergone a preeclamptic pregnancy? *Gynecol. Obstet. Invest.*, **48**, 241–6.

Pepys, M. B. and Hirschfield, G. M. (2003). C-reactive protein: a critical update. *J. Clin. Invest.*, **112**, 299.

Perry, K. G. J. and Martin, J. N. J. (1992). Abnormal hemostasis and coagulopathy in preeclampsia and eclampsia. *Clin. Obstet. Gynecol.*, **35**, 338–50.

Pickup, J. C., Chusney, G. D., Thomas, S. M. and Burt, D. (2000). Plasma interleukin-6, tumour necrosis factor alpha and blood cytokine production in type 2 diabetes. *Life Sci.*, **67**, 291–300.

Pitkin, R. M. and Witte, D. L. (1979). Platelet and leukocyte counts in pregnancy. *J. Am. Med. Ass.*, **242**, 2696–8.

Rebelo, I., Carvalho Guerra, F., Pereira Leite, L. and Quintanilha, A. (1995). Lactoferrin as a sensitive blood marker of neutrophil activation in normal pregnancies. *Eur. J. Obstet. Gynecol. Reprod. Biol.*, **62**, 189–94.

Redman, C. W. G. (1991). Current topic. Pre-eclampsia and the placenta. *Placenta*, **12**, 301–8.

Redman, C. W. G. (1992). The placenta and pre-eclampsia. In *The Human Placenta*, ed. C. W. G. Redman, I. L. Sargent and P. M. Starkey. Oxford: Blackwell Scientific Publications, pp. 433–67.

Redman, C. W. G. and Sargent, I. L. (2000). Placental debris, oxidative stress and pre-eclampsia. *Placenta*, **21**, 597–602.

Redman, C. W. G., Sacks, G. P., and Sargent, I. L. (1999). Preeclampsia, an excessive maternal inflammatory response to pregnancy. *Am. J. Obstet. Gynecol.*, **180**, 499–506.

Rein, D. T., Schondorf, T., Gohring, U. J., *et al.* (2002). Cytokine expression in peripheral blood lymphocytes indicates a switch to T(HELPER) cells in patients with preeclampsia. *J. Reprod. Immunol.*, **54**, 133–42.

Ridker, P. M. (2001). High-sensitivity C-reactive protein: potential adjunct for global risk assessment in the primary prevention of cardiovascular disease. *Circulation*, **103**, 1813–18.

Roberts, J. M., Taylor, R. N., Musci, T. J., Rodgers, G. M., Hubel, C. A. and McLaughlin, M. K. (1989). Preeclampsia, an endothelial cell disorder. *Am. J. Obstet. Gynecol.*, **161**, 1200–4.

Roberts, R. N., Henriksen, J. E. and Hadden, D. R. (1998). Insulin sensitivity in pre-eclampsia. *Br. J. Obstet. Gynaecol.*, **105**, 1095–100.

Rock, F. L., Hardiman, G., Timans, J. C., Kastelein, R. A. and Bazan, J. F. (1998). A family of human receptors structurally related to *Drosophila* Toll. *Proc. Natl Acad. Sci. USA*, **95**, 588–93.

Ros, H. S., Cnattingius, S. and Lipworth, L. (1998). Comparison of risk factors for preeclampsia and gestational hypertension in a population-based cohort study. *Am. J. Epidemiol.*, **147**, 1062–70.

Sacks, G. P., Studena, K., Sargent, I. L. and Redman, C. W. G. (1998). Normal pregnancy and pre-eclampsia both produce inflammatory changes in peripheral blood leukocytes akin to those of sepsis. *Am. J. Obstet. Gynecol.*, **179**, 80–6.

Sacks, G. P., Sargent, I. L. and Redman, C. W. G. (1999). An innate view of human pregnancy. *Immunol. Today*, **20**, 114–18.

Sacks, G. P., Redman, C. W. G. and Sargent, I. L. (2003). Monocytes are primed to express the Th1 type cytokine IL-12 in normal human pregnancy: an intracellular flow cytometric analysis of peripheral blood mononuclear cells. *Clin. Exp. Immunol.*, **131**, 490–7.

Sacks, G. P., Seyani, L., Lavery, S. and Trew, G. (2004). Maternal C-reactive protein levels are raised at 4 weeks gestation *Hum. Reprod.*, **19**, 1025–30.

Saito, S., Sakai, M., Sasaki, Y., Tanebe, K., Tsuda, H. and Michimata, T. (1999). Quantitative analysis of peripheral blood Th0, Th1, Th2 and the Th1:Th2 cell ratio during normal human pregnancy and preeclampsia. *Clin. Exp. Immunol.*, **117**, 550–5.

Sakai, M., Tsuda, H., Tanebe, K., Sasaki, Y. and Saito, S. (2002). Interleukin-12 secretion by peripheral blood mononuclear cells is decreased in normal pregnant subjects and increased in preeclamptic patients. *Am. J. Reprod. Immunol.*, **47**, 91–7.

Schena, F. P., Manno, C., Selvaggi, L., Loverro, G., Bettocchi, S. and Bonomo, L. (1982). Behaviour of immune complexes and the complement system in normal pregnancy and pre-eclampsia. *J. Clin. Lab. Immunol.*, **7**, 21–6.

Schrocksnadel, H., Daxenbichler, G., Artner, E., Steckel Berger, G. and Dapunt, O. (1993). Tumor markers in hypertensive disorders of pregnancy. *Gynecol. Invest.*, **35**, 204–8.

Sethi, J. K. and Hotamisligil, G. S. (1999). The role of TNF alpha in adipocyte metabolism. *Semin. Cell. Dev. Biol.*, **10**, 19–29.

Shanklin, D. R. and Sibai, B. M. (1989). Ultrastructural aspects of preeclampsia. I. Placental bed and uterine boundary vessels. *Am. J. Obstet. Gynecol.*, **161**, 735–41.

Shibuya, T., Izuchi, K., Kuroiwa, A., Okabe, N. and Shirakawa, K. (1987). Study on nonspecific immunity in pregnant women: increased chemiluminescence response of peripheral blood phagocytes. *Am. J. Reprod. Immunol. Microbiol.*, **15**, 19–23.

Sibai, B. M., Gordon, T., Thom, E., *et al.* (1995). Risk factors for preeclampsia in healthy nulliparous women: a prospective multicenter study. The National Institute of Child Health and Human Development Network of Maternal–Fetal Medicine Units. *Am. J. Obstet. Gynecol.*, **172**, 642–8.

Smarason, A. K., Gunnarsson, A., Alfredsson, J. H. and Valdimarsson, H. (1986). Monocytosis and monocytic infiltration of decidua in early pregnancy. *J. Clin. Lab. Immunol.*, **21**, 1–5.

Smarason, A. K., Sargent, I. L., Starkey, P. M. and Redman, C. W. G. (1993). The effect of placental syncytiotrophoblast microvillous membranes from normal and pre-eclamptic women on the growth of endothelial cells in vitro. *Br. J. Obstet. Gynaecol.*, **100**, 943–9.

Stallmach, T., Hebisch, G., Joller, H., Kolditz, P. and Engelmann, M. (1995). Expression pattern of cytokines in the different compartments of the feto-maternal unit under various conditions. *Reprod. Fertil. Dev.*, **7**, 1573–80.

Stanley, K., Fraser, R. and Bruce, C. (1998). Physiological changes in insulin resistance in human pregnancy: longitudinal study with the hyperinsulinaemic euglycaemic clamp technique. *Br. J. Obstet. Gynaecol.*, **105**, 756–9.

Strevens, H., Wide-Swensson, D., Hansen, A., *et al.* (2003). Glomerular endotheliosis in normal and pregnancy and pre-eclampsia. *Br. J. Obstet. Gynaecol.*, **110**, 831–6.

Taylor, R. N., Crombleholme, W. R., Friedman, S. A., Jones, L. A., Casal, D. C. and Roberts, J. M. (1991). High plasma cellular fibronectin levels correlate with biochemical and clinical features of preeclampsia but cannot be attributed to hypertension alone. *Am. J. Obstet. Gynecol.*, **165**, 895–901.

Tedder, R. S., Nelson, M. and Eisen, V. (1975). Effects on serum complement of normal and pre-eclamptic pregnancy and of oral contraceptives. *Br. J. Exp. Pathol.*, **56**, 389–95.

Teran, E., Escudero, C., Moya, W., Flores, M., Vallance, P. and Lopez-Jaramillo, P. (2001). Elevated C-reactive protein and pro-inflammatory cytokines in Andean women with pre-eclampsia. *Int. J. Gynaecol. Obstet.*, **75**, 243–9.

Terrone, D. A., Rinehart, B. K., May, W. L., Moore, A, Magann, E. F. and Martin, J. N. (2000). Leukocytosis is proportional to HELLP syndrome severity: evidence for an inflammatory form of preeclampsia. *South Med. J.*, **93**, 768–71.

Ukkola, O. and Bouchard, C. (2001). Clustering of metabolic abnormalities in obese individuals: the role of genetic factors. *Ann. Med.*, **33**, 79–90.

Vince, G. S., Starkey, P. M., Austgulen, D. and Redman, C. W. (1995). Interleukin-6, tumour necrosis factor and soluble tumour necrosis factor receptors in women with pre-eclampsia. *Br. J. Obstet. Gynaecol.*, **102**, 20–5.

Vitoratos, N., Salamalekis, E., Dalamaga, N., Kassanos, D. and Creatsas, G. (1999). Defective antioxidant mechanisms via changes in serum ceruloplasmin and total iron binding capacity of serum in women with pre-eclampsia. *Eur. J. Obstet. Gynecol. Reprod. Biol.*, **84**, 63–7.

Von Dadelszen, P., Hurst, G. and Redman, C. W. G. (1999). The supernatants from co-cultured endothelial cells and syncytiotrophoblast microvillous membranes activate peripheral blood leukocytes in vitro. *Hum. Reprod.*, **14**, 919–24.

Wegmann, T. G., Lin, H., Guilbert, L. and Mosmann, T. R. (1993). Bidirectional cytokine interactions in the maternal–fetal relationship: is successful pregnancy a Th2 phenomenon? *Immunol. Today*, **14**, 353–6.

Wickens, D., Wilkins, M. H., Lunec, J., Ball, G. and Dormandy, T. L. (1981). Free radical oxidation (peroxidation) products in plasma in normal and abnormal pregnancy. *Ann. Clin. Biochem.*, **18**, 158–62.

Willis, C., Morris, J. M., Danis, V. and Gallery, E. D. (2003). Cytokine production by peripheral blood monocytes during the normal human ovulatory menstrual cycle. *Hum. Reprod.*, **18**, 1173–8.

Yang, J. C., Haworth, L., Sherry, R. M., *et al.* (2003). A randomized trial of bevacizumab, an anti-vascular endothelial growth factor antibody, for metastatic renal cancer. *N. Engl. J. Med.*, **349**, 427–34.

Yoo, J. Y. and Desiderio, S. (2003). Innate and acquired immunity intersect in a global view of the acute-phase response. *Proc. Natl Acad. Sci. USA*, **100**, 1157–62.

Yudkin, J. S., Stehouwer, C. D., Emeis, J. J. and Coppack, S. W. (1999). C-reactive protein in healthy subjects: associations with obesity, insulin resistance, and endothelial dysfunction: a potential role for cytokines originating from adipose tissue? *Arterioscler. Thromb. Vasc. Biol.*, **19**, 972–8.

Yura, S., Sagawa, N., Itoh, H., *et al.* (2003). Resistin is expressed in the human placenta. *J. Clin. Endocrinol. Metab.*, **88**, 1394–7.

Zabriskie, J. R. (1963). Effect of cigarette smoking during pregnancy. Study of 2000 cases. *Obstet. Gynecol.*, **21**, 405–11.

Zarkesh-Esfahani, H., Pockley, G., Metcalfe, R. A., *et al.* (2001). High-dose leptin activates human leukocytes via receptor expression on monocytes. *J. Immunol.*, **167**, 4593–9.

Ziccardi, P., Nappo, F., Giugliano, G., *et al.* (2002). Reduction of inflammatory cytokine concentrations and improvement of endothelial functions in obese women after weight loss over one year. *Circulation*, **105**, 804–9.

Zimmerman, G. A., Prescott, S. M. and McIntyre, T. M. (1992). Endothelial cell interactions with granulocytes: tethering and signaling molecules. *Immunol. Today*, **13**, 93–100.

Zusterzeel, P. L., Mulder, T. P., Peters, W. H., Wiseman, S. A. and Steegers, E. A. (2000). Plasma protein carbonyls in nonpregnant, healthy pregnant and preeclamptic women. *Free Rad. Res.*, **33**, 471–6.

The role of oxidative stress in pre-eclampsia

M. T. M. Raijmakers and L. Poston

Abbreviations

8-iso-PGF$_{2\alpha}$	8-iso-prostaglandin F$_{2\alpha}$
GPX	Glutathione peroxidase
GST	Glutathione S-transferase
H$_2$O$_2$	Hydrogen peroxide
LDL	Low-density lipoprotein
MDA	Malondialdehyde
NO	Nitric oxide
O$_2^\bullet$	Superoxide radical
OxLDL	Oxidized form of low-density lipoprotein
ROS	Reactive oxygen species
SeGPX	Selenium-dependent glutathione peroxidase
SOD	Superoxide dismutase
TBARS	Thiobarbituric acid-reactive substances
XO	Xanthine oxidase
XOR	Xanthine oxidoreductase

Oxidative stress has been implicated in a broad spectrum of disease. This chapter provides a summary of the biochemical principles underlying oxidative stress, including the diversity of laboratory methods employed in its assessment, and will attempt to explain why free radicals are now widely considered to play a pivotal role in the placenta and in the maternal circulation of pregnancies affected by pre-eclampsia.

What is oxidative stress?

Oxidative stress is said to occur when the generation of free radicals (i.e. reactive substances with one or more unpaired electrons) exceeds the capacity of antioxidant defense. An increasing literature has lent support to the hypothesis that oxidative stress is not only an accompaniment to the disorder of pre-eclampsia, but may also contribute to the etiology of the maternal syndrome. Supporting evidence includes reports in both placenta and maternal blood of oxidative damage to lipids, proteins and DNA, decreased total antioxidant capacity and depletion of individual antioxidants (Raijmakers et al., 2005). The diversity of the methods employed reflects the lack of a "gold standard" assay for oxidative stress assessment in the laboratory (Hubel, 1999) that, as this chapter will highlight, can lead to confusion and inevitably to some misinterpretation of data.

The generation of free radicals

The most commonly produced reactive oxygen species (ROS) in the human body is superoxide (O$_2^\bullet$), but this is rapidly converted to the more stable hydrogen peroxide (H$_2$O$_2$; Table 8.1), which in turn dissociates to form the highly reactive hydroxyl anion (OH$^\bullet$). There are a variety of biological sources of (O$_2^\bullet$). In the mitochondrial respiratory chain some electrons (1–3%) "escape" so forming O$_2^\bullet$ (Lenaz et al., 2002). Uncoupling of mitochondrial oxidative phosphorylation or structural changes in the electron-transfer complexes due to oxidative damage to mitochondrial DNA may both increase mitochondrial O$_2^\bullet$ production.

Table 8.1. Potential sources of superoxide and ROS in pre-eclampsia

Source of free radical	Mechanism	Reference
Mitochondria	Leakage through the oxidative phosphorylation	(Lenaz *et al.*, 2002)
Leukocytes	Respiratory burst, $O_2^{\bullet}$ generation	(Luppi *et al.*, 2002)
NADPH oxidase	Generation of $O_2^{\bullet}$	(Griendling *et al.*, 2000b)
Xanthine oxidase	Generation of $O_2^{\bullet}$	(Harrison, 2002; Pritsos, 2000)
Superoxide dismutase	Conversion of $O_2^{\bullet}$ to H_2O_2	(Zelko *et al.*, 2002)

In excess, mitochondrial $O_2^{\bullet}$ synthesis is associated with apoptosis, processes of aging and age-related diseases, and has been linked to trophoblast oxidative damage in the placenta (Lenaz *et al.*, 2002; Wang and Walsh, 1998).

In neutrophils, vascular endothelial cells, vascular smooth muscle cells and trophoblast an important source of $O_2^{\bullet}$ is the family of closely related NAD(P)H oxidases (Griendling *et al.*, 2000a). Activation of the NAD(P)H oxidase enzyme complex and increased subunit expression occurs upon response to a range of stimuli including angiotensin II, platelet-derived growth factor, thrombin, cytokines, hemodynamic forces and local metabolic changes. Augmented $O_2^{\bullet}$ generation by NAD(P)H oxidase has been implicated in oxidative stress and the development of cardiovascular disease (Griendling *et al.*, 2000a).

Under normal conditions xanthine oxidoreductase (XOR), which is abundantly present in liver and also found in trophoblasts (Many *et al.*, 2000), exists in the xanthine dehydrogenase (XDH) form, converting hypoxanthine to xanthine and xanthine to urate (Pritsos, 2000). Cytokines increase human XOR activity, whereas hypoxia stimulates the irreversible conversion to xanthine oxidase (XO). Upon reperfusion with oxygenated blood, XO uses oxygen as the electron recipient, thus coupling the conversion of purines to the generation of $O_2^{\bullet}$ and uric acid (Many *et al.*, 2000). In a number of pathological processes XO is released into the plasma where it may bind to target tissue and be incorporated via endocytosis into a superoxide dismutase-resistant intracellular compartment.

XO-dependent $O_2^{\bullet}$ generation may then proceed unopposed, resulting in oxidative damage (Houston *et al.*, 1999).

It is now recognized that $O_2^{\bullet}$ and other ROS are involved in the regulatory pathways of both physiological (e.g. growth, proliferation, angiogenesis) and pathophysiological (e.g. inflammatory response, hypertrophy) gene expression (Griendling *et al.*, 2000a,b; Irani, 2000).

Mechanisms of defense against oxidative stress

The most abundant antioxidant defense pathways are summarized in Table 8.2. Antioxidant defense is comprised of enzymatic as well as non-enzymatic systems.

Enzymatic antioxidants

Superoxide dismutases (SOD) provide a first line defense against free radicals through conversion of $O_2^{\bullet}$, to H_2O_2 and oxygen (Zelko *et al.*, 2002). The rapid cellular response to oxidative stress leads to a defensive increase in expression of SOD (Mates *et al.*, 1999). SOD works in concordance with H_2O_2-removing enzymes such as glutathione peroxidase (GPX) and catalase (Mates *et al.*, 1999).

Selenium-dependent glutathione peroxidase (SeGPX) catalyzes the reduction of H_2O_2 and organic hydroperoxides (e.g. lipid hydroperoxides and DNA hydroperoxides) (Hayes and McLellan, 1999). In contrast, non-selenium-dependent GPX, predominantly glutathione *S*-transferase (GST)

Table 8.2. Principal antioxidant pathways

Antioxidant	Main function	Reference
	Enzymatic antioxidants	
Glutathione peroxidase	Reduction of organic hydroperoxides and H_2O_2	(Arthur, 2000)
Glutathione reductase	Regeneration of oxidized glutathione	
Glutathione S-transferase	Reduction of organic hydroperoxides	(Hayes and McLellan, 1999)
	Conjugation of glutathione in Phase II	
Superoxide dismutase	Conversion of $O_2^{\bullet}$ to H_2O_2	(Zelko *et al.*, 2002)
Catalase	Conversion of H_2O_2 to H_2O and O_2	(Mates *et al.*, 1999)
Thioredoxin	Regeneration of antioxidants	(Nordberg and Arner, 2001)
Water-soluble	*Non-enzymatic antioxidants*	
Glutathione	Co-factor for GST and GPX	(Stamler and Slivka, 1996)
	Maintenance of intracellular redox status	(Meister, 1988)
Vitamin C	Reduction of reactive nitrogen species and ROS	(Nordberg and Arner, 2001)
	Regeneration of vitamin E	
Uric acid	Scavenging of free radicals	(Sevanian *et al.*, 1991)
	Stabilization of vitamin C	
Transferrin/ferritin	Binding free iron	(Mates *et al.*, 1999)
Haptoglobin	Binding hemoglobin	(Langlois and Delanghe, 1996)
Lipid soluble		
Vitamin E	Inhibition of propagation of lipid peroxidation	(Brigelius-Flohe *et al.*, 2002)
Carotenoids	Inhibition of propagation of lipid peroxidation	(Krinsky, 1998)
	Quenching of singlet oxygen ($^1O_2$)	
Ubiquinone	Membrane-associated redox reactions	(Nohl *et al.*, 1998)
Bilirubin	Inhibition of propagation of lipid peroxidation	(Tomaro and Batlle, 2002)

isoforms, only inactivates organic hydroperoxides (Hayes and McLellan, 1999; Knapen *et al.*, 1999).

The thioredoxin system (Holmgren and Bjornstedt, 1995), although playing a lesser role in a quantitative sense, is positioned at the core of redox control and antioxidant defense, being involved in the regeneration of antioxidants (e.g. ascorbic acid, glutathione and ubiquinone), in the reduction of a variety of peroxides and in the activation of redox-sensitive transcription factors such as AP-1 and NF-κB (Nordberg and Arner, 2001).

Water-soluble antioxidants

In general, non-enzymatic antioxidants can be grouped into water- and lipid-soluble antioxidants. Glutathione is the most important water-soluble antioxidant and is widely distributed in human tissues (Hayes and McLellan, 1999; Meister, 1988). Dietary-derived ascorbic acid (vitamin C), vital for species (including man) that cannot synthesize ascorbic acid, reduces reactive nitrogen species, ROS and also the α-tocopherol radical (Nordberg and Arner, 2001). Uric acid is generally considered as a waste product of the metabolic action of XO, but shows strong antioxidant capacity toward water-soluble free radicals and stabilizes ascorbic acid at physiological concentrations. However, uric acid is ineffective against lipid-soluble radicals and forms potent radicals when oxidized (Sevanian *et al.*, 1991). Metal-binding proteins (e.g. transferrin and ferritin) as well as heme-binding proteins (e.g. haptoglobin) are also important antioxidants (Krinsky, 1998).

Lipid-soluble antioxidants

All lipid-soluble antioxidants are effective inhibitors of the propagation step of lipid peroxidation through reaction with one or more peroxyl radicals. The major lipid-soluble antioxidants are the tocopherols (vitamin E), of which α-tocopherol is the predominant form in humans (Brigelius-Flohe et al., 2002). Other potentially biologically important roles for α-tocopherol have been described (Brigelius-Flohe et al., 2002; Rimbach et al., 2002). Although the biological function of ubiquinone is not yet clear, it seems to play a pivotal role in several processes (Nohl et al., 1998). Carotenoids may quench the reactive form of oxygen, singlet oxygen (Krinsky, 1998). Bilirubin, an end product of heme metabolism, is the most potent antioxidant against lipid peroxidation known to date (Tomaro and Batlle, 2002).

Assessment of oxidative stress

A good biomarker for oxidative stress would be one that combines the two arms that contribute to the balance of the redox state (i.e. free radical generation and antioxidant defense), is simple and inexpensive to measure, and measurement is reproducible. However, no such marker is available. Most methods only measure one aspect and therefore present a single, simplified and unbalanced view of the possible presence of oxidative stress.

Many investigators have assessed total antioxidant capacity (e.g. the oxygen radical absorbance capacity and the ferric reducing ability of plasma) (Cao and Prior, 1998), individual antioxidant levels (Krinsky, 1998) or the enzyme activity of antioxidant enzymes (Hayes and McLellan, 1999; Mates et al., 1999) as indirect evidence of oxidative stress. Most relevant assays are easy, inexpensive and generally accessible, but may be misleading. For instance, measures of "total" antioxidant capacity do not include all of the major antioxidants (Cao and Prior, 1998). Additionally, enzymatic antioxidants may be over-expressed as a defensive response to oxidative stress, and the measurement of a single antioxidant is never able to reflect antioxidant defense overall. The influence of dietary intake on concentrations of individual antioxidant must also be considered.

Measurement of the products of oxidative modification presents a more direct assessment of oxidative stress. These are derived directly from free radical attack to lipids (e.g. conjugated dienes, malondialdehyde (MDA) and isoprostanes) (Conti et al., 1991; Cracowski et al., 2002; Little and Gladen, 1999), proteins (e.g. carbonyls and nitrotyrosine residues) (Adams et al., 2001; Myatt et al., 1996) and DNA (8-hydroxydeoxyguanosine) (Hong et al., 2002). The isoprostanes, a family of stable isomers generated after free radical attack on arachonidonic acid, have been heralded as the "gold standard" for oxidative modification of lipids (Roberts and Morrow, 2000). Even normal physiological situations are associated with a modest generation of the products of oxidative damage (Halliwell, 1997). Since most products require excretion, they are good candidates for measurement in either blood or urine. A major problem is that rapid synthesis can occur in vitro, after exposure to atmospheric oxygen during sample collection, preparation or storage (Hubel, 1999). Additionally, the assessment of the most stable lipid peroxidation products, the isoprostanes, is labor-intensive and technically demanding.

New techniques are now available that directly detect superoxide or other free radicals. Since free radicals are very reactive, unstable and have a very short half-life, these techniques are technically difficult and require specialized equipment such as that for electron spin trapping (Berliner et al., 2001). Assessment of the capacity to generate $O_2^{\bullet}$ by XO or NAD(P)H oxidase in blood or tissue are simpler than the spin trapping assays (Griendling et al., 2000b). However, none of these approaches assess antioxidant responses, which might be provoked by $O_2^{\bullet}$ generation in vivo. Other good approaches include the assessment of the ratio between the reduced and oxidized forms of ascorbic acid or aminothiols. The free-to-oxidized ratio for thiols as a measure of the thiol redox balance has proven to be a marker of oxidative stress in women with pre-eclampsia (Raijmakers *et al.*, 2001b).

Oxidative stress in normal pregnancy

Normal pregnancy is a mild state of oxidative stress. Despite the presence of antioxidant systems such as SOD, catalase, GPX and GSTPi, and the co-factors glutathione and cysteine that are present from early pregnancy onwards (Jauniaux *et al.*, 2000; Raijmakers *et al.*, 2001a), a low level of oxidative modification occurs in placental tissue of uncomplicated pregnancies (Qanungo *et al.*, 1999; Raijmakers *et al.*, 2002). Also maternal factors lead to increased generation of $O_2^{\bullet}$ and other ROS during pregnancy (Luppi *et al.*, 2002). Indeed, physiological pregnancy is characterized by a transient increase of ROS production that is partially counteracted by an induction of antioxidant defense mechanisms (Chappell *et al.*, 2002; Cikot *et al.*, 2001; Little and Gladen, 1999). After delivery, both the level of oxidative damage and antioxidants return to pre-conception values (Cikot *et al.*, 2001; Uotila *et al.*, 1991). Normal vaginal delivery is associated with increased oxidative stress when compared with delivery by Cesarean section (Burton and Hang, 2003). Researchers are to be warned of the importance of matching for type of delivery in placental studies related to oxidative stress.

Placental oxidative stress in pre-eclampsia

A potential source of placental oxidative stress in pre-eclampsia

The development of pre-eclampsia has been linked to abnormalities in trophoblast invasion (Figure 8.1). More recently, Jauniaux *et al.* (2000) found that the activity of several antioxidant enzymes in normal placental tissue was increased in parallel with the rise in oxygen tension which occurs at 10–12 weeks' gestation (Jauniaux *et al.*, 2000). The authors hypothesized that a diminished antioxidant response to this oxygenation stimulus would result in oxidative stress. This could lead to trophoblast degeneration and possibly contribute to impairment of trophoblast invasion. Indeed, in a later study, these authors reported increased staining for nitrotyrosine residues and heat shock protein 70 in placental tissue from missed miscarriage, indicating that oxidative stress may be a key factor in early pregnancy loss (Jauniaux *et al.*, 2003).

Burton and Hung (2003) have suggested that maintenance of the muscular coat of the spiral artery, due to impaired trophoblast invasion, would lead to intermittent placental perfusion (Burton and Hung, 2003). Together with frequent thrombotic occlusion followed by clot dissolution this may lead to chronic hypoxia/reoxygenation insults in the placenta throughout pregnancy with subsequent initiation of oxidative stress. Due to the hypoxic environment XOR, which is abundantly expressed in the placenta, would be converted to the oxidase form (Many *et al.*, 2000), leading to increased $O_2^{\bullet}$ generation upon reoxygenation. It is highly relevant that Hung *et al.* have shown that exposure of normal term placenta in vitro to a period of hypoxia followed by reperfusion leads to an increase in nitrotyrosine staining in trophoblast and activation of apoptotic pathways, which could be attenuated by addition of a free radical scavenger (Hung *et al.*, 2002).

Evidence for increased placental free radical synthesis in pre-eclampsia

Placental tissue from women with pre-eclampsia show an increased capacity to generate $O_2^{\bullet}$ (Dechend *et al.*, 2003; Sikkema *et al.*, 2001; Wang and Walsh, 2001) that, at least in part, may be related to higher expression of XO (Many *et al.*, 2000). In term placenta, NAD(P)H oxidase is reported to be present in both syncytiotrophoblast

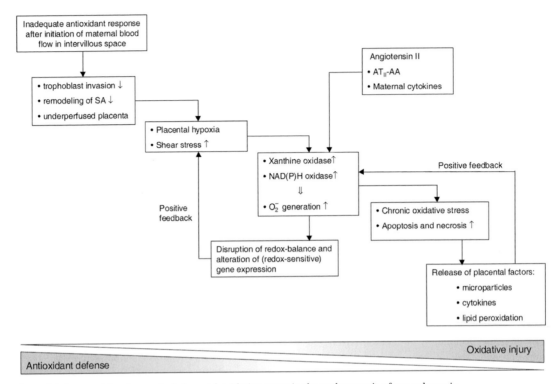

Figure 8.1 Proposed involvement of placental oxidative stress in the pathogenesis of pre-eclampsia.

and cytotrophoblast (Dechend *et al.*, 2003). Dechend *et al.* reported increased immunostaining for the NAD(P)H oxidase subunits in pre-eclamptic placentas (Dechend *et al.*, 2003). Recently, we have reported similar NAD(P)H oxidase-mediated $O_2^{\bullet}$ generation in placental tissue of women with pre-eclampsia when compared to normotensive controls and women with early-onset pre-eclampsia showed higher placental $O_2^{\bullet}$ generation. The authors' unpublished preliminary data show that NAD(P)H oxidase is functionally active as early as the first trimester of pregnancy, raising the possibility that NAD(P)H oxidase could play a role in early placental development.

Placental antioxidant status in pre-eclampsia

As a presumed adaptive response, several studies provide evidence that glutathione levels (Gülmezoglu *et al.*, 1996), GPX enzyme activity (Knapen *et al.*, 1999) or catalase activity (Wang and Walsh, 1996) are also raised. However, a decrease in placental antioxidant capacity is more frequently reported (Walsh, 1998; Zusterzeel *et al.*, 2001); vitamin E levels are reported to be lower (Wang and Walsh, 1996), whereas the expression of several important enzymatic antioxidants (e.g. SOD, GPX, GSTPi and glucose-6-phosphate dehydrogenase) appear to be down-regulated (Walsh, 1998; Wang and Walsh, 1996; Zusterzeel *et al.*, 1999).

Placental oxidative damage in pre-eclampsia

Numerous independent oxidative damage markers indicate the presence of placental oxidative stress; there is evidence for lipid peroxidation (Gülmezoglu *et al.*, 1996; Walsh *et al.*, 2000), for increased synthesis of the isoprostane, 8-iso-prostaglandin $F_{2\alpha}$ (Walsh et al., 2000), for enhanced generation of protein carbonyls (Zusterzeel et al., 2001) and for nitrotyrosine formation (Many et al., 2000; Myatt et al., 1996). The isoprostane, 8-iso-prostaglandin $F_{2\alpha}$ is in itself biologically active. Indeed, Staff et al. have shown in an in vitro model that this isoprostane reduces trophoblast invasion and matrix metalloproteinase activity (Staff et al., 2000).

Maternal oxidative stress in pre-eclampsia

The origin of systemic oxidative stress in pre-eclampsia

Placental oxidative stress may, in turn, be the origin of maternal systemic oxidative stress. As might be anticipated, women with pre-eclampsia show evidence of increased apoptosis in trophoblast and microvilli (Crocker et al., 2003). The deportation of microparticles from the placenta into the maternal circulation in normal pregnancy has been hypothesized to contribute to the exaggerated maternal inflammatory response characteristic of pre-eclampsia (Redman and Sargent, 2000) and is associated with local $O_2^\bullet$ generation (Figure 8.2).

Evidence of increased systemic free radical generation in pre-eclampsia

Stimulated $O_2^\bullet$ generation with receptor-mediated agonists is higher in isolated neutrophils from affected than normotensive pregnant women (Tsukimori et al., 1993). However, stimulation with phorbol esters that directly activate protein

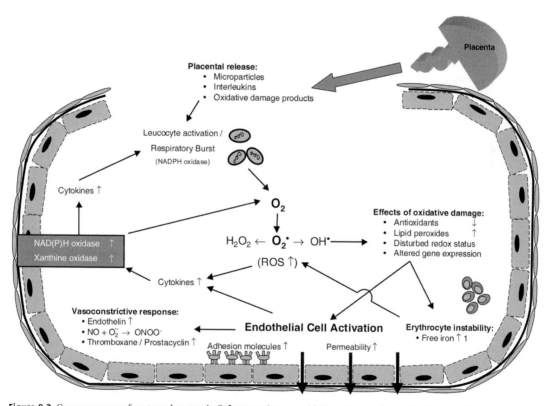

Figure 8.2 Consequences of maternal systemic $O_2^\bullet$ generation on oxidative stress and vascular function in pre-eclampsia.

kinase results either in higher (Lee *et al.*, 2003) or similar $O_2^\bullet$ generation of pre-eclamptic neutrophils when compared to normal pregnant controls (Tsukimori *et al.*, 1993).

Since NAD(P)H oxidase is present in neutrophils, this enzyme seems to be the mediator of the respiratory burst response (Lee *et al.*, 2003).

In women with gestational hypertension, an increase in plasma uric acid concentration, a product of XO activity, was associated with raised XO enzyme activity in plasma (Nemeth *et al.*, 2002). Elevated concentrations of uric acid in the blood of women with pre-eclampsia could therefore be an indirect marker of increased $O_2^\bullet$ production by XO, but may also reflect other mechanisms (Many *et al.*, 1996).

Erythrocyte membrane instability and subsequent increased red cell turnover lead to release of iron in blood of women with pre-eclampsia (Spickett *et al.*, 1998). Non-bound iron is capable of generating ROS (e.g. $O_2^\bullet$, H_2O_2, and $OH^\bullet$) (Rayman *et al.*, 2002). Women with established pre-eclampsia have differences in measures of iron metabolism, including decreased (apo)transferrin and total iron-binding capacity, whereas serum ferritin is increased, which could contribute to the raised free iron concentrations in serum (Hubel *et al.*, 1996a; Rayman *et al.*, 2002).

Maternal antioxidant status in pre-eclampsia

The total peroxyl radical-trapping ability of plasma has been found to be higher in women with pre-eclampsia (Kharb, 2000c; Uotila *et al.*, 1994), unsurprising, perhaps, since this assay includes the antioxidant uric acid, which has frequently been reported to be raised (Chappell *et al.*, 2002; Kharb, 2000c; Many *et al.*, 1996; Zusterzeel *et al.*, 2002). As explained above, this may reflect increased XO activity with subsequent generation of $O_2^\bullet$, rather than an elevation of functional antioxidant capacity. The oxygen radical absorbance capacity, based on direct quenching of free radicals (Cao and Prior, 1998), is reported to be unchanged in women with mild pre-eclampsia

(Zusterzeel *et al.*, 2002), whereas studies in more severe disease have suggested that overall antioxidant capacity, is lower (Davidge *et al.*, 1992; Sagol *et al.*, 1999). Overall, estimates of "total" antioxidants are unlikely to provide a good index of antioxidant capacity because of the dependency on the antioxidant species included or excluded in the different assays.

Many studies have investigated the role of glutathione and other aminothiols in the etiology of oxidative stress in pre-eclampsia. Total $-SH$ groups, including both amino thiols and $-SH$ moieties of protein, are reduced in plasma (Chen *et al.*, 1994; Hubel *et al.*, 1997; Uotila *et al.*, 1994) or erythrocyte lysates (Kharb, 2000a), and are indicative of a state of oxidative stress. The reports of glutathione are diverse. This may relate to the fact that erythrocyte concentrations are high compared to those in plasma, have a broad intra-individual variation, and that several different methods are used for glutathione assessment (Redegeld *et al.*, 1990; Richie Jr. *et al.*, 1996). Some studies have reported lower glutathione levels in the plasma of women with pre-eclampsia (Chen *et al.*, 1994; Kharb, 2000b), and the glutathione:hemoglobin ratio in whole blood has been found to be lower compared to normotensive control women (Knapen *et al.*, 1998).

Both iron-induced oxidation and free radical attack of the $-SH$ group of aminothiols, including cysteine, homocysteine and cysteinylglycine, results in the formation of (mixed) disulfides. This shifts the redox thiol status (i.e. the dynamic equilibrium of the reduced, oxidized and protein-bound thiol forms) to a higher oxidized state that can be measured as a decrease in the free-to-oxidized ratio (Ueland *et al.*, 1996). The main target of oxidative attack is cysteine, the aminothiol with the lowest redox potential (Stamler and Slivka, 1996); however, oxidized cysteine will quickly be reduced by subsequent oxidation of other aminothiols. We (MR) have reported that the free-to-oxidized ratios for cysteine, cysteinylglycine and homocysteine are lower in pre-eclampsia (Raijmakers *et al.*, 2001a,b). In the case of homocysteine this was maintained until 6 weeks postpartum (unpublished results). We have also observed abnormally high total plasma concentrations and a decreased free-to-oxidized ratio for homocysteine in non-pregnant women who have had pre-eclampsia previously. As approximately 60% of subsequent pregnancies were affected by hypertension, this disturbed redox balance could be a pre-disposing risk factor (Raijmakers *et al.*, 2004b).

Reports of vitamin E status, normally measured as the α-tocopherol form, in pre-eclampsia are ambiguous. Since vitamin E is transported by lipoproteins, this is most likely explained by varying degrees of associated hyperlipoproteinemia (Brigelius-Flohe *et al.*, 2002). Moreover, circulating concentrations of this lipophilic antioxidant do not give insight into cellular vitamin E status and are probably poorly indicative of functional vitamin E capacity. Plasma vitamin E concentrations, not adjusted for the lipid profile, have been reported to be lower (Madazli *et al.*, 1999; Sagol *et al.*, 1999), similar (Uotila *et al.*, 1994; Valsecchi *et al.*, 1999), or increased (Hubel *et al.*, 1997; Schiff *et al.*, 1996; Zusterzeel *et al.*, 2002) in pre-eclampsia compared with normotensive pregnancy. However, when corrected for lipids, no differences have been found (Chappell *et al.*, 2002; Hubel *et al.*, 1997; Zhang *et al.*, 2001). Pre-eclampsia is almost undoubtedly a state of vitamin C depletion, as most studies have reported lowered plasma vitamin C concentrations (Chappell *et al.*, 2002; Madazli *et al.*, 1999; Mikhail *et al.*, 1994; Sagol *et al.*, 1999; Zhang *et al.*, 2002c), although a few have found unchanged levels (Uotila *et al.*, 1994; Zusterzeel *et al.*, 2002). The deficiency in vitamin C could impact on vitamin E metabolism, as vitamin C is claimed to act in synergy with vitamin E. Impairment of the regeneration of reduced vitamin E from oxidized vitamin E (because of lowered vitamin C concentrations) could contribute to reduced free radical scavenging capacity of vitamin E.

The reduction in vitamin C could arise from reduced dietary intake as well as depletion by enhanced free radical synthesis. Two epidemiological studies have used validated food questionnaires to estimate dietary intake of vitamin C (Zhang *et al.*, 2002b) or vitamin E (Schiff *et al.*, 1996) over the year prior to pregnancy, including the pre-conception period. In a recent study, performed in a mixed population of American women with pre-eclampsia, dietary intake of vitamin C below the recommended dietary allowance (<85 mg daily) was found to double the pre-eclampsia risk (Zhang *et al.*, 2002a). However, Schiff *et al.*, who compared fewer cases from a similar American population, found no such relationship (Schiff *et al.*, 1996). A large prospective study in the USA did not find any association with pre-eclampsia and either vitamin C or vitamin E intake (Morris *et al.*, 2001). However, in this study a 24 h recall questionnaire was used, which only included dietary intake during early pregnancy, but more importantly, participants were given a daily pre-natal supplement that could have changed the participant awareness of the importance of diet during pregnancy.

Carotenoids including retinol (or vitamin A) have not been the subject of intensive investigation in pre-eclampsia and a consensus viewpoint is not attainable. In most studies several carotenoids have been measured simultaneously, and have suggested that β-carotene (Mikhail *et al.*, 1994; Palan *et al.*, 2001), lycopene (Palan *et al.*, 2001) and retinal (Zhang *et al.*, 2001) are decreased, without any notable differences in the other carotenoids.

In contrast to the non-enzymatic antioxidants, the presence and activity of enzymatic oxidants has seldom been studied in pre-eclampsia and contradictory findings have been reported in the few studies performed. The expression of SOD in subcutaneous fat vessels (Roggensack *et al.*, 1999) and the activity of the same enzyme in erythrocytes (Bayhan *et al.*, 2000; Chen *et al.*, 1994) has been observed to be lower in women with pre-eclampsia. In contrast to reduced activity of SOD in pre-eclamptic erythrocytes, GPX and catalase have been reported to be unchanged in erythrocytes (Bayhan *et al.*, 2000) or plasma (Karsdorp et al., 1998). Some studies have reported that in association with reduced erythrocyte enzyme activity of both SOD and catalase, GPX activity is paradoxically increased (Diedrich et al., 2001). However, GPX activity is largely comprised of GSTs that also play an important role in the direct metabolism of toxic products of oxidative stress (Hayes and Pulford, 1995). Both ROS and oxidative damage products induce the expression of antioxidant enzymes through activation of the "antioxidant-responsive element" in the promoter region (Hayes and McLellan, 1999). Thus it can be hypothesized that the expression of GPX is induced to prevent excessive lipid peroxidation and to metabolize oxidative damage products arising from low SOD and catalase enzyme activities.

Evidence of maternal oxidative damage in pre-eclampsia

Investigations of marker molecules in the maternal circulation in pre-eclampsia have shown varying results; however, most are indicative of oxidative stress. Reports of increased generation of peroxynitrite radicals suggest higher oxidative damage (Hubel, 1999; Roggensack et al., 1999). MDA, a major breakdown product of lipid peroxides, was one of the first biomarkers found to be raised (Ishihara, 1978). Numerous studies have confirmed that serum MDA levels or the amounts of thiobarbituric acid reactive substances, mainly consisting of MDA, are elevated in women with pre-eclampsia (Bayhan et al., 2000; Kharb, 2000c; Madazli et al., 1999; Takacs et al., 2001; Uotila et al., 1993). Only one study has not demonstrated a difference in MDA (Davidge et al., 1992).

One of the consequences of lipid peroxidation is bond migration in the hydrocarbon chain of the unsaturated fatty acid resulting in the formation of conjugated dienes (Hubel et al., 1989), which may be a specific biomarker for lipid peroxidation. Conjugated dienes are elevated in plasma or platelets of women with pre-eclampsia

(Garzetti et al., 1993; Hubel et al., 1989; Uotila et al., 1993). The most frequently assayed isoprostane in pre-eclampsia is 8-iso-prostaglandin $F_{2\alpha}$ (8-iso-$PGF_{2\alpha}$). Reliability of estimation depends on the method (GC/MS vs. ELISA) and kind of sample (plasma vs. urine) used for analysis. GC/MS provides a specific analysis of several isoprostanes, but is time-consuming in contrast to a high throughput ELISA assay but this is less reliable due to the poor specificity of some antibodies. Plasma is preferred since possible differences in renal metabolism and clearance in women with pre-eclampsia could influence concentrations in urine. Taken together, it is not surprising that reports of isoprostane concentrations in women with pre-eclampsia are ambiguous. Higher plasma 8-iso-$PGF_{2\alpha}$ concentrations than those in normal pregnancy have been detected, but in the same patients urine concentrations are lower, which may be explicable by impaired renal clearance (Barden et al., 2001). Other studies found no abnormalities in the plasma concentration of the same isoprostane (Chappell et al., 2002; Morris et al., 1998) and urine concentrations of another isomer, 8,12-iso-iPF$_{2\alpha}$-VI, have been found to be similar to those of normal pregnant women (Regan et al., 2001).

The lipid profile of women with pre-eclampsia differs from that of normotensive pregnancy (Hubel et al., 1996b; Sattar et al., 2000). In pre-eclampsia LDL decreases in particle size, which results in greater susceptibility to oxidative modification (Hubel et al., 1998; Pierucci et al., 1996). There are reports of increased antibody titers against the oxidized form of LDL and of an elevation in the ratio between this antibody and that against the native form of LDL (Branch et al., 1994; Uotila et al., 1998; Wakatsuki et al., 2000).

Proteins may be modified by ROS or reactive nitrogen species or indirectly by reactions with products of lipid peroxidation. This results in the formation of additional carbonyl groups, which as one report has suggested are elevated in plasma of women with pre-eclampsia

(Zusterzeel *et al.*, 2000). Reaction with reactive nitrogen species such as peroxynitrite results in the formation of nitrotyrosine residues, the increased expression of which has been reported in the small arteries from women with pre-eclampsia (Roggensack *et al.*, 1999).

Consequences of oxidative stress in pre-eclampsia

As discussed above, the products of oxidative stress from the placenta may contribute to the maternal inflammatory response. These will be compounded by local generation of ROS in the mother. Indeed, it is possible the characteristics of pre-eclampsia could be explained on the basis of oxidative stress (Hubel, 1999). Vascular function may be altered by oxidative stress (Davidge, 1998). Lipid peroxides can interact and alter endothelial cell function (Davidge, 1998; Hubel *et al.*, 1989; Taylor *et al.*, 1998). Some reports have suggested that NO synthase and nitric oxide are increased in the vasculature of women with pre-eclampsia (Davidge, 1998; Roggensack *et al.*, 1999). NO may rapidly react with $O_2^\bullet$ yielding peroxynitrite, which reduces the availability of NO to act as a vasorelaxant, is involved in necrosis and apoptosis, and may damage endothelial cells. Additionally, peroxynitrite together with lipid peroxides may result in overproduction of both prostacyclin and thromboxane (Davidge, 1998; Roggensack *et al.*, 1999). Extreme levels of lipid peroxides inhibit prostaglandin H synthase, resulting in decreased concentrations of prostacyclin, a vasorelaxant. Furthermore, both cell damage and oxygen radicals stimulate the release of endothelin, a potent vasoconstrictor, which is increased in women with pre-eclampsia (Slowinski *et al.*, 2002).

Both placental and systemic oxidative stress may alter gene expression. The activity of the transcription factors of the Mitogen Activated Protein Kinase family seems to be directly activated by $O_2^\bullet$ and results in the expression of proteins involved in growth, angiogenesis, matrix remodeling, apoptosis and cell proliferation. However, at high levels of $O_2^\bullet$ transcription factors including AP-1 and NFKB are activated, and lead to many of the facets of the inflammatory response and tissue hypertrophy. By the modulation of the (thiol) redox status of cell, oxidative stress may have an effect on redox-sensitive gene-expression, resulting in the expression of proteins with an antioxidant responsive element in the promoter region, including most of the antioxidant enzymes (Hayes and McLellan, 1999).

Prophylaxis of pre-eclampsia using antioxidants

Despite increased understanding of the etiology of the syndrome, there is currently no accepted method of prevention of pre-eclampsia. Studies of aspirin and calcium prophylaxis have proved disappointing (Coomarasamy *et al.*, 2003). However, the abundant evidence for oxidative stress in pre-eclampsia provides a potential avenue of hope for the development of new strategies involving antioxidant prophylaxis. The choice of antioxidant is important. Some antioxidants, particularly vitamin E, not only detoxify free radicals, but also have other properties that may benefit women with pre-eclampsia directly (Azzi *et al.*, 2002; Brigelius *et al.*, 2002). Antioxidants, by altering the cell redox status, are indirectly involved in the regulation of redox-sensitive gene expression. At levels close to those found in plasma, α-tocopherol has been shown to play a role in cell signaling by the inhibition of PKC activation (Azzi *et al.*, 2002). Via this pathway vitamin E exerts antiproliferative effects and may directly influence the reduction of $O_2^\bullet$ generation by NAD(P)H oxidase, aggregation of platelets and the inhibition of monocyte–endothelium adhesion (Azzi *et al.*, 2002). Through the down regulation of NFκB, α-tocopherol plays a role in the reduction of an inflammatory response (Rimbach *et al.*, 2002;

Weber et al., 1994). Vitamin C has been reported to inhibit apoptosis (Rossig et al., 2001) and could thereby reduce microparticle formation in the placenta. As mentioned earlier, ascorbic acid regenerates α-tocopherol by the reduction of the α-tocopherol radical. The multimode of action of α-tocopherol together with the synergistic association with ascorbic acid may be fortuitous in relation to pre-eclampsia. Together these antioxidants could not only inhibit the lipid peroxidation chain reaction, but also reduce the generation of free radicals, the inflammatory response and the procoagulant state.

To date, three studies have employed antioxidant supplementation, which all included a combination of high-dose vitamin E and vitamin C, in the prevention of pre-eclampsia (Gülmezoglu et al., 1997; Stratta et al., 1994). In these studies antioxidants were administered at onset of disease and no effect of antioxidant treatment was found. In contrast, Chappell et al. (1999) treated a high-risk population, defined by the presence of an abnormal Doppler waveform or pre-eclampsia in their previous pregnancy, from early pregnancy (18–22 weeks) until delivery with 1000 mg vitamin C and 400 IU vitamin E daily in a double-blind randomized trial. They reported not only a highly reduced risk of pre-eclampsia, but also showed that antioxidant treatment led to the improvement of biochemical markers associated with oxidative stress, an indication that antioxidant treatment reduced the level of oxidative damage (Chappell et al., 1999).

The differences between these studies may indicate that early intervention might be essential for the prevention of pre-eclampsia. In pre-eclampsia an increased oxidative pressure from the placenta and/or a poor antioxidant response in the maternal circulation could initiate a chain of events leading to rapid progression of oxidative stress. Early vitamin intervention could assist the adaptive maternal antioxidant response, thereby normalizing the effects of oxidative stress. However, with treatment after the "point-of-no-return" when the clinical syndrome is evident with multiple organ involvement, the oxidative stress may no longer be reversible corrected by antioxidant supplementation. Multicenter trials momentarily underway in the UK, the USA, and three developing countries will now determine whether antioxidant prophylaxis may be used routinely in the prevention of pre-eclampsia.

Conclusions

Oxidative stress is a result of a complex, dynamic equilibrium between (pro)oxidant generation and antioxidant protection. Several distinct pathways that contribute to the induction or propagation of oxidative stress are activated which have many detrimental effects. A single marker will never provide a clear picture and oxidative stress should ideally be estimated by new methods that include both "arms" of the oxidative stress balance.

$O_2^{\bullet}$ generation increases in normal pregnancy. Through redox-sensitive genes, $O_2^{\bullet}$ could play a role in trophoblast invasion, and placental development during pregnancy. The oxidative stress balance is delicate and disturbances in either direction could predispose to a poor pregnancy outcome. Free radical damage appears to play a major role in the maternal syndrome of pre-eclampsia. The placenta is the likely source of origin, but oxidative stress is compounded by the subsequent contribution of maternally generated superoxide. The results of large clinical trials currently underway will determine whether antioxidants may offer prophylactic benefit.

REFERENCES

Adams, S., Green, P., Claxton, R., et al. (2001). Reactive carbonyl formation by oxidative and non-oxidative pathways. Front Biosci., 6, A17–24.

Arthur, J. R. (2000). The glutathione peroxidases. Cell Mol. Life Sci., 57(13–14), 1825–35.

Azzi, A., Ricciarelli, R. and Zingg, J. M. (2002). Non-antioxidant molecular functions of alpha-tocopherol (vitamin E). FEBS Lett., 519(1–3), 8–10.

Barden, A., Ritchie, J., Walters, B., *et al.* (2001). Study of plasma factors associated with neutrophil activation and lipid peroxidation in preeclampsia. *Hypertension*, **38**(4), 803–8.

Bayhan, G., Atamer, Y., Atamer, A., Yokus, B. and Baylan, Y. (2000). Significance of changes in lipid peroxides and antioxidant enzyme activities in pregnant women with preeclampsia and eclampsia. *Clin. Exp. Obstet. Gynecol.*, **27**(2), 142–6.

Berliner, L. J., Khramtsov, V., Fujii, H. and Clanton, T. L. (2001). Unique in vivo applications of spin traps. *Free Rad. Biol. Med.*, **30**(5), 489–99.

Branch, D. W., Mitchell, M. D., Miller, E., Palinski, W. and Witztum, J. L. (1994). Pre-eclampsia and serum antibodies to oxidised low-density lipoprotein. *Lancet*, **343**(8898), 645–6.

Brigelius-Flohe, R., Kelly, F. J., Salonen, J. T., Neuzil, J., Zingg, J. M. and Azzi, A. (2002). The European perspective on vitamin E: current knowledge and future research. *Am. J. Clin. Nutr.*, **76**(4), 703–16.

Burton, G. J. and Hung, T. H. (2003). Hypoxia-reoxygenation; a potential source of placental oxidatives stress in normal pregnancy and preeclampsia. *Fetal Maternal Med. Rev.*, **14**(2), 97–117.

Cao, G. and Prior, R. L. (1998). Comparison of different analytical methods for assessing total antioxidant capacity of human serum. *Clin. Chem.*, **44**(6)(Pt. 1), 1309–15.

Chappell, L. C., Seed, P. T., Briley, A. L., *et al.* (1999). Effect of antioxidants on the occurrence of pre-eclampsia in women at increased risk: a randomised trial. *Lancet*, **345**, 810–16.

Chappell, L. C., Seed, P. T., Briley, A., *et al.* (2002). A longitudinal study of biochemical variables in women at risk of preeclampsia. *Am. J. Obstet. Gynecol.*, **187**(1), 127–36.

Chen, G., Wilson, R., Cumming, G., Walker, J. J., Smith, W. E. and McKillop, J. H. (1994). Intracellular and extracellular antioxidant buffering levels in erythrocytes from pregnancy-induced hypertension. *J. Hum. Hypertens.*, **8**(1), 37–42.

Cikot, R. J. L. M., Steegers Theunissen, R. P. M., Thomas, C. M. G., de Boo, T. M., Merkus, H. M. W. M. and Steegers, E. A. P. (2001). Longitudinal vitamin and homocysteine levels in normal pregnancy. *Br. J. Nutr.*, **85**(1), 49–58.

Conti, M., Morand, P. C., Levillain, P. and Lemonnier, A. (1991). Improved fluorometric determination of malonaldehyde. *Clin. Chem.*, **37**(7), 1273–5.

Coomarasamy, A., Honest, H., Papaioannou, S., Gee, H. and Khan, K. S. (2003). Aspirin for prevention of preeclampsia in women with historical risk factors: a systematic review. *Obstet. Gynecol.*, **101**(6), 1319–32.

Cracowski, J. L., Durand, T. and Bessard, G. (2002). Isoprostanes as a biomarker of lipid peroxidation in humans: physiology, pharmacology and clinical implications. *Trends Pharmacol. Sci.*, **23**(8), 360–6.

Crocker, I. P., Cooper, S., Ong, S. C. and Baker, P. N. (2003). Differences in apoptotic susceptibility of cytotrophoblasts and syncytiotrophoblasts in normal pregnancy to those complicated with preeclampsia and intrauterine growth restriction. *Am. J. Pathol.*, **162**(2), 637–43.

Davidge, S. T. (1998). Oxidative stress and altered endothelial cell function in preeclampsia. *Semin. Reprod. Endocrinol.*, **16**(1), 65–73.

Davidge, S. T., Hubel, C. A., Brayden, R. D., Capeless, E. C. and McLaughlin, M. K. (1992). Sera antioxidant activity in uncomplicated and preeclamptic pregnancies. *Obstet. Gynecol.*, **79**(6), 897–901.

Dechend, R., Viedt, C., Muller, D. N., *et al.* (2003). AT1 receptor agonistic antibodies from preeclamptic patients stimulate NADPH oxidase. *Circulation*, **107**(12), 1632–9.

Diedrich, F., Renner, A., Rath, W., Kuhn, W. and Wieland, E. (2001). Lipid hydroperoxides and free radical scavenging enzyme activities in preeclampsia and HELLP (hemolysis, elevated liver enzymes, and low platelet count) syndrome: no evidence for circulating primary products of lipid peroxidation. *Am. J. Obstet. Gynecol.*, **185**(1), 166–72.

Garzetti, G. G., Tranquilli, A. L., Cugini, A. M., Mazzanti, L., Cester, N. and Romanini, C. (1993). Altered lipid composition, increased lipid peroxidation, and altered fluidity of the membrane as evidence of platelet damage in preeclampsia. *Obstet. Gynecol.*, **81**(3), 337–40.

Griendling, K. K., Sorescu, D., Lassegue, B. and Ushio-Fukai, M. (2000a). Modulation of protein kinase activity and gene expression by reactive oxygen species and their role in vascular physiology and pathophysiology. *Arterioscler. Thromb. Vasc. Biol.*, **20**(10), 2175–83.

Griendling, K. K., Sorescu, D. and Ushio-Fukai, M. (2000b). NAD(P)H oxidase: role in cardiovascular biology and disease. *Circ. Res.*, **86**(5), 494–501.

Gülmezoglu, A. M., Oosthuizen, M. M. J. and Hofmeyr, G. J. (1996). Placental malondialdehyde and glutathione levels in a controlled trial of antioxidant treatment in severe preeclampsia. *Hypertens. Pregn.*, **15**(3), 287–95.

Gülmezoglu, A. M., Hofmeyr, G. J. and Oosthuizen, M. M. J. (1997). Antioxidants in the treatment of severe pre-eclampsia: an explanatory randomised controlled trial. *Br. J. Obstet. Gynaecol.*, **104**, 689–96.

Halliwell, B. (1997). Antioxidants and human disease: a general introduction. *Nutr. Rev.*, **55**(1)(Pt. 2), S44–9.

Harrison, R. (2002). Structure and function of xanthine oxidoreductase: where are we now? *Free Rad. Biol. Med.*, **33**(6), 774–97.

Hayes, J. D. and Pulford, D. J. (1995). The glutathione *S*-transferase supergene family: regulation of GST and the contribution of the isoenzymes to cancer chemo-protection and drug resistance. *Crit. Rev. Biochem. Mol. Biol.*, **30**(6), 445–600.

Hayes, J. D. and McLellan, L. I. (1999). Glutathione and glutathione-dependent enzymes represent a co-ordinately regulated defence against oxidative stress. *Free Rad. Res.*, **31**(4), 273–300.

Holmgren, A. and Bjornstedt, M. (1995). Thioredoxin and thioredoxin reductase. *Meth. Enzymol.*, **252**, 199–208.

Hong, Y. C., Lee, K. H., Yi, C. H., Ha, E. H. and Christiani, D. C. (2002). Genetic susceptibility of term pregnant women to oxidative damage. *Toxicol. Lett.*, **129**(3), 255–62.

Houston, M., Estevez, A., Chumley, P., *et al.* (1999). Binding of xanthine oxidase to vascular endothelium. Kinetic characterization and oxidative impairment of nitric oxide-dependent signaling. *J. Biol. Chem.*, **274**(8), 4985–94.

Hubel, C. A. (1999). Oxidative stress in the pathogenesis of preeclampsia. *Proc. Soc. Exp. Biol. Med.*, **222**(3), 222–35.

Hubel, C. A., Roberts, J. M., Taylor, R. N., Musci, T. J., Rogers, G. M. and McLaughlin, M. K. (1989). Lipid peroxidation in pregnancy: new perspectives on pre-eclampsia. *Am. J. Obstet. Gynecol.*, **161**(4), 1025–34.

Hubel, C. A., Kozlov, A. V., Kagan, V. E., *et al.* (1996a). Decreased transferrin and increased transferrin saturation in sera of women with preeclampsia: implications for oxidative stress. *Am. J. Obstet. Gynecol.*, **175**(3)(Pt. 1), 692–700.

Hubel, C. A., McLaughlin, M. K., Evans, R. W., Hauth, B. A., Sims, C. J. and Roberts, J. M. (1996b). Fasting serum triglycerides, free fatty acids, and malondialdehyde are increased in preeclampsia, are positively correlated, and decrease within 48 hours post partum. *Am. J. Obstet. Gynecol.*, **174**(3), 975–82.

Hubel, C. A., Kagan, V. E., Kisin, E. R., McLaughlin, M. K. and Roberts, J. M. (1997). Increased ascorbate radical formation and ascorbate depletion in plasma from women with preeclampsia: implications for oxidative stress. *Free Rad. Biol. Med.*, **23**(4), 597–609.

Hubel, C. A., Shakir, Y., Gallaher, M. J., McLaughlin, M. K. and Roberts, J. M. (1998). Low-density lipoprotein particle size decreases during normal pregnancy in association with triglyceride increases. *J. Soc. Gynecol. Invest.*, **5**(5), 244–50.

Hung, T. H., Skepper, J. N., Charnock-Jones, D. S. and Burton, G. J. (2002). Hypoxia-reoxygenation: a potent inducer of apoptotic changes in the human placenta and possible etiological factor in preeclampsia. *Circ. Res.*, **90**(12), 1274–81.

Irani, K. (2000). Oxidant signaling in vascular cell growth, death, and survival: a review of the roles of reactive oxygen species in smooth muscle and endothelial cell mitogenic and apoptotic signaling. *Circ. Res.*, **87**(3), 179–83.

Ishihara, M. (1978). Studies on lipoperoxide of normal pregant women and of patients with toxemia of pregnancy. *Clin. Chim. Acta*, **84**, 1–9.

Jauniaux, E., Watson, A. L., Hempstock, J., Bao, Y. P., Skepper, J. N. and Burton, G. J. (2000). Onset of maternal arterial blood flow and placental oxidative stress. A possible factor in human early pregnancy failure. *Am. J. Pathol.*, **157**(6), 2111–22.

Jauniaux, E., Hempstock, J., Greenwold, N. and Burton, G. J. (2003). Trophoblastic oxidative stress in relation to temporal and regional differences in maternal placental blood flow in normal and abnormal early pregnancies. *Am. J. Pathol.*, **162**(1), 115–25.

Karsdorp, V. H. M., Dekker, G. A., Bast, A., *et al.* (1998). Maternal and fetal plasma concentrations of endothelin, lipidhydroperoxides, glutathione peroxidase and fibronectin in relation to abnormal umbilical artery velocimetry. *Eur. J. Obstet. Gynecol. Reprod. Biol.*, **80**(1), 39–44.

Kharb, S. (2000a). Altered thiol status in preeclampsia. *Gynecol. Obstet. Invest.*, **50**(1), 36–8.

Kharb, S. (2000b). Low whole blood glutathione levels in pregnancies complicated by preeclampsia and diabetes. *Clin. Chim. Acta*, **294**(1–2), 179–83.

Kharb, S. (2000c). Total free radical trapping antioxidant potential in pre-eclampsia. *Int. J. Gynaecol. Obstet.*, **69**(1), 23–6.

Knapen, M. F. C. M., Mulder, T. P. J., Van Rooij, I. A. L. M., Peters, W. H. M. and Steegers, E. A. P. (1998). Low whole blood glutathione levels in pregnancies complicated by preeclampsia or the hemolysis, elevated liver enzymes, low platelets syndrome. *Obstet. Gynecol.*, **92**, 1012–15.

Knapen, M. F. C. M., Peters, W. H. M., Mulder, T. P. J., Merkus, H. M. W. M., Jansen, J. B. M. J. and Steegers, E. A. P. (1999). Glutathione and glutathione-related enzymes in decidua and placenta of controls and women with pre-eclampsia. *Placenta*, **20**(7), 541–6.

Krinsky, N. I. (1998). The antioxidant and biological properties of the carotenoids. *Ann. N. Y. Acad. Sci.*, **854**, 443–7.

Langlois, M. R. and Delanghe, J. R. (1996). Biological and clinical significance of haptoglobin polymorphism in humans. *Clin. Chem.*, **42**(10), 1589–600.

Lee, V. M., Quinn, P. A., Jennings, S. C. and Ng, L. L. (2003). Neutrophil activation and production of reactive oxygen species in pre-eclampsia. *J. Hypertens.*, **21**(2), 395–402.

Lenaz, G., Bovina, C., D'Aurelio, M., *et al.* (2002). Role of mitochondria in oxidative stress and ageing. *Ann. N. Y. Acad. Sci.*, **959**, 199–213.

Little, R. E. and Gladen, B. C. (1999). Levels of lipid peroxides in uncomplicated pregnancy: a review of the literature. *Reprod. Toxicol.*, **13**(5), 347–52.

Luppi, P., Haluszczak, C., Trucco, M. and DeLoia, J. A. (2002). Normal pregnancy is associated with peripheral leukocyte activation. *Am. J. Reprod. Immunol.*, **47**(2), 72–81.

Madazli, R., Benian, A., Gumustas, K., Uzun, H., Ocak, V. and Aksu, F. (1999). Lipid peroxidation and antioxidants in preeclampsia. *Eur. J. Obstet. Gynecol. Reprod. Biol.*, **85**(2), 205–8.

Many, A., Hubel, C. A. and Roberts, J. M. (1996). Hyperuricemia and xanthine oxidase in preeclampsia, revisited. *Am. J. Obstet. Gynecol.*, **174**(1)(Pt. 1), 288–91.

Many, A., Hubel, C. A., Fisher, S. J., Roberts, J. M. and Zhou, Y. (2000). Invasive cytotrophoblasts manifest evidence of oxidative stress in preeclampsia. *Am. J. Pathol.*, **156**(1), 321–31.

Mates, J. M., Perez-Gomez, C. and Nunez, d. C. (1999). Antioxidant enzymes and human diseases. *Clin. Biochem.*, **32**(8), 595–603.

Meister, A. (1988). Glutathione metabolism and its selective modification. *J. Biol. Chem.*, **263**(33), 17,205–8.

Mikhail, M. S., Anyaegbunam, A., Garfinkel, D., Palan, P. R., Basu, J. and Romney, S. L. (1994). Preeclampsia and antioxidant nutrients: decreased plasma levels of reduced ascorbic acid, alpha-tocopherol, and beta-carotene in women with preeclampsia. *Am. J. Obstet. Gynecol.*, **171**(1), 150–7.

Morris, C. D., Jacobson, S. L., Anand, R., *et al.* (2001). Nutrient intake and hypertensive disorders of pregnancy: evidence from a large prospective cohort. *Am. J. Obstet. Gynecol.*, **184**(4), 643–51.

Morris, J. M., Gopaul, N. K., Endresen, M. J. R., *et al.* (1998). Circulating markers of oxidative stress are raised in normal pregnancy and pre-eclampsia. *Br. J. Obstet. Gynaecol.*, **105**(11), 1195–9.

Myatt, L., Rosenfield, R. B., Eis, A. L., Brockman, D. E., Greer, I. and Lyall, F. (1996). Nitrotyrosine residues in placenta. Evidence of peroxynitrite formation and action. *Hypertension*, **28**(3), 488–93.

Nemeth, I., Talosi, G., Papp, A. and Boda, D. (2002). Xanthine oxidase activation in mild gestational hypertension. *Hypertens. Pregn.*, **21**(1), 1–11.

Nohl, H., Gille, L. and Staniek, K. (1998). The biochemical, pathophysiological, and medical aspects of ubiquinone function. *Ann. N. Y. Acad. Sci.*, **854**, 394–409.

Nordberg, J. and Arner, E. S. (2001). Reactive oxygen species, antioxidants, and the mammalian thioredoxin system. *Free Rad. Biol. Med.*, **31**(11), 1287–312.

Palan, P. R., Mikhail, M. S. and Romney, S. L. (2001). Placental and serum levels of carotenoids in preeclampsia. *Obstet. Gynecol.*, **98**(3), 459–62.

Pierucci, F., Piazze Garnica, J. J., Cosmi, E. V. and Anceschi, M. M. (1996). Oxidability of low density lipoproteins in pregnancy-induced hypertension. *Br. J. Obstet. Gynaecol.*, **103**(11), 1159–61.

Pritsos, C. A. (2000). Cellular distribution, metabolism and regulation of the xanthine oxidoreductase enzyme system. *Chem. Biol. Interact.*, **129**(1–2), 195–208.

Qanungo, S., Sen, A. and Mukherjea, M. (1999). Antioxidant status and lipid peroxidation in human feto-placental unit. *Clin. Chim. Acta*, **285**(1–2), 1–12.

Raijmakers, M. T. M., Steegers, E. A. P. and Peters, W. H. M. (2001a). Glutathione S-transferases and thiol concentrations in embryonic and early fetal tissues. *Hum. Reprod.*, **16**(11), 2445–50.

Raijmakers, M. T. M., Zusterzeel, P. L. M., Roes, E. M., Steegers, E. A. P., Mulder, T. P. J. and Peters, W. H. M. (2001b). Oxidized and total whole blood thiols in women with preeclampsia. *Obstet. Gynecol.*, **97**, 272–6.

Raijmakers, M. T. M., Bruggeman, S. W. M., Steegers, E. A. P. and Peters, W. H. M. (2002). Distribution of components of the glutathione detoxification system across the human placenta after uncomplicated vaginal deliveries. *Placenta*, **23**(6), 490–6.

Raijmakers, M. T. M., Peters, W. H. M., Steegers, E. A. P. and Poston, L. (2005). Amino thiols, detoxification and oxidative stress in pre-eclampsia and other disorders of pregnancy. *Curr. Pharmaceut. Design*, **11**(6), 711–34.

Raijmakers, M. T. M., Peters, W. H. M., Steegers, E. A. P. and Poston, L. (2004a). NAD(P)H oxidase associated superoxide production in human placenta from normotensive and pre-eclamptic women. *Placenta*, **25S**, S85–9.

Raijmakers, M. T. M., Roes, E. M., Zusterzeel, P. L. M., Steegers, E. A. P. and Peters, W. H. M. (2004b). Thiol status and antioxidant capacity in women with a history of severe pre-eclampsia. *Br. J. Obstet. Gynaecol.*, **11**(3), 207–12.

Rayman, M. P., Barlis, J., Evans, R. W., Redman, C. W. and King, L. J. (2002). Abnormal iron parameters in the pregnancy syndrome preeclampsia. *Am. J. Obstet. Gynecol.*, **187**(2), 412–18.

Redegeld, F. A. M., Koster, A. S. and van Bennekom, W. P. (1998). Determination of tissue glutathione. In *Glutathione: Metabolism and Physiological Function*, ed. J. Vina. Boca Raton, FL, CRC Press, pp. 11–20.

Redman, C. W. G. and Sargent, I. L. (2000). Placental debris, oxidative stress and pre-eclampsia. *Placenta*, **21**(7), 597–602.

Regan, C. L., Levine, R. J., Baird, D. D., *et al.* (2001). No evidence for lipid peroxidation in severe preeclampsia. *Am. J. Obstet. Gynecol.*, **185**(3), 572–8.

Richie, J. P., Jr., Skowronski, L., Abraham, P. and Leutzinger, Y. (1996). Blood glutathione concentrations in a large-scale human study. *Clin. Chem.*, **42**(1), 64–70.

Rimbach, G., Minihane, A. M., Majewicz, J., *et al.* (2002). Regulation of cell signalling by vitamin E. *Proc. Nutr. Soc.*, **61**(4), 415–25.

Roberts, L. J. and Morrow, J. D. (2000). Measurement of F(2)-isoprostanes as an index of oxidative stress in vivo. *Free Rad. Biol. Med.*, **28**(4), 505–13.

Roggensack, A. M., Zhang, Y. and Davidge, S. T. (1999). Evidence for peroxynitrite formation in the vasculature of women with preeclampsia. *Hypertension*, **33**(1), 83–9.

Rossig, L., Hoffmann, J., Hugel, B., *et al.* (2001). Vitamin C inhibits endothelial cell apoptosis in congestive heart failure. *Circulation*, **104**(18), 2182–7.

Sagol, S., Ozkinay, E. and Ozsener, S. (1999). Impaired antioxidant activity in women with pre-eclampsia. *Int. J. Gynaecol. Obstet.*, **64**(2), 121–7.

Sattar, N., Clark, P., Greer, I. A., Shepherd, J. and Packard, C. J. (2000). Lipoprotein (a) levels in normal pregnancy and in pregnancy complicated with pre-eclampsia. *Atherosclerosis*, **148**(2), 407–11.

Schiff, E., Friedman, S. A., Stampfer, M., Kao, L., Barrett, P. H. and Sibai, B. M. (1996). Dietary consumption and plasma concentrations of vitamin E in pregnancies complicated by preeclampsia. *Am. J. Obstet. Gynecol.*, **175**(4)(Pt. 1), 1024–8.

Sevanian, A., Davies, K. J. and Hochstein, P. (1991). Serum urate as an antioxidant for ascorbic acid. *Am. J. Clin. Nutr.*, **54**(6, Suppl.), 1129S–34S.

Sikkema, J. M., van Rijn, B. B., Franx, A., *et al.* (2001). Placental superoxide is increased in pre-eclampsia. *Placenta*, **22**(4), 304–8.

Slowinski, T., Neumayer, H. H., Stolze, T., Gossing, G., Halle, H. and Hocher, B. (2002). Endothelin system in normal and hypertensive pregnancy. *Clin. Sci. (Lond.)*, **103**(Suppl. 48), 446S–9S.

Spickett, C. M., Reglinski, J., Smith, W. E., Wilson, R., Walker, J. J. and McKillop, J. (1998). Erythrocyte glutathione balance and membrane stability during preeclampsia. *Free Rad. Biol. Med.*, **24**(6), 1049–55.

Staff, A. C., Ranheim, T., Henriksen, T. and Halvorsen, B. (2000). 8-Iso-prostaglandin f(2alpha) reduces trophoblast invasion and matrix metalloproteinase activity. *Hypertension*, **35**(6), 1307–13.

Stamler, J. S. and Slivka, A. (1996). Biological chemistry of thiols in the vasculature and in vascular-related disease. *Nutr. Rev.*, **54**(1), 1–30.

Stratta, P., Canavese, C., Porcu, M., *et al.* (1994). Vitamin E supplementation in preeclampsia. *Gynecol. Obstet. Invest.*, **37**(4), 246–9.

Takacs, P., Kauma, S. W., Sholley, M. M., Walsh, S. W., Dinsmoor, M. J. and Green, K. (2001). Increased circulating lipid peroxides in severe pre-eclampsia activate NF-kappaB and upregulate ICAM-1 in vascular endothelial cells. *FASEB J.*, **15**(2), 279–81.

Taylor, R. N., de Groot, C. J. M., Cho, Y. K. and Lim, K.-H. (1998). Circulating factors as markers and mediators of endothelial cell dysfunction in preeclampsia. *Semin. Reprod. Endocrinol.*, **16**(1), 17–31.

Tomaro, M. L. and Batlle, A. M. (2002). Bilirubin: its role in cytoprotection against oxidative stress. *Int. J. Biochem. Cell Biol.*, **34**(3), 216–20.

Tsukimori, K., Maeda, H., Ishida, K., Nagata, H., Koyanagi, T. and Nakano, H. (1993). The superoxide generation of neutrophils in normal and preeclamptic pregnancies. *Obstet. Gynecol.*, **81**(4), 536–40.

Ueland, P.M., Mansoor, M.A., Guttormsen, A.B., *et al.* (1996). Reduced, oxidized and protein-bound forms of homocysteine and other aminothiols in plasma comprise the redox thiol status – a possible element of the extracellular antioxidant defense system. *J. Nutr.*, **126**(4, Suppl.), 1281S–4S.

Uotila, J., Solakivi, T., Jaakkola, O., Tuimala, R. and Lehtimaki, T. (1998). Antibodies against copper-oxidised and malondialdehyde-modified low density lipoproteins in pre-eclampsia pregnancies. *Br. J. Obstet. Gynaecol.*, **105**(10), 1113–17.

Uotila, J., Tuimala, R., Aarnio, T., Pyykko, K. and Ahotupa, M. (1991). Lipid peroxidation products, selenium-dependent glutathione peroxidase and vitamin E in normal pregnancy. *Eur. J. Obstet. Gynaecol. Reprod. Biol.*, **42**(2), 95–100.

Uotila, J.T., Kirkkola, A.L., Rorarius, M., Tuimala, R.J. and Metsa-Ketela, T. (1994). The total peroxyl radical-trapping ability of plasma and cerebrospinal fluid in normal and preeclamptic parturients. *Free Rad. Biol. Med.*, **16**(5), 581–90.

Uotila, J.T., Tuimala, R.J., Aarnio, T.M., Pyykko, K.A. and Ahotupa, M.O. (1993). Findings on lipid peroxidation and antioxidant function in hypertensive complications of pregnancy. *Br. J. Obstet. Gynaecol.*, **100**(3), 270–6.

Valsecchi, L., Cairone, R., Castiglioni, M.T., Almirante, G.M. and Ferrari, A. (1999). Serum levels of alpha-tocopherol in hypertensive pregnancies. *Hypertens. Pregn.*, **18**(3), 189–95.

Wakatsuki, A., Ikenoue, N., Okatani, Y., Shinohara, K. and Fukaya, T. (2000). Lipoprotein particles in preeclampsia: susceptibility to oxidative modification. *Obstet. Gynecol.*, **96**(1), 55–9.

Walsh, S.W. (1998). Maternal–placental interactions of oxidative stress and antioxidants in preeclampsia. *Semin. Reprod. Endocrinol.*, **16**(1), 93–104.

Walsh, S.W., Vaughan, J.E., Wang, Y. and Roberts, L.J. (2000). Placental isoprostane is significantly increased in preeclampsia. *FASEB J.*, **14**(10), 1289–96.

Wang, Y. and Walsh, S.W. (1996). Antioxidant activities and mRNA expression of superoxide dismutase, catalase, and glutathione peroxidase in normal and preeclamptic placentas. *J. Soc. Gynecol. Invest.*, **3**(4), 179–84.

Wang, Y. and Walsh, S.W. (1998). Placental mitochondria as a source of oxidative stress in pre-eclampsia. *Placenta*, **19**(8), 581–6.

Wang, Y. and Walsh, S.W. (2001). Increased superoxide generation is associated with decreased superoxide dismutase activity and mRNA expression in placental trophoblast cells in pre-eclampsia. *Placenta*, **22**(2–3), 206–12.

Weber, C., Erl, W., Pietsch, A., Strobel, M., Ziegler-Heitbrock, H.W. and Weber, P.C. (1994). Antioxidants inhibit monocyte adhesion by suppressing nuclear factor-kappa B mobilization and induction of vascular cell adhesion molecule-1 in endothelial cells stimulated to generate radicals. *Arterioscler. Thromb.*, **14**(10), 1665–73.

Zelko, I.N., Mariani, T.J. and Folz, R.J. (2002). Superoxide dismutase multigene family: a comparison of the CuZn-SOD (SOD1), Mn-SOD (SOD2), and EC-SOD (SOD3) gene structures, evolution, and expression. *Free Rad. Biol. Med.*, **33**(3), 337–49.

Zhang, C., Williams, M.A., Sanchez, S.E., *et al.* (2001). Plasma concentrations of carotenoids, retinol, and tocopherols in preeclamptic and normotensive pregnant women. *Am. J. Epidemiol.*, **153**(6), 572–80.

Zhang, C., Williams, M.A., King, I.B., *et al.* (2002a). Vitamin C and the risk of preeclampsia – results from dietary questionnaire and plasma assay. *Epidemiology*, **13**(4), 409–16.

Zhang, C., Williams, M.A., King, I.B., *et al.* (2002b). Vitamin C and the risk of preeclampsia – results from dietary questionnaire and plasma assay. *Epidemiology*, **13**(4), 409–16.

Zhang, C., Williams, M.A., King, I.B., *et al.* (2002c). Vitamin C and the risk of preeclampsia – results from dietary questionnaire and plasma assay. *Epidemiology*, **13**(4), 409–16.

Zusterzeel, P.L.M., Peters, W.H.M., De Bruyn, M.A., Knapen, M.F.C.M., Merkus, H.W.J.M. and Steegers, E.A.P. (1999). Glutathione S-transferase isoenzymes in decidua and placenta of preeclamptic pregnancies. *Obstet. Gynecol.*, **94**(6), 1033–8.

Zusterzeel, P.L.M., Mulder, T.P.J., Peters, W.H.M., Wiseman, S.A. and Steegers, E.A.P. (2000). Plasma protein carbonyls in nonpregnant, healthy pregnant and preeclamptic women. *Free Rad. Res.*, **33**(5), 471–6.

Zusterzeel, P.L.M., Rutten, H., Roelofs, H.M.J., Peters, W.H.M. and Steegers, E.A.P. (2001). Protein carbonyls in decidua and placenta of pre-eclamptic women as markers for oxidative stress. *Placenta*, **22**(2–3), 213–19.

Zusterzeel, P.L.M., Steegers Theunissen, R.P.M., Harren, F.J.M., *et al.* (2002). Ethene and other biomarkers of oxidative stress in hypertensive disorders of pregnancy. *Hypertens. Pregn.*, **21**, 39–49.

9

Placental hypoxia, hyperoxia and ischemia–reperfusion injury in pre-eclampsia

Graham J. Burton, Tai-Ho Hung and Eric Jauniaux

Introduction

Oxidative stress of the placenta is a key element in the pathogenesis of pre-eclampsia, although its precise contribution remains uncertain (Hubel, 1999; Redman and Sargent, 2000). The aim of this chapter is to address the origin of that oxidative stress and, as the title suggests, to consider the effects of different oxygen concentrations on placental tissues. In the past it has widely been assumed that the vascular abnormalities in the endometrial arteries of women with pre-eclampsia result in reduced placental perfusion, and hence chronic hypoxia within the feto-placental unit. More recently, the converse has been proposed, and that in pre-eclampsia associated with intra-uterine growth restriction (IUGR) the placenta is in fact hyperoxic due to less oxygen than normal being extracted from the intervillous space by the smaller fetus (Kingdom and Kaufmann, 1997). Hypoxia and hyperoxia are relative terms, however, and these assessments have of necessity been based on data obtained at the time of delivery, which, in the majority of cases, represents the end-stage of a process that may have been developing over many weeks. It is therefore difficult to separate primary from secondary effects, and to elucidate earlier stages in the pathogenesis of the disorder. The situation is further complicated by the fact that pre-eclampsia varies widely in severity. Late onset pre-eclampsia is often associated with normal birthweight, whereas early onset of the disease is generally linked with IUGR (Douglas and Redman,

1994). A spectrum of pathological changes may therefore be expected, and it is possible that oxygen concentrations within the placenta may vary both across that spectrum and within an individual organ during the progression of the disease. As no physiological measurements of those oxygen concentrations are currently available we can only examine the evidence available and speculate on the likely state of affairs.

The maternal circulation to the placenta

Before considering oxygen concentrations within the intervillous space it is worthwhile reviewing the basic features of the maternal intraplacental circulation in order to appreciate the likely impact of the endometrial vascular abnormalities that are associated with pre-eclampsia. The main uterine arteries give off branches which extend inward for about a third of the thickness of the myometrium without significant branching and then subdivide into an arcuate wreath encircling the uterus (Ramsey and Donner, 1980). From this network arise smaller branches, the radial arteries, directed toward the uterine lumen. These arteries become the endometrial spiral arteries as they pass the myometrial–endometrial junction. Shortly after entering the endometrium, the spiral arteries give off branches which ramify in the deepest layers of the endometrium and whose role is to nourish the basal layer of the endometrium, preserving it intact as a seedbed for reconstruction after menstrual periods and parturition (Ramsey and Donner, 1980).

During early pregnancy the spiral arteries undergo physiological conversion in association with extravillous trophoblast invasion of the endometrium (Brosens *et al.*, 2002; Kam *et al.*, 1999). As a result, the distal portions of the arteries feeding into the placenta lose their endothelial lining and the smooth muscle from their walls. They become flaccid funnel-shaped conduits, dilating greatly as they approach the basal plate. This transformation in caliber is widely cited as being necessary to increase placental blood flow, although hemodynamic analysis does not support this assertion. Under normal conditions the changes extend as far as the inner third of the myometrium, but not all the way to the parent arcuate artery. Consequently, a short length of muscular radial artery of normal diameter is interposed between the funnel and the arcuate artery. During its transit through the intervillous space the maternal blood is in an open circulation, a cardiovascular phenomenon that is unique amongst higher mammals (Moll *et al.*, 1975). This has important consequences for the physical properties of that circulation, in particular removing the resistance normally imposed by a peripheral circulation. Consequently, it is the resistance offered by the arcuate, the radial and the proximal unconverted segments of the spiral arteries that will determine placental blood flow. These dilate enormously as pregnancy advances through the vasoactive effects of estrogens. As flow is proportional to the fourth power of the radius of a vessel (Poiseuille's law) these changes will have a far greater impact on placental blood flow than the slight reduction in resistance conferred by dilation of the terminal portion of the spiral artery.

By contrast with its limited effects on flow, the physiological conversion has a major impact on the pressure within the artery. Because of the large increase in caliber, and the fact that the dilated funnel communicates with the low resistance open circulation within the intervillous space, the pressure within the distal segment of a converted spiral artery will be greatly reduced. Moll *et al.* (1975) reported that in the rhesus monkey, where the uterine vascular architecture is almost identical to that of the human, the mean pressure near the opening of a spiral artery is less than 25 mmHg. This drop in perfusion pressure will ensure a low pressure within the intervillous space, a feature that is essential to prevent collapse of the fetal villous capillary system (Karimu and Burton, 1994). Hence conversion of the spiral arteries solves one of the paradoxes of hemochorial placentation, enabling the inherently low-pressure fetal circulation to perfuse a villous capillary net immersed in the normally high-pressure maternal circulation whilst allowing a thin villous membrane to be maintained between the two circulations.

Consequences of the changes seen in pre-eclampsia

Pre-eclampsia is associated with two abnormalities in the spiral arteries: incomplete conversion and acute atherosis. Conversion of the arteries is deficient both in terms of the number of vessels involved and the extent of the transformation within individual arteries (Brosens, 1988; Meekins *et al.*, 1994). Dilatation of the distal segment of the artery will be impaired, but what impact does this have on the placental circulation? On the basis of the analysis of Moll and his colleagues (1975) we would predict that the pressure at the mouths of the vessels will be higher than normal. Although no measurements are available to confirm this assumption, with ultrasound it can be seen that maternal inflow into the intervillous space is often more in the form of jet-like spurts in pre-eclampsia. These spurts are associated with the formation of intervillous blood-lakes, thrombosis and excessive fibrin-deposition (Jauniaux and Nicolaides, 1996; Jauniaux *et al.*, 1994). The effect on the volume of blood flow will be minimal, however, since as discussed these are not the flow-limiting elements in the utero-placental circulation.

Acute atherosis is characterized by the presence of foam cells in the wall of the artery and the accumulation of fibrin deposits within the lumen (Brosens, 1964; De Wolf *et al.*, 1975). In placental bed biopsies the lumens of such vessels appear conspicuously narrowed, almost to the point of occlusion in the most severe cases. Although greater dilatation may occur under physiological pressures in vivo it is likely that these lesions may significantly impair blood flow into the intervillous space. Such lesions were observed in the decidual arteries in 11% of normotensive pregnancies compared to 92% of pre-eclamptic cases (Meekins *et al.*, 1994). They have also been reported in cases of IUGR, with approximately equal frequency in normotensive and pre-eclamptic pregnancies (Sheppard and Bonnar, 1988).

Comparing these two vascular abnormalities, it would appear that incomplete conversion of the spiral arteries by itself will have little impact on the volume of placental blood flow and hence oxygenation, whereas the influence of acute atherosis is likely to be more profound.

Placental hypoxia and pre-eclampsia

Although many conditions have been associated with placental hypoxia, no physiological measurements from the intervillous space are available to confirm these assumptions. The only situation in which we can be confident that the oxygen tension of the maternal blood within the intervillous space is reduced is pregnancy at high altitude. In a recent study of Mestizos women living at 4300 m, Espinoza *et al.* (2001) reported that the peripheral arterial oxygen concentration is reduced to 53 mmHg compared with 106 mmHg at sea level. Birthweight is significantly lower in this high-altitude population (Krampl *et al.*, 2000). These results therefore argue against chronic intraplacental hypoxia in cases of late onset pre-eclampsia in which birthweight is normal, but support the concept that acute atherosis impairs placental oxygenation in early onset disease associated with IUGR.

More direct evidence relating to intervillous oxygenation in pre-eclampsia has been obtained through an analysis of placental metabolism. Tissue hypoxia and ischemia are generally associated with an increased ratio of lactate to pyruvate, and a reduction in the ratio of adenosine triphosphate to adenosine diphosphate. The constancy of these ratios in pre-eclamptic placentas again argues against chronic hypoxia, although other metabolic abnormalities may be present (Bloxham *et al.*, 1987).

Finally, placentas from uncomplicated pregnancies at high altitude do not display the high incidence of infarction that characterizes pre-eclampsia (Reshetnikova *et al.*, 1994). A reduced maternal arterial oxygen tension by itself is therefore not a sufficient cause for the placental changes observed. Also, in pre-eclampsia the villous lesions occur most commonly near the mouths of the spiral arteries, which will be the region of the highest relative oxygen concentration.

Placental hyperoxia and pre-eclampsia

The oxygen concentration within the intervillous space will be determined by the balance of supply from the spiral arteries and extraction by the fetus and the placenta. Each spiral artery delivers its blood into the central cavity of a placental lobule and the blood disperses in a classic smoke-ring pattern, passing between the villi and exchanging respiratory gases before finally entering the uterine veins. Consequently, it was proposed that an oxygen gradient exists across a lobule (Wigglesworth, 1969), and recent data describing differences in antioxidant enzyme activity support this hypothesis (Hempstock *et al.*, 2003a). Morphological and enzymatic differences have been reported in villi from the central compared to peripheral regions of a lobule, with those in the center appearing to be more immature (Critchley and Burton, 1987; Schuhmann *et al.*, 1988).

As these intralobular villous changes appear to mirror, and to be extended by, those observed between low- and high-altitude placentas (Reshetnikova *et al.*, 1994), it is tempting to conclude that they are oxygen-induced.

It has been proposed that impaired extraction of oxygen from the intervillous space in cases of IUGR associated with absent end-diastolic umbilical flow results in an increased oxygen concentration in the intervillous space (Kingdom and Kaufmann, 1997). The effect would be to extend the arterial zone of the lobule peripherally, leading to suppression of villous angiogenesis which would further impair oxygen extraction. A viscous cycle may therefore be established. This is likely to be a secondary effect and will only influence a small proportion of cases of pre-eclampsia, in particular those with early onset of the disease.

Placental ischemia–reperfusion and pre-eclampsia

An alternative approach to the pathogenesis of pre-eclampsia is that of ischemia–reperfusion. Over recent years there has been an explosion of interest in this field in relation to cerebrovascular and cardiovascular insults (Carden and Granger, 2000; Collard and Gelman, 2001; Grace and Mathie, 1999), and there is increasing evidence that much of the pathophysiology involved can also be applied to the placenta. Underlying ischemia–reperfusion injury must be intermittent perfusion, and in the case of the placenta this can occur through two mechanisms: intrinsic vasoconstriction of the spiral arteries, and external compression of the arcuate and radial arteries during uterine contractions.

The spiral and radial arteries have a thick muscular wall, and vasoconstriction of these vessels plays a key role in preventing excessive blood loss during menstruation. Because the proximal unconverted segment of the spiral artery retains its smooth muscle coat it remains vasoreactive even in normal pregnancies. This has been clearly demonstrated in the rhesus monkey, in which the intravenous administration of epinephrine or norepinephrine causes a severe reduction in placental perfusion, to the point that high doses can result in fetal asphyxia and death (Adamsons and Myers, 1975; Adamsons *et al.*, 1971). Evidence that the unconverted segment of the vessel is indeed flow-limiting is provided by the fact that despite the systemic hypertension induced the pressure in the dilated mouth of the spiral artery is decreased after administration. It has been suggested that a similar mechanism underlies the high rate of fetal loss during the second and third trimesters in women suffering from pheochromocytoma (Adamsons and Myers, 1975). Spontaneous changes in maternal catecholamine release, for example in response to stress, may therefore also influence the caliber of these vessels and hence perfusion of the intervillous space. Epidemiologically, there is an association between maternal anxiety and low birthweight, and the finding that women with high anxiety scores display increased uterine artery resistance may explain the link (Teixeira *et al.*, 1999).

More direct evidence that constriction of the proximal sections of the arteries may occur in vivo is again largely based on the rhesus monkey, in which cineradioangiography has revealed that flow from many spiral arteries into the intervillous space is intermittent (Martin *et al.*, 1964; Ramsey and Donner, 1980, 1988). When performing repeated injections of contrast medium into the aorta at intervals of 5–30 min, Martin *et al.* observed that whilst discharge occurred from some spiral arteries following each injection, discharge from other arteries occurred after some injections but not others. The proportion of the arteries demonstrating such intermittent flow ranged from 1 in 7 in one female to 14 of 28 in another, and a larger number of vessels showed variations in the size of the intervillous spurts between injections. There was no association with gestational age, although the sample size was small, and the arteries were located both centrally and peripherally within the placenta. Because the injections were timed to coincide with periods of uterine relaxation, Martin et al. concluded that the effect was due to vasoconstriction within individual arteries rather than external compression caused by myometrial contractions.

There is no doubt from observations on the rhesus monkey that uterine contractions can have a profound impact on intervillous blood flow (Ramsey and Donner, 1980). During contractions the pressure rises in the different fluid compartments of the feto-placental unit and the normal differential that drives maternal blood through the intervillous space will be disrupted. In addition, external compression of the artery during the contraction may occlude the lumen. By placing a cannula in the amniotic cavity Ramsey et al. were able to measure the pressure within the cavity and so time injections of contrast medium with relation to the cycle of uterine contractions (Ramsey et al., 1963). They observed that inflow of maternal blood into the intervillous space is either abolished or greatly reduced during contractions depending on the strength of the latter. Thus in one animal at 64 days of gestation entry was observed from 18 spiral arteries following injection during the relaxation phase. By contrast, entry was observed only from two arteries after injection during a strong contraction, and from six during a milder contraction. The strength of the contractions varied with gestational age, being strongest in early and late pregnancy when they either abolished or severely reduced inflow, and weaker during mid-pregnancy when they had little effect.

Such detailed experiments are not possible for the human, but there is limited evidence from the literature that intermittent perfusion of the intervillous space does occur. Separating the phenomena of individual arterial constriction and external compression during uterine contractions is difficult, as serial imaging cannot be performed. None the less, evidence for the latter was provided by Borell and colleagues. These authors performed angiography at 17–20 weeks of gestation in patients prior to termination of pregnancy, and induced uterine contractions with oxytocin or intra-amniotic injections of saline (Borell et al., 1965a). Contrast medium introduced into the aorta entered the intervillous space within 4–5 s in the relaxed state, whereas during contractions entry was only observed in around 50% of cases. Furthermore, the number of entry sites was reduced during contractions, as was the volume of contrast medium discharged. The same group performed similar investigations on three women carrying severely malformed fetuses at or near term (Borell et al., 1965b). They observed both local and generalized narrowing of large and small arterial branches within the uterine wall during contractions. No definite changes in the diameter of the spiral arteries could be detected, a feature that the authors attributed to the fact that these lie predominantly within the endometrium where local external pressure does not occur.

These data are therefore in accord with those from the rhesus monkey. More recently, magnetic resonance imaging techniques have been applied to the human, both in normal and growth restricted pregnancies (Francis et al., 1998). As studies have only been performed at a single time point they cannot provide information on the constancy of intervillous blood flow. None the less, they have revealed significant regional differences in flow in both groups, indicating that intervillous flow is not homogeneous throughout the organ.

Incomplete conversion of the spiral arteries will most likely exacerbate this situation, for the retention of a greater length of vasoreactive muscular spiral artery must predispose to more spasmodic intervillous flow. We suggest that this effect will have a more profound impact in the pathogenesis of pre-eclampsia than the diminished caliber of the terminal funnel.

The effect of intermittent perfusion on intraplacental oxygen concentration

Each lobule within the human and primate placenta acts as an individual materno-fetal exchange unit. This was confirmed by cineradioangiography in the rhesus monkey, which demonstrated that there is little or no overlap in the maternal perfusion of adjacent lobules (Richart et al., 1964). Hence if inflow is restricted temporarily from a particular spiral artery there will be maternal vascular stasis within the lobule supplied. In view of the high oxygen consumption by the placental tissues in vivo (Carter, 2000), coupled with continuing fetal extraction, it is likely that the oxygen concentration within the intervillous space will fall during this period. When the circulation is re-established it will rise again, so constituting an ischemia–reperfusion type event. The magnitude of the fluctuation in concentration will depend on the duration of the period of stasis, the oxygen reserves within the intervillous space and the rate of extraction and consumption by the fetal and placental tissues.

Values for these parameters are difficult to obtain. On the fetal side of the equation fetal weight rises rapidly during the second half of gestation, and so oxygen extraction might be expected to follow a similar pattern. On the maternal side it is now well established that the maternal circulation to the placenta is only fully established at 10–12 weeks of pregnancy. Consequently, the oxygen concentration in the intervillous space rises from <20 mmHg at 8–10 weeks to >50 mmHg at 12–14 weeks (Jauniaux et al., 2000; Rodesch et al., 1992) (Figure 9.1). As extraction will be low at this time we speculate that oxygen reserves within the intervillous space will exceed fetal demands, and so the placenta will be relatively hyperoxic at the start of the second trimester. Later in gestation, as fetal extraction increases the mean oxygen concentration within the intervillous space declines (Soothill et al., 1986), and the placenta becomes progressively hypoxic. Periods of maternal stasis will therefore have a more profound effect on the oxygen concentration toward term when fetal extraction is at its greatest. The point in gestation when the placenta switches from being relatively hyperoxic to hypoxic is difficult to predict, but is likely to be around the start of the third trimester. Other factors may influence this timing – for example, it may be brought forward in multiple pregnancies due to the higher rate of fetal oxygen extraction.

The pathophysiology of hypoxia, hyperoxia and ischemia–reperfusion

In most cell types a period of prolonged hypoxia results in the cessation of mitochondrial oxidative phosphorylation and so, despite activation of anaerobic glycolytic pathways, to a profound reduction in the cell's ability to synthesize high-energy phosphates, including adenosine triphosphate (ATP). Cell functions that consume large amounts of energy, such as ion pumping and protein synthesis, are impaired, favoring the influx of calcium, sodium and water into the cytoplasm. Swelling occurs and the activation of calcium-dependent proteases leads to loss of cytoskeletal and membrane integrity, culminating in cell death (Majno and Joris, 1995). Despite their high oxygen consumption in vivo placental tissues appear remarkably resistant to hypoxia in vitro (Schneider, 2000). This may reflect the efficacy of anaerobic pathways upon which the placenta largely depends during the first trimester when the oxygen concentration within the feto-placental unit is physiologically low (Jauniaux et al., 2001). Alternatively, the placenta may demonstrate partial metabolic arrest during periods of low oxygenation, down-regulating ATP turnover by reducing the activity of ion pumps and the rate of protein synthesis, which together are estimated to account for 50–80% of placental oxygen consumption (Carter, 2000; Schneider, 2000). The precise mechanisms are far from clear, and there may be complex alterations in the balance between fetal extraction and placental consumption when uterine perfusion is impaired (Schneider, 2000). None the less, in a detailed study of the energetics of placental tissues at various time points following vaginal delivery it was found that the concentration of lactate began to rise, and that of ATP to fall,

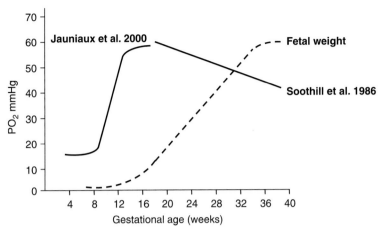

Figure 9.1 Oxygen concentrations within the intervillous space vary with gestational age, being low initially, rising at the start of the second trimester as the maternal circulation becomes fully established and then falling progressively as fetal extraction increases. No data are available for the latter, but as fetal weight increases exponentially fetal oxygen extraction may do the same. Hence, imbalances between maternal supply and fetal demand are likely to be greatest toward the end of pregnancy, increasing the risk of placental hypoxia–reoxygenation injury.

immediately after delivery (Serkova *et al.*, 2003). These differences first reached statistical significance at the 11–14 min time point, and by 21–24 min the ATP concentration had fallen to $29 \pm 18\%$ of the original value. Whilst it is clear from these data that profound changes occur rapidly after cessation of the maternal circulation the techniques unfortunately cannot distinguish between different tissue types. Thus it is not known whether all cellular components are affected to the same degree. Maintenance of term placental villi under hypoxic conditions leads to necrosis of the syncytiotrophoblast while other cell types remain viable, suggesting the tissue may have an increased susceptibility (Hung *et al.*, 2004; Huppertz *et al.*, 2003).

Hypoxia can also influence cells through the increased generation of oxygen free radical species (Halliwell and Gutteridge, 1999). During aerobic metabolism electrons are passed along the enzymes of the mitochondrial respiratory chain before they are finally combined with oxygen to form water. The enzymatic reactions are not totally efficient, however, and electrons may "leak" on to

molecular oxygen to form the superoxide anion $O_2^{\cdot-}$, particularly from Complex III (Raha *et al.*, 2000). It is estimated that under normal conditions 1–2% of oxygen consumed is diverted into the formation of superoxide radicals, but this figure is increased paradoxically during hypoxia. The lack of oxygen restricts the activity of Complex III, causing electrons to build up on the earlier enzymes in the chain and so increasing the risk of "leakage" on to what molecular oxygen is available. The free radicals generated will attack all categories of biological molecules in the immediate vicinity, resulting in DNA damage, protein misfolding and lipid peroxidation (Halliwell and Gutteridge, 1999). It is notable that evidence of the latter was observed in the postpartum placenta 21–24 min after delivery (Serkova *et al.*, 2003).

Generation of oxygen free radicals is also increased during hyperoxic conditions due to increased activity of the respiratory chain and the greater availability for oxygen to combine non-catalytically with electrons to form superoxide anions (Freeman and Crapo, 1981). Using the fluorescent intracellular probe dichlorofluorescein diacetate we have demonstrated increased formation of reactive oxygen species within first trimester villi maintained under 21% oxygen rather than the more physiological 5% (Watson *et al.*, 1999). Formation was particularly pronounced within the syncytiotrophoblast, which at this stage of gestation contains low levels of antioxidant enzymes, and was associated with rapid degeneration of the tissue (Watson *et al.*, 1998). Exposure to such high concentrations of oxygen is clearly unphysiological, but equivalent, although less severe, changes are observed in normal placentas during onset of the maternal circulation when the intraplacental oxygen concentration rises approximately threefold (Jauniaux *et al.*, 2003). Using immunohistochemistry it can be observed that the oxidative stress is particularly strong in the syncytiotrophoblast and the endothelial cells. Indeed, the elevated oxygen concentration associated with onset of blood flow in the peripheral regions of the placenta may be responsible for villous regression and formation of the chorion laeve over the abembryonic pole of the chorionic sac (Jauniaux *et al.*, 2003).

Villous regression is also observed in cases of missed miscarriage, in which there is precocious maternal blood flow and evidence of severe oxidative stress throughout the placenta (Hempstock *et al.*, 2003b). Hyperoxia can therefore have profound adverse effects on the placental tissues in early gestation, but it is doubtful whether increases of oxygenation of equivalent magnitude occur later in pregnancy. As discussed previously, even if fetal extraction is reduced due to severe IUGR the oxygen concentration in the intervillous space can only rise to that which occurs normally in the central cavity of the lobule. Subtle changes in villous vascularization may be induced through influences on the expression of hypoxically regulated growth factors such as vascular endothelial growth factor, but the end result can only be greater "arterialization" of the lobule (Burton, 1997).

Whilst both hypoxia and hyperoxia can induce the formation of free radicals, a much more potent stimulus is ischemia–reperfusion. During the ischemic phase of the insult electrons accumulate on the enzymes of the respiratory chain in the absence of oxygen as a recipient for Complex III. When oxygen is reintroduced during the reperfusion phase many of these electrons "leak" onto oxygen, causing a burst of superoxide production. The situation may be exacerbated by the activity of xanthine dehydrogenase/oxidase. Under normal conditions this enzyme exists in the dehydrogenase form, converting hypoxanthine to xanthine and xanthine to uric acid. In the process it donates electrons to NAD^+. Under hypoxic conditions it can be converted to the xanthine oxidase form, either through oxidation of critical –SH groups or partial proteolytic cleavage by proteases activated by calcium influx into the cell (Halliwell and Gutteridge, 1999). In this form the enzyme donates electrons to oxygen, so forming superoxide anions (Figure 9.2). Activity of the enzyme is stimulated during the reperfusion phase by the accumulation of hypoxanthine that arises due to the increased breakdown of ATP in the ischemic period. The finding that the activity of xanthine oxidase is increased following vaginal delivery as compared with Cesarean delivery confirms that oxidative

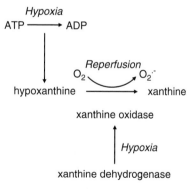

Figure 9.2 Conversion of the enzyme xanthine dehydrogenase to the oxidase form during the period of hypoxia plays a key role in the generation of superoxide radicals when oxygen is reintroduced in ischemia–reperfusion injury.

stress can be generated in the placenta through this mechanism (Many and Roberts, 1997).

Other cellular oxidases may also contribute to free radical generation at sites of ischemia–reperfusion. In particular, local activation of maternal neutrophils by a stress-induced change in the expression of cell adhesion molecules on the apical surface of the syncytiotrophoblast can lead to a respiratory burst of superoxide generation through NADPH oxidase. This effect will reinforce and disseminate the placental oxidative stress. NADPH oxidase is also present on the apical surface of the syncytiotrophoblast (Manes, 2001; Matsubra and Tamada, 1991), although its contribution in the pathogenesis of pre-eclampsia is still unclear.

Comparison of the effects of hypoxia and ischemia–reperfusion on placental tissues in vitro

All three insults, hypoxia, hyperoxia and ischemia–reperfusion, can therefore have similar effects on tissues through their capacity to generate oxidative stress. One of the major differences between hypoxia alone and ischemia–reperfusion is the extent to which energy reserves within the cells are depleted. If the period of ischemia is relatively short then ATP levels may be able to be restored during the reperfusion phase and cell function maintained. In general the severity of the insult determines the outcome in terms of cell death, with severe insults favoring primary necrosis and milder ones favoring apoptosis (Crompton, 1999; Hockenbery, 1995). Apoptosis is an energy-dependent process, and T-lymphocytes can be switched between these two pathways following treatment with staurosporine by prior depletion of ATP (Leist et al., 1997).

In order to investigate the potential effects of ischemia–reperfusion on placental tissues we have developed an in vitro model in which villi from normal term placentas are subjected to a period of hypoxia followed by reoxygenation (Hung et al., 2001). A burst of free radical production was observed using the dye dichlorofluorescein diacetate when villi that had been maintained under hypoxic conditions for 20 min were reoxygenated. The signal was particularly intense within the endothelial cells, but was also present to a lesser degree in the syncytiotrophoblast. Immunohistochemistry using antibodies to nitrotyrosine and hydroxynonenal confirmed the presence of oxidative stress in these tissues, and in the periarterial smooth muscle cells of stem villi, in equivalent samples subjected to 2 h reoxygenation with either 5 or 21% oxygen. The distribution of these markers was identical to that reported for pre-eclamptic placentas (Many et al., 2000; Myatt et al., 1996), and the intensity of staining could be reduced in a dose-dependent fashion by the administration of free radical scavengers. Control samples maintained under constant hypoxia for 2 h demonstrated only a minimal rise in staining intensity (Hung et al., 2001).

The downstream consequences of this stress are only beginning to be explored. Increased apoptosis in the trophoblast has been reported in placentas from pre-eclampsia and IUGR (Allaire et al., 2000; Ishihara et al., 2002; Leung et al., 2001). In our in vitro system maintenance of villi under constant hypoxic conditions (dissolved PO_2 in the medium $= 12$–16 mmHg) induced a higher rate of apoptosis within the syncytiotrophoblastic nuclei compared to controls under normoxia (dissolved $PO_2 = 45$–62 mmHg), but the rate was almost doubled following hypoxia–reoxygenation (Hung et al., 2004). A somewhat similar pattern was observed regarding the production of tumor necrosis factor (TNFα). Thus the mRNA concentration was increased under hypoxic conditions, but the rise was more sustained following hypoxia–reoxygenation and was associated with increased secretion of the cytokine into the culture medium (Hung et al., 2004). Previous work by Malek and colleagues compared the effects of hypoxia and oxidative stress generated using the xanthine/xanthine oxidase system on cytokine production by villous explants (Malek et al., 2001). They found that whilst hypoxia increased the production of interleukin 1β it had no effect on other cytokines or prostanoids. The generation of oxidative stress, however, led to increased production of TNFα, interleukin 1α, interleukin 1β, prostaglandins and thromboxane. These are potentially powerful mediators of the coagulation cascade, and their release could explain the increased incidence of infarction that characterizes the placenta in severe pre-eclampsia.

Overview

The considerable overlap between the pathophysiology of hypoxia, hyperoxia and ischemia–reperfusion makes it difficult to separate the effects of these respective insults in delivered material at term. In addition, the normal delivery process would appear to be an excellent basis for a classical ischemia–reperfusion injury, with periodic strong uterine contractions reducing uterine blood flow. The recent observation that maternal and fetal concentrations of the antioxidant vitamin C are reduced following vaginal delivery compared to Cesarean section suggests that significant oxidative stress is induced during the delivery (Woods et al., 2002). This stress may confound the interpretation of data arising from examination of postpartum placentas, and their attribution to pathological processes occurring in utero.

In the absence of longitudinal physiological measurements of the oxygen concentrations within the intervillous space in normal and pre-eclamptic pregnancies we have to consider the various strands of evidence reviewed and speculate on what is the most likely scenario. In uncomplicated pregnancies we must assume that the blood flow to the placenta is generally adequate to support normal placental and fetal development. None the less, there is a rational basis for believing that some element of intermittent perfusion may occur, either through constriction of individual vessels or during uterine contractions. As the latter become stronger and more frequent toward term, and fetal oxygen extraction continues to rise, it is not unreasonable to assume that fluctuations in intervillous oxygen concentration will be greatest toward term. These may cause the low level of oxidative stress observed in supposedly normal placentas (Hung et al., 2001), and may even play a physiological role in signaling processes as delivery approaches.

In late-onset pre-eclampsia, when birthweight is within the normal range, there would seem to be little evidence to support the concept of chronic intraplacental hypoxia. Placental development is normal (Mayhew et al., 2003; Teasdale, 1985), although there is irrefutable evidence of increased oxidative stress (Hubel, 1999). From the in vitro data it is clear that although both hypoxia and hypoxia–reoxygenation can cause oxidative stress, the latter is a much more potent stimulus and so likely to be more important under physiological conditions. Hence, we speculate that either the magnitude of the fluctuations in oxygen concentration seen in normal pregnancies is greater in these patients, and incomplete conversion of the spiral arteries may contribute significantly here by leaving more of the vessel vasoreactive, or that their placental tissues are more susceptible through deficiencies in antioxidant defences (Figure 9.3). Again, the effects will only become apparent near term when fetal oxygen extraction from the intervillous space is at its highest, and a spectrum of severity is to be expected between the normal and pre-eclamptic situations. Clinical data demonstrating considerable overlap in the values of many parameters between normal and pre-eclamptic pregnancies confirm that pre-eclampsia is not an all-or-nothing phenomenon (Redman and Sargent, 2000).

Pre-eclampsia associated with IUGR is obviously a more aggressive disorder with a more complex pathophysiology. The case for chronic hypoxia in this condition is stronger, although this is most likely a secondary effect, caused by the severe narrowing of the spiral arteries through acute atherosis, that develops during the third trimester (Figure 9.3). The origin of the atherosis is not known, but as ischemia–reperfusion is a potent

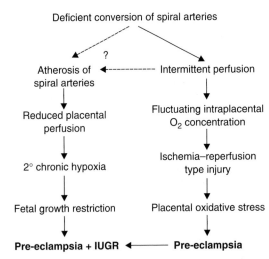

Figure 9.3 Proposed pathway by which incomplete conversion of the spiral arteries may lead to placental oxidative stress in pre-eclampsia. Atherosis of the spiral arteries may develop as a secondary effect, possibly through an ischemia–reperfusion injury in the walls of the distal parts of the arteries, as indicated by the dashed lines. This may lead to occlusion of the vessels, reduced placental perfusion and hence superimposed intrauterine growth restriction.

inducer of atherosclerotic changes in other vessels it is possible that it plays a role in this location too. Hence, we speculate that severe impairment of trophoblast invasion leads to minimal conversion of the spiral arteries, and so increased intermittent vasoconstriction in their proximal segments. This may lead to an ischemia–reperfusion type injury in the distal segments that would normally be converted into flaccid conduits, as well as initiating oxidative stress within the placenta at an earlier stage than in pre-eclampsia alone. Placental development may be disrupted by that stress in a similar, but milder, fashion to that by which villi regress to form the chorion laeve (Jauniaux *et al.*, 2003). As a result, villous volume and surface area will be reduced at delivery (Mayhew *et al.*, 2003; Teasdale, 1987). Placental perfusion will be impaired by the atherotic changes in the spiral arteries leading to chronic hypoxia and IUGR later in pregnancy.

Although there are many aspects of this hypothesis that remain to be tested we believe that ischemia–reperfusion provides a more physiological approach to the understanding of pre-eclampsia than hypoxia alone. Viewing the syndrome in this light will hopefully lead to the introduction of more effective interventions and therapies that will reduce the burden of the disease on human reproduction.

REFERENCES

Adamsons, K. and Myers, R. E. (1975). Circulation in the intervillous space; obstetrical considerations in fetal deprivation. In *The Placenta and its Maternal Supply Line. Effects of Insufficiency on the Fetus*, ed. P. Gruenwald. Lancaster: Medical and Technical Publishing Co. Ltd., pp. 158–77.

Adamsons, K., Mueller-Heubach, E. and Myers, R. E. (1971). Production of fetal asphyxia in the rhesus monkey by administration of catecholamines to the mother. *Am. J. Obstet. Gynecol.*, **109**, 248–62.

Allaire, A. D., Ballenger, K. A., Wells, S. R., McMahon, M. J. and Lessey, B. A. (2000). Placental apoptosis in preeclampsia. *Obstet. Gynecol.*, **96**, 271–6.

Bloxham, D. L., Bullen, B. E., Walters, B. N. J. and Lao, T. T. (1987). Placental glycolysis and energy metabolism in preeclampsia. *Am. J. Obstet. Gynecol.*, **157**, 97–101.

Borell, U., Fernström, I., Ohlson, L. and Wiqvist, N. (1965a). An arteriographic study of the blood flow through the uterus and the placenta at midpregnancy. *Acta Obstet. Gynecol. Scand.*, **44**, 22–31.

Borell, U., Fernström, I., Ohlson, L. and Wiqvist, N. (1965b). Influence of uterine contractions on the uteroplacental blood flow at term. *Am. J. Obstet. Gynecol.*, **93**, 44–57.

Brosens, I. (1964). A study of the spiral arteries of the decidua basalis in normotensive and hypertensive pregnancies. *J. Obstet. Gynaecol. Br. Commonwlth*, **71**, 222–30.

Brosens, I. A. (1988). The utero-placental vessels at term – the distribution and extent of physiological changes. *Trophoblast Res.*, **3**, 61–7.

Brosens, J. J., Pijnenborg, R. and Brosens, I. A. (2002). The myometrial junctional zone spiral arteries in normal and abnormal pregnancies. *Am. J. Obstet. Gynecol.*, **187**, 1416–23.

Burton, G. J. (1997). On 'Oxygen and placental villous development: origins of fetal hypoxia'. *Placenta*, **18**, 625–6.

Carden, D. L. and Granger, D. N. (2000). Pathophysiology of ischaemia–reperfusion injury. *J. Pathol.*, **190**, 255–66.

Carter, A. M. (2000). Placental oxygen consumption. Part I: in vivo studies – a review. *Placenta*, **21** (Suppl A), S31–7.

Collard, C. D. and Gelman, S. (2001). Pathophysiology, clinical manifestations, and prevention of ischemia–reperfusion injury. *Anesthesiology*, **94**, 1133–8.

Critchley, G. R. and Burton, G. J. (1987). Intralobular variations in barrier thickness in the mature human placenta. *Placenta*, **8**, 185–94.

Crompton, M. (1999). The mitochondrial permeability transition pore and its role in cell death. *Biochem. J.*, **341**, 233–49.

De Wolf, F., Robertson, W. B. and Brosens, I. (1975). The ultrastructure of acute atherosis in hypertensive pregnancy. *Am. J. Obstet. Gynecol.*, **123**, 164–74.

Douglas, K. A. and Redman, C. (1994). Eclampsia in the United Kingdom. *Br. Med. J.*, **309**, 1395–400.

Espinoza, J., Sebire, N. J., McAuliffe, F., Krampl, E. and Nicolaides, K. H. (2001). Placental villus morpholgy in relation to maternal hypoxia at high altitude. *Placenta*, **22**, 606–8.

Francis, S. T., Duncan, K. R., Moore, R. J., Baker, P. N. and Johnson, I. R. (1998). Non-invasive mapping of placental perfusion. *Lancet*, **351**, 1397–9.

Freeman, B. A. and Crapo, J. D. (1981). Hyperoxia increases oxygen radical production in rat lungs and lung mitochondria. *J. Biol. Chem.*, **256**, 10,986–92.

Grace, P. A. and Mathie, R. T. (1999). *Ischaemia–Reperfusion Injury*. Oxford: Blackwell Science. 384 pp.

Halliwell, B. and Gutteridge, J. M. C. (1999). *Free Radicals in Biology and Medicine*. Oxford: Oxford Science Publications. 936 pp.

Hempstock, J., Bao, Y.-P., Bar-Issac, M., *et al.* (2003a). Intralobular differences in antioxidant enzyme expression and activity reflect oxygen gradients within the human placenta. *Placenta*, **24**, 517–23.

Hempstock, J., Jauniaux, E., Greenwold, N. and Burton, G. J. (2003b) The contribution of placental oxidative stress to early pregnancy failure. *Hum. Pathol.*, **34**, 1265–75.

Hockenbery, D. (1995). Defining apoptosis. *Am. J. Pathol.*, **146**, 16–19.

Hubel, C. A. (1999). Oxidative stress in the pathogenesis of preeclampsia. *Proc. Soc. Exp. Biol. Med.*, **222**, 222–35.

Hung, T.-H., Charnock-Jones, D. S., Skepper, J. N. and Burton, G. J. (2004). Secretion of tumour necrosis factor-α from human placental tissues induced by hypoxia–reoxygenation causes endothelial cell activation in vitro: a potential mediator of the inflammatory response in preeclampsia. *Am. J. Pathol.*, **164**, 1049–61.

Hung, T.-H., Skepper, J. N. and Burton, G. J. (2001). In vitro ischemia–reperfusion injury in term human placenta as a model for oxidative stress in pathological pregnancies. *Am. J. Pathol.*, **159**, 1031–43.

Hung, T.-H., Skepper, J. N., Charnock-Jones, D. S. and Burton, G. J. (2002). Hypoxia/reoxygenation. A potent inducer of apoptotic changes in the human placenta and possible etiological factor in preeclampsia. *Circ. Res.*, **90**, 1274–81.

Huppertz, B., Kingdom, J., Caniggia, I., *et al.* (2003). Hypoxia favours necrotic versus apoptotic shedding of placental syncytiotrophoblast into the maternal circulation. *Placenta*, **24**, 181–90.

Ishihara, N., Matsuo, H., Murakoshi, H., Laoag-Fernandez, J., Samoto, T. and Maruo, T. (2002). Increased apoptosis in the syncytiotrophoblast in human term placentas complicated by either preeclampsia or intrauterine growth retardation. *Am. J. Obstet. Gynecol.*, **186**, 158–66.

Jauniaux, E. and Nicolaides, K. H. (1996). Placental lakes, absent umbilical artery diastolic flow and poor fetal growth in early pregnancy. *Ultras. Obstet. Gynecol.*, **7**, 141–4.

Jauniaux, E., Ramsay, B. and Campbell, S. (1994). Ultra-sonographic investigation of placental morphologic characteristics and size during the second trimester of pregnancy. *Am. J. Obstet. Gynecol.*, **170**, 130–7.

Jauniaux, E., Watson, A. L. and Burton, G. J. (2001). Evaluation of respiratory gases and acid-base gradients in fetal fluids and uteroplacental tissue between 7 and 16 weeks. *Am. J. Obstet. Gynecol.*, **184**, 998–1003.

Jauniaux, E., Hempstock, J., Greenwold, N. and Burton, G. J. (2003). Trophoblastic oxidative stress in relation to temporal and regional differences in maternal placental blood flow in normal and abnormal early pregnancies. *Am. J. Pathol.*, **162**, 115–25.

Jauniaux, E., Watson, A. L., Hempstock, J., Bao, Y.-P., Skepper, J. N. and Burton, G. J. (2000). Onset of maternal arterial bloodflow and placental oxidative stress; a possible factor in human early pregnancy failure. *Am. J. Pathol.*, **157**, 2111–22.

Kam, E. P. Y., Gardner, L., Loke, Y. W. and King, A. (1999). The role of trophoblast in the physiological change in decidual spiral arteries. *Hum. Reprod.*, **14**, 2131–8.

Karimu, A. L. and Burton, G. J. (1994). The effects of maternal vascular pressure on the dimensions of the placental capillaries. *Br. J. Obstet. Gynaecol.*, **101**, 57–63.

Kingdom, J. C. P. and Kaufmann, P. (1997). Oxygen and placental villous development: origins of fetal hypoxia. *Placenta*, **18**, 613–21.

Krampl, E., Lees, C., Bland, J. M., Espinoza Dorado, J., Moscoso, G. and Campbell, S. (2000). Fetal biometry at 4300 m compared to sea level Peru. *Ultras. Obstet. Gynaecol.*, **16**, 9–18.

Leist, M., Single, B., Castoldi, A. F., Kühnle, S. and Nicotera, P. (1997). Intracellular adenosine triphosphate (ATP) concentration: a switch in the decision between apoptosis and necrosis. *J. Exp. Med.*, **185**, 1481–6.

Leung, D. N., Smith, S. C., To, K. F., Sahota, D. S. and Baker, P. N. (2001). Increased placental apoptosis in pregnancies complicated by preeclampsia. *Am. J. Obstet. Gynecol.*, **184**, 1249–50.

Majno, G. and Joris, I. (1995). Apoptosis, oncosis, and necrosis. An overview of cell death. *Am. J. Pathol.*, **146**, 3–15.

Malek, A., Sager, R. and Schneider, H. (2001). Effect of hypoxia, oxidative stress and lipopolysaccharides on the release of prostaglandins and cytokines from human term placental explants. *Placenta*, **22** (Suppl A), S45–50.

Manes, C. (2001). Human placental NAD(P)H oxidase: solubilization and properties. *Placenta*, **22**, 58–63.

Many, A. and Roberts, J. M. (1997). Increased xanthine oxidase during labour-implications for oxidative stress. *Placenta*, **18**, 725–6.

Many, A., Hubel, C. A., Fisher, S. J., Roberts, J. M. and Zhou, Y. (2000). Invasive cytotrophoblasts manifest evidence of oxidative stress in preeclampsia. *Am. J. Pathol.*, **156**, 321–31.

Martin, C. B., McGaughey, H. S., Kaiser, I. H., Donner, M. W. and Ramsey, E. M. (1964). Intermittent functioning of the uteroplacental arteries. *Am. J. Obstet. Gynecol.*, **90**, 819–23.

Matsubra, S. and Tamada, T. (1991). Ultracytochemical localisation of NAD(P)H oxidase activity in the human placenta. *Acta Obstet. Gynaecol. Jap.*, **43**, 117–21.

Mayhew, T. M., Ohadike, C., Baker, P. N., Crocker, I. P., Mitchell, C. and Ong, S. S. (2003). Stereological investigation of placental morphology in pregnancies complicated by pre-eclampsia with and without intrauterine growth restriction. *Placenta*, **24**, 219–26.

Meekins, J. W., Pijnenborg, R., Hanssens, M., McFadyen, I. R. and Van Assche, F. A. (1994). A study of placental bed spiral arteries and trophoblast invasion in normal and severe pre-eclamptic pregnancies. *Br. J. Obstet. Gynaecol.*, **101**, 669–74.

Moll, W., Künzel, W. and Herberger, J. (1975). Hemodynamic implications of hemochorial placentation. *Eur. J. Obstet. Gynecol. Reprod. Biol.*, **5**, 67–74.

Myatt, L., Rosenfield, R. B., Eis, A. L. W., Brockman, D. E., Greer, I. and Lyall, F. (1996). Nitrotyrosine residues in placenta. Evidence of peroxynitrite formation and action. *Hypertension*, **28**, 488–93.

Raha, S., McEachern, G. E., Myint, A. T. and Robinson, B. H. (2000). Superoxides from mitochondrial complex III: the role of manganese superoxide dismutase. *Free Radi. Biol. Med.*, **29**, 170–80.

Ramsey, E. M. and Donner, M. W. (1980). *Placental Vasculature and Circulation. Anatomy, Physiology, Radiology, Clinical Aspects, Atlas and Textbook.* Stuttgart: Georg Thieme. 101 pp.

Ramsey, E. M. and Donner, M. W. (1988). Placental vasculature and circulation in primates. *Trophoblast Res.*, **3**, 217–33.

Ramsey, E. M., Corner, G. W. and Donner, M. W. (1963). Serial and cineradiographic visualization of the maternal circulation in the primate (hemochorial) placenta. *Am. J. Obstet. Gynecol.*, **86**, 213–25.

Redman, C. W. G. and Sargent, I. L. (2000). Placental debris, oxidative stress and pre-eclampsia. *Placenta*, **21**, 597–602.

Reshetnikova, O. S., Burton, G. J. and Milovanov, A. P. (1994). Effects of hypobaric hypoxia on the feto-placental unit; the morphometric diffusing capacity of the villous membrane at high altitude. *Am. J. Obstet. Gynecol.*, **171**, 1560–5.

Richart, R. M., Doyle, G. B. and Ramsay, G. C. (1964). Visualisation of the entire maternal placental circulation in the rhesus monkey. *Am. J. Obstet. Gynecol.*, **90**, 334–9.

Rodesch, F., Simon, P., Donner, C. and Jauniaux, E. (1992). Oxygen measurements in endometrial and trophoblastic tissues during early pregnancy. *Obstet. Gynecol.*, **80**, 283–5.

Schneider, H. (2000). Placental oxygen consumption. Part II: in vitro studies – a review. *Placenta*, **21** (Suppl A), S38–44.

Schuhmann, R., Stoz, F. and Maier, M. (1988). Histometric investigations in placentones (materno-fetal circulation units) of human placentae. *Trophoblast Res.*, **3**, 3–16.

Serkova, N., Bendrick-Peart, J., Alexander, B. and Tissot van Patot, M. C. (2003). Metabolite concentrations in human term placentae and their changes due to delayed collection after delivery. *Placenta*, **24**, 227–35.

Sheppard, B. L. and Bonnar, J. (1988). The maternal blood supply to the placenta in pregnancy complicated by intrauterine fetal growth retardation. *Trophoblast Res.*, **3**, 69–81.

Soothill, P. W., Nicolaides, K. H., Rodeck, C. H. and Campbell, S. (1986). Effect of gestational age on fetal and intervillous blood gas and acid–base values in human pregnancy. *Fetal Therapy*, **1**, 168–75.

Teasdale, F. (1985). Histomorphometry of the human placenta in maternal preeclampsia. *Am. J. Obstet. Gynecol.*, **152**, 25–31.

Teasdale, F. (1987). Histomorphometry of the human placenta in pre-eclampsia associated with severe intra-uterine growth retardation. *Placenta*, **8**, 119–28.

Teixeira, J. M., Fisk, N. M. and Glover, V. (1999) Association between maternal anxiety in pregnancy and increased uterine artery resistance index: cohort based study. *Br. Med. J.*, **318**, 153–7.

Watson, A. L., Skepper, J. N., Jauniaux, E. and Burton, G. J. (1998). Susceptibility of human placental syncytiotrophoblastic mitochondria to oxygen-mediated damage in relation to gestational age. *J. Clin. Endocrinol. Metab.*, **83**, 1697–705.

Watson, A. L, Skepper, J. N., Jauniaux, E. and Burton, G. J. (1999). Reducing oxidative stress effects in early human placental villi during in vitro culture. *Placenta*, **20**, A69.

Wigglesworth, J. S. (1969). Vascular anatomy of the human placenta and its significance for placental pathology. *J. Obstet. Gynaecol. Br. Commonwlth*, **76**, 979–89.

Woods, J. R. Jr., Cavanaugh, J. L., Norkus, E. P., Plessinger, M. A. and Miller, R. K. (2002). The effect of labor on maternal and fetal vitamins C and E. *Am. J. Obstet. Gynecol.*, **187**, 1179–83.

10

Tenney–Parker changes and apoptotic versus necrotic shedding of trophoblast in normal pregnancy and pre-eclampsia

Peter Kaufmann and Berthold Huppertz

Two-dimensional morphology of a three-dimensional organ

Histopathology of the human placenta is mostly based on the light-microscopical evaluation of paraffin sections. Therefore, the three-dimensional features of normal and pathological placental villi are usually described in terms of the two-dimensional description analysed by light microscopy. Remarkably, the two-dimensional findings often do not reflect the underlying three-dimensional characteristics of villi. This is particularly true when nuclear accumulations (syncytial sprouts, knots, bridges, Tenney–Parker changes) are involved which partly represent true sprouts, knots and bridges (Figure 10.1a,b); however, more often are the result of trophoblastic flat sectioning (Figure 10.1c) (Burton 1986a,b; Cantle et al., 1987; Kaufmann et al., 1987; Kuestermann, 1981).

The histological features of syncytial knotting have different origins

Historically, fungus-shaped, multinucleated protrusions of placental villous surfaces have been interpreted as (a) signs of villous sprouting (Boyd and Hamilton, 1970), as well as (b) signs of nuclear aging (Schiebler and Kaufmann, 1969; Martin and Spicer, 1973) and nuclear shedding (Ikle, 1964).

However, the interpretation became more difficult when it was reported that the multinucleated knots, sprouts and bridges found in two-dimensional paraffin sections very often did not reflect the three-dimensional characteristics of the structures that had been cut. In 1981 Kuestermann used serial paraffin sections to reconstruct the villous tree and found that the seeming sprouts and bridges are mostly flat sections of branches of the villous tree. Similar results were obtained by Burton (1986a,b, 1987) using plastic serial sections and by Cantle et al. (1987) and Kaufmann et al. (1987) using plastic sections of villi which were previously studied by scanning electron microscopy. All of the above groups came to the conclusion that tangential sections of the syncytial surface of villi result in various features of syncytial nuclear accumulation that mimic true syncytial knots, sprouts and bridges.

Syncytial knotting (also called Tenney–Parker changes) is the usual histopathological term to describe the histological appearance of increased numbers of seemingly multinucleated trophoblastic outgrowths at the villous surfaces. Sometimes these outgrowths reach the neighboring villi resulting in congested conglomerates of villi linked to each other by multinucleated bridges and flanges of syncytium. Almost all of those are flat sections of the trophoblastic surface due to the irregularly shaped and branched villous trees (Cantle et al., 1987; Kaufmann et al., 1987). Under specific

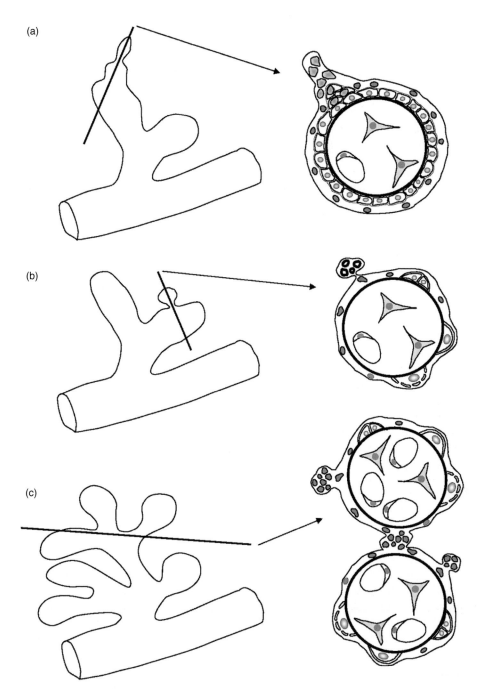

Figure 10.1 Schematic representation of the three-dimensional organization of villi and the resulting villous cross-sections. In (a), a villus of a first-trimester placenta has been cut and demonstrates the formation of a new villus, represented by a syncytial sprout. In (b), a villus of a term placenta is ready to pinch off a true apoptotic syncytial knot; the same can be seen in the cross-section. In (c), the cut has been made through a highly branched pattern of villi resulting in a cross-section with various sites of accumulated nuclei inside the syncytiotrophoblast. These Tenney–Parker changes are all flat sections through parts of the syncytiotrophoblast.

pathological conditions (see below) the outer shape of the villi becomes more and more irregular and thus increases the chance of trophoblastic flat sections (syncytial knotting, Tenney–Parker changes).

For the placental pathologist it is of considerable importance to correctly interpret such features since the histological feature of aggregated syncytial nuclei, "syncytial knotting" is widely accepted as diagnostic markers of placental ischemia and pre-eclampsia (Alvarez *et al.*, 1969, 1970; Schuhmann and Geier, 1972; Tenney and Parker, 1940). These features are derived from

(a) true syncytial and villous sprouting, that is the accumulation of nuclei freshly incorporated into the syncytium by syncytial fusion (Figure 10.1a), or

(b) simple flat-sectioning of distorted but otherwise normal syncytial surfaces with seeming accumulation of normal nuclei (Figure 10.1c), or

(c) "syncytial degeneration" with "nuclear aging" including necrotic, aponecrotic or apoptotic (Figure 10.1b) processes within the villous syncytiotrophoblast, resulting in nuclear shedding into the maternal blood.

In spite of the phenotypic similarities among these different modes of nuclear aggregation, there are clear structural hints that help us to identify the underlying mechanism even in conventionally stained paraffin sections.

True syncytial sprouting

Syncytial sprouts serve as first steps of villous sprouting and thus are early precursors of new villi (Boyd and Hamilton, 1970; Cantle *et al.*, 1987; Castellucci *et al.*, 1990). They result from proliferation of cytotrophoblast underneath with subsequent syncytial fusion. During early pregnancy larger aggregates of such freshly incorporated trophoblastic nuclei arch into the intervillous space and form mushroom-like syncytial structures (Figure 10.2a). True syncytial sprouts are characterized by loosely distributed, large ovoid nuclei that possess little heterochromatin and never show signs of apoptosis. In the surroundings of the nuclei high numbers of free ribosomes can be found together with ample and well-developed rough endoplasmic reticulum. The smooth surface of the sprouts is covered with well developed microvilli (Figure 10.2b). Often, the sprouts are located close to villous tips and continue in slender segments of villi (villous sprouts), which just have been invaded by mesenchyme (Castellucci *et al.*, 1990).

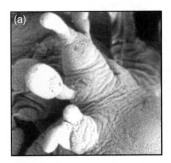 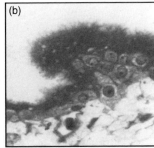 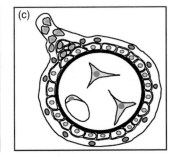

Figure 10.2 True syncytial sprouts. (a) The scanning electron microscopical picture shows the drumstick-like appearance of the sprouts. (b) The semi-thin section depicts the increased number of cytotrophoblast cells below and the microvillous brush border at the apical surface of the syncytiotrophoblast. (c) The scheme shows the newly fused and larger nuclei of the syncytiotrophoblast only in the sprout while the other nuclei are more condensed. a: ×130; b: ×400.

The syncytial sprouts are found exclusively along the surfaces of mesenchymal villi and immature intermediate villi. Together with the latter villous types, they prevail in the first half of pregnancy (Figure 10.2c). Throughout the last trimester true sprouts and the producing immature villous types are restricted to the centers of villous trees where they form the growth zones of the latter (Benirschke and Kaufmann, 2000).

Trophoblastic flat-sectioning, syncytial knotting, Tenney–Parker changes

Syncytial knotting, also called Tenney–Parker changes, is characterized by aggregated villi (Figure 10.3). Their cross-sections are covered with numerous knots of accumulated syncytial nuclei, and are connected to each other by numerous syncytial bridges again containing accumulated syncytial nuclei (Figure 10.3b–e). The intervillous space in between is particularly narrow (Figure 10.3d). As has been shown by several groups (Burton, 1986a,b; Cantle et al., 1987; Kaufmann et al., 1987; Kuestermann, 1981; for review see Benirschke and Kaufmann, 2000) the underlying structural correlates are trophoblastic flat sections due to increased branching of villi or to otherwise distorted villous surfaces (Figure 10.3a). Moreover, it has been shown that the incidence of knotting/trophoblastic flat-sectioning increases with sectional thickness due to geometric reasons (Benirschke and Kaufmann, 2000; Cantle et al., 1987). It is a rare event in ultra-thin sections (~0.1 μm) for electron microscopy (Figure 10.3b), it can be seen more often in semi-thin plastic sections (0.5–1 μm) for light microscopy (Figure 10.3c), and is a usual event in 5–10 μm paraffin

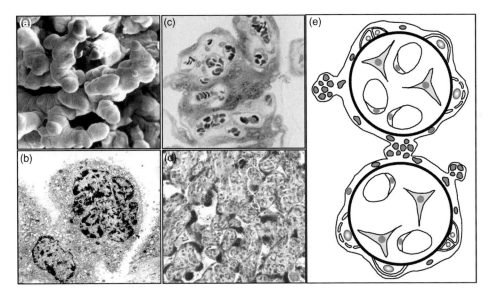

Figure 10.3 Tenney–Parker changes. (a) The scanning electron microscopical picture shows the densely packed and highly branched villi. (b) The electron microscopical picture reveals that the nuclei within such a flat section have the same heterogeneous chromatin distribution compared to the nucleus underneath in the syncytiotrophoblast.
(c) The semi-thin section depicts the dense package of villi and the increased number of syncytial cross-sections between the villi. (d) The paraffin section reveals a high number of syncytial flat sections, the typical Tenney–Parker changes.
(e) The scheme shows the seeming bridges between villi and the protrusions at the villous surfaces. They all resemble simply flat sections of a highly branched villous tree. a: ×80; b: ×3,100; c: ×300; d: ×60.

sections (Figure 10.3d). Accordingly, when evaluating sections one should be aware that the degree of knotting always depends on two factors, irregularity of villous surfaces and sectional thickness.

Several authors have pointed out that syncytial knotting is related to pregnancy complications such as placental ischemia and pre-eclampsia (Alvarez et al., 1969, 1970; Schuhmann and Geier, 1972; Tenney and Parker, 1940; Todros et al., 1999; for review see Benirschke and Kaufmann, 2000). It was speculated by the above authors that hypoxia is the underlying pathogenetic cause. On first glance, hypoxia is not a very likely cause for a sectional artefact. However, when bearing in mind that (a) hypoxia stimulates branching angiogenesis of villi (Kaufmann and Kingdom, 2000), and (b) that the type of angiogenesis shapes the villi since the syncytial cover behaves like a tight elastic glove around the underlying capillaries, it becomes reasonable that increased capillary coiling and branching results in increased villous branching and villous surface irregularities (Todros et al., 1999). Consequently, it is well-established that placental conditions (IUGR with preserved end-diastolic flow in the umbilical arteries – PED, with or without pre-eclampsia) resulting from low pO_2 coincide with branching angiogenesis and richly branched terminal villi and increased syncytial knotting in paraffin sections (Todros et al., 1999). On the other hand, pregnancy conditions with abnormally high intraplacental pO_2 (IUGR with absent or reversed end-diastolic flow in the umbilical arteries – ARED with or without pre-eclampsia) produce long filiform terminal villi with unbranched capillary loops and scarcity of syncytial knotting (Macara et al., 1996).

Taking a closer look on the morphology of the syncytial nuclei inside these flat sections, it becomes clear that neither apoptosis nor necrosis can be detected here. The nuclei show their typical irregularly shaped morphology of mature syncytiotrophoblast and an irregular distribution of heterochromatin (Figure 10.3b).

Most syncytial bridges found in histological sections are sectional artefacts as described above. However, as has been shown by Cantle et al. (1987), in rare cases also true syncytial bridges do exist. They are thought to serve as simple mechanical aids to establish junctions between neighboring villi. Langhans (1870) was the first to describe these structures. And more than 100 years later Burton (1986a, 1987) and Cantle et al. (1987) made clear that besides a huge number of artificial two-dimensional structures real syncytial bridges do exist. These bridges are very likely the result of a prolonged intimate contact of adjacent villous surfaces. First small areas of both syncytial surfaces come into contact, become bridged by desmosomes, and finally the separating apical membranes of both parts of the syncytiotrophoblast disintegrate (Benirschke and Kaufmann, 2000). Since the underlying mechanisms do not lead to changes in nuclear morphology, the nuclei in these areas show the normal characteristics of heterogeneous shapes and chromatin distribution that are typical for syncytiotrophoblast nuclei.

Shedding of aged or degenerative nuclei

True syncytial knots serve as a mechanism to extrude old syncytial nuclei (Jones and Fox, 1977; Martin and Spicer, 1973). They are true bulbous or even mushroom-like protrusions of the syncytial surface (Figure 10.4) characterized by a dense package of nuclei separated from each other only by slender strands of cytoplasm. The cytoplasm already exhibits degenerative changes and is usually void of ribosomes.

Syncytial knots are sites of shedding of aged syncytiotrophoblast into the intervillous space. Following accumulation of nuclei, the protrusions become pinched off into the maternal blood. Here they have been detected in uterine vein blood (Johansen et al., 1999) and in the lung capillaries of the mother (Ikle, 1964). Since they do not regularly appear in peripheral blood of pregnant women they are believed to be engulfed by lung macrophages.

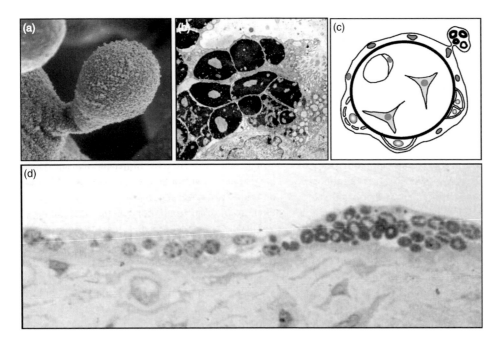

Figure 10.4 True syncytial knots. (a) The scanning electron microscopical picture shows the bulbous appearance of the knot. (b) The electron microscopical picture shows the annular chromatin condensation of accumulated syncytial nuclei and the cover with an apical plasma membrane that is mostly void of the microvillous brush border. (c) The scheme depicts the normal turnover of villous trophoblast from proliferation and differentiation of cytotrophoblast to syncytial fusion of the stem cell with the overlying syncytiotrophoblast. Within the syncytium the differentiation continues finalizing in package of old material into syncytial knots and extrusion of these structures into the maternal circulation. (d) The semi-thin section shows a piece of syncytial surface with largely normal nuclei (left) which show increasing chromatin condensation as they accumulate to the right. a: ×1000; b: ×3000; d: ×450.

Regarding nuclear size, nuclear structure, organization of the covering plasma membrane and underlying pathogenic mechanisms, different types of syncytial knots and different types of shedding of aged or degenerative syncytiotrophoblast can be observed:

(a) **Knot-like apoptotic shedding:** in true apoptotic shedding the nuclei are reduced in size (Mayhew and Barker, 2001; Mayhew et al., 1999) and their chromatin is more or less condensed, sometimes showing an annular chromatin condensation (Figure 10.4b–d). The apical syncytial membrane is intact, very smooth and mostly devoid of microvilli (Figure 10.4b). These morphological features place the syncytial knots at the site of late syncytiotrophoblast apoptosis. Detailed studies of the underlying apoptosis mechanisms have made it clear that these apoptotic knots represent the morphological correlate of apoptotic bodies of mononucleated cells at the end of the apoptosis cascade including DNA strand breaks identified by the TUNEL test (terminal deoxynucleotidyl transferase-mediated dUTP nick-end labeling) (Huppertz et al., 1998; Nelson, 1996; Smith et al., 1997).

As described before, syncytial fusion of villous trophoblast involves early steps of the apoptosis cascade (for a review see Huppertz et al., 1999). Under normal conditions, upon successful fusion activation of execution caspases and thus continuation of the cascade is interrupted by inhibitory proteins such as Mcl-1 and Bcl-2 which are transferred in excess amounts from the fusing cytotrophoblast into the syncytiotrophoblast (Huppertz et al., 2003). Three to four weeks later, the cascade is re-started (Benirschke and Kaufmann, 2000; Huppertz et al., 2002); cleavage of cytoskeletal proteins enables nuclear movement and formation of nuclear aggregates (syncytial knots) that are finally pinched off as membrane-sealed structures, a kind of giant apoptotic bodies. Typical for membrane-sealed apoptotic material, they do not induce an inflammatory response. Thus syncytial knots are thought to be trapped in the lung capillaries where they are phagocytosed by lung macrophages without starting an inflammatory reaction.

This is considered the normal way of trophoblastic shedding as the endpoint of normal trophoblast turnover (Figure 10.4c). In a normal term placenta 3 g of trophoblast are shed apoptotically daily into the maternal blood (Benirschke and Kaufmann, 2000; Huppertz et al., 2002), an amount that represents the daily trophoblastic proliferation and fusion rate (3.6 g per day) minus the growth rate of syncytiotrophoblast (about 0.6 g per day).

(b) **Wave-like apoptotic shedding:** in a specific subset of cases with severe IUGR (IUGR with absent end-diastolic flow in the umbilical arteries) without pre-eclampsia we found a dramatic reduction in the number of cytotrophoblast cells in combination with a clearly reduced thickness of the syncytiotrophoblast (Figure 10.5a–d). In these cases the syncytiotrophoblast showed a specific ring-like pattern of nuclear distribution. The aggregated apoptotic syncytial nuclei accumulated in ring-like waves around the vertical axis of the villi. In longitudinal sections this can be visualized by multiple cross-sections of nuclear accumulations (Figure 10.5a). In flat sections through the longitudinal axis of villi as well as by

scanning electron microscopy the wave-like pattern is clearly identifiable (Figure 10.5b–d). The underlying pathogenic mechanisms remain in the dark that link the pathogenesis of IUGR to this special form of trophoblast turnover with apoptotic shedding of nuclei.

(c) **Arrested apoptotic shedding:** another rare variation of apoptotic trophoblast turnover was also found in cases of severe IUGR (with absent end-diastolic flow in the umbilical arteries) without pre-eclampsia. In these cases trophoblast turnover ended up with the knot-like accumulation of clearly apoptotic TUNEL-positive nuclei, suggesting that a more or less normal apoptosis cascade triggered the process. But its final event, shedding of the mushroom-like sprouts into the intervillous space seemed to be arrested: hundreds of clearly apoptotic nuclei accumulated in these knots, and enormous numbers of such giant knots were formed throughout the placenta (Figure 10.5e–g). Sometimes the sites with accumulated nuclei were even larger than the cross-section of the producing villus. Also in this case, it can only be speculated that deficits in the apoptotic cleavage of the syncytial cytoskeleton that is linked to the formation of sealed bodies, prevented regular delivery of the apoptotic material into the intervillous space.

(d) **Aponecrotic shedding:** in the material available to us, the above two forms of pathologic apoptotic turnover were combined with IUGR, but never with symptoms of pre-eclampsia. Also in the latter case (c) we found signs of apoptotic trophoblast turnover and apoptotic trophoblast shedding, but this time mixed with signs of syncytial necrosis (so-called aponecrosis). However, it needs to be pointed out that to a lesser degree signs of necrosis/aponecrosis can also be found in every normal placenta.

Continuation of the apoptosis cascade by necrotic events with damage of the plasma membrane, water influx, secondary hydropic

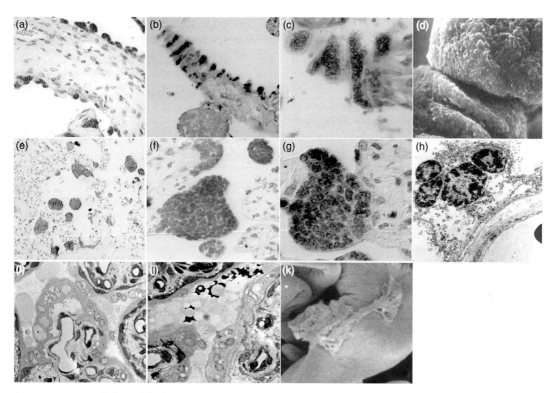

Figure 10.5 Histopathological findings of the syncytiotrophoblast. Wave-like apoptotic shedding (a–d). The aggregated apoptotic nuclei inside the syncytiotrophoblast show a specific ring-like pattern around the vertical axis of villi. This can be visualized in longitudinal paraffin sections (a–c) as well as in scanning electron microscopy (d). Arrested apoptotic shedding (e–g). Apoptotic syncytial nuclei accumulate in knot-like structures, while the normal extrusion of the knots into the intervillous space seems to be arrested. In paraffin sections enormous numbers of such giant knots can be found throughout the placenta. Aponecrotic shedding (h). The electron microscopical picture shows that nuclei inside the knot reveal the first stages of annular chromatin condensation, while the cytoplasm is edematous and the plasma membrane shows local defects. Necrotic shedding (i–l). In semi-thin sections necrosis can be visualized by edematous nuclei with a complete absence of chromatin condensation in a hydropic cytoplasm with membrane defects (i, k). The scanning electron microscopical picture reveals that these sites are characterized by fibrin clots covering membrane defects (l). a, b, e: ×25; c, f: ×100; d: ×1000; g: ×200; h: ×3800; i, k, l: ×300.

changes of cellular structures and release of cytoplasmic contents, are well-known as secondary necrosis or aponecrosis (Formigli *et al.*, 2000). Since apoptosis is an energy-dependent type of cell death, the lack of energy in later stages of apoptosis has been accused as one factor responsible for this abortive type of apoptosis, the so-called aponecrosis.

In in vitro experiments with villous explants mimicking conditions of pre-eclampsia with increased turnover (proliferation and apoptosis), not only the rate of apoptosis increased but signs of necrosis appeared in parallel: the conditioned media of these explants contained cell-free DNA and cell-free actin besides membrane-wrapped nuclei (apoptotic syncytial knots). Figure 10.5h shows a respective aponecrotic syncytial knot from a patient with pre-eclampsia: the nuclei reveal an early stage of annular chromatin condensation, but the cytoplasm is edematous and the plasma membrane shows local defects.

The placentas derived from patients with pre-eclampsia available to us, showed evidence of increased syncytial apoptosis and of increased syncytiotrophoblast shedding in general. The most prominent difference when compared to cases without preeclampsia was the increase in aponecrotic shedding and thus the altered balance from predominant apoptotic shedding to predominant aponecrotic shedding.

(e) **Necrotic shedding:** Pure necrotic alterations of villous syncytiotrophoblast without signs of apoptotic death, i.e. edematous nuclei in a hydropic cytoplasm with membrane defects (Figure 10.5i,k), are a rather rare event. We have seen such features in severe cases of pre-eclampsia as well as in severe cases of rhesus incompatibility. The complete absence of chromatin condensation within the syncytial nuclei (Figure 10.5i) suggests that the apoptosis cascade upon syncytial fusion has been successfully blocked by inhibitory proteins, but has not been restarted to complete normal syncytial shedding.

Continuous incorporation of new cytotrophoblast but absence of syncytial shedding will lead to intrasyncytial accumulation of aged trophoblastic components and finally to local or general breakdown of syncytiotrophoblast. Using scanning electron microscopy respective sites are characterized by membrane defects together with fibrin clots (Figure 10.5l). Histological, nuclear and cytoplasmic edema together with blebbing of the syncytial surface are typical features.

In the human, the continuous necrotic and aponecrotic release of intrasyncytial contents will very likely lead to a maternal inflammatory response. Experimentally we have produced the same features by complete blockage of the energy metabolism of the trophoblast in pregnant guinea pigs by administration of monoiodine acetate or sodium fluoride, both potent inhibitors of glycolysis (Kaufmann *et al.*, 1974).

Conclusions

Aggregations of nuclei within the syncytiotrophoblast of human placental villi, the former syncytial knots and sprouts, are phenotypically rather similar only at first glance. When studying the external shape of the aggregate, nuclear morphology and integrity of the plasma membrane in more detail (Figure 10.6), it is possible to differentiate a series of different structures with different functional and pathohistological significance. (a) True syncytial sprouts with large euchromatic nuclei prevail in the first half of pregnancy and are early stages of formation of new villi. (b) Syncytial knotting (Tenney–Parker changes) is characterized by accumulated mushroom-like protrusions of normally structured nuclei and syncytial bridges connecting neighboring villi; these are sectional artefacts caused by flat-sectioning across distorted and highly branched villous surfaces. (c) True apoptotic knots are mushroom-like syncytial protrusions containing nuclei in more or less advanced stages of apoptotic chromatin condensation; they represent normal final stages of extrusion of aged syncytiotrophoblast (Figure 10.6a). (d) Wave-like apoptotic knots are histologically similar structures which, however, form multiple ring-like bands around the villi (Figure 10.6e). They are closely related to severe cases of IUGR without pre-eclampsia. (e) Arrested apoptotic knots accumulate hundreds of apoptotic nuclei without subsequent shedding into the maternal circulation (Figure 10.6b); this phenomenon is also linked to cases of severe IUGR without pre-eclampsia. (f) Aponecrotic knots resemble apoptotic knots (c) but additionally show edematous changes and defects of the plasma membrane (Figure 10.6c). They can be found in normal pregnancies but prevail in pre-eclampsia. (g) Necrotic shedding is characterized by severe edematous damages

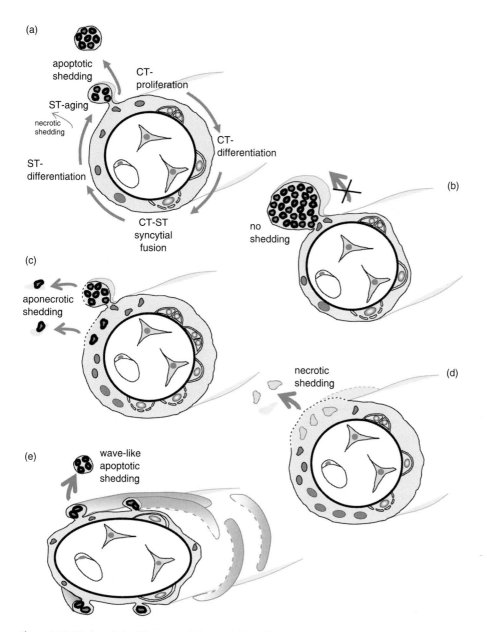

Figure 10.6 Modes of shedding syncytial material into the maternal circulation. (a) Knot-like apoptotic shedding. Under normal conditions turnover of villous trophoblast comprises proliferation and differentiation of cytotrophoblast (CT), fusion of cytotrophoblast with the overlying syncytiotrophoblast (ST), further differentiation inside the syncytiotrophoblast with subsequent aging and package of old material into apoptotic syncytial knots that are extruded into the maternal circulation. (b) Arrested apoptotic shedding. If extrusion of the syncytial knots is blocked, the number of nuclei inside the knots increases dramatically. (c) Aponecrotic shedding. If the apoptosis cascade does not progress to its very end but is interrupted and stopped, necrotic release of apoptotic material may take place. This aponecrotic material may induce inflammation in the mother. (d) Necrotic shedding. If no apoptosis takes place parts of the syncytium may undergo necrosis, resulting in the release of necrotic material and thus inducing an inflammatory reaction of the mother. (e) Wave-like apoptotic shedding. A dramatic reduction in the number of cytotrophoblast cells is combined with a clearly reduced thickness of the syncytiotrophoblast. Here the syncytial nuclei accumulate in specific ring-like waves around the vertical axis of the villi.

of syncytiotrophoblast with defects of the plasma membrane and absence of signs of apoptosis (Figure 10.6d). Nuclei may be aggregated and form knots but may also be evenly distributed. Also this is mainly a pathological phenomenon.

REFERENCES

Alvarez, H., Morel, R. L., Benedetti, W. L. and Scavarelli, M. (1969). Trophoblast hyperplasia and maternal arterial pressure at term. *Am. J. Obstet. Gynecol.*, **105**, 1015–21.

Alvarez, H., Benedetti, W. L., Morel, R. L. and Scavarelli, M. (1970). Trophoblast development gradient and its relationship to placental hemodynamics. *Am. J. Obstet. Gynecol.*, **106**, 416–20.

Benirschke, K. and Kaufmann, P. (2000). *Pathology of the Human Placenta* (4th edn). New York: Springer.

Boyd, J. D. and Hamilton, W. J. (1970). *The Human Placenta*. Cambridge: Heffer.

Burton, G. J. (1986a). Intervillous connections in the mature human placenta: instances of syncytial fusion or section artefacts? *J. Anat.*, **145**, 13–23.

Burton, G. J. (1986b). Scanning electron microscopy of intervillous connections in the mature human placenta. *J. Anat.*, **147**, 245–54.

Burton, G. J. (1987). The fine structure of the human placental villus as revealed by scanning electron microscopy. *Scannings Microsc.*, **1**, 1811–28.

Cantle, S. J., Kaufmann, P., Luckhardt, M. and Schweikhart, G. (1987). Interpretation of syncytial sprouts and bridges in the human placenta. *Placenta*, **8**, 221–34.

Castellucci, M., Scheper, M., Scheffen, I., Celona, A. and Kaufmann, P. (1990). The development of the human placental villous tree. *Anat. Embryol.*, **181**, 117–28.

Formigli, L., Papucci, L., Tani, A., *et al.* (2000). Aponecrosis: morphological and biochemical exploration of a syncretic process of cell death sharing apoptosis and necrosis. *J. Cell Physiol.*, **182**, 41–9.

Huppertz, B., Frank, H. G., Kingdom, J. C. P., Reister, F. and Kaufmann, P. (1998). Villous cytotrophoblast regulation of the syncytial apoptotic cascade in the human placenta. *Histochem. Cell Biol.*, **110**, 495–508.

Huppertz, B., Frank, H. G. and Kaufmann, P. (1999). The apoptosis cascade – morphological and immuno-histochemical methods for its visualization. *Anat. Embryol.*, **200**, 1–18.

Huppertz, B., Kaufmann, P. and Kingdom, J. (2002). Trophoblast turnover in health and disease. *Fetal Maternal Med. Rev.*, **13**, 103–18.

Huppertz, B., Kingdom, J., Caniggia, I., *et al.* (2003). Hypoxia favours necrotic versus apoptotic shedding of placental syncytiotrophoblast into the maternal circulation. *Placenta*, **24**, 181–90.

Ikle, F. A. (1964). Trophoblastzellen im strömenden Blut. *Schweiz. Med. Wochenschr.*, **91**, 934–45.

Johansen, M., Redman, C. W., Wilkins, T. and Sargent, I. L. (1999). Trophoblast deportation in human pregnancy – its relevance for pre-eclampsia. *Placenta*, **20**, 531–9.

Jones, J. P. and Fox, H. (1977). Syncytial knots and intervillous bridges in the human placenta: an ultrastructural study. *J. Anat.*, **124**, 275–86.

Kaufmann, P. and Kingdom, J. (2000). Development of the vascular system in the placenta. In *Morphogenesis of Endothelium*, ed. W. Risau and G. Rubanyi. Reading, UK: Harwood Academic, pp. 255–75.

Kaufmann, P., Thorn, W. and Jenke, B. (1974). Die Morphologie der Meerschweinchenplacenta nach Monojodacetat- und Fluoridvergiftung. *Arch. Gynecol.*, **216**, 185–203.

Kaufmann, P., Luckhardt, M., Schweikhart, G. and Cantle, S. J. (1987). Cross-sectional features and three-dimensional structure of human placental villi. *Placenta*, **8**, 235–47.

Kuestermann, W. (1981). Über Proliferationsknoten und Syncytialknoten der menschlichen Placenta. *Anat. Anz.*, **150**, 144–57.

Langhans, T. (1870). Zur Kenntnis der menschlichen Placenta. *Arch. Gynäkol.*, **1**, 317–34.

Macara, L., Kingdom, J. C., Kaufmann, P., *et al.* (1996). Structural analysis of placental terminal villi from growth-restricted pregnancies with abnormal umbilical artery Doppler waveforms. *Placenta*, **17**, 37–48.

Martin, B. J. and Spicer, S. S. (1973). Ultrastructural features of cellular maturation and aging in human trophoblast. *J. Ultrastruct. Res.*, **43**, 133–49.

Mayhew, T. M. and Barker, B. L. (2001). Villous trophoblast: morphometric perspectives on growth, differentiation, turnover and deposition of fibrin-type fibrinoid during gestation. *Placenta*, **22**, 628–38.

Mayhew, T. M., Leach, L., McGee, R., Ismail, W. W., Myklebust, R. and Lammiman, M. J. (1999). Proliferation, differentiation and apoptosis in villous trophoblast at 13–41 weeks of gestation (including observations on annulate lamellae and nuclear pore complexes). *Placenta*, **20**, 407–22.

Nelson, D. M. (1996). Apoptotic changes occur in syncytiotrophoblast of human placental villi where fibrin type fibrinoid is deposited at discontinuities in the villous trophoblast. *Placenta*, **17**, 387–91.

Schiebler, T. H. and Kaufmann, P. (1969). Reife Plazenta. In *Die Plazenta des Menschen*, ed. V. Becker, T. H. Schiebler and F. Kubli. Stuttgart: Georg Thieme-Verlag, pp. 51–100.

Schuhmann, R. and Geier, G. (1972). Histomorphologische Placentabefunde bei EPH-Gestose. *Arch. Gynäkol.*, **213**, 31–47.

Smith, S. C., Baker, P. N. and Symonds, E. M. (1997). Placental apoptosis in normal human pregnancy. *Am. J. Obstet. Gynecol.*, **177**, 57–65.

Tenney, B. and Parker, F. (1940). The placenta in toxaemia of pregnancy. *Am. J. Obstet. Gynecol.*, **39**, 1000–5.

Todros, T., Sciarrone, A., Piccoli, E., Guiot, C., Kaufmann, P. and Kingdom, J. (1999). Umbilical Doppler waveforms and placental villous angiogenesis in pregnancies complicated by fetal growth restriction. *Obstet. Gynecol.*, **93**, 499–503.

11

Dyslipidemia and pre-eclampsia

Carl A. Hubel

Introduction

The causes of the pregnancy syndrome pre-eclampsia are multifactorial and poorly understood. According to current concepts, the disorder has two principal stages (Redman *et al.*, 1999; Roberts and Hubel, 1999). The first stage is reduced placental perfusion, frequently secondary to abnormal implantation and insufficient remodeling of spiral arteries feeding the intervillous space. The second stage is the maternal response to this condition, modulated by maternal constitution and heredity, and characterized by widespread inflammation and endothelial cell dysfunction. The link between the two stages is an area of intense investigation. It is clear that placental factors are not solely accountable for the maternal manifestations of pre-eclampsia. Intrauterine growth restriction and preterm birth are commonly associated with abnormalities in Stage 1 but without the occurrence of a maternal syndrome. Maternal factors, including pre-pregnancy obesity and insulin resistance, predispose to development of pre-eclampsia. Evidence is accumulating that maternal constitutional predisposition to cardiovascular disease, unmasked or accentuated during the stress of pregnancy, is a key component in the development of pre-eclampsia. Data also suggest that women with a history of pre-eclampsia are at increased risk of cardiovascular disease in later life. Dyslipidemia may play an important role in these interrelationships. This chapter reviews the changes in lipid metabolism that occur with normal pregnancy and pre-eclampsia, and develops the hypothesis that dyslipidemia contributes to both the pathogenesis of preeclampsia and risk of later-life cardiovascular disease.

Pregnancy-induced changes in lipid metabolism

The diverse effects of pregnancy include a profound impact upon lipid metabolism. Several comprehensive reviews deal with the changes in lipid metabolism that occur with normal pregnancy and their importance for fetal development (Herrera, 2002). This section summarizes some of these aspects to provide a framework for discussion of lipid abnormalities and pre-eclampsia.

Maternal metabolism is disposed toward adipose tissue fat accumulation during early gestation. In marked contrast, a shift to a state of net breakdown/mobilization of adipose lipid depots occurs during the second half of pregnancy (Alvarez *et al.*, 1996; Herrera *et al.*, 1988). One of the more striking results is an increase in free (non-esterified) fatty acid (FFA) concentrations in maternal plasma with advancing gestation. Maternally derived essential fatty acids and long chain polyunsaturated fatty acids are important for fetal development and growth. At 12–14 weeks of normal pregnancy, insulin sensitivity is slightly increased but then decreases during the rest of pregnancy (Catalano *et al.*, 1991). The decline in insulin sensitivity (increase in peripheral insulin resistance) peaks during the last third of pregnancy, and is a physiological adaptation that helps to ensure availability of glucose and FFA for the fetus.

Circulating FFAs are regulated partly by hormone-sensitive lipase in maternal adipocytes. One action of insulin is to inhibit this enzyme, decreasing adipocyte triglyceride hydrolysis and thus limiting serum FFA and glycerol concentrations. Gestational insulin resistance, therefore, is likely to be partly responsible for increased release of FFA and glycerol from adipocytes (Figure 11.1) (Alvarez et al., 1996). Suggesting a feed-forward process, the high levels of plasma FFA typically observed during the last half of pregnancy may actually cause some of the insulin resistance that occurs during this period (Sivan et al., 1998). Tumor necrosis factor-α and leptin probably also foster gestational insulin resistance (Kirwan et al., 2002). The lipolytic action of human placental lactogen, which reaches very high levels during late gestation, also appears to contribute to the increase in FFA (Murai et al., 1997).

Much of the glycerol and FFA released from fat are taken up by the liver and re-esterified for synthesis of very-low-density lipoprotein (VLDL) triglycerides (Figure 11.1). Increased estrogen

and decreased hepatocyte B-oxidation also lead to increased hepatocyte VLDL production. By term, plasma triglycerides increase by 50–300% over pre-pregnant levels, at which time increased amounts of triglycerides are found not only in VDL but also in intermediate density lipoprotein (IDL), low-density lipoprotein (LDL) and high-density lipoprotein (HDL) (Hubel and Roberts, 1999; Montelongo et al., 1992). Lipoprotein lipase, tethered to the luminal side of capillaries and arteries of extrahepatic tissues, hydrolyzes lipoprotein triglycerides to produce FFA and monoacyl-glycerol (Figure 11.1). These lipolysis products are predominantly taken up by tissue locally to meet the needs of that tissue. This promotes triglyceride clearance from the circulation. However, adipose tissue lipoprotein lipase activity decreases substantially during the last third of pregnancy due to insulin resistance and other hormonal influences. The result is a decrease in the rate of removal of triglyceride-rich lipoproteins from the circulation (Alvarez et al., 1996). Thus, both increased production and decreased removal probably contribute to the dramatic increase in postprandial and fasting triglycerides evident by late gestation (Alvarez et al., 1996).

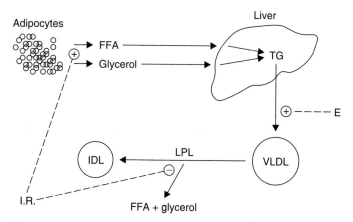

Figure 11.1 Representation of a few of the interactions of lipoprotein metabolism with insulin resistance and estrogen during pregnancy. Key: +, activation; −, inhibition; I.R., insulin resistance; E, estrogen; TG, triglyceride; FFA, free fatty acid; LPL, lipoprotein lipase; VLDL, very low-density lipoprotein; IDL, intermediate-density lipoprotein. See text and also Alvarez et al. (1996) and Herrera (2002) for more details.

Circulating triglycerides do not cross the placenta (Coleman, 1989). However, an elaborate placental transport process ensures that adequate amounts of fatty acids, originally packaged in maternal lipoprotein triglycerides, are delivered to the fetus. Components of this transport process include LDL and VLDL/apo E receptors in the placenta, placental lipoprotein lipase (not suppressed during pregnancy), placental phospholipase A2, and intracellular placental lipases (Bonet et al., 1992; Herrera, 2002; Winkler et al., 2003; Wittmaack et al., 1995). Lipoprotein lipase, present only on the maternal surface of the placenta, makes FFA available by hydrolyzing triglycerides carried by maternal VLDL (Coleman, 1989). After uptake by trophoblast cells, fatty acids are re-esterified to provide a fat reservoir. After intracellular hydrolysis releases fatty acids to fetal plasma, they bind α-fetoprotein and are transported to the fetal liver (Herrera, 2002). The placenta delivers as much as 50% of the total daily fatty acid requirement of the fetus, all of the essential fatty acids, the fat soluble vitamins, and cholesterol-derived precursors of steroid hormones to the fetus. A direct relationship between maternal triglycerides and birthweight has been found in humans. Severe correction of maternal hypertriglyceridemia (as with hypolipidemic drugs) has negative effects on fetal growth and development (Herrera, 2002).

Interestingly, lipoprotein lipase plays a key role in the transport of vitamin E. The vitamin is carried by triglyceride-rich lipoproteins and enters cells as triglycerides are hydrolyzed. Vitamin E is also incorporated into cells via receptor-bound LDL (Coleman, 1989). However, unlike the maternal circulation, vitamin E levels do not increase in fetal plasma with advancing gestation because fetal concentrations of the major lipoprotein carriers remain low.

Maternal cholesterol levels increase during pregnancy, with a 50–60% rise over prepregnant levels by term (Lorentzen and Henriksen, 1998). Maternal cholesterol is important for the fetus during early pregnancy, but its importance lessens by late pregnancy owing to the ability of fetal tissues to synthesize cholesterol (Herrera, 2002). Reversal of the "physiologic hyperlipidemia" of pregnancy begins within hours of delivery and is essentially complete by 6–10 weeks postpartum (Potter and Nestel, 1979).

Changes in circulating lipids with pre-eclampsia

Marked dyslipidemia occurs with pre-eclampsia (Hubel, 1998; Hubel and Roberts, 1999; Kaaja, 1998; Lorentzen and Henriksen, 1998). In some respects, this represents an accentuation of normal pregnancy changes. Mean plasma triglyceride and FFA concentrations increase about twofold on average in women with pre-eclampsia relative to women with uncomplicated pregnancy (Figures 11.2 and 11.3) (Endresen et al., 1992; Hubel et al., 1996; Lorentzen et al., 1995). About one-third of women with pre-eclampsia develop plasma triglyceride values above $400\,mg\,dL^{-1}$ (Hubel et al., 1996), greater than the 90th percentile measured in randomly selected women at 36 weeks of gestation. This reflects markedly increased concentrations of triglyceride-rich lipoproteins (especially $VLDL_1$) (Sattar et al., 1997a). The hypertriglyceridemia of pre-eclampsia is accompanied by a decrease in cardioprotective HDL cholesterol relative to normal pregnancy (Kaaja et al., 1995; Sattar et al., 1997a). It is noteworthy, however, that not all women with pre-eclampsia develop gestational dyslipidemia and that some women with profound dyslipidemia have an uncomplicated pregnancy outcome. This fits with the concept that the syndrome is multifactorial and heterogeneous (Ness and Roberts, 1996).

Case-control differences in circulating levels of the major fatty acids are unlikely to be solely attributable to differences in dietary fat intake even if dietary histories were to be dissimilar. Nevertheless, diet may impart certain differences. For example, women with low concentrations of erythrocyte membrane omega-3 (marine oil)

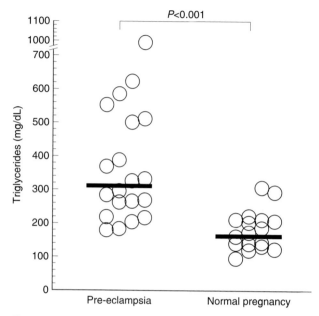

Figure 11.2 Scatterplot of serum triglyceride concentrations during late pregnancy. Each symbol corresponds to a different individual. Thick horizontal bars correspond to median values for each group. $P < 0.001$, pre-eclampsia vs. normal pregnant by Mann–Whitney U test. Data redrawn from Hubel *et al.* (1998a).

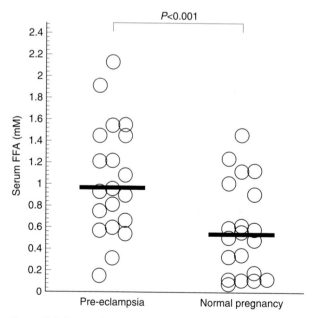

Figure 11.3 Scatterplot of serum free fatty acid concentrations during late pregnancy. Each symbol corresponds to a different individual. Thick horizontal bars correspond to median values for each group. $P < 0.01$, pre-eclampsia vs. normal pregnant by Mann–Whitney U test. Data redrawn from Hubel *et al.* (1998a).

fatty acids are reportedly more likely to have had pre-eclamptic pregnancies compared with women with high levels of erythrocyte omega-3 fatty acids (Williams *et al.*, 1995). Since erythrocyte turnover is approximately 120 days, erythrocyte fatty acid profiles probably reflect differences in dietary intake (Williams *et al.*, 1995).

The relative content of linoleic acid, a polyunsaturated fatty acid, is decreased in both the triglyceride and phospholipid fractions in women with pre-eclampsia (Lorentzen and Henriksen, 1998; Lorentzen *et al.*, 1995). The most likely explanation for this is that polyunsaturated fatty acids are prone to peroxidation with conversion to lipid peroxides. Thus, the reduced content of polyunsaturated fatty acids in lipoprotein triglycerides and phospholipids may result from free radical modification related to increased oxidative stress during the disease (Lorentzen and Henriksen, 1998; Lorentzen *et al.*, 1995).

Of particular significance, dyslipidemia becomes evident during the first and second trimester, far preceding the clinical manifestations of pre-eclampsia (Arbogast *et al.*, 1996; Chappell *et al.*, 2002; Gratacos *et al.*, 1996; Lorentzen *et al.*, 1994, 1995). HDL-cholesterol ("good cholesterol") is reduced at earliest measurement (20 weeks gestation) and then throughout gestation in women who later develop the disease, again implicating dyslipidemia in the disease process (Chappell *et al.*, 2002). Decreased HDL may result from increased triglycerides since the two are metabolically linked (Hubel *et al.*, 1998b; Lamarche *et al.*, 1999). Increases in mean concentrations of the major FFAs (oleic, linoleic, palmitic) are detectable by 16–20 weeks of gestation in groups of women who later develop pre-eclampsia (Lorentzen *et al.*, 1994, 1995). Abnormal elevations in fasting triglycerides occur as early as 10 weeks of gestation (Gratacos *et al.*, 1996). Interestingly, early hypertriglyceridemia is associated with increased risk of early onset pre-eclampsia (pre-eclampsia developing before 36 weeks of gestation) but not late onset pre-eclampsia (Clausen *et al.*, 2001). This adds to evidence that early- and late-onset variants of

the disease are pathogenically distinguishable and is consistent with the notion of multiple pathways to pre-eclampsia.

Relative to normal pregnancy, total cholesterol and LDL cholesterol levels are generally not altered during pre-eclampsia (Hubel *et al.*, 1998a). According to two reports, however, women with raised total cholesterol during the first trimester are at increased risk of pre-eclampsia (Elzen *et al.*, 1996; Solomon *et al.*, 1999). Serum cholesterol is also increased, months postpartum in many women with a history of pre-eclampsia (Barden *et al.*, 1999). These data suggest that pre-eclampsia is associated with chronically abnormal cholesterol metabolism that becomes transiently masked by the physiologic hypercholesterolemia of late pregnancy.

The finding of early lipid changes fits with the notion that dyslipidemia promotes dysfunction of the maternal vascular endothelium. The early lipid changes also beg the question of whether lipid abnormalities are present before pregnancy in women who later develop pre-eclampsia, perhaps in a latent form that becomes unmasked or amplified by the stress of pregnancy. These lipid markers might also herald an opportunity for therapeutic intervention to ameliorate or prevent pre-eclampsia. Considering the direct relationship between maternal triglyceride concentration and newborn weight, however, the potential for adverse effects of lipid-lowering agents on fetal health must be kept in mind. It is biologically plausible that, in some women, exaggerated hyperlipidemia occurs as a response to signals (leptin, human placental lactogen, etc.) from the feto-placental unit to mobilize more substrate for the poorly perfused placenta and fetus. Although intrauterine fetal growth restriction (IUGR) is a common complication of pre-eclampsia, many babies born of pre-eclamptic pregnancies are not small for gestational age. Pregnancies complicated by IUGR without pre-eclampsia have placental lesions similar to pre-eclampsia but without a maternal syndrome (no hypertension or proteinuria). Women with IUGR pregnancies without the maternal syndrome do not develop hypertriglyceridemia (Sattar *et al.*, 1999). Furthermore, as a group they actually have lower VLDL$_2$, IDL, and cholesterol concentrations than healthy pregnant controls (Sattar *et al.*, 1999). One might surmise that failure to mobilize/synthesize lipids in the face of inadequate placental perfusion contributes to fetal growth restriction. A robust hyperlipidemic response (possibly good for the baby) might put the maternal vascular endothelium at risk of dysfunction (bad for the mother).

Mechanisms of altered lipid metabolism in pre-eclampsia

It is likely that both maternal and placental factors cause dyslipidemia in pre-eclampsia. The insulin resistance syndrome, a cluster of metabolic abnormalities associated with reduced insulin sensitivity, is a strong predisposing factor for cardiovascular disease (Kahn and Flier, 2000; Reaven, 1994). Pre-eclampsia is associated with accentuation of many features of the metabolic syndrome, including insulin resistance, hypertriglyceridemia, elevated FFA, low HDL cholesterol, hyperuricemia, and abnormalities in the fibrinolytic system, usually in the absence of frank diabetes (Kaaja, 1998; Kaaja *et al.*, 1995; Lorentzen *et al.*, 1998; Solomon *et al.*, 1994; Solomon *et al.*, 1999; Sowers *et al.*, 1995; Wolf *et al.*, 2002). Accompanying abnormalities include increased serum concentrations of leptin, C-reactive protein, tumor necrosis factor-α, testosterone, and plasminogen activator-inhibitor-1 (Sattar and Greer, 2002; Wolf *et al.*, 2001).

Evidence has been accruing that insulin resistance actually precedes the development of pre-eclampsia, consistent with a role in pathogenesis (Solomon *et al.*, 1994, 1999; Wolf *et al.*, 2002). Furthermore, high prepregnancy body mass index (obesity), a component of the insulin resistance syndrome, is a strong, independent risk factor for pre-eclampsia (Barden *et al.*, 1999; Ness and Roberts, 1996; Sibai *et al.*, 1997; Wolf *et al.*, 2001).

As described in more detail later in this review, dyslipidemia, obesity and hyperinsulinemia have also been noted years after delivery in women with a history of pre-eclampsia, consistent with the hypothesis that these metabolic abnormalities predate pregnancy, often in latent form, and that they predispose to the disease (Barden *et al.*, 1999; Chambers *et al.*, 2001; Hubel *et al.*, 2000; Nisell *et al.*, 1999). However, prospective studies are needed to actually test the hypothesis that lipid/insulin abnormalities exist before pregnancy in women who later develop pre-eclampsia.

Heightened gestational insulin resistance (Kaaja, 1998; Lorentzen and Henriksen, 1998), or abnormally increased concentrations of TNF-α or human placental lactogen (Murai *et al.*, 1997) are candidate promoters of increased lipolytic activity in maternal adipocytes, leading to liberation of excessive amounts of FFA into the circulation of women with (or destined to develop) pre-eclampsia. Increased serum FFA provide substrate to increase liver VLDL triglyceride synthesis.

In addition to increased synthesis, decreased clearance probably contributes to hypertriglyceridemia in pre-eclamptic women. VLDL and LDL receptor expression is decreased in placentas of women with pre-eclampsia, which might reduce the clearance of maternal circulating triglycerides (Murata *et al.*, 1996). However, the relationship of these lipoprotein receptor changes to fetal growth remains unclear. Insulin resistance can decrease peripheral triglyceride clearance by suppressing adipose tissue lipoprotein lipase activity. In addition to hormones, genetic variation influences lipoprotein lipase activity. Two reports indicate that inhibitory mutations in the lipoprotein lipase gene are more prevalent in women with pre-eclampsia compared to normal pregnancy and population controls (Hubel *et al.*, 1999; Zhang *et al.*, 2006). The differences in allele frequency are small, however, in keeping with the concept of polygenic inheritance. Another carefully conducted study, however, reported no difference in frequency of lipoprotein lipase mutations among pre-eclamptics and controls (Kim *et al.*, 2001).

One interpretation is that genetic lipoprotein lipase deficiency is associated with pre-eclampsia in some populations but not others. To date, however, adipose tissue lipoprotein lipase mass and post-heparin activity have not been examined in women with pre-eclampsia.

Free fatty acids, oxidative stress and vascular dysfunction

Increased serum FFA, as a facet of the metabolic syndrome, adversely alters vascular function and constitutes an independent risk factor for coronary disease (Sattar et al., 1998). Experiments on endothelial cells in culture and on rat femoral artery segments in vitro suggest that physiologically relevant concentrations of FFA cause reductions in vasodilator prostacyclin and nitric oxide and reductions in vascular relaxation responsiveness (Davda et al., 1995; Endresen et al., 1994). In lean, insulin-sensitive subjects, manipulations to increase circulating FFA levels to the range observed in insulin-resistant patients (two- to ninefold elevations) impair relaxation to the endothelium-dependent vasodilator methacholine as measured by leg blood flow (Steinberg et al., 1997, 2000). Endogenous FFA correlate well with adverse vascular function in vivo (Steinberg et al., 1996, 1997, 2000). As discussed by these authors, elevated FFA may induce formation of reactive oxygen species which could destroy NO and thus attenuate NO-dependent vasodilation. The vascular superoxide-producing NAD(P)H oxidase, an enzyme that can be activated by FFA, may be of paramount importance in this regard (Bilodeau and Hubel, 2003; Griendling et al., 2000).

There is currently no direct evidence for a role of FFA in the attenuated vascular relaxation responses that typify pre-eclampsia. There are data, however, that FFA cause relevant alterations to the behavior of endothelial cells in culture. Endothelial monolayers exposed to pre-eclampsia plasma take up FFA in proportion to the excessive plasma FFA concentration, whereupon they synthesize triglycerides and become laden with triglyceride-rich lipid droplets. The increase in intracellular triglyceride is associated with decreased release of prostacyclin (Endresen et al., 1994).

The endogenous transition metals, iron (Fe) and copper (Cu) can catalyze the production of reactive oxygen species such as hydroxyl radical and thus promote oxidative stress. Albumin and ceruloplasmin are the major Cu-binding proteins in plasma. When sequestered by albumin or ceruloplasmin, Cu is usually redox-inactive (incapable of producing reactive oxygen species). However, plasma samples from at least a subset of women with pre-eclampsia (compared to normal pregnancy) display an elevated endogenous redox-cycling activity of Cu that can be inhibited by the copper (II) chelator, cuprizone I (Kagan et al., 2001). This activity may result from increased FFA in the circulation (Figure 11.4). Circulating FFAs are complexed with albumin. The molar ratio of FFA to albumin is two- to threefold greater in pre-eclampsia than normal pregnancy (Endresen et al., 1992, 1994; Vigne et al., 1997). The excess binding of fatty acids to albumin results in a conformational change in the albumin molecule accompanied by an isoelectric shift (from pI 5.6 to pI 4.8) (Vigne et al., 1997). These changes are also accompanied by an alteration in Cu/albumin interactions with the appearance of "loosely bound" Cu capable of generating reactive oxygen species (Figure 11.4) (Kagan et al., 2001). Indeed, model experiments show that Cu-dependent redox-cycling activity of purified human serum albumin is bolstered by excess FFA (Kagan et al., 2001). In this manner, FFAs convert albumin from an antioxidant to a pro-oxidant. Since elevated levels of plasma FFA are not unique to pre-eclampsia, there should be other conditions in which dysregulated copper/albumin interactions result in enhanced oxidative stress. One example is diabetes, where not only FFAs but also glycation of albumin may be responsible for its erroneous binding of Cu and high redox-cycling activity (Bourdon et al., 1999; Yuan et al., 1996). The reactive oxygen species generated after FFA

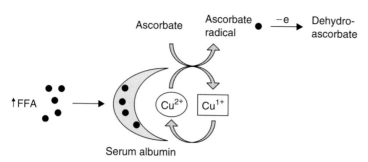

Figure 11.4 A mechanism of fatty acid-induced oxidative stress. Excess binding of fatty acids (FFA) to human serum albumin results in a conformational shift in the albumin molecule accompanied by an alteration in copper (Cu)-albumin interactions with the appearance of "loosely bound" Cu capable of redox cycling. This redox cycling oxidizes ascorbate to ascorbate radical which further decomposes to dehydroascorbate. (Adapted from a drawing by Valerian Kagan, Ph.D., by personal permission.)

binding to Cu-albumin are capable of destroying vitamin C and nitric oxide in vitro, and might do so in vivo (Bilodeau and Hubel, 2003; Kagan et al., 2001).

Triglycerides, oxidative stress and vascular dysfunction

There is strong support for a causal relationship between cholesterol and coronary artery disease. Nevertheless, up to half of patients with coronary artery disease have cholesterol levels in the normal range, suggesting involvement of other factors (Lamarche and Lewis, 1998; Lamarche et al., 1998). Hypertriglyceridemia is emerging as a major risk factor (Krauss, 1991, 1997; Lamarche et al., 1998; Lewis and Steiner, 1996; Reaven, 1994). Elevated triglycerides compromise vascular function in several ways. Triglyceride-rich lipoproteins have prothrombotic activity (Lewis and Steiner, 1996). Functional assays have revealed that human VLDL is toxic to human umbilical vein endothelial cells in culture and that this toxicity is prevented by the addition of pI 5.6, but not fatty acid-laden pI 4.8, albumin to the culture medium (Vigne et al., 1997). Triglyceride-rich lipoprotein remnant particles, identified as atherogenic in other settings, are

increased in women with pre-eclampsia (Winkler et al., 2003).

Triglyceride-rich lipoproteins in the form of a single high-fat meal impair endothelium-dependent vasodilation in a reversible manner (Plotnick et al., 1997; Vogel et al., 1997). Hypertriglyceridemia may increase the prevalence of reactive oxygen species by stimulation of leukocyte NAD(P)H oxidase, by lowering concentrations of protective HDL, or by increasing the formation of smaller, peroxidation-susceptible LDL particles (reviewed in Hubel, 1999). Reactive oxygen species, in turn, can decrease the bioavailability of NO, either directly by destruction or indirectly by formation of oxidized lipids that subsequently destroy NO or decrease NO synthase (Bilodeau and Hubel, 2003). Intraperitoneal injection of the nontoxic surfactant, poloxamer 407 in rats results in sustained elevations of triglycerides, cholesterol and FFA (Ramirez et al., 2001). Mesenteric arteries isolated from pregnant rats treated with poloxamer 407 (but not non-lipemic pluronic F-88) display increased constrictor responses to step increases in intraluminal pressure (myogenic constriction). This increase in myogenic constriction is due to selective attenuation of a modulatory, NO-mediated, vasodilator component of the myogenic response (Ramirez et al., 2001). These data are consistent with the notion that dyslipidemia can adversely affect NO homeostasis.

Hypertriglyceridemia shifts the spectrum of LDL subclasses toward predominance of LDL particles that are smaller in diameter, denser, and more prone to oxidative modification. Several prospective studies have shown that a preponderance of small dense LDL is associated with increased risk of coronary heart disease (Gardner et al., 1996; Lamarche et al., 1997, 1998; Stampfer et al., 1996). The small dense LDL ("pattern B") phenotype is associated with impaired NO-dependent forearm vasodilation in non-insulin-dependent diabetes mellitus (NIDDM) (O'Brien et al., 1997). As measured by nondenaturing polyacrylamide gradient gel electrophoresis, the rise in plasma triglyceride during normal pregnancy is accompanied by a progressive shift from predominantly large diameter LDL to predominantly intermediate and small-sized LDL, with reversal by 6 weeks postpartum (Hubel et al., 1998b; Silliman et al., 1994). Three studies using gradient gel electrophoresis have reported that the diameter of the principal LDL subclass is significantly decreased in pre-eclampsia relative to normal pregnancy (Belo et al., 2002; Hubel et al., 1998a; Ogura et al., 2002). Studies using density gradient ultracentrifugation in which LDL is separated primarily by floatation rate into three subfractions indicate that LDL becomes denser with advancing pregnancy once a serum triglyceride concentration threshold is crossed (Sattar et al., 1997b). LDL is reportedly even denser in women with pre-eclampsia (Sattar et al., 1997a). Taken together, these data suggest that potentially atherogenic, smaller, denser LDL predominates in pre-eclampsia. However, the floatation rate of lipoproteins depends on both particle buoyancy and size. Using a method purported to separate LDL particles strictly by virtue of their density, another group has reported accumulation of buoyant LDL with advancing gestation and depletion of the most dense LDL subfractions in pre-eclampsia (Winkler et al., 2000, 2003). Perhaps NMR spectroscopy or scanning electron microscopy will help to clarify whether this discrepancy reflects methodological flaws or biology, i.e. formation of a buoyant (conceivably a unique small buoyant) LDL subtype during pregnancy that is accentuated during pre-eclampsia. LDL isolated from plasma of women with pre-eclampsia is more susceptible to oxidation upon exposure to exogenous free radicals than normal pregnancy LDL (Wakatsuki et al., 2000). This is consistent with a subtype of LDL capable of disrupting NO homeostasis and impairing endothelial cell function.

Lipid peroxidation and the placenta

Lipid peroxidation products may have a role in the pathogenesis of pre-eclampsia (Hubel, 1998; Lorentzen and Henriksen, 1998; Walsh, 1998). The pathologic lesions of the decidual arterioles in pre-eclampsia ("acute atherosis") include fibrinoid necrosis of the vessel wall, aggregates of platelets, and accumulation of lipid-laden macrophages (foam cells) (DeWolf et al., 1975; Sheppard and Bonnar, 1981). The morphology of these vessels suggests parallels with the atherogenic process in which LDL lipid peroxidation with foam cell formation has a paramount role (Branch et al., 1994; Lorentzen and Henriksen, 1998). Pre-eclamptic decidual tissue has an increased content of lipid peroxides (oxidized polyunsaturated fatty acids) (Staff et al., 1999a, 1999b). Consistent with a hypothesized role for lipid peroxides, immediate postpartum curettage (removal of decidual tissue) accelerates the recovery from pre-eclampsia (Henriksen, 2000).

Can dyslipidemia during pregnancy flag later-life cardiovascular risk?

Recent data have linked maternal vascular, metabolic, and inflammatory complications of pregnancy (including gestational diabetes, pre-eclampsia, and low birthweight) with an increased risk of cardiovascular disease in later life (Hubel *et al.*, 2000; Sattar and Greer, 2002). As mentioned previously, the insulin resistance syndrome is a key factor underlying non-pregnancy cardiovascular disease. The maternal physiologic response to normal pregnancy includes a transient excursion into several aspects of this metabolic syndrome, i.e. insulin resistance, hyperlipidemia, and an increase in coagulation factors (Herrera *et al.*, 1988; Hubel *et al.*, 1998b; Martin *et al.*, 1999; Montes *et al.*, 1984; Sattar and Greer, 2002). Normal pregnancy also involves upregulation of the inflammatory cascade including activation of peripheral white blood cells (Sacks *et al.*, 1998, 1999). Upregulation of the inflammatory cascade in non-pregnant women is a strong risk factor for adverse cardiovascular events and diabetes (Ross, 1999). Several lines of evidence suggest that pregnancy represents a "stress test" of maternal carbohydrate, lipid, and inflammatory pathways, and vascular function (Agatisa *et al.*, 2004; Barden *et al.*, 1999; Hubel *et al.*, 1999; Kaaja *et al.*, 1999; Ma *et al.*, 1994; Montes *et al.*, 1984; Sattar and Greer, 2002; Wolf *et al.*, 2001). Accordingly, abnormal accentuation of these metabolic changes during pregnancy, even in women with normal pregnancy outcome, may be a harbinger of later-life cardiovascular problems.

Although glucose tolerance decreases during normal pregnancy the majority of women remain euglycemic. However, approximately 2–3% of pregnant women cannot overcome the peripheral insulin resistance and hence develop gestational diabetes (Kuhl, 1991). These women undergo a deterioration of glucose homeostasis under the stress of pregnancy but appear to revert to normal after delivery. The risk for later-life NIDDM is high in women with gestational diabetes, however, and its diagnosis during pregnancy is an important indicator of future health risk (Gregory *et al.*, 1993).

Although not well studied at this point, there are indications that a supra-physiologic rise in plasma lipids serves as a marker of "prelipemia" in the same way that gestational diabetes is a marker for prediabetes (Montes *et al.*, 1984). In women with extreme hypertriglyceridemia (>95th percentile)

during pregnancy, HDL cholesterol is concurrently abnormally low and does not revert to normal postpartum even after triglycerides return to within the 95th percentile; this suggests that extreme hypertriglyceridemia of pregnancy is a true pathophysiologic disorder. In addition, non-pregnant family members of women with supraphysiologic pregnancy triglycerides also show evidence of hyperlipidemia (Montes *et al.*, 1984). These data are consistent with an underlying prelipemic trait unmasked by the "stress-test" of pregnancy.

Several variations within the coding region of the lipoprotein lipase gene are common in the general population and are associated with alterations in lipoprotein lipase mass and activity. By decreasing lipoprotein lipase activity, these mutations promote the dyslipidemic triad of increased triglyceride, decreased HDL cholesterol, and predominance of atherogenic small dense LDL. Heterozygous lipoprotein lipase deficiency is thought to play an important role in the pathogenesis of coronary artery disease. Interestingly, heterozygous lipoprotein lipase deficiency is often insufficient to cause overt dyslipidemia in nonpregnant, premenopausal women. However, dyslipidemia is promoted by factors such as pregnancy, obesity, or diabetes, which challenge the lipolytic system by increasing hepatic secretion of VLDL. Lipoprotein lipase heterozygotes can thus become severely hypertriglyceridemic during pregnancy (Hubel *et al.*, 1999; Ma *et al.*, 1994). High triglycerides during pregnancy in these women reveal, often for the first time, a genotype known to predispose to coronary artery disease. As noted earlier, inhibitory mutations in the lipoprotein lipase gene are more prevalent in some populations of women with pre-eclampsia.

Women with an abnormal lipemic response to pregnancy but with normal pregnancy outcome may have advantages (such as superior placentation or genes favoring endothelial resistance) that protect from endothelial dysfunction in the setting of pregnancy. Further studies are needed to determine the extent to which an abnormal carbohydrate or lipoprotein response to pregnancy can "flag" women at risk of cardiovascular dysfunction after pregnancy. Identification of women who display these risk markers during or after pregnancy might allow for early interventions (i.e. exercise, antioxidants) to diminish or delay future cardiovascular morbidity and mortality (Figure 11.5).

Pre-eclampsia, later-life dyslipidemia and cardiovascular risk

Several studies have shown that an association between pre-eclampsia and later-life hypertension or ischemic heart disease is strongly supported, especially (but not only) when the hypertension in pregnancy was recurrent or developed before 30 weeks of gestation (Hannaford et al., 1997; Jonsdottir et al., 1995; Ness et al., 2003; Sattar and Greer, 2002; Sibai et al., 1986). On the other hand, there is some evidence of a decreased frequency of

adverse cardiovascular outcomes in women with a normal pregnancy history compared with the overall female population (Fisher et al., 1981). Women whose pregnancies were normal may comprise a population more representative of a healthy phenotype than the female population at large. Evaluation of women before, during and after their reproductive history is needed to clarify these associations and evaluate their mechanisms.

Women with pre-eclampsia frequently develop dyslipidemia as early as 10 weeks of gestation. This dyslipidemia peaks during late pregnancy and reverts by 6–10 weeks after delivery. To what baseline, however? Subtle dyslipidemia persists after pregnancy in non-pregnant women with prior pre-eclampsia, at least in some populations, consistent with a hypothesized contribution to adverse remote prognosis.

A retrospective comparison of 62 women with pre-eclampsia and 84 with normal pregnancy, seen antenatally and at 6 weeks and 6 months

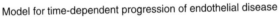

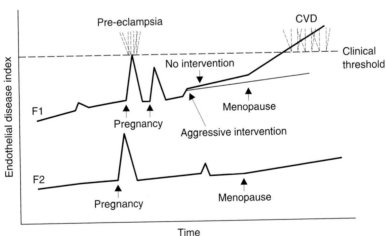

Figure 11.5 Intervention strategies against time-dependent progression of endothelial disease. F1, female 1 (high-risk); F2, female 2 (low-risk); CVD, cardiovascular disease. Genetic factors contribute to both the endothelial health baseline and the susceptibility to negative environmental factors (slope). Risk factors for endothelial disease are identifiable during the "stress-test" of pregnancy. Clinically evident disease manifests once a threshold is crossed (as is the case for F1 during first pregnancy and post-menopause). Interventions such as antioxidant vitamins or statin drugs may significantly delay progression of endothelial disease.

postpartum, revealed persistent dyslipidemia (increased triglycerides total cholesterol and LDL cholesterol), increased blood pressure, and a high prevalence of obesity in women with prior pre-eclampsia (Barden *et al.*, 1999). In this study, women with previous pre-eclampsia reported a greater incidence of family history of hypertension (65% versus 35%). Intriguingly, these authors have also reported that 8-isoprostane, an indicator of oxidative stress, is increased in pre-eclampsia and is still increased 6 weeks postpartum (Barden *et al.*, 2001).

Aberrations indicative of dyslipidemia and insulin resistance (higher fasting insulin, glucose, HOMA index of insulin resistance, triglycerides, uric acid and blood pressure) have been reported in women 6 months to 2.5 years after pre-eclamptic pregnancy (Nisell *et al.*, 1999). Another study examined women 2–5 years after pre-eclampsia, matched (by age, parity at index pregnancy, and time of delivery) to controls with prior normal index pregnancies. Plasma vWF concentrations were higher in the women with a history of pre-eclampsia, suggestive of endothelial dysfunction. Dyslipidemia was also noted, presenting as higher cholesterol, total triglycerides, and VLDL triglycerides, but only in luteal phase samples (He *et al.*, 1999). In a study of Finnish women, mild hyperinsulinemia and higher blood pressures, but no significant lipid changes (triglycerides, or total-HDL-, and LDL-cholesterol), were observed in women 17 years after pre-eclamptic pregnancy (Laivuori *et al.*, 1996).

Elevated plasma apolipoprotein B (greater than 120 mg dL^{-1}) and a decrease in mean LDL particle diameter (a combination that indicates high concentrations of atherogenic, small-sized LDL particles) confers an especially high cardiovascular risk in the general population (Lamarche and Lewis, 1998; Lamarche *et al.*, 1998). Icelandic women who had undergone a pregnancy with eclampsia (convulsions with pre-eclampsia), 50–67 years old at re-examination, show this abnormal lipid profile (Figure 11.6) (Hubel *et al.*, 2000). In this study cases and controls were individually matched for date of birth, age at pregnancy and parity. All were without evidence of pre-pregnancy disease. The percentage of cases on blood pressure medication (33%) was significantly greater than controls (6.7%). The subset of postmenopausal women with history of hypertensive complications in at least one other pregnancy in addition to the index eclamptic pregnancy (recurrent subgroup) displayed significantly increased diastolic blood pressures, and a more diverse profile of atherogenic lipids (smaller-sized LDL, increased apolipoprotien B, decreased HDL$_2$ cholesterol, and increased ratio of total cholesterol to HDL cholesterol) compared to their controls (Hubel *et al.*, 2000).

LDL isolated from women with a history of pre-eclampsia, 1–3 years postpartum, reportedly shows an increase in intrinsic susceptibility to oxidative modification upon exposure to exogenous copper compared to LDL from women with a history of normal pregnancy. LDL cholesterol and triglycerides were also increased in these postpartum women who had had the pregnancy syndrome (Gratacos *et al.*, 2003). This profile suggests increased susceptibility to oxidative stress postpartum, a state that might predispose to future cardiovascular disease.

Impairment of endothelial vasodilatory function exists years after pre-eclamptic pregnancy (Agatisa *et al.*, 2004; Chambers *et al.*, 2001). One study has shown that this impairment is reversed by intravenous administration of the supremely important antioxidant nutrient, vitamin C (ascorbic acid) (Chambers *et al.*, 2001). Multivariable analysis suggested that the impairment was not explained by the significantly increased body mass index, blood pressure, family history of hypertension or increased total cholesterol to HDL-cholesterol ratio evidenced by these women. Dyslipidemia-induced endothelial dysfunction in non-pregnant, insulin-resistant patients is reversed by vitamin C (Pleiner *et al.*, 2002). The potential benefit of antioxidants toward amelioration of dyslipidemia-mediated vascular dysfunction in the setting of

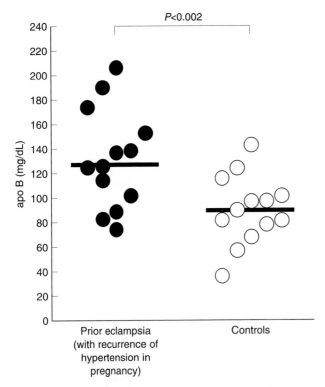

Figure 11.6 Scatterplot of serum apolipoprotein B concentrations in postmenopausal women with a history of eclampsia or history of uncomplicated pregnancies. Each symbol corresponds to a different individual. Thick horizontal bars correspond to median values for each group. $P < 0.02$ by Wilcoxon signed-rank test, postmenopausal women with prior eclampsia (with recurrence of hypertension in at least one other pregnancy) vs. postmenopausal women with a history of only normal pregnancy (matched pair design). Data redrawn from Hubel *et al.* (2000).

pregnancy, and postpartum, warrants further analysis.

As suggested by Chesley (1978), it seems unlikely that pre-eclampsia or eclampsia actually causes later-life cardiovascular disease. One might propose that a life-long (possibly inherited) predisposition to the metabolic syndrome leads to exaggerated insulin resistance and dyslipidemia during pregnancy that, in susceptible women, fosters endothelial cell dysfunction and other maternal manifestations of pre-eclampsia. This constitutional predisposition may also increase the likelihood of future cardiovascular disease. Further research is clearly needed regarding interrelationships of pregnancy history, lipids, and endothelial cell-related disease in later stages of life.

Concluding remarks

Dyslipidemia, detectable during early pregnancy and in many studies years postpartum, is a possible contributor to both the development of pre-eclampsia and future cardiovascular disease. One cannot exclude the possibility that pre-eclampsia causes postpartum problems as opposed to being caused by an underlying predisposition that preceded pregnancy. This distinction is less important, however, if dyslipidemia or other factors can identify patients at risk of future disease. Given the epidemiological association between pre-eclampsia and future cardiovascular disease, and the emerging evidence of early postpartum pathophysiology, aggressive risk factor modifications may prove to especially benefit these women (Figure 11.5).

Adipose tissue is a metabolically active endocrine and paracrine organ, and hence more than just a repository for fat. Experimentation on this tissue would undoubtedly increase our understanding of the pre-eclampsia phenotype. Abdominal fat biopsied from women with normal pregnancy exhibits an increase in basal and hormone-stimulated rates of lipolysis in vitro compared to abdominal fat from non-pregnant women (Williams and Coltart, 1978). To date, however, there has been little study of adipose tissue of women with normal, pre-eclamptic, or fetal growth-restricted pregnancy. The role of novel lipid-regulatory factors such as peroxisome proliferator-activated receptors, resistin, and adiponectin in pregnancy adaptation and pathogenesis also await evaluation. Fascinating interactions between adipogenesis and angiogenesis have been noted (Fukumura et al., 2003). Circulating endothelial progenitor cells likely contribute to ongoing endothelial maintenance and repair in the adult peripheral circulation (Hill et al., 2003). The influence of cardiovascular risk factors on these processes in the setting of pregnancy and postpartum may provide new horizons for research.

REFERENCES

Agatisa, P., Ness, R., Roberts, J., Costantino, J., Kuller, L. and McLaughlin, M. (2004). Impairment of endothelial function in women with a history of preeclampsia: an indicator of cardiovascular risk. Am. J. Physiol., 286, 1389–93.

Alvarez, J.J., Montelongo, A., Iglesias, A., Lasuncion, M.A. and Herrera, E. (1996). Longitudinal study on lipoprotein profile, high density lipoprotein subclass, and postheparin lipases during gestation in women. J. Lipid Res., 37, 299–308.

Arbogast, B.W., Leeper, S.C., Merrick, R.D., Olive, K.E. and Taylor, R.N. (1996). Plasma factors that determine endothelial cell lipid toxicity in vitro correctly identify women with preeclampsia in early and late pregnancy. Hypertens. Pregn., 15, 263–79.

Barden, A., Ritchie, J., Walters, B., et al. (2001). Study of plasma factors associated with neutrophil activation and lipid peroxidation in preeclampsia. Hypertension, 38, 803–8.

Barden, A.E., Beilin, L.J., Ritchie, J., Walters, B.N. and Michael, C. (1999). Does a predisposition to the metabolic syndrome sensitize women to develop pre-eclampsia? J. Hypertens., 17, 1307–15.

Belo, L., Caslake, M., Gaffney, D., et al. (2002). Changes in LDL size and HDL concentration in normal and preeclamptic pregnancies. Atherosclerosis, 162, 425–32.

Bilodeau, J.-F. and Hubel, C. (2003). Current concepts in the use of antioxidants for the treatment of preeclampsia. J. Obstet. Gynecol. Can., 25, 742–50.

Bonet, B., Brunzell, J.D., Gown, A.M. and Knopp, R.H. (1992). Metabolism of very-low-density lipoprotein triglyceride by human placental cells: the role of lipoprotein lipase. Metabolism, 41, 596–603.

Bourdon, E., Loreau, N. and Blache, D. (1999). Glucose and free radicals impair the antioxidant properties of serum albumin. FASEB J., 13, 233–44.

Branch, D.W., Mitchell, M.D., Miller, E., Palinski, W. and Witztum, J.L. (1994). Pre-eclampsia and serum antibodies to oxidised low-density lipoprotein. Lancet, 343, 645–6.

Catalano, P., Tyzbir, E., Roman, N., Amini, S. and Sims, E. (1991). Longitudinal changes in insulin release and insulin resistance in non-obese pregnant women. Am. J. Obstet. Gynecol., 165, 1667–72.

Chambers, J., Fusi, L., Malik, I., Haskard, D., De Swiet, M. and Kooner, J. (2001). Association of maternal endothelial dysfunction with preeclampsia. J. Am. Med. Ass., 285, 1607–12.

Chappell, L., Seed, P., Briley, A., et al. (2002). A longitudinal study of biochemical variables in women at risk of pre-eclampsia. Am. J. Obstet. Gynecol., 187, 127–36.

Chesley, L.C. (1978). Eclampsia: the remote prognosis. Semin. Perinatol., 2, 99–111.

Clausen, T., Djurovic, S. and Henriksen, T. (2001). Dyslipidemia in early second trimester is mainly a feature of women with early onset pre-eclampsia. Br. J. Obstet. Gynaecol., 108, 1081–7.

Coleman, R.A. (1989). The role of the placenta in lipid metabolism and transport. Semin. Perinatol., 13, 180–91.

Davda, R., Stepniakowski, K. T., Lu, G., Ullian, M. E., Goodfriend, T. L. and Egan, B. M. (1995). Oleic acid inhibits nitric oxide synthase by a protein kinase C-independent mechanism. *Hypertension*, **26**, 764–70.

Dewolf, F., Robertson, W. B. and Brosens, I. (1975). The ultrastructure of acute atherosis in hypertensive pregnancy. *Am. J. Obstet. Gynecol.*, **123**(2), 164–74.

Elzen, H. v. d., Waldimiroff, J., Cohen-Overbeek, T., Bruijn, A. d. and Grobbee, D. (1996). Serum lipids in early pregnancy and risk of preeclampsia. *Br. J. Obstet. Gynaecol.*, **103**, 117–22.

Endresen, M. J., Lorentzen, B. and Henriksen, T. (1992). Increased lipolytic activity and high ratio of free fatty acids to albumin in sera from women with preeclampsia leads to triglyceride accumulation in cultured endothelial cells. *Am. J. Obstet. Gynecol.*, **167**, 440–7.

Endresen, M. J., Tosti, E., Heimli, H., Lorentzen, B. and Henriksen, T. (1994). Effects of free fatty acids found increased in women who develop pre-eclampsia on the ability of endothelial cells to produce prostacyclin, cGMP and inhibit platelet aggregation. *Scand. J. Clin. Lab. Invest.*, **54**, 549–57.

Fisher, K. A., Lluger, A., Spargo, B. H. and Lindheimer, M. D. (1981). Hypertension in pregnancy: clinical–pathological correlations and remote prognosis. *Medicine*, **60**, 267–76.

Fukumura, D., Ushiyama, A., Duda, D., *et al.* (2003). Paracrine regulation of angiogenesis and adipocyte differentiation during in vivo adipogenesis. *Circ. Res.*, **93**, e88–e97.

Gardner, C. D., Fortmann, S. P. and Krauss, R. M. (1996). Association of small low-density lipoprotein particles with the incidence of coronary artery disease in men and women. *J. Am. Med. Ass.*, **276**, 875–81.

Gratacos, E., Casals, E., Sanllehy, C., Cararach, V., Alonso, P. L. and Fortuny, A. (1996). Variation in lipid levels during pregnancy in women with different types of hypertension. *Acta Obstet. Gynecol. Scand.*, **75**, 896–901.

Gratacos, E., Casals, E., Gomez, O., *et al.* (2003). Increased susceptibility to low density lipoprotein oxidation in women with a history of pre-eclampsia. *Br. J. Obstet. Gynaecol.*, **110**, 400–4.

Gregory, K., Kjos, S. and Peters, R. (1993). Cost of non-insulin-dependent diabetes in women with a history of gestational diabetes: implications for prevention. *Obstet. Gynecol.*, **81**, 782–6.

Griendling, K. K., Sorescu, D. and Ushio-Fukai, M. (2000). NAD(P)H oxidase – role in cardiovascular biology and disease. *Circ. Res.*, **86**, 494–501.

Hannaford, P., Ferry, S. and Hirsch, S. (1997). Cardiovascular sequelae of toxaemia of pregnancy. *Heart*, **77**, 154–8.

He, S., Silveira, A., Hamsten, A., Blomback, M. and Bremme, K. (1999). Haemostatic, endothelial and lipoprotein parameters and blood pressure levels in women with a history of preeclampsia. *Thromb. Haemost.*, **81**, 538–42.

Henriksen, T. (2000). The role of lipid oxidation and oxidative lipid derivatives in the development of preeclampsia. *Semin. Perinatol.*, **24**, 29–32.

Herrera, E. (2002). Lipid metabolism in pregnancy and its consequences in the fetus and newborn. *Endocrine*, **19**, 43–55.

Herrera, G., Lasuncion, M. A., Coronado, D. G., Aranda, P., Lona, P. L. and Maier, I. (1988). Role of lipoprotein lipase activity on lipoprotein metabolism and the fate of circulating triglycerides in pregnancy. *Am. J. Obstet. Gynecol.*, **158**, 1575–83.

Hill, J., Zalos, G., Hacox, J., *et al.* (2003). Circulating endothelial progenitor cells, vascular function, and cardiovascular risk. *N. Engl. J. Med.*, **348**, 593–600.

Hubel, C. (1999). Oxidative stress in the pathogenesis of preeclampsia. *Proc. Soc. Exp. Biol. Med.*, **222**, 222–35.

Hubel, C. A. (1998). Dyslipidemia, iron, and oxidative stress in preeclampsia: assessment of maternal and feto-placental interactions. *Semin. Reprod. Endocrinol.*, **16**, 75–92.

Hubel, C. A. and Roberts, J. M. (1999). Lipid metabolism and oxidative stress. In *Chesley's Hypertensive Disorders in Pregnancy*, ed. M. D. Lindheimer, J. M. Roberts and F. G. Cunningham. Stamford, CT: Appleton & Lange, pp. 453–86.

Hubel, C. A., McLaughlin, M. K., Evans, R. W., Hauth, B. A., Sims, C. J. and Roberts, J. M. (1996). Fasting serum triglycerides, free fatty acids, and malondialdehyde are increased in preeclampsia, are positively correlated, and decrease within 48 hours post partum. *Am. J. Obstet. Gynecol.*, **174**, 975–82.

Hubel, C. A., Lyall, F., Weissfeld, L., Gandley, R. E. and Roberts, J. M. (1998a). Small low-density lipoproteins and vascular cell adhesion molecule (VCAM-1) are increased in association with hyperlipidemia in pre-eclampsia. *Metabolism*, **47**, 1281–8.

Hubel, C. A., Shakir, Y., Gallaher, M. J., McLaughlin, M. K. and Roberts, J. M. (1998b). Low-density lipoprotein particle size decreases during normal pregnancy in association with triglyceride increases. *J. Soc. Gynecol. Invest.*, **5**, 244–50.

Hubel, C.A., Roberts, J.M. and Ferrell, R.E. (1999). Association of pre-eclampsia with common coding sequence variations in the lipoprotein lipase gene. *Clin. Genet.*, **56**, 289–96.

Hubel, C.A., Snaedal, S., Ness, R.B., *et al.* (2000). Dyslipoproteinemia in postmenopausal women with a history of eclampsia. *Br. J. Obstet. Gynaecol.*, **107**, 776–84.

Jonsdottir, L.S., Arngrimsson, R., Geirsson, R.T., Sigvaldason, H. and Sigfusson, N. (1995). Death rates from ischemic heart disease in women with a history of hypertension in pregnancy. *Acta Obstet. Gynecol. Scand.*, **74**, 772–6.

Kaaja, R. (1998). Insulin resistance syndrome in pre-eclampsia. *Semin. Reprod. Endocrinol.*, **16**, 41–6.

Kaaja, R., Tikkanen, M.J., Viinikka, L. and Ylikorkala, O. (1995). Serum lipoproteins, insulin, and urinary prostanoid metabolites in normal and hypertensive pregnant women. *Obstet. Gynecol.*, **85**, 353–6.

Kaaja, R., Laivuori, H., Laakso, M., Tikkanen, M.J. and Ylikorkala, O. (1999). Evidence of a state of increased insulin resistance in preeclampsia. *Metabolism*, **48**, 892–6.

Kagan, V., Tyurin, V., Borisenko, G., *et al.* (2001). Mishandling of copper by albumin: role in redox-cycling and oxidative stress in preeclampsia plasma. *Hypertens. Pregn.*, **20**, 221–42.

Kahn, B.B. and Flier, J.S. (2000). Obesity and insulin resistance. *J. Clin. Invest.*, **106**, 473–81.

Kim, Y.J., Williamson, R.A., Chen, K., Smith, J.L., Murray, J.C. and Merrill, D.C. (2001). Lipoprotein lipase gene mutations and the genetic susceptibility of preeclampsia. *Hypertension*, **38**, 992–6.

Kirwan, J., Hauguel-Demouzon, S., Leqercq, J., *et al.* (2002). TNFα is a predictor of insulin resistance in human pregnancy. *Diabetes*, **51**, 2207–13.

Krauss, R.M. (1991). The tangled web of coronary risk factors. *Am. J. Med.*, **90**, 2a–36s.

Krauss, R.M. (1997). Genetic, metabolic, and dietary influences on the atherogenic lipoprotein phenotype. In *Genetic Variation and Dietary Response. World Rev. Nutr. Diet*, vol. **80**, ed. A.P. Simopoulos and P.J. Nestel. Basel: Karger, pp. 2–43.

Kuhl, C. (1991). Insulin secretion and insulin resistance in pregnancy and GDM. Implications for diagnosis and management. *Diabetes*, **40**, 18–24.

Laivuori, H., Tikkanen, M.J. and Ylikorkala, O. (1996). Hyperinsulinemia 17 years after preeclamptic first pregnancy. *J. Clin. Endocrinol. Metab.*, **81**, 2908–11.

Lamarche, B. and Lewis, G. (1998). Atherosclerosis prevention for the next decade: risk assessment beyond low density lipoprotein cholesterol. *Can. J. Cardiol.*, **14**, 841–51.

Lamarche, B., Tchernof, A., Moorjani, S., *et al.* (1997). Small, dense low-density lipoprotein particles as a predictor of the risk of ischemic heart disease in men. *Circulation*, **95**, 69–75.

Lamarche, B., Tchernof, A., Mauriege, P., *et al.* (1998). Fasting insulin and apolipoprotein B levels and low-density lipoprotein particle size as risk factors for ischemic heart disease. *J. Am. Med. Ass.*, **279**, 1955–61.

Lamarche, B., Rashid, S. and Lewis, G.F. (1999). HDL metabolism in hypertriglyceridemic states: an overview. *Clin. Chim. Acta*, **286**, 145–61.

Lewis, G.F. and Steiner, G. (1996). Hypertriglyceridemia and its metabolic consequences as a risk factor for atherosclerotic cardiovascular disease in non-insulin-dependent diabetes mellitus. *Diabetes Metab. Rev.*, **12**, 37–56.

Lorentzen, B. and Henriksen, T. (1998). Plasma lipids and vascular dysfunction in preeclampsia. *Semin. Reprod. Endocrinol.*, **16**, 33–9.

Lorentzen, B., Endresen, M.J., Clausen, T. and Henriksen, T. (1994). Fasting serum free fatty acids and triglycerides are increased before 20 weeks of gestation in women who later develop preeclampsia. *Hypertens. Pregn.*, **13**, 103–9.

Lorentzen, B., Drevon, C.A., Endressen, M.J. and Henriksen, T. (1995). Fatty acid pattern of esterfied and free fatty acids in sera of women with normal and pre-eclamptic pregnancy. *Br. J. Obstet. Gynaecol.*, **102**, 530–7.

Lorentzen, B., Birkeland, K.I., Endresen, M.J. and Henriksen, T. (1998). Glucose intolerance in women with preeclampsia. *Acta Obstet. Gynecol. Scand.*, **77**, 22–7.

Ma, Y., Ooi, T.C., Liu, M.S., *et al.* (1994). High frequency of mutations in the human lipoprotein lipase gene in pregnancy-induced chylomicronemia: possible association with apolipoprotein E2 isoform. *J. Lipid. Res.*, **35**, 1066–75.

Martin, U., Davies, C., Hayavi, S., Hartland, A. and Dunne, F. (1999). Is normal pregnancy atherogenic? *Clin. Sci.*, **96**, 421–5.

Montelongo, A., Lasuncion, M.A., Pallardo, L.F. and Herrera, E. (1992). Longitudinal study of plasma lipoproteins and hormones during pregnancy in normal and diabetic women. *Diabetes*, **41**, 1651–9.

Montes, A., Walden, C. E., Knopp, R. H., Cheung, M., Chapman, M. B. and Albers, J. J. (1984). Physiologic and supraphysiologic increases in lipoprotein lipids and apoproteins in late pregnancy and postpartum. Possible markers for the diagnosis of "prelipemia". *Arteriosclerosis*, **4**, 407–17.

Murai, J. T., Muzykanskiy, E. and Taylor, R. N. (1997). Maternal and fetal modulators of lipid metabolism correlate with the development of preeclampsia. *Metabolism*, **46**, 963–7.

Murata, M., Kodama, H., Goto, K., Hirano, H. and Tanaka, T. (1996). Decreased very-low-density lipoprotein and low-density lipoprotein receptor messenger ribonucleic acid expression in placentas from preeclamptic pregnancies. *Am. J. Obstet. Gynecol.*, **175**, 1551–6.

Ness, R. B. and Roberts, J. M. (1996). Heterogeneous causes constituting the single syndrome of preeclampsia: a hypothesis and its implications. *Am. J. Obstet. Gynecol.*, **175**, 1365–70.

Ness, R., Markovic, N., Bass, D., Harger, G. and Roberts, J. (2003). Family history of hypertension, heart disease, and stroke among women who develop hypertension in pregnancy. *Obstet. Gynecol.*, **102**, 1366–71.

Nisell, H., Erikssen, C., Persson, B. and Carlstrom, K. (1999). Is carbohydrate metabolism altered among women who have undergone a preeclamptic pregnancy? *Gynecol. Obstet. Invest.*, **48**, 241–6.

O'Brien, S. F. O., Watts, G. F., Playford, D. A., Burke, V., O'Neal, D. N. and Best, J. D. (1997). Low-density lipoprotein size, high density lipoprotein-concentration, and endothelial dysfunction in non-insulin-dependent diabetes. *Diabetic Med.*, **14**, 974–8.

Ogura, K., Miyatake, T., Fukui, O., Nakamura, T., Kameda, T. and Yoshino, G. (2002). Low-density lipoprotein particle diameter in normal pregnancy and preeclampsia. *J. Atheroscler. Thromb.*, **9**, 42–7.

Pleiner, J., Schaller, G., Mittermayer, F., Bayerle-Eder, M., Roden, M. and Wolzt, M. (2002). FFA-induced endothelial dysfunction can be corrected by vitamin C. *J. Clin. Endocrinol. Metab.*, **87**, 2913–17.

Plotnick, G. D., Corretti, M. C. and Vogel, R. A. (1997). Effect of antioxidant vitamins on the transient impairment of endothelium-dependent brachial artery vasoactivity following a single high-fat meal. *J. Am. Med. Ass.*, **278**, 1682–6.

Potter, J. M. and Nestle, P. J. (1979). The hyperlipidemia of pregnancy in normal and complicated pregnancies. *Am. J. Obstet. Gynecol.*, **133**, 165–70.

Ramirez, R. J., Novak, J., Johnston, T. P., Gandley, R. E., McLaughlin, M. K. and Hubel, C. A. (2001). Endothelial function and myogenic reactivity in small mesenteric arteries of hyperlipidemic pregnant rats. *Am. J. Physiol.*, **281**, R1330–7.

Reaven, G. M. (1994). Syndrome X: 6 years later. *J. Internal. Med.*, **236**, 13–22.

Redman, C. W. G., Sacks, G. P. and Sargent, I. L. (1999). Preeclampsia: an excessive maternal inflammatory response to pregnancy. *Am. J. Obstet. Gynecol.*, **180**, 499–506.

Roberts, J. M. and Hubel, C. A. (1999). Is oxidative stress the link in the two-stage model of pre-eclampsia? *Lancet*, **354**, 788–9.

Ross, R. (1999). Atherosclerosis – an inflammatory disease. *N. Engl. J. Med.*, **340**, 115–26.

Sacks, G. P., Studena, K., Sargent, I. I. and Redman, C. W. G. (1998). Normal pregnancy and preeclampsia both produce inflammatory changes in peripheral blood leukocytes akin to those of sepsis. *Am. J. Obstet. Gynecol.*, **179**, 80–6.

Sacks, G., Sargent, I. and Redman, C. (1999). An innate view of human pregnancy. *Immunol. Today*, **20**, 114–18.

Sattar, N. and Greer, I. A. (2002). Pregnancy complications and maternal cardiovascular risk: opportunities for intervention and screening? *Br. Med. J.*, **325**, 157–60.

Sattar, N., Bedomir, A., Berry, C., Shepherd, J., Greer, I. A. and Packard, C. J. (1997a). Lipoprotein subfraction concentrations in preeclampsia: pathogenic parallels to atherosclerosis. *Obstet. Gynecol.*, **89**, 403–8.

Sattar, N., Greer, I. A., Louden, J., Lindsay, G., McConnell, M., Shepherd, J. and Packard, C. J. (1997b). Lipoprotein subfraction changes in normal pregnancy: threshold effect of plasma triglyceride on appearance of small, dense low density lipoprotein. *J. Clin. Endocrinol. Metab.*, **82**, 2483–91.

Sattar, N., Petrie, J. R. and Jaap, A. J. (1998). The atherogenic lipoprotein phenotype and vascular endothelial dysfunction. *Atherosclerosis*, **138**, 229–35.

Sattar, N., Greer, I. A., Galloway, P. J., *et al.* (1999). Lipid and lipoprotein concentrations in pregnancies complicated by intrauterine growth restriction. *J. Clin. Endocrinol. Metab.*, **84**, 128–30.

Sheppard, B. L. and Bonnar, J. (1981). An ultrastructural study of utero-placental spiral arteries in hypertensive and normotensive pregnancy and fetal growth retardation. *Br. J. Obstet. Gynaecol.*, **88**, 695–705.

Sibai, B., El-Nazer, A. and Gonzalez-Ruiz, A. (1986). Severe preeclampsia–eclampsia in young primigravid women: subsequent pregnancy outcome and remote prognosis. *Am. J. Obstet. Gynecol.*, **155**, 1011–16.

Sibai, B.M., Ewell, M., Levine, R.J., *et al.* (1997). Risk factors associated with preeclampsia in healthy nulliparous women. The Calcium for Preeclampsia Prevention (CPEP) Study Group. *Am. J. Obstet. Gynecol.*, **177**, 1003–10.

Silliman, K., Shore, V. and Forte, T.M. (1994). Hypertriglyceridemia during late pregnancy is associated with the formation of small dense low-density lipoproteins and the presence of large buoyant high-density lipoproteins. *Metabolism*, **43**, 1035–41.

Sivan, E., Homko, C.J., Whittaker, P.G., Reece, E.A., Chen, X. and Boden, G. (1998). Free fatty acids and insulin resistance during pregnancy. *J. Clin. Endocrinol. Metab.*, **83**, 2338–42.

Solomon, C., Carroll, J., Okamura, K., Graves, S. and Seeley, E. (1999). Higher cholesterol and insulin levels in pregnancy are associated with increased risk for pregnancy-induced hypertension. *Am. J. Hypertens.*, **12**, 276–82.

Solomon, C.G., Graves, S.W., Greene, M.F. and Seely, E.W. (1994). Glucose intolerance as a predictor of hypertension in pregnancy. *Hypertension*, **23**, 717–21.

Sowers, J.R., Saleh, A.A. and Sokol, R.J. (1995). Hyperinsulinemia and insulin resistance are associated with preeclampsia in African-Americans. *Am. J. Hypertens.*, **8**, 1–4.

Staff, A.C., Halvorsen, B., Ranheim, T. and Henriksen, T. (1999a). Free 8-iso-prostaglandin F2α is elevated in decidua basalis in women with preeclampsia. *Am. J. Obstet. Gynecol.*, **181**, 1211–15.

Staff, A.C., Ranheim, T., Khoury, J. and Henriksen, T. (1999b). Increased contents of phospholipids, cholesterol, and lipid peroxides in decidua basalis in women with preeclampsia. *Am. J. Obstet. Gynecol.*, **180**, 587–92.

Stampfer, M.J., Krauss, R.M., Ma, J., *et al.* (1996). A prospective study of triglyceride level, low-density lipoprotein particle diameter, and risk of myocardial infarction. *J. Am. Med. Ass.*, **276**, 882–8.

Steinberg, H.O., Chaker, H., Leaming, R., Johnson, A., Brechtel, G. and Baron, A.D. (1996). Obesity/insulin resistance is associated with endothelial dysfunction. *J. Clin. Invest.*, **97**, 2601–10.

Steinberg, H.O., Paradisi, G., Hook, G., Crowder, K., Cronin, J. and Baron, A.D. (2000). Free fatty acid elevation impairs insulin-mediated vasodilation and nitric oxide production. *Diabetes*, **49**, 1231–8.

Steinberg, H.O., Tarshoby, M., Monestel, R., *et al.* (1997). Elevated circulating free fatty acid levels impair endothelium-dependent vasodilation. *J. Clin. Invest.*, **100**, 1230–9.

Vigne, J.L., Murai, J.T., Arbogast, B.W., Jia, W., Fisher, S.J. and Taylor, R.N. (1997). Elevated nonesterified fatty acid concentrations in severe preeclampsia shift the isoelectric characteristics of plasma albumin. *J. Clin. Endocrinol. Metab.*, **82**, 3786–92.

Vogel, R.A., Corretti, M.C. and Plotnick, G.D. (1997). Effect of a single high-fat meal on endothelial function in healthy subjects. *Am. J. Cardiol.*, **79**, 350–4.

Wakatsuki, A., Ikenoue, N., Okatani, Y., Shinohara, K. and Fukaya, T. (2000). Lipoprotein particles in preeclampsia: susceptibility to oxidative modification. *Obstet. Gynecol.*, **96**, 55–9.

Walsh, S.W. (1998). Maternal–placental interactions of oxidative stress and antioxidants in preeclampsia. *Semin. Reprod. Endocrinol.*, **16**, 93–104.

Williams, C. and Coltart, T.M. (1978). Adipose tissue metabolism in pregnancy: the lipolytic effect of human placental lactogen. *Br. J. Obstet. Gynaecol.*, **85**, 43–6.

Williams, M., Zingheim, R., King, I. and Zebelman, A. (1995). Omega-3 fatty acids in maternal erythrocytes and risk of preeclampsia. *Epidemiology*, **6**, 232–7.

Winkler, K., Wetzka, B., Hoffmann, M.M., *et al.* (2000). Low density lipoprotein (LDL) subfractions during pregnancy: accumulation of buoyant LDL with advancing gestation. *J. Clin. Endocrinol. Metab.*, **85**, 4543–50.

Winkler, K., Wetzka, B., Hoffmann, M.M., *et al.* (2003). Triglyceride-rich lipoproteins are associated with hypertension in preeclampsia. *J. Clin. Endocrinol. Metab.*, **88**, 1162–6.

Wittmaack, F., Gafvels, M., Bronner, M., *et al.* (1995). Localization and regulation of the human very low density lipoprotein/apolipoprotein-E receptor: trophoblast expression predicts a role for the receptor in placental lipid transport. *Endocrinology*, **136**, 340–8.

Wolf, M., Kettyle, E., Sandler, L., Ecker, J.L., Roberts, J. and Thadhani, R. (2001). Obesity and preeclampsia: the potential role of inflammation. *Obstet. Gynecol.*, **98**, 757–62.

Wolf, M., Sandler, L., Munoz, K., Hsu, K., Ecker, J. and Thadhani, R. (2002). First trimester insulin resistance and subsequent preeclampsia: a prospective study. *J. Clin. Endocrinol. Metab.*, **87**, 1563–8.

Yuan, H., Antholine, W. E., Subczynski, W. K. and Green, M. A. (1996). Release of CuPTSM from human serum albumin after addition of fatty acids. *J. Inorg. Biochem.*, **61**, 251–9.

Zhang, C., Austin, M., Edwards, K., *et al.* (2006). Functional variants of the lipoprotein lipase gene and the risk of preeclampsia among non-Hispanic Caucasian women. *Clin. Genet.*, **69**, 33–9.

12

Pre-eclampsia a two-stage disorder: what is the linkage? Are there directed fetal/placental signals?

Jim Roberts

Introduction

Several years ago Chris Redman formalized the concept that pre-eclampsia could be best thought of as a two-stage disorder (Redman, 1991) (Figure 12.1). The first stage was reduced placental perfusion and the second stage the maternal syndrome. This model emphasizes that, although the placenta is the important component causing pre-eclampsia and that reduced placental perfusion, the relevant insult, there was clearly more to pre-eclampsia than simply reduced placental perfusion. Somehow the reduction of oxygen and/or nutrients to the placenta results in a multisystemic maternal syndrome. Furthermore, not all pregnancies with reduced placental perfusion result in pre-eclampsia. Elucidating the process of implantation, which is frequently the origin of reduced placental perfusion, and increasing knowledge of the proximate pathophysiological changes of the maternal syndrome are vital to the

understanding of pre-eclampsia. Determining how these two stages are linked will provide special insight especially relevant to disease management. In this presentation we will provide an overview of the two-stage model, discuss maternal interactions with reduced placental perfusion and address potential linkages. We will give special attention to the possibility that the linkage of the two stages involves directed fetal placental signals. The implications of these concepts will be addressed.

Stage 1

Almost 60 years ago Ernest Page formalized the concept that reduced placental perfusion is the important initiating cause of pre-eclampsia (Page, 1939). One line of evidence supporting this was the failed vascular modeling of the maternal vessels supplying the intervillus space that was present in women with pre-eclampsia (Pijnenborg *et al.*, 1991;

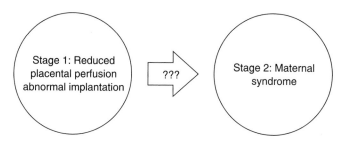

Figure 12.1 Two-stage model of pre-eclampsia: pre-eclampsia is posited to be initiated by reduced fetal/placental perfusion. Reduced perfusion is linked by the production of a placental product (unknown) to the maternal syndrome of pre-eclampsia.

Brosens *et al.*, 1979). In pre-eclamptic women these vessels do not increase in diameter nor do they lose their vascular smooth muscle, as is characteristic of normal implantation. Since blood flow increases in proportion to the fourth power of the radius, intervillus blood flow is reduced enormously. Also, while in normal pregnancy spiral artery remodeling of the smooth muscle of the vessels is lost, in pre-eclampsia this does not take place, thereby rendering these vessels potentially responsive to vasoconstrictors.

Further evidence for reduced perfusion comes from medical conditions that predispose to pre-eclampsia such as hypertension and diabetes. These and several other medical conditions that increase the risk of pre-eclampsia are known to manifest microvascular disease and could therefore reduce uterine and subsequently placental perfusion (Roberts, 1998b). Obstetrical conditions with large placentas also predispose to pre-eclampsia (Page, 1939). This is proposed to result in "relative placental hypoperfusion", as it would not be possible for even a normal intervillus blood supply to adequately perfuse this increased placental mass. Additional support comes from animal experiments in which several strategies to decrease blood flow to the placenta result in a pre-eclampsia-like syndrome (Roberts, 1998b). In addition, assessment of intervillus blood flow, either by direct wash out studies (Roberts, 1998b) or more recently by uterine artery Doppler velocimetry, supports reduced flow (Papageorghiou *et al.*, 2002).

Stage 2

Although pre-eclampsia is diagnosed by increased blood pressure and proteinuria, it is a complex multiorgan syndrome of reduced organ blood flow and striking metabolic modification (Roberts and Lain, 2002). This reduced organ blood flow is secondary to vasoconstriction, activation of the coagulation cascade, presumably with microthrombae and reduced intravascular volume. The reduced intravascular volume is at least partially explained by leakage of fluid from the intravascular compartment. The vasoconstriction is likely primarily due to increased vascular sensitivity to pressor agents (Chesley, 1966).

This constellation of findings suggests that endothelial activation might be a central pathophysiological feature with altered endothelial function increasing pressor sensitively, activating the coagulation cascade, and leading to loss of fluid from the intravascular space (Roberts *et al.*, 1989). This hypothesis has been extensively supported over the last decade (Roberts, 1998a). Women with pre-eclampsia have increased markers of endothelial activation in their circulation, while vessels from these women manifest altered endothelial function ex vivo. Furthermore, women who have had pre-eclampsia manifest blunted endothelial mediated vasodilatation years after a pre-eclamptic pregnancy (Chambers *et al.*, 2001). The concept of increased endothelial activation in pre-eclampsia has been extended to suggest that the endothelial dysfunction is only one of a constellation of changes brought about by excessive activation of inflammatory responses in the syndrome (Redman *et al.*, 1999). These ideas have redirected the study of pre-eclampsia from attempting to understand almost exclusively factors that altered blood pressure to a more generalized assessment of agents that can alter endothelial function and/or activate inflammatory responses.

It is important to point out that the increased inflammatory response/endothelial activation with subsequent vasoconstriction and reduced blood flow to systemic organs also decreases uterine blood flow with subsequent further reduction of placental blood flow. This model predicts pre-eclampsia as including a feed forward loop, which is quite consistent with the natural history. Pre-eclampsia, once manifest, never abates; once the clinical condition begins to worsen the progression may be extremely rapid.

The vascular changes of pre-eclampsia are accompanied by profound metabolic changes (Roberts and Lain, 2002). These consist largely of the changes of the metabolic syndrome.

Thus, increased insulin resistance, LDL cholesterol, triglycerides, uric acid, and reduced HDL cholesterol are all present in pre-eclampsia. These have suggested a similarity between pre-eclampsia and later-life atherosclerosis (Roberts and Lain, 2002). Leptin and sympathetic output that increase fat mobilization are also increased in women with pre-eclampsia. As with the physiological changes, many of these differences can be demonstrated in very early pregnancy and can be detected years postpartum (Hubel *et al.*, 1998; Laivuori *et al.*, 1996, 1998, 2000; Lorentzen *et al.*, 1994). Several of these alterations could be secondary to increased activation of the inflammatory response. Interestingly, these metabolic modifications all increase potential nutrient availability for the fetus.

Maternal fetal interactions in pre-eclampsia

Although reduced placental perfusion may be necessary, it is certainly not sufficient to invariably result in stage 2 of pre-eclampsia. Reduced uterine perfusion also accompanies intrauterine growth restriction (IUGR) not associated with infection or chromosomal anomalies. Despite the reduced perfusion, most women with IUGR infants do not manifest the maternal syndrome of pre-eclampsia. Perhaps the most compelling evidence that reduced placental perfusion does not invariably result in pre-eclampsia is the observation that the failed remodeling of the placental bed vascular characteristic of pre-eclampsia is also present in pregnancies complicated by IUGR (Khong *et al.*, 1986), and in one-third of pregnancies delivering preterm (Arias *et al.*, 1993). These facts have led to the suggestion that stage 2 of pre-eclampsia may also require maternal susceptibilities. These differences in "maternal constitution" result in increased sensitivity of the mother to the consequences of reduced placental perfusion. The maternal constitution is the genetic, behavioral and environmental set that the mother brings into pregnancy. Thus, it includes not only genetic polymorphisms and behavioral

factors such as obesity but also diet, toxin exposures and perhaps even pre-existing infection.

Maternal factors predisposing to pre-eclampsia are strikingly similar to those that increase the risk for cardiovascular disease in later life. This has been reviewed by Sattar and Greer (2002). Obesity, hypertension, dyslipidemia, abnormal endothelial function, diabetes, and hyperhomocysteinemia contribute to both disorders. Pre-eclampsia and atherosclerosis manifest increased evidence of inflammation, endothelial dysfunction and oxidative stress. An intriguing observation is that whereas these insults result in endothelial dysfunction and the maternal syndrome, pre-eclampsia, during pregnancy, the pathophysiological changes of pre-eclampsia abate with delivery despite the persistence of the insult. Decades must ensue before this insult results in the endothelial dysfunction of atherosclerosis. This suggests that there is enhanced endothelial sensitivity to these insults during pregnancy.

The hypothesis of maternal fetal/placental interactions, which is illustrated in Figure 12.2, has several implications. First, the maternal constitution may, as discussed above, directly affect placental blood flow either by vascular effects or by microthrombae secondary to thrombophilias occluding intervillus blood flow. However, maternal factors also contribute to the syndrome by interacting with the consequences of reduced placental blood flow to increase inflammatory response and endothelial dysfunction. As discussed, the effects of the maternal constitution can be amplified by pregnancy specific changes. These include not only the well-recognized physiological and metabolic changes of pregnancy, but also the increased inflammatory activation during pregnancy that might, for example, render endothelial cells more sensitive to injury. It is also evident that the particular maternal predisposition or combinations of predispositions is not the same in all women. This is exceptionally well illustrated by studies of candidate genes as indicators of susceptibility to pre-eclampsia. Angiotensinogen polymorphisms are associated with pre-eclampsia in

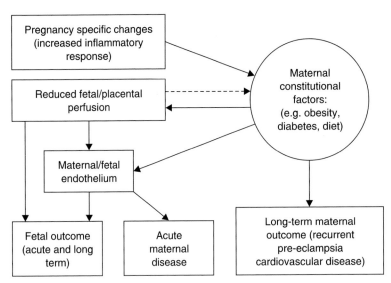

Figure 12.2 Maternal fetal placental interactions in the genesis of pre-eclampsia. This model proposes that reduced placental perfusion is not adequate for the development of pre-eclampsia. The reduction in placental perfusion interacts with maternal constitutional factors to result in acute maternal disease and to contribute to fetal disease. The maternal constitutional factors are those that predispose to maternal disease in later life while the reduced placental perfusion may result in fetal disease. Quite importantly, the maternal factors that the woman brings to the pregnancy are modified by pregnancy-specific physiological changes and of these, the inflammatory response is of paramount importance. Maternal thrombophilias with consequent microthrombae, and pre-existing vascular disease may further reduce placental perfusion. The dotted line suggests that the materials produced by the placenta in response to reduced placental perfusion may include directed fetal signals that further modify maternal physiology and metabolism.

Utah (Ward *et al.*, 1993) and Japan (Kobashi *et al.*, 1999), but not England (Morgan *et al.*, 1995), China (Bai *et al.*, 2002), Australia (Guo *et al.*, 1997), or in Hispanic Americans (Bashford *et al.*, 2001). A similar discrepancy is also evident for other genetic polymorphisms suggested as relevant to pre-eclampsia (Roberts and Cooper, 2001).

Another implication is that reduced placental perfusion and the maternal constitution can contribute different "proportions" of the insult in different women. Thus, in some women the major contribution is the reduced placental perfusion that could, for example, be severe enough that almost all women would develop the maternal syndrome. Alternatively, a particular woman could be so sensitive to the insult that minimally reduced perfusion would result in stage 2. An open question is whether this maternal sensitivity could be great

enough that even normal placental perfusion would result in pre-eclampsia. That is, reduced placental perfusion is not only insufficient to cause the maternal syndrome, but in some cases it may not be necessary.

Linkage of stage 1 and stage 2

An extremely important question is how reduced perfusion results in the maternal syndrome, pre-eclampsia. What is the stimulus engendered by reduced placental perfusion and what is the linkage? Placental and/or fetal hypoxia has been the usual candidate stimulus. Recent information indicating that nutrients such as amino acids can influence intestinal protein synthesis raises the interesting possibility that nutrients other than

Table 12.1. Evidence of oxidative stress in pre-eclampsia

Circulating markers
  Nonlipid
    Antibodies to LDL (Uotila *et al.*, 1998)
    Ascorbate oxidizing activity (Hubel *et al.*, 1997)
    Increased nitrosothiols (Tyurin *et al.*, 2001)
  Lipid markers
    Lipid oxidation products (Hubel and Roberts, 1999)
    Antibodies to oxidized LDL (Uotila *et al.*, 1998)
In maternal tissues
  Increased nitrotyrosine residues in blood vessels (Roggensack *et al.*, 1999)
  Activated neutrophils and monocytes (von Dadelszen *et al.*, 1999)
In decidua
  Atherosis with lipid-laden macrophages (Zeek and Assali, 1950)
  Increased lipid peroxides (Staff *et al.*, 1999b)
  Increased isoprostanes (8-iso-PGF2alpha) (Staff *et al.*, 1999a)
  Protein carbonyls (Zusterzeel *et al.*, 2001)
In placenta
  Non-lipid markers
    Increased xanthine oxidase in invading trophoblast cells (Many *et al.*, 2000)
    Increased nitrotyrosine resides in fetal blood vessel (Myatt *et al.*, 1996)
  Antioxidants
    Reduced superoxide dismutase (Many *et al.*, 2000; Wang and Walsh, 2001)
    Reduced glutathione peroxidase (Walsh and Wang, 1993)
  Lipid markers
    Increased malondialdehyde (Cester *et al.*, 1994)
    Increased lipid peroxides (Wang *et al.*, 1992)
    Protein carbonyls (Zusterzeel *et al.*, 2001)
    Increased isoprostane (8-iso-PGF2alpha) (Walsh *et al.*, 2000)

oxygen could also generate fetal/placental signals (Meijer, 2003).

Whatever the stimulus, a fetal/placental signal must result that alters maternal systemic response. There are several consequences of hypoxia with the potential to transport information from the placenta to the systemic circulation. Cytokines such as TNF alpha can be induced by hypoxia and released into the circulation to increase systemic inflammatory responses and induce endothelial dysfunction (Benyo *et al.*, 1997; Conrad and Benyo, 1997). Placental apoptosis (Ishihara *et al.*, 2002) and syncytiotrophoblast necrosis (Huppertz *et al.*, 2003) are increased in pre-eclampsia and lead to increased shedding of syncytiotrophoblast microparticles. There is

evidence that these microparticles are increased in the blood of women with pre-eclampsia, and further evidence that these microparticles can, at least in vitro, alter endothelial function and activate inflammatory cells (Redman and Sargent, 2000). Recently, the endogenous antagonist of VEGF and PlGF, s-Flt, has been proposed as a linkage (Maynard *et al.*, 2003).

A unifying hypothesis is that oxidative stress is the ultimate signal (Roberts and Hubel, 1999). There is abundant evidence for increased systemic oxidative stress in women with pre-eclampsia (Table 12.1). Lipid and protein markers of oxidative stress are increased in blood and maternal tissues of women with pre-eclampsia. There is also evidence of oxidative stress at the maternal–fetal interface. Increased interaction of superoxide and nitric oxide resulting in the formation of the free radical, peroxynitrite, is indicated by increased nitrotyrosine staining in the placenta (Myatt et al., 1996). In addition, isoprostanes, lipid markers of oxidative stress, are increased in the placenta (Walsh et al., 2000) and decidual tissues (Staff et al., 1999a) of women with pre-eclampsia. Furthermore, the enzyme activity of xanthine oxidase is increased in the cytotrophoblast of women with pre-eclampsia (Many et al., 2000). This enzyme generates the reactive oxygen species, superoxide, and uric acid. Oxidative stress in the placenta can lead to the formation of stable oxidation products such as malondialdehyde or isoprostanes that could interact with endothelium systemically. In addition, there is evidence of activation of circulating blood products in pre-eclampsia. Neutrophils and monocytes could be activated by the oxidative stress as they pass through the intervillus space and subsequently interact with endothelium and release reactive oxygen species (von Dadelszen et al., 1999). It is also possible that the apoptosis, leading to microvillus particle shedding, the increased synthesis of placental s-Flt and increased placental cytokines are secondary to increased oxidative stress. In addition, activated neutrophils and monocytes interact with vascular endothelium to release reactive oxygen species. It is likely that microvillus particles generated in a setting of increased oxidative stress contain oxidized lipids that can interact with endothelial cell membranes to oxidize lipids, and proteins.

Another intriguing possibility is that uric acid, long known to be increased in pre-eclampsia, is more than a consequence of disease. There is, for example, evidence that adverse outcomes increase with increasing uric acid. Infant death (Redman et al., 1976), eclampsia (Wakwe and Abudu, 1999), frequency of intrauterine growth restriction (D'Anna et al., 2000) and time to resolution post-partum (Ferrazzani et al., 1994) all correlate with increasing uric acid. Recent information indicates that uric acid itself may increase blood pressure in

animal experiments (Mazzali et al., 2001). The role of placental uric acid produced by xanthine oxidase as a response to reduced placental perfusion as the linkage of stage 1 and stage 2 of pre-eclampsia deserves further attention.

Directed fetal placental signals and fetal/placental maternal interactions

Recently we have been testing the hypothesis that the fetal/placental signals in pre-eclampsia may not merely be "toxic side effects" but rather a directed fetal response to reduced placental perfusion. This hypothesis proposes that the poorly perfused placenta generates signals that attempt to overcome the reduced fetal/placental nutrient availability. These signals function to modify maternal metabolism and physiology in a manner that increases nutrient availability. We further posited that the signal(s) may also modify placental transport to increase nutrient availability. An extension of this hypothesis is that some women because of their constitution cannot tolerate these changes and pre-eclampsia results (Figure 12.3).

The hypothesis is consistent with the heritability of pre-eclampsia. The survival value of the condition is not the pre-eclampsia but the directed fetal/placental signal(s) that increases fetal nutrient availability (and in women with constitutional risk factors, pre-eclampsia). It could also explain why abnormal vascular remodeling is present in the vast majority of placental bed biopsies of pre-eclamptic women but growth restriction in only 30%. Furthermore, it is consistent with the excess of large for gestational age infants in women with pre-eclampsia delivered after 37 weeks gestational age (Xiong et al., 2000).

It is also possible that the reduced nutrient availability resulting in the putative fetal/placental signal is mediated not solely by reduced placental perfusion but also by reduced maternal stores or reduced intake of appropriate nutrients. This could explain why the role of maternal nutrition, long suspected as having a role in growth restriction,

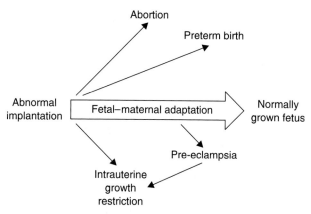

Figure 12.3 Fetal maternal adaptation to reduced placental perfusion: reduced placental perfusion may result in abortion, preterm birth pre-eclampsia or growth restriction. This model posits another possibility, that there are fetal–maternal adaptive responses that result in normally grown fetuses and that the relationship to pre-eclampsia is not direct. The model proposes that an appropriate response to reduced placental perfusion is the generation of fetal/placental signals that modify maternal metabolism and physiology to increase nutrient delivery to the poorly perfused placenta. Some women cannot tolerate the response and pre-eclampsia is the result. In two-thirds of women with pre-eclampsia this does not result in intrauterine growth restriction, but in one-third of the cases, either because of profoundly reduced perfusion that cannot be overcome by the fetal signal or with maternal adverse physiological responses further reducing perfusion, growth restriction results. The model also posits intrauterine growth restriction in the absence of pre-eclampsia as a failure of production of the putative fetal/placental signal. It further predicts normally grown infants despite reduced placental perfusion.

has been so difficult to establish. The reduced nutrient intake could be countered by fetal/placental signals that in rare women would result in pre-eclampsia.

This hypothesis predicts that there will be women with reduced fetal/placental nutrient availability who, because of the fetal/placental signal which they are able to tolerate, have normally grown infants. This concept is supported by findings that 10% of women with normally grown infants will have abnormal uterine artery Dopplers at term accompanied by failed vascular bed remodeling on placental bed biopsy (Aardema et al., 2001). Also it is consistent with the observation that 50% of women with abnormal uterine artery Dopplers in early pregnancy will have normal pregnancy outcomes despite evidence of oxidative stress in many of them (Chappell et al., 2002; Morris et al., 1998; Savvidou et al., 2003).

Determination of the fetal signal could have therapeutic implications for pre-eclampsia and IUGR. What are the possible candidates? The placenta produces a number of molecules that might potentially modify maternal physiology and metabolism and placental function. These include norepinephrine (Manyonda et al., 1998; Sarkar et al., 2001; Sodha et al., 1984), acetylcholine (Sastry, 1997), CRH (Fadalti et al., 2000; Karteris et al., 2001, 2003) and leptin (Ashworth et al., 2000; Domali and Messinis, 2002; Mantzoros, 2000; Poston, 2002; Sagawa et al., 2002) to name a few.

We believe that of the placental hormones listed, leptin holds special promise as one of the putative signals to modify maternal and placental function to augment nutrient delivery. Leptin has numerous effects to alter energy metabolism and influence adiposity (Harris, 2000). Many of these are quite relevant to the metabolic adaptations of pregnancy that are accentuated in pre-eclampsia. Leptin acts centrally to increase sympathetic outflow, increasing the breakdown of triglycerides and glycogen and also resulting in generalized increased sympathetic activity, as seen pre-eclampsia (Haynes *et al.*, 1997). Leptin interacts with insulin, increasing insulin sensitivity in brown fat and muscle but reducing insulin sensitivity of white fat (Wang *et al.*, 1999).

The prime tissue for the production of leptin in humans is adipose tissue. The placenta is the only other tissue with a concentration of mRNA equivalent to that of adipose tissue in humans (Ashworth *et al.*, 2000). Leptin concentration doubles during normal pregnancy and drops dramatically post delivery consistent with a placental origin (McCarthy *et al.*, 1999). Leptin produced by the placenta can be upregulated by hypoxia (Mise *et al.*, 1998) and in vitro perfusion studies indicate secretion almost exclusively to the maternal compartment (Linnemann *et al.*, 2000).

Consistent with the effect of hypoxia to increase placental leptin, placental mRNA (Mise *et al.*, 1998) and maternal circulating leptin are increased in pre-eclampsia (McCarthy *et al.*, 1999). Paradoxically, leptin is not increased in maternal blood in pregnancies complicated by SGA (Chappell *et al.*, 2002). Leptin receptors are present on the maternal (villus) surface of syncytiotrophoblast (Bodner *et al.*, 1999). Recent data indicates that exposure of villus fragments to leptin increases amino acid uptake (Jansson *et al.*, 2003).

Leptin has effects in several tissues to modify energy metabolism and uptake; in the placenta leptin can increase amino acid uptake. Leptin is produced by the placenta and increased by hypoxia, as might be expected in placental and fetal tissues with poor placental perfusion. In keeping with the effect of hypoxia, leptin is increased in the blood of women with pre-eclampsia and in the placentas from these pregnancies (McCarthy *et al.*, 1999; Mise *et al.*, 1998; Teppa *et al.*, 2000). Paradoxically and consistent with a fetal signal not expressed in response to reduced nutrient and oxygen delivery in IUGR,

leptin is not increased in mothers destined to have SGA pregnancies (Chappell *et al.*, 2002).

Clinical and research implications of the two-stage model

The two-stage model of pre-eclampsia proposes that there is more to pre-eclampsia than reduced placental perfusion. It is clear that reduced perfusion of the intervillus space is not sufficient for the development of pre-eclampsia and that a maternal contribution is also necessary. The identification of such maternal factors raises the possibility of preventive therapy for pre-eclampsia directed at countering specific abnormalities present in specific women. Is it possible, for example, that therapy to either reduce obesity or counter the consequences of obesity would be useful in women with high BMI? Furthermore, since many of the risk factors for pre-eclampsia are risk factors for later-life cardiovascular disease, women with a history of pre-eclampsia should be recognized as women at increased risk for cardiovascular disease. This information should encourage healthy lifestyle interventions to reduce risk.

The concept that the interaction of maternal and fetal factors converge to generate the maternal syndrome suggests that therapy directed at this convergence point might be useful for all women destined to develop pre-eclampsia. Currently, the concept that this interaction converges to generate oxidative stress with subsequent inflammatory activation and endothelial dysfunction has directed large studies of antioxidant prophylaxis. The success of these trials is the ultimate test of the hypothesis. However, increased understanding of the steps leading to and subsequent to the convergences will also provide useful insights. Is it possible that overt pre-eclampsia which has long been considered as untreatable other than by palliative therapy and delivery could be reversed?

The two-stage model provides a unifying theory to explain the widely disparate outcomes in pre-eclampsia ranging from findings in the 10% of cases that occur prior to 34 weeks and are associated with increased maternal and fetal morbidity and mortality to the vast majority of cases that occur near to term. The cases at term range from those associated with bad maternal and fetal outcome in the absence of expeditious delivery to cases with minimal consequence to mother and baby and an excess of large babies (Xiong *et al.*, 2000). The relative contribution of fetal–placental factors and maternal risk factors (sensitivities) would dictate this variable outcome.

The possibility that the response to the reduced placental perfusion of stage 1 may generate not merely toxic signals but signals secondary to a fetal/placental adaptive response to reduced nutrient/oxygen availability has important implications. Certainly identifying these fetal/placental adaptive signals could suggest strategies for therapy for growth restriction. More immediately, it dictates that any therapy for pre-eclampsia must be assessed not only in terms of maternal effectiveness but at least short-term and preferably long-term effects on the fetus/infant.

REFERENCES

Aardema, M. W., Oosterhof, H., Timmer, A., van Rooy, I. and Aarnoudse, J. G. (2001). Uterine artery Doppler flow and uteroplacental vascular pathology in normal pregnancies and pregnancies complicated by pre-eclampsia and small for gestational age fetuses. *Placenta*, **22**, 405–11.

Arias, F., Rodriquez, L., Rayne, S. C. and Kraus, F. T. (1993). Maternal placental vasculopathy and infection: two distinct subgroups among patients with preterm labor and preterm ruptured membranes. *Am. J. Obstet. Gynecol.*, **168**, 585–91.

Ashworth, C. J., Hoggard, N., Thomas, L., Mercer, J. G., Wallace, J. M. and Lea, R. G. (2000). Placental leptin. *Rev. Reprod.*, **5**, 18–24.

Bai, H., Liu, X., Liu, R., Liu, Y., Li, M. and Liu, B. (2002). Angiotensinogen and angiotensin-I converting enzyme gene variations in Chinese pregnancy induced hypertension. *Hua-Hsi i Ko Ta Hsueh Hsueh Pao (Journal of West China University of Medical Sciences)*, **33**, 233–7.

Bashford, M. T., Hefler, L. A., Vertrees, T. W., Roa, B. B. and Gregg, A. R. (2001). Angiotensinogen and endothelial nitric oxide synthase gene polymorphisms among Hispanic patients with preeclampsia. *Am. J. Obstet. Gynecol.*, **184**, 1345–50; discussion 1350–1.

Benyo, D. F., Miles, T. M. and Conrad, K. P. (1997). Hypoxia stimulates cytokine production by villous explants from the human placenta. *J. Clin. Endocrinol. Metab.*, **82**, 1582–8.

Bodner, J., Ebenbichler, C. F., Wolf, H. J., *et al.* (1999). Leptin receptor in human term placenta: in situ hybridization and immunohistochemical localization. *Placenta*, **20**, 677–82.

Brosens, I. A., Robertson, W. B., and Dixon, H. G. (1979). The role of the spiral arteries in the pathogenesis of preeclampsia. In *Obstetrics and Gynecology Annual*, ed. R. Wynn. pp. 177–91.

Cester, N., Staffolani, R., Rabini, R. A., *et al.* (1994). Pregnancy induced hypertension: a role for peroxidation in microvillus plasma membranes. *Mol. Cell. Biochem.*, **131**, 151–5.

Chambers, J. C., Fusi, L., Malik, I. S., Haskard, D. O., De Swiet, M. and Kooner, J. S. (2001). Association of maternal endothelial dysfunction with preeclampsia. *J. Am. Med. Ass.*, **285**, 1607–12.

Chappell, L. C., Seed, P. T., Briley, A., *et al.* (2002). A longitudinal study of biochemical variables in women at risk of preeclampsia. *Am. J. Obstet. Gynecol.*, **187**, 127–36.

Chesley, L. C. (1966). Vascular reactivity in normal and toxemic pregnancy. *Clin. Obstet. Gynecol.*, **9**, 871–81.

Conrad, K. P. and Benyo, D. F. (1997). Placental cytokines and the pathogenesis of preeclampsia. *Am. J. Reprod. Immun.*, **37**, 240–9.

D'Anna, R., Baviera, G., Scilipoti, A., Leonardi, I. and Leo, R. (2000). The clinical utility of serum uric acid measurements in pre-eclampsia and transient hypertension in pregnancy. *Panminerva Medica*, **42**, 101–3.

Domali, E. and Messinis, I. E. (2002). Leptin in pregnancy. *J. Maternal–Fetal Neonatal Med.*, **12**, 222–30.

Fadalti, M., Pezzani, I., Cobellis, L., *et al.* (2000). Placental corticotropin-releasing factor. An update. *Ann. N. Y. Acad. Sci.*, **900**, 89–94.

Ferrazzani, S., De Carolis, S., Pomini, F., Testa, A. C., Mastromarino, C. and Caruso, A. (1994). The duration of hypertension in the puerperium of preeclamptic women: relationship with renal impairment and week of delivery. *Am. J. Obstet. Gynecol.*, **171**, 506–12.

Guo, G., Wilton, A. N., Fu, Y., Qiu, H., Brennecke, S. P. and Cooper, D. W. (1997). Angiotensinogen gene variation in a population case-control study of preeclampsia/eclampsia in Australians and Chinese. *Electrophoresis*, **18**, 1646–9.

Harris, R. B. S. (2000). Leptin – much more than a satiety signal. *Ann. Rev. Nutr.*, **20**, 45–75.

Haynes, W. G., Morgan, D. A., Walsh, S. A., Mark, A. L. and Sivitz, W. I. (1997). Receptor-mediated regional sympathetic nerve activation by leptin. *J. Clin. Invest.*, **100**, 270–8.

Hubel, C. and Roberts, J. (1999). In *Chesley's Hypertensive Disorders in Pregnancy*, ed. F. Cunningham. Appleton & Lange, pp. 453–86.

Hubel, C., Snaedal, S., Geirsson, R., Roberts, J. and Arngrímsson, R. (1998). Women with a history of eclampsia manifest dyslipidemia during later life. *J. Soc. Gynecol. Invest.*, **5**(Suppl.), 40A–41A.

Hubel, C. A., Kagan, V. E., Kisin, E. R., McLaughlin, M. K. and Roberts, J. M. (1997). Increased ascorbate radical formation and ascorbate depletion in plasma from women with preeclampsia – implications for oxidative stress. *Free Rad. Biol. Med.*, **23**, 597–609.

Huppertz, B., Kingdom, J., Caniggia, I., *et al.* (2003). Hypoxia favours necrotic versus apoptotic shedding of placental syncytiotrophoblast into the maternal circulation. *Placenta*, **24**, 181–90.

Ishihara, N., Matsuo, H., Murakoshi, H., Laoag-Fernandez, J. B., Samoto, T. and Maruo, T. (2002). Increased apoptosis in the syncytiotrophoblast in human term placentas complicated by either preeclampsia or intrauterine growth retardation. *Am. J. Obstet. Gynecol.*, **186**, 158–66.

Jansson, N., Greenwood, S. L., Johansson, B. R., Powell, T. L. and Jansson, T. (2003). Leptin stimulates the activity of the system. A amino acid transporter in human placental villous fragments. *J. Clin. Endocrinol. Metab.*, **88**, 1205–11.

Karteris, E., Grammatopoulos, D. K., Randeva, H. S. and Hillhouse, E. W. (2001). The role of corticotropin-releasing hormone receptors in placenta and fetal membranes during human pregnancy. *Mol. Genet. Metab.*, **72**, 287–96.

Karteris, E., Goumenou, A., Koumantakis, E., Hillhouse, E. W. and Grammatopoulos, D. K. (2003). Reduced expression of corticotropin-releasing hormone receptor type-1 alpha in human preeclamptic and growth-restricted placentas. *J. Clin. Endocrinol. Metab.*, **88**, 363–70.

Khong, T. Y., De Wolf, F., Robertson, W. B. and Brosens, I. (1986). Inadequate maternal vascular response to placentation in pregnancies complicated by pre-eclampsia and by small-for-gestational age infants. *Br. J. Obstet. Gynaecol.*, **93**, 1049–59.

Kobashi, G., Hata, A., Shido, K., *et al.* (1999). Association of a variant of the angiotensinogen gene with pure type of hypertension in pregnancy in the Japanese: implication of a racial difference and significance of an age factor. *Am. J. Med. Genet.*, **86**, 232–6.

Laivuori, H., Tikkanen, M. J. and Ylikorkala, O. (1996). Hyperinsulinemia 17 years after preeclamptic first pregnancy. *J. Clin. Endocrinol. Metab.*, **81**, 2908–11.

Laivuori, H., Kaaja, R., Rutanen, E. M., Viinikka, L. and Ylikorkala, O. (1998). Evidence of high circulating testosterone in women with prior preeclampsia. *J. Clin. Endocrinol. Metab.*, **83**, 344–7.

Laivuori, H., Kaaja, R., Koistinen, H., *et al.* (2000). Leptin during and after preeclamptic or normal pregnancy: its relation to serum insulin and insulin sensitivity. *Metab. – Clin. Exp.*, **49**, 259–63.

Linnemann, K., Malek, A., Sager, R., Blum, W. F., Schneider, H. and Fusch, C. (2000). Leptin production and release in the dually in vitro perfused human placenta. *J. Clin. Endocrinol. Metab.*, **85**, 4298–301.

Lorentzen, B., Endresen, M. J., Clausen, T. and Henriksen, T. (1994). Fasting serum free fatty acids and triglycerides are increased before 20 weeks of gestation in women who later develop preeclampsia. *Hypertens. Pregn.*, **13**, 103–9.

Mantzoros, C. S. (2000). Role of leptin in reproduction. *Ann. N. Y. Acad. Sci.*, **900**, 174–83.

Many, A., Hubel, C. A., Fisher, S. J., Roberts, J. M. and Zhou, Y. (2000). Invasive cytotrophoblasts manifest evidence of oxidative stress in preeclampsia. *Am. J. Pathol.*, **156**, 321–31.

Manyonda, I. T., Slater, D. M., Fenske, C., Hole, D., Choy, M. Y. and Wilson, C. (1998). A role for noradrenaline in pre-eclampsia: towards a unifying hypothesis for the pathophysiology. *Br. J. Obstet. Gynaecol.*, **105**, 641–8.

Maynard, S. E., Min, J. Y., Merchan, J., *et al.* (2003). Excess placental soluble fms-like tyrosine kinase 1 (sFlt1) may contribute to endothelial dysfunction, hypertension, and proteinuria in preeclampsia. Comment. *J. Clin. Invest.*, **111**, 649–58.

Mazzali, M., Hughes, J., Kim, Y. G., *et al.* (2001). Elevated uric acid increases blood pressure in the rat by a novel crystal-independent mechanism. *Hypertension*, **38**, 1101–6.

McCarthy, J. F., Misra, D. N. and Roberts, J. M. (1999). Maternal plasma leptin is increased in preeclampsia and positively correlates with fetal cord concentration. *Am. J. Obstet. Gynecol.*, **180**, 731–6.

Meijer, A. J. (2003). Amino acids as regulators and components of nonproteinogenic pathways. *J. Nutr.*, **133**, 2057S–62S.

Mise, H., Sagawa, N., Matsumoto, T., *et al.* (1998). Augmented placental production of leptin in preeclampsia: possible involvement of placental hypoxia. *J. Clin. Endocrinol. Metab.*, **83**, 3225–9.

Morgan, L., Baker, P., Pipkin, F. B. and Kalsheker, N. (1995). Pre-eclampsia and the angiotensinogen gene. *Br. J. Obstet. Gynaecol.*, **102**, 489–90.

Morris, J., Fay, R. and Ellwood, D. (1998). Abnormal uterine artery waveforms in the second trimester are associated with adverse pregnancy outcome in high risk women. *J. Maternal–Fetal Invest.*, **8**, 82–4.

Myatt, L., Rosenfield, R., Eis, A., Brockman, D., Greer, I. and Lyall, F. (1996). Nitrotyrosine residues in placenta evidence of peroxynitrite formation and action. *Hypertension*, **28**, 488–93.

Page, E. W. (1939). The relation between hydatid moles, relative ischemia of the gravid uterus, and the placental origin of eclampsia. *Am. J. Obstet. Gynecol.*, **37**, 291–3.

Papageorghiou, A. T., Yu, C. K., Cicero, S., Bower, S. and Nicolaides, K. H. (2002). Second-trimester uterine artery Doppler screening in unselected populations: a review. Comment. *J. Maternal–Fetal Neonatal Med.*, **12**, 78–88.

Pijnenborg, R., Anthony, J., Davey, D. A., *et al.* (1991). Placental bed spiral arteries in the hypertensive disorders of pregnancy. *Br. J. Obstet. Gynaecol.*, **98**, 648–55.

Poston, L. (2002). Leptin and preeclampsia. *Semin. Reprod. Med.*, **20**, 131–8.

Redman, C. W., Beilin, L. J., Bonnar, J. and Wilkinson, R. H. (1976). Plasma-urate measurements in predicting fetal death in hypertensive pregnancy. *Lancet*, **1**, 1370–3.

Redman, C. W., Sacks, G. P. and Sargent, I. L. (1999). Preeclampsia: an excessive maternal inflammatory response to pregnancy. *Am. J. Obstet. Gynecol.*, **180**, 499–506.

Redman, C. W. G. (1991). Current topic: pre-eclampsia and the placenta. *Placenta*, **12**, 301–8.

Redman, C. W. G. and Sargent, I. L. (2000). Placental debris, oxidative stress and pre-eclampsia. *Placenta*, **21**, 597–602.

Roberts, J. M. (1998a). Endothelial dysfunction in pre-eclampsia. *Semin. Reprod. Endocrinol.*, **16**, 5–15.

Roberts, J. M. (1998b). In *Maternal Fetal Medicine*, ed. R. Resnik. Philadelphia: W. B. Saunders, pp. 833–72.

Roberts, J. M. and Hubel, C. A. (1999). Is oxidative stress the link in the two-stage model of pre-eclampsia? Comment. *Lancet*, **354**, 788–9.

Roberts, J. M. and Cooper, D. W. (2001). Pathogenesis and genetics of pre-eclampsia. *Lancet*, **357**, 53–6.

Roberts, J. M. and Lain, K. Y. (2002). Recent insights into the pathogenesis of pre-eclampsia. *Placenta*, **23**, 359–72.

Roberts, J. M., Taylor, R. N., Musci, T. J., Rodgers, G. M., Hubel, C. A. and McLaughlin, M. K. (1989). Preeclampsia: an endothelial cell disorder. *Am. J. Obstet. Gynecol.*, **161**, 1200–4.

Roggensack, A. M., Zhang, Y. and Davidge, S. T. (1999). Evidence for peroxynitrite formation in the vasculature of women with preeclampsia. *Hypertension*, **33**, 83–9.

Sagawa, N., Yura, S., Itoh, H., *et al.* (2002). Role of leptin in pregnancy – a review. *Placenta*, **23**, S80–6.

Sarkar, S., Tsai, S. W., Nguyen, T. T., Plevyak, M., Padbury, J. F. and Rubin, L. P. (2001). Inhibition of placental 11 beta-hydroxysteroid dehydrogenase type 2 by catecholamines via alpha-adrenergic signaling. *Am. J. Physiol. Regul. Integr. Compar. Physiol.*, **281**, R1966–74.

Sastry, B. V. (1997). Human placental cholinergic system. *Biochem. Pharmacol.*, **53**, 1577–86.

Sattar, N. and Greer, I. A. (2002). Pregnancy complications and maternal cardiovascular risk: opportunities for intervention and screening? *Br. Med. J.*, **325**, 157–60.

Savvidou, M. D., Hingorani, A. D., Tsikas, D., Frolich, J. C., Vallance, P. and Nicolaides, K. H. (2003). Endothelial dysfunction and raised plasma concentrations of asymmetric dimethylarginine in pregnant women who subsequently develop pre-eclampsia. *Lancet*, **361**, 1511–17.

Sodha, R. J., Proegler, M. and Schneider, H. (1984). Transfer and metabolism of norepinephrine studied from maternal-to-fetal and fetal-to-maternal sides in the in vitro perfused human placental lobe. *Am. J. Obstet. Gynecol.*, **148**, 474–81.

Staff, A. C., Halvorsen, B., Ranheim, T. and Henriksen, T. (1999a). Elevated level of free 8-iso-prostaglandin F-2 alpha in the decidua basalis of women with preeclampsia. *Am. J. Obstet. Gynecol.*, **181**, 1211–15.

Staff, A. C., Ranheim, T., Khoury, J. and Henriksen, T. (1999b). Increased contents of phospholipids, cholesterol, and lipid peroxides in decidua basalis in women with preeclampsia. *Am. J. Obstet. Gynecol.*, **180**, 587–92.

Teppa, R. J., Ness, R. B., Crombleholme, W. R. and Roberts, J. M. (2000). Free leptin is increased in normal pregnancy and further increased in preeclampsia. *Metab. – Clin. Exp.*, **49**, 1043–8.

Tyurin, V. A., Liu, S. X., Tyurina, Y. Y., *et al.* (2001). Elevated levels of S-nitrosoalbumin in preeclampsia plasma. Comment. *Circ. Res.*, **88**, 1210–15.

Uotila, J., Solakivi, T., Jaakkola, O., Tuimala, R. and Lehtimaki, T. (1998). Antibodies against copper-oxidised and malondialdehyde-modified low density lipoproteins in pre-eclamptic pregnancies. *Br. J. Obstet. Gynaecol.*, **105**, 1113–17.

von Dadelszen, P., Wilkins, T. and Redman, C. W. G. (1999). Maternal peripheral blood leukocytes in normal and pre-eclamptic pregnancies. *Br. J. Obstet. Gynaecol.*, **106**, 576–81.

Wakwe, V. C. and Abudu, O. O. (1999). Estimation of plasma uric acid in pregnancy induced hypertension (PIH). Is the test still relevant? *Afr. J. Med. Medic. Sci.*, **28**, 155–8.

Walsh, S. W. and Wang, Y. (1993). Deficient glutathione peroxidase activity in preeclampsia is associated with increased placental production of thromboxane and lipid peroxides. *Am. J. Obstet. Gynecol.*, 1456–61.

Walsh, S. W., Vaughan, J. E., Wang, Y. and Roberts, L. J. (2000). Placental isoprostane is significantly increased in preeclampsia. *FASEB J.*, **14**, 1289–96.

Wang, J. L., Chinookoswong, N., Scully, S., Qi, M. and Shi, Z. Q. (1999). Differential effects of leptin in regulation of tissue glucose utilization in vivo. *Endocrinology*, **140**, 2117–24.

Wang, Y. and Walsh, S. W. (2001). Increased superoxide generation is associated with decreased superoxide dismutase activity and mRNA expression in placental trophoblast cells in pre-eclampsia. *Placenta*, **22**, 206–12.

Wang, Y., Walsh, S. W. and Kay, H. H. (1992). Placental lipid peroxides and thromboxane are increased and prostacyclin is decreased in women with preeclampsia. *Am. J. Obstet. Gynecol.*, **167**, 945–9.

Ward, K., Hata, A., Jeunemaitre, X., *et al.* (1993). A molecular variant of angiotensinogen associated with preeclampsia. *Nature Genetics*, **4**, 59–61.

Xiong, X., Demianczuk, N. N., Buekens, P. and Saunders, L. D. (2000). Association of preeclampsia with high birth weight for gestational age. *Am. J. Obstet. Gynecol.*, **183**, 148–55.

Zeek, P. and Assali, N. (1950). Vascular changes in the decidua associated with eclamptogenic toxemia of pregnancy. *Am. J. Clin. Pathol.*, **20**, 1099–109.

Zusterzeel, P. L., Rutten, H., Roelofs, H. M., Peters, W. H. and Steegers, E. A. (2001). Protein carbonyls in decidua and placenta of pre-eclamptic women as markers for oxidative stress. *Placenta*, **22**, 213–19.

13

High altitude and pre-eclampsia

Stacy Zamudio

Introduction

Most well-described risk factors for pre-eclampsia are constitutional maternal attributes, such as primiparity, obesity, ethnicity, chronic hypertension, renal disease, etc. (Eskenazi *et al.*, 1991; Saftlas *et al.*, 1990; Sibai *et al.*, 1995; Stone *et al.*, 1994), or behavioral attributes such as contraceptive practices or smoking (or the lack thereof) (Klonoff-Cohen *et al.*, 1989, 1993; Sibai *et al.*, 1995). Residence at high altitude (>2700 m) is the only external environmental factor that, to date, has been consistently linked with an increased incidence of pre-eclampsia (Keyes *et al.*, 2003; Mahfouz *et al.*, 1994; Moore *et al.*, 1982; Palmer *et al.*, 1999). Far from being a problem limited to only isolated human populations, more than 40 million people reside at elevations >2700 m, with their numbers increasing rapidly (Moore *et al.*, 1998). The primary effect of high altitude is lowered arterial oxygen tension (PO_2). Thus, of the several competing hypotheses concerning the etiology of pre-eclampsia, the data from high altitude support that hypoxia (presumably of the fetoplacental unit) is an underlying cause or at the very least contributes to the development of the syndrome. The high-altitude data additionally support altered immunological function, impaired placentation (shallow invasion) and ischemia or ischemia/reperfusion injury as possible etiological factors. This review considers the impact of lowered maternal arterial PO_2 on pregnancy physiology and the development of pre-eclampsia.

High altitude and hypertension during pregnancy

The first published report indicating that residence at high altitude may be associated with an increased risk for pre-eclampsia was by Colorado researchers in 1982. Pregnancy-induced hypertension, noted as a diagnosis within medical records, occurred in 12%, 4% and 3% of pregnancies at 3100 m, 2410 m and 1600 m, respectively. Proteinuria greater than 1+ was noted in 28% and 9% of pregnancies at 3100 m and 1600 m, respectively. Blood pressure was generally higher in all pregnant women at high altitude based on medical records review. Further, in a small group of prospectively studied women with pregnancy-induced hypertension (PIH, hypertension without proteinuria or other organ system involvement), arterial oxygen saturation (which is largely determined by maternal arterial PO_2) was inversely correlated with blood pressure. Thus women with the lowest saturations had the highest mean arterial pressures (Moore *et al.*, 1982). Support for the idea that lowered maternal arterial oxygen pressure is associated with an increased risk of pre-eclampsia can also be found in the disease literature: women with a variety of congenital heart diseases associated with poor cardiac output or impaired lung transfer of oxygen to blood also have a markedly increased risk for pre-eclampsia (Shime *et al.*, 1987). The Colorado group continued to pursue (in animal studies) the relationship between pregnancy, hypoxia and hypertension (Harrison and Moore, 1990; Harrison *et al.*, 1986), uterine artery structure and growth (Rockwell *et al.*, 2000), vascular reactivity (Harrison and Moore, 1989; Keyes *et al.*, 1998; Mateev *et al.*, 2003; Sillau *et al.*, 2002; White *et al.*, 1998, 2000) and the incidence and physiological correlates of pre-eclampsia in retrospective and prospective human studies (Jensen and Moore, 1997; Palmer *et al.*, 1999; Zamudio *et al.*, 1995a, b, c). Using a variety of research designs, including cohort studies, birth-certificate analyses and prospective longitudinal physiological analyses, the data have consistently shown anywhere from a two- to a fourfold elevation in the incidence of pre-eclampsia at high altitude using both strict criteria (primiparas with documented proteinuria and hypertension that resolved following delivery) and less strict, but clinically relevant criteria (e.g. hypertension plus evidence of other organ system involvement, such as neurological symptoms, abnormal liver function tests or platelet consumption). While strictly anecdotal, it is our impression that neurological symptoms are more common at high altitude, although the numbers of residents at >2700 m and the limitations of epidemiological databases such as birth certificates preclude formal testing of this relationship. However, the general finding that pre-eclampsia is increased at high altitude has been replicated in Saudi Arabia, in women long resident at 3000 m, and in Bolivia, in women residing at 3600 m. In these larger-scale epidemiological analyses, there is a near twofold elevation in the incidence of pre-eclampsia at high altitude, independent of other risk factors, in both Saudi Arabia and Bolivia (Keyes *et al.*, 2003; Mahfouz *et al.*, 1994).

Maternal physiology in high-altitude pregnancy

In this section we consider that one of the possible explanations for the link between maternal hypoxia (lowered arterial oxygen pressure) and an increased risk for pre-eclampsia lies in the impact of hypoxia on multiple physiological systems (see Figures 13.1 and 13.2). In this model it is not just one effect of hypoxia that "causes" pre-eclampsia, rather it is the impact of hypoxic stress on several important adjustments to pregnancy that shifts the general population risk such that more women eventually develop the disease (Figure 13.1).

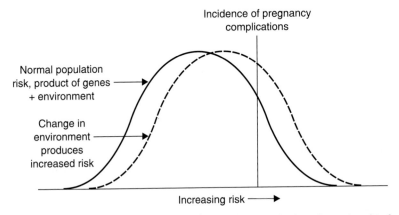

Figure 13.1 The solid bell-shaped curve represents the distribution of any given biochemical or physiological risk factor within a normal population under normal (in this case sea-level) environmental conditions. The hatched bell-shaped curve represents the shift in the value of this factor with a change in the environment. Thus under normal sea-level conditions the risk factor may lead to a 5–10% incidence of a given pregnancy complication, while the shift in the value of risk factor "x" with a change in environment (in this case high altitude) leads to more cases of the syndrome.

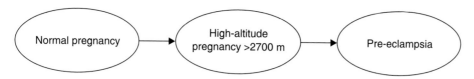

Physiological changes in pregnancy at high relative to low altitude
↑ Blood pressure
↓ Plasma volume
↑ Catecholamines
↑ Pro-inflammatory relative to anti-inflammatory cytokines
↓ Uteroplacental vascular remodeling
↓ Uterine blood flow

Figure 13.2 A model of physiological changes in pregnancy in which the normal state is represented by sea-level normal pregnancies on the left side, and intermediate state of adaptation is represented by high-altitude pregnancies in the middle, and the extremes of physiological mal-adaptation are present in pre-eclampsia, the far right side. The list below the model are the data published to date in high-altitude pregnancy showing the direction of the changes observed relative to sea-level normal pregnancies.

Maternal oxygen consumption increases by a minimum of 20% and carbon dioxide production by 25% in human pregnancy at sea level. This increase is accomplished by a 35% increase in ventilation, which in turn is due to increased tidal volume as opposed to breathing frequency. The increase in oxygen consumption is not just due to increased weight and metabolic rate; at term oxygen consumption and carbon dioxide per kilogram of body weight are still 10% higher than in the non-pregnant condition (Moore et al., 1987). At least part of the increased drive to breathe stems from a general doubling of hypoxic ventilatory response. But, as with any normally distributed variable, there must be women at the upper and lower ends of the bell-shaped curve who have greater or lesser capacity for increasing their tidal volume and hence oxygen transport. Likewise, humans are remarkably variable in their ventilatory sensitivity to hypoxia and hypercarbia, and women with low responsiveness in pregnancy do not increase their breathing as much as those with higher responses (Moore et al., 1986, 1987). In the model presented in Figure 13.1, we suggest that most physiological variables have a normal distribution, and that perturbation of the environment (e.g. by lowered oxygen pressure and hence

availability) can shift a greater proportion of individuals into a higher-risk category for the development of a syndrome such as pre-eclampsia. In Figure 13.2, based on the published literature, we emphasize that for many physiological variables known to be associated with an increased risk of pre-eclampsia, high-altitude women tend be shifted towards higher risk.

Blood pressure fails to fall mid-trimester at high altitude, and is increased relative to low altitude from week 16 forward (Palmer et al., 1999). While studies testing whether isolated mean arterial pressures can predict the development of pre-eclampsia lack specificity (Moutquin et al., 1985; Sibai et al., 1995; Villar and Sibai, 1989), it has long been known that even small increments in blood pressure in an otherwise normal pregnancy are associated with increased risk of adverse outcomes, including pre-eclampsia and lower birthweight (Page and Christianson, 1976). That mean arterial pressure in pregnancy at high altitude was inversely related to maternal arterial oxygen saturation, and, in a later study, to plasma volume expansion, supports the idea that maternal oxygen transport and blood pressure during pregnancy are related (Moore et al., 1982; Zamudio et al., 1993). Disturbed oxygen extraction/metabolism has also been observed at sea level in pre-eclampsia (Belfort *et al.*, 1993), and the extensive literature on oxidative stress as a potential contributor cannot even begin to be covered here.

Plasma volume expansion is a well-known correlate of fetal growth (Longo and Hardesty, 1984), and is impaired in a variety of pregnancy complications ranging from oligohydramnios to diabetes to IUGR in the absence of pre-eclampsia (Goodlin *et al.*, 1981). Hypovolemia is therefore a general marker of risk for pregnancy complications, and one that has been argued, both past and present, as an indicator of abnormal vascular responsiveness (Bernstein *et al.*, 1998a; Croall *et al.*, 1978). In our studies at 3100 m women with the lowest arterial oxygen saturations had the highest mean arterial pressures and the least increase in plasma volume late in pregnancy (Zamudio *et al.*, 1993). Of interest here is that the only sex difference known in long-term high-altitude residents appears to be an important contributor to the risk for developing pre-eclampsia. Men residing at high altitude increase their red cell mass and have plasma volumes only slightly lower than at sea level (Hurtado *et al.*, 1945; Sanchez *et al.*, 1970). An increase in red cell mass leads to an increase in oxygen carrying capacity per unit of blood. In contrast, women living at high altitude have lower plasma volumes and a similar red cell mass when compared to women living at low altitude (Zamudio *et al.*, 1993). The same net effect is accomplished – hemoconcentration increases oxygen carrying capacity, but at the cost of a lowered plasma volume, and, presumably, venoconstriction, since the veins house the majority of plasma volume at any given moment. A low non-pregnant plasma volume is associated with an increased risk for pre-eclampsia and/or intrauterine growth restriction (Bernstein *et al.*, 1998a; Croall *et al.*, 1978; Gibson, 1973). The chronic reduction in plasma volume noted in women residing at high altitude could be due to either arterial or venous vasoconstriction. The former is supported by the observation that plasma volume decreases as

peripheral vascular resistance rises (Dustan *et al.*, 1973) and the latter by decreased venous distensibility and by the increased ratio of central to total blood volume in hypertensive subjects and in acute high-altitude exposure (Ulrych *et al.*, 1969; Weil *et al.*, 1971; Zamudio *et al.*, 2001). We favor venoconstriction as the cause, as blood pressure does not differ in women who are not pregnant at high versus low altitude (Palmer *et al.*, 1999), nor is there any evidence that more women are constitutionally hypertensive or at the high end of the normal range of blood pressure when not pregnant. In our long-term residents of 3100 m altitude in Colorado, we found that while the increase in plasma volume was normal in women who remained normotensive during pregnancy at high altitude, plasma volume at 36 weeks was similar to that of non-pregnant women living at low altitude, and volume expansion was more often disrupted, with a third trimester fall in women who developed PIH, and failure to expand altogether in women who eventually developed pre-eclampsia (Table 13.1) (Zamudio *et al.*, 1993). It should be noted that these data are entirely consistent with what has been observed in pre-eclampsia at low altitude, and that the relationship between volume expansion and infant birth weight ($r = 0.58$) was similar or greater than that reported in previous studies (Longo and Hardesty, 1984).

Systemic vascular resistance/response to pressor agents has not been measured in pregnant women at high altitude, although as noted above, a considerable literature on animals exists, and is thoroughly reviewed in White and Zhang with respect to the most relevant animal models, sheep and guinea pigs (White and Zhang, 2003). However, the relative lack of fall in blood pressure and impaired blood volume expansion noted in pregnant women at high altitude suggest that systemic vascular resistance may be elevated relative to normal pregnancy at low altitude. While the formation of a new uteroplacental circuit contributes to the decrease in vascular resistance observed in normal pregnancy, the residual systemic (non-uteroplacental) circulation accounts

Table 13.1. Abnormal plasma volume expansion in hypertensive pregnancies at high altitude

	1600 m Normotensive ($n=11$)	3100 m Normotensive ($n=22$)	3100 m PIH ($n=5$)	3100 m Pre-eclampsia ($n=8$)
Plasma volume nonpregnant (ml)	2523 ± 109	2112 ± 42	2292 ± 180	2464 ± 157
Plasma volume nonpregnant (ml/kg)	$42.4 \pm 1.2^*$	33.2 ± 0.8	31.9 ± 4.9	36.2 ± 2.3
Δ Plasma volume nonpregnant to wk 36 (ml)	1363 ± 178	1111 ± 120	564 ± 456	$216 \pm 203^\dagger$
Δ Plasma volume, wk 24 to wk 36 (ml)		404 ± 67	$-194 \pm 100^\dagger$	$-227 \pm 61^\dagger$

$^*p < 0.05$ high vs. low altitude.

$^\dagger p < 0.05$ normotensive vs. pre-eclampsia at 3100 m.

for the majority ($>70\%$) of the fall in resistance observed in pregnant animals (Curran-Everett et al., 1991). Hence, change in vascular responsiveness of the non-uteroplacental circulation and/or changes in the levels of circulating pressors must be present in human pregnancy. A substantial literature supports the former, i.e. that attenuated systemic vascular response to a number of pressor agents, including catecholamines, contributes to the fall in systemic vascular resistance, which, in turn, facilitates the normal increase in cardiac output and redistribution of blood flow to favor the uteroplacental circuit (Chapman et al., 1998; Chesley, 1978; Gant et al., 1973; Nisell et al., 1985a; Palmer et al., 1992). These changes in vasoreactivity are, in part, mediated by increases in estrogen and progesterone as reviewed (White et al., 1995). Pregnancy attenuates the vascular response to norepinephrine in pelvic and hindlimb vascular beds, as well as contractile responses in isolated aortic, mesenteric, femoral, caudal and uterine arteries (Crandall et al., 1990; Dogterom and DeJong, 1973; McLaughlin et al., 1989; Magness and Rosenfeld, 1986; Parent et al., 1990). Pregnancy also diminishes venous sensitivity to norepinephrine, although sensitivity can be increased several fold by increasing intraluminal pressure (Hohmann et al., 1990). This latter finding supports that pregnancy-induced changes in venous volume may be important contributors to venous reactivity. Since it is the venous system that houses 80% of plasma volume at any given moment, aberration of

venous vascular reactivity may be an underlying cause of the widely observed relationship between impaired plasma volume expansion and pre-eclampsia (Bernstein et al., 1998a), and consistent with genetic data indicating polymorphisms of relevance to angiotensin are associated with the syndrome (Bernstein et al., 1998b).

Several lines of evidence support that women who develop pre-eclampsia have greater activation of the sympathetic nervous system, in particular the alpha limb. Arterial norepinephrine levels are increased by $>40\%$ in pre-eclamptic women over their own nonpregnant values (Nisell et al., 1985a). Arterial norepinephrine levels are several-fold higher in pre-eclamptic than normal women, and while venous levels do not differ, this is most likely due to increased arterial to venous extraction in pre-eclamptic women (Nisell et al., 1985a; Oian et al., 1986; Pedersen et al., 1982). Increased urinary excretion of catecholamines in pre-eclampsia is consistent with greater circulating concentrations (Coussons-Read et al., 2002; Zuspan, 1976). Enhanced pressor and systemic vascular resistance response to catecholamines are noted in hypertensive pregnancy (Nisell et al., 1985b,c; Raab et al., 1956; Talledo et al., 1968). Moreover, circulating norepinephrine and epinephrine levels correlate with elevated blood pressure, reduced plasma volume and elevated heart rate in pre-eclamptic, but not normotensive pregnant women (Nisell et al., 1985a). More recently, directly measured sympathetic neural outflow (muscle

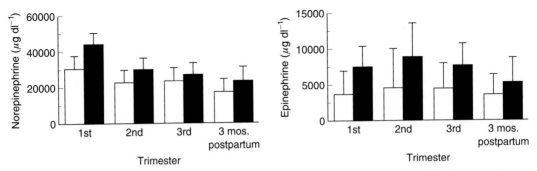

Figure 13.3 Norepinephrine (left side) and epinephrine concentrations were measured using HPLC (Mazzeo *et al.*, 1991) at 1600 m (white bars) and 3100 m (solid black bars) during each trimester of pregnancy and 3 months postpartum in nine women at 1600 m and women at 3100 m. Values are elevated for both catecholamines in women at high altitude throughout pregnancy, although high variability and small sample sizes precludes significance within any given trimester of pregnancy or postpartum. (Data adapted from Coussons-Read *et al.*, 2002.)

sympathetic nerve activity – MSNA) is markedly greater in women who develop pre-eclampsia or PIH when compared with normal pregnant women (Greenwood *et al.*, 1998, 2001; Schobel *et al.*, 1996). Moreover, a pre-eclampsia-like syndrome can be induced in animals by inducing sympathetic over-reactivity (Kanayama *et al.*, 1997), and eclamptic seizures can occur in pre-eclamptic women given anticholinergics (Kobayashi *et al.*, 2002), suggesting that diminution of para-sympathetic activity potentiates an already hyperreactive sympathetic vascular stimulation. While this particular theory concerning the etiology of pre-eclampsia waxes and wanes in popularity, and is sometimes spoken of somewhat derisively as a hypothesis about "a case of nerves," there is far too much evidence of SNS disruption and dysregulation to simply ignore the possibility (Greenwood *et al.*, 2003; Khatun *et al.*, 2000; Lewinsky and Riskin-Mashiah, 1998; Nisell and Lunell, 1984; Schobel *et al.*, 1996; Zuspan, 1977, 1979). Taken together, the data support that alpha-sympathetic activity in pre-eclamptic women is enhanced compared with normal pregnant women.

It is well known that acute altitude-induced hypoxia stimulates the sympathoadrenal system (Mazzeo *et al.*, 1991; Reeves *et al.*, 1992). While epinephrine rises early during acclimatization, and is associated with increases in metabolic rate, heart

rate and cardiac output, levels decline rapidly after a few days in conjunction with rises in arterial oxygen tension and content (Grover *et al.*, 1986; Mazzeo *et al.*, 1991, 1998). In contrast, norepinephrine, an indicator of alpha-adrenergic stimulation, rises later in acclimatization, plateaus in about a week, but remains higher even with 12–21 days of altitude exposure. Such rises parallel increases in blood pressure (Mazzeo *et al.*, 1991), venoconstriction, increased peripheral vascular resistance and a decrease in plasma volume (Mazzeo *et al.*, 2001a; Stokke *et al.*, 1986; Weil *et al.*, 1971; Wolfel *et al.*, 1991). Reasoning by analogy, we suspected that catecholamine levels might be elevated in high altitude pregnancy. Twenty-four hour urinary excretion of catecholamines were measured in a limited number of women pregnant at high vs. low altitude (Coussons-Read *et al.*, 2002). As predicted, urinary excretion of catecholamines was elevated at high altitude when all trimesters were considered together (Figure 13.3). Altitude-associated differences in both norepinephrine and epinephrine were most pronounced early in pregnancy (46% and 109% greater, respectively), although even non-pregnant values were 37% (norepinephrine) and 47% (epinephrine) greater among the high-altitude women. However, the high variability in the measurements and the small sample size precluded significant differences within specific trimesters or 3 months postpartum (Coussons-Read *et al.*, 2002).

Previous work suggests that switching from Th1-type (pro-inflammatory) to Th2-type immunity (suppression of the inflammatory response) during pregnancy is one way the maternal immune system prevents rejection of the fetoplacental unit as an allograft (Piccinni and Romagnani, 1996; Piccinni *et al.*, 2000). Moreover, increased Th1 type activity in pregnancy is associated with complications, including pre-eclampsia and premature labor and delivery (Greer *et al.*, 1994; Kupferminc *et al.*, 1994; Omu *et al.*, 1999; Redman, 1991; Saito and Sakai, 2003; Veith and Rice, 1999; Vives *et al.*, 1999). More proinflammatory cytokines are produced by lymphocytes from pre-eclamptic women than from women with normal pregnancies (Darmochwal-Kolarz *et al.*, 2002; Saito *et al.*, 1999a, 1999b). While infection during pregnancy stimulates production of these cytokines, there is no evidence whatsoever that women pregnant at high altitude have a greater incidence of infections, despite substantial evidence that they have an increased incidence of pregnancy complications (Jensen and Moore, 1997; Moore *et al.*, 1998; Palmer *et al.*, 1999).

Catecholamines modulate immune function in humans and animals and thus catecholamines may contribute to the altered cytokine profiles observed in complicated pregnancies (Elenkov and Chrousos, 1999, 2002; Minagawa *et al.*, 1999). For example, catecholamines can induce an increase in the pro-inflammatory cytokines IL-6 and IL-8, while they tend to decrease TNF-alpha, but such responses vary by the tissue sites of production and whether or not other external stressors are present or absent (Elenkov and Chrousos, 2002). Acute high-altitude exposure leads to an increase in IL-6 and other indicators of an immune system inflammatory response (Bailey *et al.*, 2003; Kubo *et al.*, 1998; Mazzeo *et al.*, 2001b). Therefore in the same women in whom catecholamines were monitored, the hypothesis that pro-inflammatory cytokines would be elevated during high-altitude pregnancy was tested.

We found that maternal circulating concentrations of the pro-inflammatory cytokines IL-6, TNF-alpha, and IL-8 were all elevated late in pregnancy in women residing at high altitude, but did not differ even marginally in the non-pregnant state. The same subjects failed to increase their levels of anti-inflammatory (Th-2) IL-10 during pregnancy, causing a marked reduction in circulating concentrations relative to low altitude control subjects that was, again, most pronounced in the third trimester when pregnancy complications develop (Coussons-Read *et al.*, 2002). The complexity of the systems involved can support a number of different explanations. It may be that pregnant women at high altitude do not make as complete a switch from Th1 to Th2-type immune responsiveness as women residing at lower altitude (Coussons-Read *et al.*, 2002). It may be that the overall profile of cytokine production during pregnancy at high altitude is altered by sympathoadrenal activation secondary to the interaction of hypoxia and pregnancy (a general stress) and therefore favors the development of complications at the extremes of the normal range of variation. Alternatively, altered cytokine production or degradation may be a reflection of underlying mechanisms that contribute both to the observed alterations in circulating concentrations and the development of complications without one necessarily causing the other.

Placental factors

Consistently noted in pre-eclampsia is a relative failure of trophoblast to invade and remodel the maternal spiral arteries to the level of the first third of the maternal myometrium (Meekins *et al.*, 1994; Pijnenborg *et al.*, 1991; Robertson *et al.*, 1986). The role played by oxygen in the differentiation of trophoblast is thoroughly reviewed elsewhere, as are the effects of high altitude on placental development (Kingdom and Kaufmann, 1997, 1999;

Zamudio, 2003). However, in order to test the hypothesis that high-altitude placentas would show a phenotype intermediate between that reported for normal pregnancy at sea level and pre-eclampsia, we examined the decidual ends of uteroplacental arteries in placentas from high (3100 m) vs. low (1600 m) altitude. We found that while individually variable, remodeling was absent in 67% of all arteries examined in the high-altitude placentas vs. 27% of the arteries examined in low altitude placentas (Tissot van Patot *et al.*, 2003). The latter contrasts with findings from sea level, wherein 100% of arteries from normal placentas were remodeled (Labarrere and Faulk, 1994). Unexpected was the finding that there were more uteroplacental arteries at the level of the decidua in the high-altitude placentas, although this has been noted before in placental bed biopsies from pre-eclamptic pregnancies (Starzyk *et al.*, 1997). Remodeled or not, these data suggest that angiogenesis was increased and perhaps a compensatory response to hypoxia. None the less, the infants, despite being the product of normal, healthy pregnancies, were still smaller than the lower altitude controls.

These data are consistent with a variety of studies indicating that failed remodeling contributes to reduced uteroplacental blood flow and fetoplacental ischemia (Aardema *et al.*, 2001; Kreczy *et al.*, 1995; Lin *et al.*, 1995; Macara *et al.*, 1996). It should be stressed here that ischemia is generally suspected where uteroplacental artery resistance indices are elevated. We found reduced uterine artery blood flow in a small number of subjects in whom quantitative, Doppler based flow and diameter measurements were obtained. However, a 33% reduction in unilateral uterine artery blood flow existed in near-term pregnant women residing at 3100 m without any evidence of increased vascular resistance being present (Zamudio *et al.*, 1995a). This is perhaps because in contrast to intrauterine growth restriction (without pre-eclampsia), in which reduced villous vascular development is often noted (Kingdom and Kaufmann, 1997), a pronounced effect of altitude

on placental morphology is increased fetal capillary density (Zamudio, 2003). This may account for why Doppler ultrasound data do not support that there is increased resistance to flow in the normal high altitude placenta (Krampl *et al.*, 2001; Zamudio *et al.*, 1995a). It does not, however, preclude a reduction in overall uteroplacental blood flow, which would reduce both oxygen and substrate delivery and thereby contribute to reduced fetal growth, if not to the development of pre-eclampsia. Estimates of blood flow in the subset of subjects who developed pre-eclampsia at 3100 m suggested a 60% reduction in blood flow was present, but the reduction was due not to increased resistance to flow, but rather to a failure of blood flow velocity within the uterine arteries to increase between 24 and 36 week of pregnancy (Zamudio *et al.*, 1995b, d). The magnitude of the overall reduction is consistent with invasive measurements obtained in pre-eclamptic women (Lunell *et al.*, 1982; Nylund *et al.*, 1983), but differs in that there was no evidence of increased impedance to flow, at least in the uterine arteries, until symptoms such as hypertension were already present. Whether this is an artifact of small sample size or whether the degree to which impaired decidual and maternal arterial remodeling vs. impaired villous vascular development effects resistance to flow within the uteroplacental arteries cannot be addressed with the present data.

There are, finally, recent data derived from high-altitude pregnancies, but published only in abstract form that bear on several additional theories concerning the etiology of pre-eclampsia. The laboratory of Dr. Fiona Lyall has been investigating markers of endothelial cell activation and placental vascular reactivity. The laboratory of Dr. Isabella Caniggia has been investigating oxygen-mediated trophoblast differentiation and function via studies of the regulation, expression and activity of the nuclear transcription factor hypoxia-inducible factor 1 alpha (HIF-1α). It is worth noting, if only briefly, that the model of chronic hypoxia in pregnancy offered by high-altitude residence is proving fruitful in distinguishing unique circulating and molecular markers of pre-eclampsia from those which may be due to hypoxia alone, without pathological consequences (Caniggia *et al.*, 2002; Lyall *et al.*, 2002, 2003; Marks *et al.*, 2002, 2006; Soleymanlou *et al.*, 2005; Zamudio *et al.*, 2002, 2007).

Summary

In a series of investigations spanning more than a decade, the hypothesis that maternal physiological changes of pregnancy at high altitude would be intermediate between those observed in normal sea level pregnancy, and those observed in pre-eclampsia has been largely supported. What is important to remember is that none of the variables discussed above, in and of themselves, are sufficient to cause pre-eclampsia. Rather, they are correlates of the syndrome, perhaps markers of a single underlying cause, but far more likely to represent the range of variability present in human pregnancy. Dr. Chris Redman has elegantly argued that the range of variation present in any single attribute associated with pre-eclampsia demonstrates that the disease is both multifactorial in origin, and that univariate associations are no more than manifestations of extremes in multiple domains as opposed to indicative of a single cause. Recall here the statistical plot advocated by Dr. Jim Roberts, which is now almost universally used to display data points regarding factor *x*, *y* or *z* obtained from pre-eclamptics vs. normal controls. The plot shows the scatter of all individual data points with a bar indicating the mean. Means for innumerable univariate measures are elevated (or depressed) in pre-eclampsia, but invariably there is significant overlap with the individual values observed in normal controls, i.e. there is no cutoff at which the development of pre-eclampsia is inevitable with the presence of any single variable studied to date. The model of chronic hypoxia in pregnancy in the natural environmental experiment presented by voluntary residence at high altitude clearly supports the idea that pre-eclampsia is associated with extremes of variation, but that there is virtually always overlap with the normal range. The question remains to be answered that IF, and that is a big if, there is a single cause, or a final common pathway by which pre-eclampsia is induced, why would it be more common at high altitude?

REFERENCES

Aardema, M. W., Oosterhof, H., Timmer, A., van Rooy, I. and Aarnoudse, J. G. (2001). Uterine artery Doppler flow and uteroplacental vascular pathology in normal pregnancies and pregnancies complicated by pre-eclampsia and small for gestational age fetuses. *Placenta*, **22**, 405–11.

Bailey, D. M., Kleger, G. R., Holzgraefe, M., Ballmer, P. E. and Bartsch, P. (2004). Pathophysiological significance of peroxidative stress, neuronal damage and membrane permeability in acute mountain sickness. *J. Appl. Physiol.*, **96**, 1459–63.

Belfort, M. A., Anthony, J., Saade, G. R., *et al.* (1993). The oxygen consumption/oxygen delivery curve in severe preeclampsia: evidence for a fixed oxygen extraction state. *Am. J. Obstet. Gynecol.*, **169**, 1448–55.

Bernstein, I. M., Meyer, M. C., Osol, G. and Ward, K. (1998a). Intolerance to volume expansion: a theorized mechanism for the development of preeclampsia. *Obstet. Gynecol.*, **92**, 306–8.

Bernstein, I. M., Ziegler, W., Stirewalt, W. S., Brumsted, J. and Ward, K. (1998b). Angiotensinogen genotype and plasma volume in nulligravid women. *Obstet. Gynecol.*, **92**, 171–3.

Caniggia, I., Wu, Y. Y. and Zamudio, S. (2002). Overexpression of HIF-1 alpha in placentas from high altitude pregnancies. *Placenta*, **23**, A49.

Chapman, A. B., Abraham, W. T., Zamudio, S., *et al.* (1998). Temporal relationships between hormonal and hemodynamic changes in early human pregnancy. *Kidney Int.*, **54**, 2056–63.

Chesley, L. (1978). *Hypertensive Disorders of Pregnancy*. New York: Appleton-Century-Crofts.

Coussons-Read, M. E., Mazzeo, R. S., Whitford, M. H., Schmitt, M., Moore, L. G. and Zamudio, S. (2002). High altitude residence during pregnancy alters cytokine and catecholamine levels. *Am. J. Reprod. Immunol.*, **48**, 344–54.

Crandall, M. E., Keve, T. M. and McLaughlin, M. K. (1990). Characterization of norepinephrine sensitivity in the maternal splanchnic circulation during pregnancy. *Am. J. Obstet. Gynecol.*, **162**, 1296–301.

Croall, J., Sherrif, S. and Matthews, J. (1978). Non-pregnant maternal plasma volume and fetal growth retardation. *Br. J. Obstet. Gynaecol.*, **85**, 90–5.

Curran-Everett, D., Morris, K. G., Jr. and Moore, L. G. (1991). Regional circulatory contributions to increased systemic vascular conductance of pregnancy. *Am. J. Physiol.*, **261**, H1842–7.

Darmochwal-Kolarz, D., Rolinski, J., Leszczynska-Goarzelak, B. and Oleszczuk, J. (2002). The expressions of intracellular cytokines in the lymphocytes of preeclamptic patients. *Am. J. Reprod. Immunol.*, **48**, 381–6.

Dogterom, J. and DeJong, W. (1973). Diminished pressor response to noradrenaline of the perfused tail artery of pregnant rats. *Eur. J. Pharmacol.*, **25**, 267–9.

Dustan, H., Tarazi, R., Bravo, E. and Dart, R. (1973). Plasma and extracellular fluid volumes in hypertension. *Circ. Res. Suppl.*, **1**, I73–81.

Elenkov, I. J. and Chrousos, G. P. (1999). Stress hormones, Th1/Th2 patterns, pro/anti-inflammatory cytokines and susceptibility to disease. *Trends Endocrinol. Metab.*, **10**, 359–68.

Elenkov, I. J. and Chrousos, G. P. (2002). Stress hormones, proinflammatory and antiinflammatory cytokines, and autoimmunity. *Ann. N. Y. Acad. Sci.*, **966**, 290–303.

Eskenazi, B., Fenster, L. and Sidney, S. (1991). A multivariate analysis of risk factors for preeclampsia. *J. Am. Med. Ass.*, **266**, 237–41.

Gant, N. F., Daley, G. L., Chand, S., Whalley, P. J. and MacDonald, P. C. (1973). A study of angiotensin II pressor response throughout primigravid pregnancy. *J. Clin. Invest.*, **52**, 2682–9.

Gibson, H. (1973). Plasma volume and glomerular filtration rate in pregnancy and their relation to differences in fetal growth. *J. Obstet. Gynaecol. Br. Com.*, **80**, 1067–74.

Goodlin, R., Quaife, M. and Dirksen, J. (1981). The significance, diagnosis and treatment of maternal hypovolemia as associated with fetal/maternal illness. *Semin. Perinatol.*, **5**, 163–74.

Greenwood, J. P., Stoker, J. B., Walker, J. J. and Mary, D. A. (1998). Sympathetic nerve discharge in normal pregnancy and pregnancy-induced hypertension. *J. Hypertens.*, **16**, 617–24.

Greenwood, J. P., Scott, E. M., Stoker, J. B., Walker, J. J. and Mary, D. A. (2001). Sympathetic neural mechanisms in normal and hypertensive pregnancy in humans. *Circulation*, **104**, 2200–4.

Greenwood, J. P., Scott, E. M., Walker, J. J., Stoker, J. B. and Mary, D. A. (2003). The magnitude of sympathetic hyperactivity in pregnancy-induced hypertension and preeclampsia. *Am. J. Hypertens.*, **16**, 194–9.

Greer, I. A., Lyall, F., Perera, T., Boswell, F. and Macara, L. M. (1994). Increased concentrations of cytokines interleukin-6 and interleukin-1 receptor antagonist in plasma of women with preeclampsia: a mechanism for endothelial dysfunction? *Obstet. Gynecol.*, **84**, 937–40.

Grover, R. F., Weil, J. V. and Reeves, J. T. (1986). Cardiovascular adaptations to hypoxia. In *Exercise Sports Science Reviews*, ed. K. B. Pandolf. New York: Macmillan, pp. 269–302.

Harrison, G. L. and Moore, L. G. (1989). Blunted vasoreactivity in pregnant guinea pigs is not restored by meclofenamate. *Am. J. Obstet. Gynecol.*, **160**, 258–64.

Harrison, G. L. and Moore, L. G. (1990). Systemic vascular reactivity during high-altitude pregnancy. *J. Appl. Physiol.*, **69**, 201–6.

Harrison, G. L., McMurtry, I. F. and Moore, L. G. (1986). Meclofenamate potentiates vasoreactivity to alpha-adrenergic stimulation in chronically hypoxic guinea pigs. *Am. J. Physiol.*, **251**, H496–501.

Hohmann, M., Keve, T. M., Osol, G. and McLaughlin, M. K. (1990). Norepinephrine sensitivity of mesenteric veins in pregnant rats. *Am. J. Physiol.*, **259**, R753–9.

Hurtado, A., Merino, C. and Delgado, E. (1945). Influence of anoxemia on hematopoietic activity. *Arch. Intern. Med.*, **75**, 284–323.

Jensen, G. M. and Moore, L. G. (1997). The effect of high altitude and other risk factors on birthweight: independent or interactive effects? *Am. J. Public Health*, **87**, 1003–7.

Kanayama, N., Tsujimura, R., She, L., Maehara, K. and Terao, T. (1997). Cold-induced stress stimulates the sympathetic nervous system, causing hypertension and proteinuria in rats. *J. Hypertens.*, **15**, 383–9.

Keyes, L., Rodman, D. M., Curran-Everett, D., Morris, K. and Moore, L. G. (1998). Effect of K+ATP channel inhibition on total and regional vascular resistance in guinea pig pregnancy. *Am. J. Physiol.*, **275**, H680–8.

Keyes, L. E., Armaza, J. F., Niermeyer, S., Vargas, E., Young, D. A. and Moore, L. G. (2003). Intrauterine growth restriction, preeclampsia, and intrauterine mortality at high altitude in Bolivia. *Pediatr. Res.*, **54**, 20–5.

Khatun, S., Kanayama, N., Belayet, H. M., *et al.* (2000). Increased concentrations of plasma neuropeptide Y in patients with eclampsia and preeclampsia. *Am. J. Obstet. Gynecol.*, **182**, 896–900.

Kingdom, J. and Kaufmann, P. (1999). Oxygen and placental vascular development. *Adv. Exp. Med. Biol.*, **474**, 259–75.

Kingdom, J. C. P. and Kaufmann, P. (1997). Oxygen and placental villous development. *Placenta*, **18**, 613–21.

Klonoff-Cohen, H., Edelstein, S. and Savitz, D. (1993). Cigarette smoking and preeclampsia. *Obstet. Gynecol.*, **81**, 541–4.

Klonoff-Cohen, H. S., Savitz, D. A., Cefalo, R. C. and McCann, M. F. (1989). An epidemiologic study of contraception and preeclampsia. Comments. *J. Am. Med. Ass.*, **262**, 3143–7.

Kobayashi, T., Sugimura, M., Tokunaga, N., *et al.* (2002). Anticholinergics induce eclamptic seizures. *Semin. Thromb. Hemost.*, **28**, 511–14.

Krampl, E. R., Espinoza-Dorado, J., Lees, C. C., Moscoso, G., Bland, J. M. and Campbell, S. (2001). Maternal uterine artery Doppler studies at high altitude and sea level. *Ultrasound Obstet. Gynecol.*, **18**, 578–82.

Kreczy, A., Fusi, L. and Wigglesworth, J. S. (1995). Correlation between umbilical arterial flow and placental morphology. *Int. J. Gynecol. Pathol.*, **14**, 306–9.

Kubo, K., Hanaoka, M., Hayano, T., *et al.* (1998). Inflammatory cytokines in BAL fluid and pulmonary hemodynamics in high-altitude pulmonary edema. *Respir. Physiol.*, **111**, 301–10.

Kupferminc, M. J., Peaceman, A. M., Wigton, T. R., Rehnberg, K. A. and Socol, M. L. (1994). Tumor necrosis factor-alpha is elevated in plasma and amniotic fluid of patients with severe preeclampsia. *Am. J. Obstet. Gynecol.*, **170**, 1752–7; discussion 1757–9.

Labarrere, C. A. and Faulk, W. P. (1994). Antigenic identification of cells in spiral artery trophoblastic invasion: validation of histologic studies by triple-antibody immunocytochemistry. *Am. J. Obstet. Gynecol.*, **171**, 165–71.

Lewinsky, R. M. and Riskin-Mashiah, S. (1998). Autonomic imbalance in preeclampsia: evidence for increased sympathetic tone in response to the supine-pressor test. *Obstet. Gynecol.*, **91**, 935–9.

Lin, S., Shimizu, I., Suehara, N., Nakayama, M. and Aono, T. (1995). Uterine artery Doppler velocimetry in relation to trophoblast migration in to the myometrium of the placental bed. *Obstet. Gynecol.*, **85**, 760–5.

Longo, L. and Hardesty, J. (1984). Maternal blood volume: measurement, hypothesis of control and clinical considerations. *Rev. Perinat. Med.*, **5**, 35–59.

Lunell, N., Nylund, L., Lewander, R., Sarby, B. and Thornstrom, S. (1982). Uteroplacental blood flow in pre-eclampsia measurements with indium-113m and a computer-linked gamma camera. *Clin. Exp. Hypertens. Pregn.*, **B1**(1), 105–17.

Lyall, F., Myatt, L., Cousins, F., Barber, A. and Zamudio, S. (2002). Abnormal expression of hemeoxygenase in placentae from high altitude pregnancies. *J. Soc. Gynecol. Invest.*, **9**, 223A.

Lyall, F., Cousins, F., Duffie, L. and Zamudio, S. (2003). VCAM-1 concentrations are reduced in the maternal circulation in high altitude pregnancies. *J. Soc. Gynecol. Invest.*, **10**, 308A.

Macara, L., Kingdom, J. C., Kaufmann, P., *et al.* (1996). Structural analysis of placental terminal villi from growth-restricted pregnancies with abnormal umbilical artery Doppler waveforms. *Placenta*, **17**, 37–48.

Magness, R. R. and Rosenfeld, C. R. (1986). Systemic and uterine responses to alpha-adrenergic stimulation in pregnant and nonpregnant ewes. *Am. J. Obstet. Gynecol.*, **155**, 897–904.

Mahfouz, A. A. R., El-Aid, M. M., Alakija, W. and Al-Erian, R. A. G. (1994). Altitude and socio-biological determinants of pregnancy-associated hypertension. *Int. J. Obstet. Gynecol.*, **44**, 135–8.

Marks, L., Zamudio, S. and Lyall, F. (2002). MMP-9 expression is abnormal in placentae at high altitude: a link to chronic hypoxia. *Hypertens. Pregn.*, **21**, 111.

Marks, L., Zamudio, S., Cousins, F., Duffie, E. and Lyall, F. (2006). Endothelial activation and cell adhesion molecule concentrations in pregnant women living at high altitude. *J. Soc. Gynecol. Invest.*, **13**, 399–403.

Mateev, S., Sillau, A. H., Mouser, R., *et al.* (2003). Chronic hypoxia opposes pregnancy-induced increase in uterine artery vasodilator response to flow. *Am. J. Physiol. Heart Circ. Physiol.*, **284**, H820–9.

Mazzeo, R. S., Bender, P. R., Brooks, G. A., *et al.* (1991). Arterial catecholamine responses during exercise with acute and chronic high altitude exposure. *Am. J. Physiol.*, **261**, E419–24.

Mazzeo, R. S., Child, A., Butterfield, G. E., Mawson, J. T., Zamudio, S. and Moore, L. G. (1998). Catecholamine response during 12 days of high-altitude exposure (4300 m) in women. *J. Appl. Physiol.*, **84**, 1151–7.

Mazzeo, R. S., Carroll, J. D., Butterfield, G. E., *et al.* (2001a). Catecholamine responses to alpha-adrenergic blockade during exercise in women acutely exposed to altitude. *J. Appl. Physiol.*, **90**, 121–6.

Mazzeo, R. S., Donovan, D., Fleshner, M., *et al.* (2001b). Interleukin-6 response to exercise and high-altitude exposure: influence of alpha-adrenergic blockade. *J. Appl. Physiol.*, **91**, 2143–9.

McLaughlin, M. K., Keve, T. M. and Cooke, R. (1989). Vascular catecholamine sensitivity during pregnancy in the ewe. *Am. J. Obstet. Gynecol.*, **160**, 47–53.

Meekins, J. W., Pijnenborg, R., Hanssens, M., McFadyen, I. R. and van Asshe, A. (1994). A study of placental bed spiral arteries and trophoblast invasion in normal and severe pre-eclamptic pregnancies. *Br. J. Obstet. Gynaecol.*, **101**, 669–74.

Minagawa, M., Narita, J., Tada, T., *et al.* (1999). Mechanisms underlying immunologic states during pregnancy: possible association of the sympathetic nervous system. *Cell Immunol.*, **196**, 1–13.

Moore, L. G., Hershey, D. W., Jahnigen, D. and Bowes, W., Jr. (1982). The incidence of pregnancy-induced hypertension is increased among Colorado residents at high altitude. *Am. J. Obstet. Gynecol.*, **144**, 423–9.

Moore, L. G., Brodeur, P., Chumbe, O., D'Brot, J., Hofmeister, S. and Monge, C. (1986). Maternal hypoxic ventilatory response, ventilation, and infant birth weight at 4,300 m. *J. Appl. Physiol.*, **60**, 1401–6.

Moore, L. G., McCullough, R. E. and Weil, J. V. (1987). Increased HVR in pregnancy: relationship to hormonal and metabolic changes. *J. Appl. Physiol.*, **62**, 158–63.

Moore, L. G., Niermeyer, S. and Zamudio, S. (1998). Human adaptation to high altitude: regional and life-cycle perspectives. *Am. J. Phys. Anthropol.* (Suppl.), 25–64.

Moutquin, J. M., Rainville, C., Giroux, L., *et al.* (1985). A prospective study of blood pressure in pregnancy: prediction of preeclampsia. *Am. J. Obstet. Gynecol.*, **151**, 191–6.

Nisell, H. and Lunell, N. O. (1984). Sympatho-adrenal activity in different hypertensive disorders in pregnancy. A short review. *Acta Obstet. Gynecol. Scand. Suppl.*, **118**, 13–16.

Nisell, H., Hjemdahl, P. and Linde, B. (1985a). Cardiovascular responses to circulating catecholamines in normal pregnancy and in pregnancy-induced hypertension. *Clin. Physiol.*, **5**, 479–93.

Nisell, H., Hjemdahl, P., Linde, B. and Lunell, N. O. (1985b). Sympatho-adrenal and cardiovascular reactivity in pregnancy-induced hypertension. I. Responses to isometric exercise and a cold pressor test. *Br. J. Obstet. Gynaecol.*, **92**, 722–31.

Nisell, H., Hjemdahl, P., Linde, B. and Lunell, N. O. (1985c). Sympathoadrenal and cardiovascular reactivity in pregnancy-induced hypertension. II. Responses to tilting. *Am. J. Obstet. Gynecol.*, **152**, 554–60.

Nylund, L., Lunell, N., Lewander, R. and Sarby, B. (1983). Uteroplacental blood flow index in intrauterine growth retardation of fetal or maternal origin. *Br. J. Obstet. Gynaecol.*, **90**, 16–20.

Oian, P., Kjeldsen, S. E., Eide, I. and Maltau, J. M. (1986). Increased arterial catecholamines in pre-eclampsia. *Acta Obstet. Gynecol. Scand.*, **65**, 613–16.

Omu, A. E., Al-Qattan, F., Diejomaoh, M. E. and Al-Yatama, M. (1999). Differential levels of T helper cytokines in preeclampsia: pregnancy, labor and puerperium. *Acta Obstet. Gynecol. Scand.*, **78**, 675–80.

Page, E. W. and Christianson, R. (1976). Influence of blood pressure changes with and without proteinuria upon outcome of pregnancy. *Am. J. Obstet. Gynecol.*, **126**, 821–33.

Palmer, S. K., Zamudio, S., Coffin, C., Parker, S., Stamm, E. and Moore, L. G. (1992). Quantitative estimation of human uterine artery blood flow and pelvic blood flow redistribution in pregnancy. *Obstet. Gynecol.*, **80**, 1000–6.

Palmer, S. K., Moore, L. G., Young, D. A., Cregger, B., Berman, J. C. and Zamudio, S. (1999). Altered blood pressure course during normal pregnancy and increased preeclampsia at high altitude (3100 meters) in Colorado. *Am. J. Obstet. Gynecol.*, **180**, 1161–8.

Parent, A., Schiffrin, E. L. and St-Louis, J. (1990). Role of the endothelium in adrenergic responses of mesenteric artery rings of pregnant rats. *Am. J. Obstet. Gynecol.*, **163**, 229–34.

Pedersen, E. B., Rasmussen, A. B., Christensen, N. J., *et al.* (1982). Plasma noradrenaline and adrenaline in pre-eclampsia, essential hypertension in pregnancy and normotensive pregnant control subjects. *Acta Endocrinol. (Copenh.)*, **99**, 594–600.

Piccinni, M. P. and Romagnani, S. (1996). Regulation of fetal allograft survival by a hormone-controlled Th1- and Th2-type cytokines. *Immunol. Res.*, **15**, 141–50.

Piccinni, M. P., Maggi, E. and Romagnani, S. (2000). Role of hormone-controlled T-cell cytokines in the maintenance of pregnancy. *Biochem. Soc. Trans.*, **28**, 212–15.

Pijnenborg, R., Anthony, J., Davey, D. A., *et al.* (1991). Placental bed spiral arteries in the hypertensive disorders of pregnancy. *Br. J. Obstet. Gynaecol.*, **98**, 648–55.

Raab, W., Schroeder, G., Wagner, R. and Gigee, W. (1956). Vascular reactivity and electrolytes in normal and toxemic pregnancy. *J. Clin. Endocrinol.*, **16**, 1196–213.

Redman, C. W. (1991). Immunology of preeclampsia. *Semin. Perinatol.*, **15**, 257–62.

Reeves, J., Moore, L., Wolfel, E., Mazzeo, R., Cymerman, A. and Young, A. (1992). Activation of the sympathoadrenal system at high altitude. In *High Altitude Medicine*, ed. G. Ueda, S. Kusama and N. Voelkel. Matsumoto, Japan: Shinshu University Press, pp. 10–23.

Robertson, W., Brosens, I., DeWolf, F., Sheppard, B., Bonnar, J. and Khong, T. (1986). The placental bed biopsy: review from three European centers. *Am. J. Obstet. Gynecol.*, **155**, 401–12.

Rockwell, L. C., Keyes, L. E. and Moore, L. G. (2000). Chronic hypoxia diminishes pregnancy-associated DNA synthesis in guinea pig uteroplacental arteries. *Placenta*, **21**, 313–19.

Saftlas, A. F., Olson, D. R., Franks, A. L., Atrash, H. K. and Pokras, R. (1990). Epidemiology of preeclampsia and eclampsia in the United States, 1979–1986. *Am. J. Obstet. Gynecol.*, **163**, 460–5.

Saito, S. and Sakai, M. (2003). Th1/Th2 balance in preeclampsia. *J. Reprod. Immunol.*, **59**, 161–73.

Saito, S., Sakai, M., Sasaki, Y., Tanebe, K., Tsuda, H. and Michimata, T. (1999a). Quantitative analysis of peripheral blood Th0, Th1, Th2 and the Th1:Th2 cell ratio during normal human pregnancy and preeclampsia. *Clin. Exp. Immunol.*, **117**, 550–5.

Saito, S., Umekage, H., Sakamoto, Y., *et al.* (1999b). Increased T-helper-1-type immunity and decreased T-helper-2-type immunity in patients with pre-eclampsia. *Am. J. Reprod. Immunol.*, **41**, 297–306.

Sanchez, C., Merino, C. and Figallo, M. (1970). Simultaneous measurement of plasma volume and red cell mass in polycythemia of high altitude. *J. Appl. Physiol.*, **28**, 776–8.

Schobel, H. P., Fischer, T., Heuszer, K., Geiger, H. and Schmieder, R. E. (1996). Preeclampsia – a state of sympathetic overactivity. *N. Engl. J. Med.*, **335**, 1480–5.

Shime, J., Mocarski, E. J., Hastings, D., Webb, G. D. and McLaughlin, P. R. (1987). Congenital heart disease in pregnancy: short- and long-term implications. *Am. J. Obstet. Gynecol.*, **156**, 313–22. Erratum appears in *Am. J. Obstet. Gynecol.* 1987, **156**(5): 1361.

Sibai, B. M., Gordon, T., Thom, E., *et al.* (1995). Risk factors for preeclampsia in healthy nulliparous women: a prospective multicenter study. The National Institute of Child Health and Human Development Network of Maternal–Fetal Medicine Units. *Am. J. Obstet. Gynecol.*, **172**, 642–8.

Sillau, A. H., McCullough, R. E., Dyckes, R., White, M. M. and Moore, L. G. (2002). Chronic hypoxia increases MCA contractile response to U-46619 by reducing NO production and/or activity. *J. Appl. Physiol.*, **92**, 1859–64.

Soleymanlou, N., Jurisica, I., Nevo, O., *et al.* (2005). Molecular evidence of placental hypoxia in preeclampsia. *J. Clin. Endocrinol. Metab.*, **90**, 4299–308.

Starzyk, K. A., Salafia, C. M., Pezzullo, J. C., *et al.* (1997). Quantitative differences in arterial morphometry define the placental bed in preeclampsia. *Hum. Pathol.*, **28**, 353–8.

Stokke, K. T., Rootwell, K., Wergeland, R. and Vale, J. R. (1986). Changes in plasma and red cell volume during exposure to high altitude. *Scand. J. Clin. Lab. Invest.*, **46**, 113–17.

Stone, J. L., Lockwood, C. J., Berkowitz, G. S., Alvarez, M., Lapinski, R. and Berkowitz, R. L. (1994). Risk factors for severe preeclampsia. *Obstet. Gynecol.*, **83**, 357–61.

Talledo, O. E., Chesley, L. C. and Zuspan, F. P. (1968). Renin–angiotensin system in normal and toxemic pregnancies. III. Differential sensitivity to angiotensin II and norepineprhine in toxemia of pregnancy. *Am. J. Obstet. Gynecol.*, **100**, 218–21.

Tissot van Patot, M., Grilli, A., Chapman, P., *et al.* (2003). Remodelling of uteroplacental arteries is decreased in high altitude placentae. *Placenta*, **24**, 326–35.

Ulrych, M., Frolich E., Tarazi, R. C., Dustan, H. P. and Page, I. H. (1969). Cardiac output and distribution of blood volume in central and peripheral circulations in hypertensive and normotensive man. *Br. Heart J.*, **31**, 570–4.

Veith, G. L. and Rice, G. E. (1999). Interferon gamma expression during human pregnancy and in association with labour. *Gynecol. Obstet. Invest.*, **48**, 163–7.

Villar, M. A. and Sibai, B. M. (1989). Clinical significance of elevated mean arterial blood pressure in second trimester and threshold increase in systolic or diastolic blood pressure during third trimester. *Am. J. Obstet. Gynecol.*, **160**, 419–23.

Vives, A., Balasch, J., Yague, J., Quinto, L., Ordi, J. and Vanrell, J. A. (1999). Type-1 and type-2 cytokines in human decidual tissue and trophoblasts from normal and abnormal pregnancies detected by reverse transcriptase polymerase chain reaction (RT-PCR). *Am. J. Reprod. Immunol.*, **42**, 361–8.

Weil, J., Byrne-Quinn, E., Battock, D., Grover, R. and Chidsey, C. (1971). Forearm circulation in man at high altitude. *Clin. Sci.*, **40**, 234–46.

White, M. M. and Zhang, L. (2003). Effects of chronic hypoxia on maternal vasodilation and vascular reactivity in guinea pig and ovine pregnancy. *High Alt. Med. Biol.*, **4**, 157–69.

White, M. M., Zamudio, S., Stevens, T., *et al.* (1995). Estrogen, progesterone, and vascular reactivity: potential cellular mechanisms. *Endocrine Rev.*, **16**, 739–51.

White, M. M., McCullough, R. E., Dyckes, R., Robertson, A. D. and Moore, L. G. (1998). Effects of pregnancy and chronic hypoxia on contractile responsiveness to alpha1-adrenergic stimulation. *J. Appl. Physiol.*, **85**, 2322–9.

White, M. M., McCullough, R. E., Dyckes, R., Robertson, A. D. and Moore, L. G. (2000). Chronic hypoxia, pregnancy, and endothelium-mediated relaxation in guinea pig uterine and thoracic arteries. *Am. J. Physiol. Heart Circ. Physiol.*, **278**, H2069–75.

Wolfel, E. E., Groves, B. M., Brooks, G. A., *et al.* (1991). Oxygen transport during steady-state submaximal exercise in chronic hypoxia. *J. Appl. Physiol.*, **70**, 1129–36.

Zamudio, S. (2003). The placenta at high altitude. *High Alt. Med. Biol.*, **4**, 171–91.

Zamudio, S., Palmer, S. K., Dahms, T. E., *et al.* (1993a). Blood volume expansion, preeclampsia, and infant birth weight at high altitude. *J. Appl. Physiol.*, **74**, 1566–73.

Zamudio, S., Palmer, S., Droma, T., Stamm, E., Coffin, C. and Moore, L. (1995a). Effect of altitude on uterine artery blood flow during normal pregnancy. *J. Appl. Physiol.*, **79**, 7–14.

Zamudio, S., Palmer, S. K., Dahms, T. E., Berman, J. C., Young, D. and Moore, L. G. (1995b). Alterations in uterine blood flow velocity and pelvic blood flow distribution precede the onset of of hypertension during pregnancy at high altitude. *J. Appl. Physiol.*, **79**, 15–22.

Zamudio, S., Palmer, S. K., Regensteiner, J. G. and Moore, L. G. (1995e). High altitude and hypertension during pregnancy. *Am. J. Human. Biol.*, **7**, 182–93.

Zamudio, S., Palmer, S. K., Stamm, E., Coffin, C. and Moore, L. G (1995f). Uterine blood flow at high altitude. In *Hypoxia and the Brain*, ed. J. R. Sutton and C. S. Houston. Burlington, VT: Queen City Press, pp. 112–24.

Zamudio, S., Douglas, M., Mazzeo, R. S., *et al.* (2001). Women at altitude: forearm hemodynamics during acclimatization to 4,300 m with alpha(1)-adrenergic blockade. *Am. J. Physiol. Heart Circ. Physiol.*, **281**, H2636–44.

Zamudio, S., Wheeler, T., Anthony, F. and Moore, L. G. (2002). Vascular endothelial growth factor (VEGF), vascular resistance and villous angiogenesis at high altitude (3100 m). *J. Soc. Gynecol. Invest.*, **9**, 141A.

Zamudio, S., Kovalenko, O., Vanderlelie, J., *et al.* (2007). Chronic hypoxia in vivo reduces placental oxidative stress. *Placenta*, in press.

Zuspan, F. P. (1976). Urinary amine excretion in pregnancy-induced hypertension. In *Hypertension in Pregnancy*, ed. M. D. Lindheimer, A. I. Katz and F. P. Zuspan. New York: John Wiley and Sons, pp. 339–46.

Zuspan, F. P. (1977). Pregnancy induced hypertension. 1. Role of sympathetic nervous system and adrenal gland. *Acta Obstet. Gynecol. Scand.*, **56**, 283–6.

Zuspan, F. P. (1979). Catecholamines. Their role in pregnancy and the development of pregnancy-induced hypertension. *J. Reprod. Med.*, **23**, 143–50.

14

The use of mouse models to explore fetal–maternal interactions underlying pre-eclampsia

James C. Cross

While the disease has been studied for decades, the pathogenesis of pre-eclampsia remains mysterious. However, studies of the disease in humans are confounded by the fact that while the disease manifests in the second and third trimester its origins likely begin in the first trimester (Cross, 1996; Roberts and Cooper, 2001; Roberts and Lain, 2002). This makes defining both the etiology and the subsequent pathological events rather difficult, and researchers are limited to making inferences from pathological specimens, and distinguishing between primary and secondary events can be impossible. Despite these challenges, the fact that pre-eclampsia is strictly a disease of pregnancy indicates that the fetus and/or placenta interact with maternal factors to produce the disease. Indeed, several lines of evidence support the idea that placental development and/or function are abnormal in pre-eclampsia (Cross, 1996; Roberts and Cooper, 2001; Roberts and Lain, 2002). The strict requirement for a fetal–maternal interaction has led to the hypothesis that both feto-placental defects and maternal susceptibility to hypertensive and/or renal disease are required in order to initiate the disease (Cross, 1996; Lachmeijer et al., 2002; Roberts and Cooper, 2001; Roberts and Lain, 2002). However, as reviewed here, emerging evidence from mouse and rat models shows that pre-eclampsia can be initiated by multiple means, each producing all of the pathognomonic features of the disease – gestational hypertension, proteinuria and renal glomerular lesions (Davisson et al., 2002; Faas et al., 1995; Kanayama et al., 2002; Maynard et al., 2003; Sakawi et al., 2000;

Wardle, 1976). In general, these data support a model in which pre-eclampsia can be initiated by either a feto-placental or a maternal susceptibility, and that there is not a strict requirement for both (Cross, 2003). The advantage of this model is that it predicts that not all forms of pre-eclampsia will show the same types of pathological changes, and therefore it can explain the heterogeneity of pathological changes that have been described in humans (Roberts and Lain, 2002).

Comparison of pregnancy in rodents and humans

Many of the features of pregnancy in rodents are different than in humans, such as a gestation length of 3 weeks versus 9 months and the fact that rodents usually give birth to litters rather than singletons. Despite these obvious differences, however, the fact that rodents can develop pre-eclampsia shows that there is more in common between rodents and humans than is widely appreciated. A number of anatomical and physiological features of pregnancy are similar in humans and rodents (Table 14.1). At a structural level, the conceptus in rodents, as in humans, invades into the uterine wall after implantation and promotes increased maternal blood flow to the implantation site by promoting both increased blood vessel formation (angiogenesis) and vasodilation (Cross et al., 2002). The outermost cells of the rodent placenta (trophoblast giant cells) are analogous to extravillous cytotrophoblast cells in humans invade

Table 14.1. Comparison of pregnancy and placental structure in humans and mice

	Human	Mouse
Length of gestation	9 months	20 days
Stage of implantation (post-fertilization)	7 days	4.5 days
Initiation of fetal heartbeat	21 days	8.5 days
Vascularization of placental villi	25 days	10 days
Hemochorial blood flow through placenta	Yes	Yes
Chorionic villi lined by syncytiotrophoblast	Yes	Yes
Invasive trophoblast cell subtype entering uterine spiral arteries	Extravillous cytotrophoblast	Trophoblast giant cells

into the spiral arteries and replace their endothelial linings, promoting the transition from endothelial lined artery to trophoblast-lined (hemochorial) blood space. The bulk of the mature placenta is a villous tree-like structure, called the labyrinth, that forms the surface for nutrient and gas exchange (Cross, 2000; Cross *et al.*, 2003; Rossant and Cross, 2001). The labyrinth is covered by three trophoblast layers (two layers of syncytiotrophoblast), and has an inner core with a dense capillary network. At a physiological level, rodents and humans show a similar fall in blood pressure during late gestation that is likely initiated by feto-placental factors (Davisson *et al.*, 2002; Wong *et al.*, 2002).

Studying development and the physiology of pregnancy in rodents obviously has considerable advantages because of the ability to carefully control both genetic and environmental influences. Indeed, in mice, it is possible to alter gene function using transgenic and knockout mouse approaches, and by control of the way in which mice are bred or embryo transfer between normal (wildtype) and mutant strains it is possible to control whether the

altered gene is present in the feto-placental unit, the mother or both. In addition, because gestation is short and the reproductive tract is relatively small in rodents, it is possible to analyze the events of pregnancy in great detail.

Rodent models of pre-eclampsia: insights into the diverse origins of the disease

In the last few years, a number of rodent models have been reported in which pregnant females develop the classic signs of pre-eclampsia including hypertension, proteinuria and renal glomerulosclerosis, and several others that show at least some of the associated features such as fetal growth restriction (Table 14.2). While each of the models is interesting in its own way, collectively they give us insights into what factors are and are not sufficient to initiate the pathogenesis of pre-eclampsia.

Hypertension as a predisposing factor for pre-eclampsia

In humans, the risk factors of essential hypertension and pre-eclampsia overlap considerably and, indeed, pre-existing hypertension increases the risk of pre-eclampsia (Eskenazi *et al.*, 1991; Sibai *et al.*, 1995). It is therefore not surprising that some genes that have been implicated as risk factors for pre-eclampsia, *AGT* (encoding angiotensinogen, a precursor of the vasoconstrictor angiotensin) (Ward *et al.*, 1993) and *NOS3* (encoding endothelial nitric oxide synthetase, eNOS) (Arngrimsson *et al.*, 1997), are also risk factors for essential hypertension. Notably, the associations with the *AGT* and *NOS3* genes have not been confirmed in all affected families (Lachmeijer *et al.*, 2002; Roberts and Cooper, 2001), implying that *AGT* and *NOS3* mutations likely do not explain all cases of pre-eclampsia. Based on these human studies alone it is difficult to say whether hypertension alone is sufficient to promote the development of pre-eclampsia. However, recent work in mice suggests that it is.

Table 14.2. Rodent models of pre-eclampsia and intrauterine growth restriction

Model	Primary defect	High BP	Proteinuria	Renal lesions	Placental changes	IUGR
BPH/5 strain	Hypertension	Yes	Yes	Yes	?	?
REN–AGT transgenic	Gestational hypertension	Yes	Yes	Yes	?	?
p57^{Kip2} mutant	Placental development	Yes	Yes	Yes	Labyrinth, giant cells	No
Endotoxin-induced	Inflammatory disease	Yes	Yes	Yes	?	?
Soluble Flt1 administration	Endothelial dysfunction	Yes	Yes	Yes	?	?
Esx1 mutant	Placental development	?	?	?	Vascularization of labyrinth	Yes
Igf2 mutant	Placental transport	?	?	?	Reduced nutrient transport	Yes
Rag2/γc null	NK cell-deficient	?	?	?	Constricted spiral arteries	?

The BPH/5 strain of mice was identified as a borderline hypertensive line that in follow up studies was found to develop high blood pressure during pregnancy. Whereas the mean arterial blood pressure in normal mice falls during mid to late gestation, it increases in BPH/5 pregnant females (Davisson *et al.*, 2002). This implies that a pregnancy-specific factor interacts with and exacerbates the propensity for increased blood pressure. Interestingly, the BPH/5 mice also develop renal glomerulosclerosis and proteinuria in late pregnancy. While the gene underlying the defect is unknown, the data are consistent with the hypothesis that hypertension, at least during pregnancy (even an otherwise normal pregnancy), is sufficient to initiate the full spectrum of clinical signs of pre-eclampsia. Notably, proteinuria and glomerulosclerosis are also observed when the renin–angiotensin system (RAS) is constitutively activated in transgenic mice even in the non-pregnant state (Caron *et al.*, 2002). Overexpression of angiotensinogen alone is not sufficient to produce pre-eclampsia, even though blood pressure is higher than in wildtype mice due to a failure to decline during pregnancy (Hefler *et al.*, 2001), indicating that placental renin is required to cause the full spectrum of disease.

Placental contribution to maternal hypertension

The normal drop in blood pressure during healthy pregnancy in humans and rodents implies that the feto-placental unit regulates maternal blood pressure. The placenta is a major source of vasoactive compounds such as nitric oxide, adrenomedullin, prostaglandins and prostacyclins (Cross, 1996; Cross *et al.*, 2002), as well as renin (Cooper *et al.*, 1999; Xia *et al.*, 2002), an enzyme that cleaves angiotensinogen to produce the vasoconstrictor angiotensin II. Therefore, through these and potentially other factors, the placenta is likely to be a direct regulator of maternal cardiovascular function though formal proof for most factors is largely missing. Female mice that are deficient for *NOS3* (eNOS) show higher blood pressure throughout pregnancy even if they are carrying non-mutant conceptuses (Hefler *et al.*, 2001), but no attempt has yet been made to assess the relative roles of feto-placental production. Adrenomedullin appears to have an essential role in blood pressure regulation (Shindo *et al.*, 2001), although homozygous mutant embryos die in utero precluding a thorough analysis of placentally derived adrenomedullin in regulating maternal cardiovascular function. The role of placental renin has been demonstrated in a transgenic mouse model in which females carrying an angiotensinogen (*AGT*) transgene are mated to males that are transgenic for a renin (*REN*) gene. The females develop gestational hypertension as a result of placental expression of renin and also proteinuria and glomerulosclerosis (Takimoto *et al.*, 1996), implying that hypertension can initiate pre-eclampsia as in the BPH/5 mouse model.

Feto-placental defects leading to pre-eclampsia

Mice that are deficient for the cyclin-dependent kinase inhibitor, p57^{Kip2}, are the basis of an interesting model of pre-eclampsia because placental lesions are observed and because the maternal disease is secondary to the placental defects (Kanayama *et al.*, 2002; Takahashi *et al.*, 2000). In this model, females that carry p57^{Kip2}-deficient pups develop pre-eclampsia, even though they have normal p57^{Kip2} function and, as such, the maternal disease is due to the mutation impacting feto-placental development. The mutant pups are often growth-restricted and show a significantly reduced villous surface area in the placenta (Takahashi *et al.*, 2000), and these changes are sufficient to account for the fact that mutant embryos either die in utero or, even if they survive to term, are growth-restricted. An important feature of this model is that pre-eclampsia develops even if not all of the conceptuses in a litter are mutant. It is unclear if the onset of the disease is correlated with the absolute number of mutant conceptuses or with the relative proportion of mutant and wildtype ones. It would be fruitful to explore this issue in order to distinguish between two main hypotheses that concern how abnormal placental function may contribute to the disease: that the maternal disease is initiated by failure of specific placental functions related to vascular adaptation to pregnancy, or that feto-placental undernutrition/hypoxia leads to production of "toxic" compounds.

Intrauterine growth restriction due to placental defects

There are several mouse models in which placental function is compromised in different ways resulting in fetal growth restriction or even death (Table 14.2). *Esx1* mutants show a defect in the vascularization of the labyrinth layer of the placenta (Li and Behringer, 1998). Mice in which placental expression of *Igf2* is reduced by gene knockout (Constancia *et al.*, 2002) or in transgenics overexpressing an IGF binding protein have reduced placental transport function (Crossey *et al.*, 2002). *Rag2/γc* mutant mice lack natural killer cells and show a relative constriction of the spiral arteries presumably leading to "pre-placental" undernutrition of the fetuses (Croy *et al.*, 2000). None of these models have been examined in detail to determine if the females develop pre-eclampsia, though it would be interesting to do so in order to compare the outcomes of these mice with the *p57^{Kip2}* mutants.

Systemic endothelial dysfunction

There is now considerable evidence of systemic endothelial activation during pre-eclampsia, at least during the end stages of disease (Roberts and Lain, 2002). In rats, systemic administration of low-dose endotoxin (Faas *et al.*, 1995; Sakawi *et al.*, 2000; Wardle, 1976) or soluble-Flt1 (an antagonist of vascular endothelial growth factor, VEGF) (Maynard *et al.*, 2003) results in endothelial dysfunction and development of hypertension, proteinuria and glomerulosclerosis. Interestingly, the dose of endotoxin that is required to induce these pathologies in pregnancy animals is considerably lower than in non-pregnant females (Faas *et al.*, 1995). This suggests that the systemic endothelium may be more sensitive during pregnancy. Alternatively, the difference in sensitivity may be that the primary target of the endotoxin may be the feto-placental unit and not the maternal system per se. The latter possibility should be explored by careful histological examination of the placenta.

Conclusions and implications for understanding pre-eclampsia in humans

The results from the rodent studies suggest two important conclusions that are consistent with the human disease. First, pre-eclampsia can be initiated by several different means. These data are consistent with recent human genetic studies that rule out simple genetic mechanisms (Arngrimsson *et al.*, 1995; Lachmeijer *et al.*, 2001, 2002; Roberts and Cooper, 2001; Treloar *et al.*, 2001), and actually implicate more than one locus (Lachmeijer *et al.*, 2002; Roberts and Cooper, 2001). Collectively these studies should give pause to investigators who may be trying to find the "one cause" of pre-eclampsia. Second, either a strict maternal susceptibility to hypertension or a feto-placental defect is sufficient to cause pre-eclampsia. This idea is supported by a study of pregnancy outcomes in twin sisters that indicated that pre-eclampsia is unlikely to have a strictly maternal basis (Treloar *et al.*, 2001). These studies highlight the need to classify the disease into different types (e.g. maternal versus feto-placental origin) when trying to assign etiologies.

While the rodent models have been very useful to date in defining the maternal and feto-placental contributions to pre-eclampsia, and in highlighting specific factors that precipitate the disease, these models should prove equally useful in outlining the progression of the disease. It is interesting that the events of later development that take the last 8 months of gestation in humans occur in only the last 9 days in mice, and yet this short time is sufficient for the clinical signs to develop. This is a huge theoretical advantage when trying to identify feto-placental factors that contribute to normal cardiovascular adaptations to pregnancy and to disease, because it considerably narrows the window during which to look. It should therefore allow investigators to more likely identify markers of disease onset rather than simply the ongoing disease itself.

Acknowledgements

The work from the author's laboratory was supported by grants from the Canadian Institutes of Health Research (CIHR).

REFERENCES

Arngrimsson, R., Bjornsson, H. and Geirsson, R. T. (1995). Analysis of different inheritance patterns in preeclampsia/eclampsia syndrome. *Hypertens. Pregn.*, **14**(1), 27–38.

Arngrimsson, R., Hayward, C., Nadaud, S., *et al.* (1997). Evidence for a familial pregnancy-induced hypertension locus in the eNOS-gene region. *Am. J. Hum. Genet.*, **61**(2), 354–62.

Caron, K. M., James, L. R., Kim, H. S., *et al.* (2002). A genetically clamped renin transgene for the induction of hypertension. *Proc. Natl Acad. Sci. U.S.A.*, **99**(12), 8248–52.

Constancia, M., Hemberger, M., Hughes, J., *et al.* (2002). Placental-specific IGF-II is a major modulator of placental and fetal growth. *Nature*, **417**(6892), 945–8.

Cooper, A. C., Robinson, G., Vinson, G. P., Cheung, W. T. and Broughton Pipkin, F. (1999). The localization and expression of the renin–angiotensin system in the human placenta throughout pregnancy. *Placenta*, **20**(5–6), 467–74.

Cross, J. C. (1996). Trophoblast function in normal and preeclamptic pregnancy. *Fet. Mat. Med. Rev.*, **8**, 57–66.

Cross, J. C. (2000). Genetic insights into trophoblast differentiation and placental morphogenesis. *Semin. Cell Dev. Biol.*, **11**, 105–13.

Cross, J. C. (2003). The genetics of pre-eclampsia: a feto-placental or maternal problem? *Clin. Genet.*, **64**(2), 96–103.

Cross, J. C., Baczyk, D., Dobrik, N., *et al.* (2003). Genes, development and evolution of the placenta. *Placenta*, **24**(2–3), 123–30.

Cross, J. C., Hemberger, M., Lu, Y., *et al.* (2002). Trophoblast functions, angiogenesis and remodeling of the maternal vasculature in the placenta. *Mol. Cell Endocrinol.*, **187**(1–2), 207–12.

Crossey, P. A., Pillai, C. C. and Mrell, J. P. (2002). Altered placental development and intrauterine growth restriction in IGF binding protein-1 transgenic mice. *J. Clin. Invest.* **110**(3), 411–18.

Croy, B. A., Di Santo, J. P., Greenwood, J. D., Chantakru, S. and Ashkar, A. A. (2000). Transplantation into genetically alymphoid mice as an approach to dissect the roles of uterine natural killer cells during pregnancy – a review. *Placenta*, **21** (Suppl. A), S77–80.

Davisson, R. L., Hoffmann, D. S., Butz, G. M., *et al.* (2002). Discovery of a spontaneous genetic mouse model of preeclampsia. *Hypertension*, **39**(2, Pt. 2), 337–42.

Eskenazi, B., Fenster, L. and Sidney, S. (1991). A multivariate analysis of risk factors for preeclampsia. *J. Am. Med. Ass.*, **266**(2), 237–41.

Faas, M. M., Schuiling, G. A., Baller, J. F. and Bakker, W. W. (1995). Glomerular inflammation in pregnant rats after infusion of low dose endotoxin. An immunohistological study in experimental pre-eclampsia. *Am. J. Pathol.*, **147**(5), 1510–18.

Hefler, L. A., Tempfer, C. B., Moreno, R. M., O'Brien, W. E. and Gregg, A. R. (2001). Endothelial-derived nitric oxide and angiotensinogen: blood pressure and metabolism during mouse pregnancy. *Am. J. Physiol. Regul. Integ. Comp. Physiol.*, **280**, R174–82.

Kanayama, N., Takahashi, K., Matsuura, T., *et al.* (2002). Deficiency in p57Kip2 expression induces preeclampsia-like symptoms in mice. *Mol. Hum. Reprod.*, **8**(12), 1129–35.

Lachmeijer, A. M., Arngrimsson, R., Bastiaans, E. J., *et al.* (2001). A genome-wide scan for preeclampsia in the Netherlands. *Eur. J. Hum. Genet.*, **9**(10), 758–64.

Lachmeijer, A. M., Dekker, G. A., Pals, G., *et al.* (2002). Searching for preeclampsia genes: the current position. *Eur. J. Obstet. Gynecol. Reprod. Biol.*, **105**(2), 94–113.

Li, Y. and Behringer, R. R. (1998). Esx1 is an X-chromosome-imprinted regulator of placental development and fetal growth. *Nat. Genet.*, **20**(3), 309–11.

Maynard, S. E., Min, J. Y., Mergham, J., *et al.* (2003). Excess placental soluble fms-like tyrosine kinase 1 (sFlt1) may contribute to endothelial dysfunction, hypertension, and proteinuria in preeclampsia. *J. Clin. Invest.*, **111**(5), 649–58.

Roberts, J. M. and Cooper, D. W. (2001). Pathogenesis and genetics of pre-eclampsia. *Lancet*, **357**(9249), 53–6.

Roberts, J. M. and Lain, K. Y. (2002). Recent insights into the pathogenesis of pre-eclampsia. *Placenta*, **23**(5), 359–72.

Rossant, J. and Cross, J. C. (2001). Placental development: lessons from mouse mutants. *Nat. Rev. Genet.*, **2**(7), 538–48.

Sakawi, Y., Tarpey, M., Chen, Y. F., *et al.* (2000). Evaluation of low-dose endotoxin administration during pregnancy as a model of preeclampsia. *Anesthesiology*, **93**(6), 1446–55.

Shindo, T., Kurihara, Y., Nishimatsu, H., *et al.* (2001). Vascular abnormalities and elevated blood pressure in mice lacking adrenomedullin gene. *Circulation*, **104**(16), 1964–71.

Sibai, B. M., Gordon, T., Thom, E., *et al.* (1995). Risk factors for preeclampsia in healthy nulliparous women: a prospective multicenter study. The National Institute of Child Health and Human Development Network of Maternal–Fetal Medicine Units. *Am. J. Obstet. Gynecol.*, **172**(2, Pt. 1), 642–8.

Takahashi, K., Kobayashi, T. and Kanayama, N. (2000). p57(Kip2) regulates the proper development of labyrinthine and spongiotrophoblasts. *Mol. Hum. Reprod.*, **6**(11), 1019–25.

Takimoto, E., Ishida, J., Sugiyama, F., Horiguchi, H., Murakami, K. and Fukamizu, A. (1996). Hypertension induced in pregnant mice by placental renin and maternal angiotensinogen. *Science*, **274**(5289), 995–8.

Treloar, S. A., Cooper, D. W., Brennecke, S. P., Grehan, M. M. and Martin, N. G. (2001). An Australian twin study of the genetic basis of preeclampsia and eclampsia. *Am. J. Obstet. Gynecol.*, **184**(3), 374–81.

Ward, K., Hata, A., Jeunemaitre, X., *et al.* (1993). A molecular variant of angiotensinogen associated with preeclampsia. *Nat. Genet.*, **4**(1), 59–61.

Wardle, E. N. (1976). The functional role of intravascular coagulation renal disease. *Scott. Med. J.*, **21**(2), 83–91.

Wong, A. Y., Kulandavelu, S., Whiteley, K. J., Qu, D., Langille, B. L. and Adamson, S. L. (2002). Maternal cardiovascular changes during pregnancy and postpartum in mice. *Am. J. Physiol. Heart Circ. Physiol.*, **282**(3), H918–25.

Xia, Y., Wen, H., Prashner, H. R., *et al.* (2002). Pregnancy-induced changes in renin gene expression in mice. *Biol. Reprod.*, **66**(1), 135–43.

15

Prediction of pre-eclampsia

Leslie Myatt and Lavenia B. Carpenter

Summary

Pre-eclampsia is associated with significant maternal and fetal morbidity and mortality worldwide. While provision of adequate antenatal care would significantly reduce morbidity and mortality in third-world countries, in first-world countries efforts are being focused on identification of at-risk patients and on targeted therapies. Pre-eclampsia can be distinguished as early (<34 weeks gestation) and late (>34 weeks) onset phenotypes. While these have been thought traditionally to be synonymous with severe and mild disease phenotypes, respectively, recent analyses show that an appreciable amount of severe disease is also late onset. There is evolving evidence that there are different underlying etiologies that ultimately lead to this syndrome defined by hypertension, proteinuria and edema. It is unlikely that one single biomarker will identify all individuals destined to develop pre-eclampsia. Rather, panels of biomarkers specific for the different phenotypes may identify those at risk for pre-eclampsia prior to the appearance of overt disease. Importantly, these measurements may also provide different (biochemical) definitions of disease. In order to have a significant impact on clinical or economic outcome it is vital to identify women who will develop early onset disease or severe disease, as these phenotypes are those associated with significant morbidity and mortality. Similarly, therapies must be targeted at these same outcomes and not just the appearance of hypertension and proteinuria at term. While there is abundant evidence in the literature for changes in expression or concentration of many biomarkers in established disease, there is still a dearth of prospective studies with well-defined clinical outcomes in which prospective measurement of biomarkers have been made. Evidence is presented for selection of genetic, placental, vascular, immunologic and coagulation markers that together with clinical history may be useful in identifying those individuals at risk of developing pre-eclampsia and to whom therapy can be targeted.

Introduction

Pre-eclampsia is a syndrome unique to humans and is one of the most common complications of pregnancy worldwide (ACOG Bulletin, 1996), being associated with significant fetal and maternal morbidity and mortality. Whereas the most significant consequences of pre-eclampsia in first-world countries are neonatal morbidity and mortality associated with delivery of preterm fetuses, in third-world countries maternal morbidity and mortality are the most significant consequences. Thus in the third-world, provision of, and improvements in, antenatal care would significantly ameliorate the consequences of pre-eclampsia, whereas in the first-world prevention and/or treatment of early onset severe pre-eclampsia is the objective. In first-world countries, the majority (75%) of pre-eclampsia in nulliparous individuals is mild with onset at term, when prompt delivery of the fetus alleviates problems. Indeed, in this low-risk population, only 25% of all pre-eclampsias occur prior to 37 weeks gestation (Myatt *et al.*, 2001) and only 10% occur before 34 weeks gestational age.

The syndrome of pre-eclampsia is defined by hypertension, proteinuria, and edema evident after 20 weeks gestation and resolving after delivery. The pathophysiology of pre-eclampsia is, however, complex and it is naïve to believe that therapies that directly seek to lower blood pressure or prevent proteinuria will alleviate pre-eclampsia. Rather, therapy should be aimed at pathophysiologic pathways that impact clinically significant endpoints including reduction of fetal morbidity and mortality. The search for markers that predict the occurrence of pre-eclampsia is instinctively linked to our understanding of pathophysiology. Indeed, both facets go hand in hand. As pre-eclampsia is a heterogeneous disorder, it is unlikely that a test with perfect discrimination for those patients who will develop pre-eclampsia will be found. We need to understand pathophysiology. A test that will identify individuals who may develop pre-eclampsia with a reasonable degree of probability is useful in several ways. First, it will enable surveillance to be directed at those patients who are high-risk to develop pre-eclampsia as distinct from those in whom extensive surveillance is not required. Ideally it will also identify those who may develop clinically significant disease and may help identify those patients for targeted prophylaxis once a therapy is identified. Predictive tests can also help in the search for prophylaxis by defining patients at risk and who should be studied in clinical trials

Whilst many biomarkers have been found to be altered in individuals with established pre-eclampsia, these have mainly been small-scale cross-sectional studies of patients at term. There is an absence of studies in patients with early onset and/or severe disease to distinguish if they are of a different pathophysiology from late onset mild disease. It has been suggested that these are two distinct etiologies or phenotypes (Table 15.1). However, analysis of data from NIH trials of

Table 15.1. Pre-eclampsia phenotypes

Temporal
  Early onset (<34 weeks gestation)
  Late onset (>34 weeks gestation)
Disease severity
  Mild
  Severe
Etiology
  Placental
  Vascular
  Immunologic
  Coagulation

low-dose aspirin to prevent pre-eclampsia (Caritis *et al.*, 1998; Sibai *et al.*, 1993) does not provide evidence of temporally distinct early vs. late onset disease, although the onset of disease is significantly earlier in high-risk patient groups, and those who develop severe disease do so significantly earlier than those who develop mild disease (Myatt *et al.*, 2001, 2002). There is also a lack of prospective longitudinal studies of biomarkers that can be used to study pathophysiology and disease progression. Studies with retrospective analysis of samples collected in the first trimester and several prospective longitudinal studies are underway.

The central thrust of this chapter is that as a heterogeneous disorder the syndrome of pre-eclampsia may have differing phenotypes with differing underlying etiologies and variable involvement of different organ systems. Thus there is likely more than one cause of pre-eclampsia and therefore more than one single biomarker or set of biomarkers will be needed to identify all individuals at risk of pre-eclampsia. Thus, one can envision that whereas individuals with multifetal gestation may primarily have a trophoblast-related disease (placental phenotype), those with previous pre-eclampsia diabetes, or chronic hypertension may have a major maternal vascular or endothelial component to their disease (vascular phenotype, Table 15.1). Different biomarkers or sets of biomarkers for fetal/placental or maternal factors will

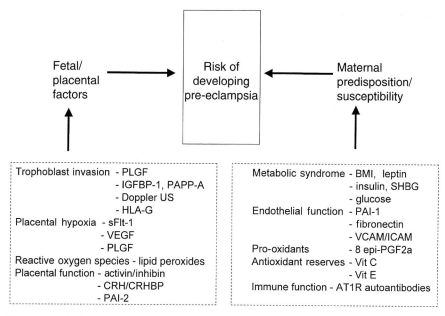

Figure 15.1 Biochemical and biophysical markers defining fetal/placental and maternal etiologies that determine the risk of developing pre-eclampsia.

identify different at-risk groups or phenotypes (Figure 15.1). They may also serve as alternate (biochemical) definitions of disease or of these pre-eclamptic phenotypes.

Etiology of pre-eclampsia

Pre-eclampsia affects 5% of all pregnancies in the USA (7% of nulliparous), but the incidence is much higher in certain high-risk groups. Pre-eclampsia can occur even in the absence of a fetus, showing that only the presence of trophoblast is necessary. Removal of trophoblastic tissue alleviates pre-eclampsia, and with increased placental mass an increased incidence is seen (Anderson and Sibai, 1986). Pregnancies complicated by pre-eclampsia and/or by fetal growth restriction are reported to have inadequate maternal vascular responses to placentation (see the chapter by Pijnenborg). Dogma has it that this defective vascular response to placentation was due to the failure of a second wave of endovascular trophoblast migration

(Pijnenborg et al., 1983). It is unlikely, though, that trophoblast invasion occurs in two distinct phases or is an all-or-none phenomenon, rather there may be a range of invasion from adequate to defective. Recent studies have shown that while invasion of interstitial trophoblast into decidua may be close to normal in pre-eclampsia, there is both a reduced amount and depth of trophoblast invasion of myometrium (Lyall, 2002; Naicker et al., 2003), and there is an absence of endovascular trophoblast in myometrial spiral arteries in pre-eclampsia (Naicker et al., 2003). The adequacy of trophoblast invasion can be measured by biophysical means (Doppler ultrasound of uterine artery flow) or biochemically (assay of VEGF, PLGF, IGFBP-1 or PAPP-A).

The endothelium is now recognized to have a pivotal role in pre-eclampsia (Roberts et al., 1989). Alterations in endothelial function have also been linked to the common theme of oxidative stress (see the chapter by Redman). This may explain in part the increased incidence of pre-eclampsia in the individual with pre-existing vascular disease (the vascular phenotype, Table 15.1).

In addition, the development of pre-eclampsia may then be determined additionally by maternal predisposition or susceptibility. We have previously presented a model where those most at risk might be those with suboptimal perfusion and the highest level of maternal susceptibility, e.g. with defective trophoblast invasion or a large placental mass coupled with pre-existing maternal vascular dysfunction (Myatt and Miodovnik, 1999).

Clinical risk factors

Several large-scale prospective prophylactic studies of pre-eclampsia have now been completed and despite being disappointing in regard to successful prophylaxis, have yielded useful data in relation to the clinical epidemiology of pre-eclampsia. The low-dose aspirin study of 1995 (Sibai *et al.*, 1995) revealed that systolic blood pressure at entry, prepregnancy obesity, the number of previous abortions or miscarriage and smoking history were risk factors for development of pre-eclampsia. Cigarette smoking during pregnancy was associated with a reduced incidence of pre-eclampsia. However, race was not a risk factor for pre-eclampsia in this study. A multivariate logistic regression equation based on these four factors could define a tenth of the population at very high risk and another tenth of the population at very low risk. In the subsequent CPEP study (Sibai *et al.*, 1997) risk factors for pre-eclampsia were found to be body mass index, systolic blood pressure and diastolic blood pressure. However, maternal age, blood group and rhesus factor, alcohol use, previous abortion or miscarriage, private insurance and calcium supplementation were not associated with significant risk of development of pre-eclampsia. In a recent review of 13 cohort studies comprising 1.4 million women, O'Brien *et al.* (2003) found that the risk of developing pre-eclampsia doubled for every $5-7 \, \text{kg m}^{-2}$ increase in prepregnancy body mass index. A family history of

pre-eclampsia has long been known to be associated with increased risk of developing it (Chesley *et al.*, 1968). It has been estimated (Cincotta and Brennecke, 1998) that a positive family history has a 20–30% risk of developing pre-eclampsia. These risk factors may be of value in counseling women but importantly target those women for detailed biochemical investigation or inclusion in clinical trials.

The prospective low-dose aspirin in high-risk pregnancy study (Caritis *et al.*, 1998) showed that the incidence of pre-eclampsia in women with chronic hypertension was 25%, pregestational diabetes 22%, multifetal gestations 16% and previous pre-eclampsia 19%. Although the rate of pre-eclampsia in these at-risk women is great, the calculated contribution of these conditions to the overall numbers of pre-eclampsia can be calculated to be 14% in nullipara, 45% among women of all parities, but would account for the majority of pre-eclampsia in multiparous women (R. Levine, personal communication). Hence, most nulliparous women, a group which contributes to the majority of cases of pre-eclampsia, are at low risk of developing it from these conditions.

Consequences of pre-eclampsia

Women who develop pre-eclampsia are at increased risk of developing recurrent pre-eclampsia, chronic hypertension (Sibai *et al.*, 1986), and maternal coronary heart disease later in life, suggesting they carry risk factors (genetic?) which may predispose them to pre-eclampsia when pregnant. A recent study of women who had developed pre-eclampsia 18–28 years previously found them to have a significantly higher diastolic blood pressure and increased concentrations of VCAM-1 and ICAM-1 but not lipoprotein (Sattar *et al.*, 2003). They also had higher glycosylated hemoglobin levels but not fasting insulin. Pregnancy can thus be considered a stress test for the maternal cardiovascular system, certainly it will never be subjected to such change again, and may therefore identify individuals such as those at risk for developing cardiovascular disease later in life or those with the metabolic syndrome. Being able to identify such risk at the time of pregnancy and applying interventions may have life-long consequences

Genetic factors

The role of genetic factors in the etiology of pre-eclampsia is well accepted, yet there is no consensus for the mode of inheritance (see the chapter by Ward). Currently, pre-eclampsia is accepted as a polygenic or multifactorial disease. Recent research has focused on maternal genes that are permissive for the development of pre-eclampsia, but there has been increasing awareness of the role of the fetal genotype. As an example, there are anecdotal reports of recurrent miscarriage resolving with a new partner (Pearson, 2002). The unique interplay of maternal and fetal genes in addition to any paternal contribution has been described by Haig (1993) as a genetic conflict between fetal gene selection to increase the transfer of nutrients and maternal gene selection to limit transfer in excess of a maternal optimum.

Increased vascular resistance is characteristic of pre-eclampsia. Abnormalities in the endothelial nitric oxide system are believed to contribute to the vasospasm seen in pre-eclampsia. The endothelial nitric oxide synthase Glu298Asp polymorphism is associated with equal enzymatic activity to the normal protein, but reduced steady-state levels due to an increase in degradation. The GLU298Asp polymorphism has not, however, been consistently linked to pre-eclampsia (Yoshimura et al., 2003). Given its role in hypertension alterations in the renin−angiotensin system have also been studied (discussed in the chapter by Ward).

Pre-eclampsia has also been described as an atherogenic state, and obesity is a risk factor for pre-eclampsia (O'Brien et al., 2003). This has prompted the evaluation of genes involved in lipid metabolism such as leptin. In a microarray analysis of placental tissue from pre-eclamptic pregnancies compared to normal, the obese gene was one of the most up-regulated transcripts (43.6-fold), correlating with increased leptin protein levels (Reimer et al., 2002). In contrast, apolipoprotein E alleles and a polymorphism in peroxisome proliferator-activated receptor-gamma gene were not associated with pre-eclampsia (Laasanen et al., 2002; Makkonen et al., 2001).

Activation of the coagulation system is another characteristic of pre-eclampsia. Attention has focused on the Leiden Factor V mutation, which causes resistance to activated protein C as a candidate gene (see the chapter by Walker). Most of these studies have focused on maternal thrombophilias, but a few have included fetal thrombophilias. Livingston et al. found no association for either maternal or fetal thrombophilia and the development of severe pre-eclampsia (Livingston et al., 2001). In contrast, there have been positive associations noted with pre-eclampsia and maternal polymorphisms in plasminogen activator inhibitor-1 (PAI-1) gene (Yamada et al., 2000).

There are recent provocative studies suggesting that variations in fetal HLA genes play a significant role in early implantation; failures at this stage resulting in miscarriage or contributing to the subsequent development of pre-eclampsia. HLA-G is a non-classical class I antigen expressed in invasive cytotrophoblast where it is believed to inhibit activation of maternal T and NK cells in the decidua. Expression of HLA-G is correlated with increased invasiveness (O'Brien et al., 2000). However, polymorphisms in this gene have not been noted in increased frequency with pre-eclampsia (Aldrich et al., 2000). Possibly, polymorphisms in HLA-G are additive to additional insults such as cytomegalovirus infection (Le Bouteiller et al., 2003).

The classic method of evaluating the genetics of a disease has been by linkage analysis. A familial pregnancy-induced hypertension locus in the region of chromosome 7q36 encoding the endothelial isoform of the nitric oxide synthase gene has been reported (Arngrimsson *et al.*, 1997). The presence of such associations does not provide direct evidence for the involvement of a particular gene in pre-eclampsia but may indeed be markers for a neighboring gene. Evidence has been presented for a pre-eclampsia/eclampsia susceptibility locus between D45450 and D45610 of the long arm of chromosome 4 (Harrison *et al.*, 1997). Chromosome 2 has also been identified as a possible locus for pre-eclampsia/eclampsia (Moses *et al.*, 2000). A recent comprehensive review of the molecular epidemiology of pre-eclampsia has been published (Wilson *et al.*, 2003). Overall, DNA analysis for potential genetic markers may serve to screen for risks of pre-eclampsia and other adverse pregnancy outcomes.

Since the human genome project, gene arrays are being used to compare genome-wide variations in pre-eclamptic pregnancies to normal pregnancies. Associations have been made with altered expression of trophoblast invasion genes, obesity-related genes and cytokine receptor genes (Pang and Xing, 2003; Reimer *et al.*, 2002). This approach is limited in the ability to differentiate "causative" from "reactive" gene up-regulation as these studies typically compare serum or placentas from third trimester patients with and without the clinical diagnosis of pre-eclampsia.

In summary, it is currently believed that pre-eclampsia is a polygenic disorder, with polymorphisms in several genes contributing to risk. These genes may differ between different populations or ethnic groups. In addition to the two temporal phenotypes (early onset vs. late onset), the placental phenotype (abnormal trophoblast invasion) and the vascular phenotypes (endothelial dysfunction/oxidative stress) (Table 15.1) probably have different genotypes. It is also important to recognize the interaction between the fetal genotype (controlling placental development) and the maternal genotype (controlling immune adaptation and decidual and vascular reaction to implantation) and the potential for one to influence the other. The fact that most pre-eclamptic pregnancies will be followed by normal pregnancies suggests that,

for most patients, such polymorphisms will not play a significant role and questions their use as a general reliable screening tool. However, for the severe pre-eclampsia phenotype it may be useful. Nebert described the use of the "discordant phenotype" in pharmacogenetics in which differences in gene expression between the two extremes in response to a drug, e.g. <5th% and >95th%, are made (Nebert, 2000). In the low-dose aspirin study (Sibai *et al.*, 1995), multivariate logistic regression based upon four risk factors defined a tenth of the population at very low risk for pre-eclampsia and a tenth of the population at very high risk. Retrospective analysis of genotypes in such studies could, therefore, enhance current knowledge.

Coagulation and fibrinolytic systems in pre-eclampsia

Pregnancy is a state of chronic intravascular coagulation (McKay, 1981) and pre-eclampsia appears to be an exaggerated state of this phenomenon. Pre-eclampsia is accompanied by endothelial injury, increased platelet activation with platelet consumption in the microvasculature and enhanced clotting (Saleh *et al.*, 1992). Activated protein C resistance (caused by the Leiden factor V mutation) has been implicated (Lindoff *et al.*, 1997). Increases in cellular fibronectin concentrations and platelet activation have been reported and may precede the onset of pre-eclampsia (Chavarria *et al.*, 2002) as do levels of C reactive (Tjoa *et al.*, 2003).

Potential markers for platelet activation in pre-eclampsia include platelet surface expression of CD63 (a fibrinogen binding site; Konijnenberg *et al.*, 1997). Activation of platelets leads to an altered thromboxane/prostacyclin ratio (Fitzgerald *et al.*, 1987a). This decrease in prostacyclin may precede the clinical manifestation of pre-eclampsia.

Mean platelet volume reportedly corresponds to the severity of hypertensive disorders of pregnancy and may have some predictive value (Hutt *et al.*, 1994).

In pre-eclampsia, PAI-1 activity is significantly increased (Estelles *et al.*, 1991) and may be another marker for endothelial dysfunction (Caron *et al.*, 1991). The ratio of PAI-1/PAI-2 has been used to test the efficacy of treatment with antioxidants on endothelial and placental function in a recent trial (Chappell *et al.*, 2002).

Endothelial dysfunction in pre-eclampsia

Pre-eclampsia is characterized by generalized vascular endothelial dysfunction (Roberts *et al.*, 1989). The link to oxidative stress, markers of oxidative stress as predictive indices and possible treatments for oxidative stress are discussed in other chapters (Hubel, Raijmakkers and Poston, Redman and Sargent, Burton). While there are generic markers of oxidative stress, e.g. increased malondialdehyde (the chapter by Hubel), a marker of lipid peroxidation that can be utilized in women with pre-eclampsia, more system-specific markers could be employed. These include antiocardiolipin antibodies. Homocysteine which acts to increase oxidant stress by forming superoxide is also increased in women with clinically manifest pre-eclampsia (Dekker *et al.*, 1995). However, when homocysteine has been measured in relation to subsequent development of pre-eclampsia, contradictory results have been obtained (Cotter *et al.*, 2001; Hietala *et al.*, 2001). Homocysteine concentrations are, however, influenced by many other factors limiting their utility.

Protection of endothelial cells against injury can be provided by the PI 5.6 isoelectric form of serum albumin. Addition of non-esterified fatty acid causes PI 5.6 albumin to become PI 4.8 albumin, which has no protective activity. Decreases in PI 5.6 albumin concentrations occur from early to late gestation in both normal and pre-eclamptic women (Arborgast *et al.*, 1996), but concentrations were always lower in women destined to become pre-eclamptic in a longitudinal study.

A preliminary study (Arborgast *et al.*, 1996) showed that measurement of PI 5.6 albumin in early pregnancy was 88% accurate in detecting pre-eclampsia by discriminant analysis.

Insulin resistance/glucose intolerance

Increased insulin resistance is seen in pregnancy and is greatest in the third trimester when hypertension typically presents. Obesity, which is a risk factor for hypertension in pregnancy (Eskenazi *et al.*, 1991) is associated with decreased insulin sensitivity. Gestational diabetics also have an increased risk of hypertension in pregnancy (Suhonen and Teramo, 1993). A strong association has been shown between glucose intolerance and subsequent development of hypertension in pregnancy (Solomon *et al.*, 1994). No absolute glucose level can distinguish between women who will remain normotensive and those who will develop new onset hypertension in pregnancy. However, only 9% of normotensives had glucose loading tests of 7.8 mmol or greater compared to 27% of women who develop hypertension. Fasting plasma insulin at 20 weeks gestation in African-American women who became pre-eclamptic was significantly greater than those who remain normotensive (Sowers *et al.*, 1995). Using discriminant analysis, mean blood pressure and fasting insulin levels were predictors of pre-eclampsia. Hence, measurement of glucose tolerance may serve as a useful predictor, alone or in combination with other markers of pre-eclampsia. Very recently, serum SHBG has been studied as a marker of insulin resistance in pregnancy (Wolf *et al.*, 2002). SHBG has potential as a marker of insulin resistance as it has minimal variability between fasting and postprandial states (Key *et al.*, 1990). Increased first trimester SHBG (increased insulin resistance) was independently associated with increased risk of pre-eclampsia, an association that strengthened in lean women (Wolf *et al.*, 2002).

Renal markers of pre-eclampsia

In pre-eclampsia both renal perfusion and glomerular filtration rate are decreased and plasma uric acid and urinary sodium are increased, whereas urinary calcium excretion is decreased due to increased tubular reabsorption. It has been suggested that these changes may be determined prior to clinical disease being manifest. Recent reports have shown limited utility of measurement of serum uric acid (Lim *et al.*, 1998) and of urinary calcium–creatinine ratios in early pregnancy (Izumi *et al.*, 1997) as predictors of pre-eclampsia. The generation of vasodilatory kinins and stimulation of prostaglandin biosynthesis by renal kallikrein may play a paracrine role in regulation of blood pressure. Excretion of active and inactive kallikrein in urine reflects renal production. An inactive urinary kallikrein/creatinine ratio of 170 or less at 16–20 weeks gestation predicted nonproteinuric or proteinuric pre-eclampsia with a sensitivity of 70% and a specificity of 86% (Millar *et al.*, 1996), suggesting this measurement might be a simple and practical test for prediction of pre-eclampsia.

Prostaglandins in pre-eclampsia

The reduction in vascular endothelial prostacyclin production, seen in pregnancy-induced hypertension (Fitzgerald *et al.*, 1987a) may be another indicator of endothelial dysfunction. Thromboxane A_2 biosynthesis is also increased in normal pregnancy, but increased further in hypertensive pregnancy. This may arise from activated platelets (Fitzgerald *et al.*, 1987b) and give the altered thromboxane/prostacyclin ratio associated with pre-eclampsia which formed the basis for prophylactic studies with low-dose aspirin (Sibai *et al.*, 1995). The reduction in prostacyclin synthesis in pre-eclampsia is present as early as the first trimester of pregnancy (Fitzgerald *et al.*, 1987a) and could be used as a predictor for development of disease. However, measurement of urinary

prostaglandin metabolites is complicated (the chapter by Raijmakers). In initial studies total plasma 8-isoprostane was not found to be significantly different in pre-eclamptics versus controls, whereas plasma free 8-isoprostane was significantly increased and urine 8-isoprostane was significantly decreased in pre-eclampsia, suggesting urinary clearance is impaired (Barden *et al.*, 1996). Therefore, alterations in plasma free 8-isoprostane could be due to increased lipid peroxidation, increased phospholipase activity or decreased renal clearance. Utility of isoprostane measurements is limited by the complexity of metabolites and lack of simplicity in assay. A retrospective analysis of 8,12 iso-iPGF$_{2\alpha}$-VI, a major urinary isoprostane (Regan *et al.*, 2001) showed no variation with presence of disease or gestational age. Longitudinal prospective studies may clarify the progression of pre-eclampsia in relation to 8-isoprostane production.

Nitric oxide in pre-eclampsia

The nitric oxide radical is a potent vasodilator synthesized by endothelial cells. Measurement of nitrate, a breakdown product of nitric oxide, in urine shows that whole body production increases during pregnancy (Myatt *et al.*, 1992). However, the many papers on cross-sectional data on plasma or urine nitrate in pre-eclampsia are somewhat conflicting, being increased, reduced or unaltered. This may reflect alterations in both renal excretion as well as synthesis. A major influence on plasma and urinary nitrite concentrations is dietary intake of nitrite/nitrate which may confound measurements of endogenous synthesis and probably renders this unsuitable as a predictive marker unless patients are subject to dietary control.

The immunology of pre-eclampsia

An immunologic cause of pre-eclampsia was proposed in 1902 and profound alterations in immunologic function in women with pre-eclampsia have been shown (see the Moffett chapter). Alterations in T cell and macrophage function during pre-eclampsia may result in altered regulation of cytokine production. There are many reports of alterations of cytokines in pre-eclampsia, for example increased concentrations of tumor necrosis factor α, interleukin-6 and tumor necrosis factor receptors (Vince *et al.*, 1995). TNFα may act to link endothelial dysfunction to placental disease as TNFα activates endothelial cells and increased TNFα has been found in the placenta of pre-eclamptics (Nevils and Conrad, 1995). Recently TNFα has been suggested to be a specific marker for pre-eclampsia but only in the third trimester (Serin *et al.*, 2002). Interleukin-6 has an endocrine function in mediating the acute phase response by the liver. IL-12 is critical to the development of a Th1 T cell response, and pregnancy appears to be characterized by being a Th2-type condition (Saito *et al.*, 1999). Elevations of IL-12 in the serum of women with pre-eclampsia lead to the speculation that pre-eclampsia may represent a shift from a Th2- to a Th1-like immune response (Sakai *et al.*, 2002). Hence, investigations into the role of IL-12 in the pathogenesis of PE would be interesting. Recently (Ohkuchi *et al.*, 2001) reported that the fraction of Th1 cells and T cytotoxic type 1 (Tc1) cells was increased in pre-eclampsia. Again, longitudinal studies are needed to assess the utility of these markers.

Doppler ultrasound blood flow velocity measurements

Uteroplacental blood flow is reduced and vascular resistance increased in pre-eclampsia due to the absence of the normal physiologic of spiral arteries (Pijnenborg *et al.*, 1983). Doppler flow velocity waveform measurements of the uterine arteries are an index of the physiologic change and have been used as an early screening test for pre-eclampsia (Fleischer *et al.*, 1986). The early studies were not encouraging due to low sensitivity and variabilities

in methodology and definition. The inclusion of an early diastolic notch in the definition of abnormal flow velocity was reported to have improved the sensitivity of predicting pre-eclampsia, but did not reduce the high false positive rate as an early diastolic notch may persist in normal pregnancy up to 24–26 weeks gestation (Fleischer *et al.*, 1986). However, including a second screening test for persistent diastolic notch at 24 weeks reportedly increased the specificity of the test (Bower *et al.*, 1993). The relative risk of developing pre-eclampsia was claimed to be increased 68-fold if a persistent notch was seen at 24 weeks. The test also has a high negative predictive value for pre-eclampsia of up to 99% (Phupong *et al.*, 2003). This gives the test utility in identifying individuals in whom interventions are not useful.

A recent meta-analysis has suggested that 35% of patients with abnormal uterine artery waveform indices develop pre-eclampsia, promoting the utility of this technique as a preliminary screening tool (Chien *et al.*, 2000). The addition of a biochemical technique (such as second trimester inhibin A) to estimate trophoblast invasion or abnormalities of placental perfusion may give further specificity (Aquilina *et al.*, 2001). Large scale prospective studies are warranted. Recent studies have found the risk of developing pre-eclampsia is increased in those patients who show additional abnormalities in the vascular component including altered concentrations of asymmetric dimethyl L-arginine (Savvidou *et al.*, 2003) or of platelet function (Missfelder-Lobos *et al.*, 2002). This is again suggestive of an interaction between placental and maternal vascular components in development of the disease.

Proteins associated with trophoblast invasion and angiogenesis

Measurement of placental proteins which regulate trophoblast invasion may help predict pre-eclampsia. The insulin-like growth factor IGFII and the binding protein IGFBP-1 are involved in extravillous trophoblast cell migration and invasion. IGFII is produced by invading trophoblast whereas IGFBP-1 is produced by decidua and together they may serve as molecular signals for trophoblast–decidual interactions. Several longitudinal studies have shown that in early pregnancy reduced IGFBP-1 levels are found from 16 weeks onwards in women destined to develop pre-eclampsia (Grobman and Kazer, 2001) and that only in late gestation (36 weeks) are they greater than in controls (Anim-Nyame *et al.*, 2000). Decreased decidual IGFBP-1 mRNA was found in the pre-eclamptic placenta (Gratton *et al.*, 2002). Measurement of Pregnancy Associated Plasma Protein A (PAPP-A), a protease specific for IGF binding proteins, has also been reported to be useful for predicting adverse pregnancy outcome (Smith *et al.*, 2002). In the same study, levels of ßhCG were not predictive of later outcomes in a multivariate analysis. As both IUGR and pre-eclampsia share the same abnormal trophoblast invasion yet with differing maternal outcomes, measurements of biochemical markers of trophoblast invasion may not be specific for pre-eclampsia but may be a marker for bad pregnancy outcome, itself a useful screen.

Trophoblast invasion and placental development may be regulated by angiogenic molecules such as vascular endothelial growth factor (VEGF) and placenta-like growth factor (PLGF) and this regulation may be disrupted in pre-eclampsia (Zhou *et al.*, 2002). VEGF may play a role in disruption of vascular systems in pregnancy but several reports on placental VEGF expression (Ranheim *et al.*, 2001) and plasma VEGF in pre-eclamptics have been inconsistent (Baker *et al.*, 1995; Lyall *et al.*, 1997). The latter discrepancies are due to the use of different assay kits measuring either total or free VEGF. Assays for PLGF, another angiogenic factor produced by the trophoblast measure free PLGF. Decreased levels of free PLGF have been reported in women who have developed PE (Torry *et al.*, 1998). This may represent decreased production of this pro-angiogenic factor linked to trophoblast invasion.

VEGF acts via two high affinity receptors, fms-like tyrosine kinase (Flt1 or VEGFR1) and kinase domain receptor (KDR or VEGFR2). The soluble form of Flt-1 (sFlt-1) which circulates in plasma, binds VEGF and PLGF and reduces their biologic activity. It is now becoming apparent that pre-eclampsia is characterized by normal or high total VEGF but low free VEGF and PLGF due to excess production of sFlt. Production of VEGF or VEGFR-1 is increased with pre-eclampsia. Plasma from women with pre-eclampsia reduces myometrial vessel contractility in vitro, an effect that could be mimicked by incubation of vessels with VEGF (Brockelsby *et al.*, 1999). However, anti-Flt antibodies block the effect of VEGF and of plasma from pre-eclamptic women suggesting VEGF acting through the Flt-1 receptor may be involved in the pathophysiology. In normal gestations, serum sFlt-1 concentrations increase with advancing gestational age. However, levels are sixfold higher in pre-eclampsia (Koga *et al.*, 2003), perhaps diminishing VEGF function. Inhibition of VEGF binding to receptors on trophoblast reduces invasion in vitro (Zhou *et al.*, 2002). Although sFlt-1 levels decrease following delivery of the placenta, there is a suggestion that there may be extra-placental sources of sFlt-1 in PE (Koga *et al.*, 2003). Indeed, sFlt-1 is increased in patients with essential hypertension (Belgore *et al.*, 2001). Recently, Sugimoto *et al.* (2003) found that neutralization of VEGF caused glomerular endothelial detachment and hypertrophy suggesting neutralization of VEGF may play a role in induction of proteinuria.

Maynard *et al.* (2003) reported elevated levels of sFlt-1 in individuals with pre-eclampsia prior to the onset of disease and further correlated this with the severity of disease. Increased sFlt-1 expression by the placenta was found in this and other studies (Zhou *et al.*, 2002). Over-expression of sFlt-1 in pregnant rats caused hypertension and pre-eclampsia (Maynard *et al.*, 2003). The stimulus to increased sFlt-1 expression by the placenta may be hypoxia (Hornig *et al.*, 2000). Further prospective studies to confirm this data on sFlt-1 together with other hypoxia-induced proteins are needed.

Measurement of peptide hormones as markers of placental function

The ischemic/hypoxic injury suffered by trophoblast in pre-eclampsia may alter its functional activity manifest as changes in production of peptide or steroid hormones and help predict the disease. While there are potential circulating markers of trophoblast invasion that can be measured as yet none have been correlated with invasion hence hormone measurements in maternal plasma more likely reflect villous trophoblast function. Concentrations of corticotrophin-releasing hormone (CRH) synthesized by trophoblast increase exponentially throughout gestation, but the effect of CRH is negated by a 34 kda CRH binding protein in maternal plasma. CRH concentrations are increased in individuals with pre-eclampsia and are accompanied by a decrease in CRH binding protein (CRHbp) (Perkins et al., 1995). Interestingly, trophoblast production of CRH, unlike maternal CRH, can be stimulated by cortisol, the increase in CRH in pre-eclampsia may be due to increased fetal cortisol, itself a reflection of fetal stress. Therefore, longitudinal measurements of CRH and CRHbp may be able to detect changes to indicate the presence of pre-eclampsia.

The concentration of activin A, a placentally derived peptide was increased in plasma of pre-eclamptic patients (Petraglia et al., 1995). Serum concentrations of inhibin A, proα C containing inhibins and total activin A were significantly increased in serum of pre-eclamptic patients (Muttukrishna et al., 1997) indicating they could be sensitive markers. This is interpreted as further evidence for trophoblast dysfunction in pre-eclampsia. While Muttukrishna et al. (2000) and others claim to see a significant elevation of inhibin A early in gestation other groups, Grobman and Wang (2000) do not see early increases in inhibin A or activin A in women who develop pre-eclampsia. Muttukrishna et al. (2000) also reported from a nested case control study that early elevation of activin A might predict early onset pre-eclampsia.

This needs to be tested in prospective longitudinal studies with well-defined patient outcomes.

Normally maternal plasma concentrations of βhCG peak in the first trimester, but decline afterwards. Early work (Vaillant et al., 1996) reporting that βhCG concentrations > two times median concentrations at 17 weeks gestation was a good criteria for selecting patients likely to develop PIH with proteinuria and an SGA baby have been challenged by others (Pouta et al., 1998). Increases of βhCG, total hCG and total hCGα have been found in patients with severe pre-eclampsia in the third trimester compared to normotensive controls and taken to indicate a secretory reaction of the placenta in pre-eclampsia (Hsu et al., 1994). As hCG is secreted by the differentiated syncytiotrophoblast, alterations in βhCG may reflect alterations in trophoblast differentiation or function in pre-eclampsia. The end product of hCG metabolism in the kidney is the hCGβ core fragment. Bahado-Singh et al. (1998) found a positive correlation between urinary β core fragment concentrations and risk of pre-eclampsia in singleton pregnancies.

Leptin which is produced and secreted by the adipocyte is also synthesized in the placenta (Masuzaki et al., 1997) and production increases throughout gestation perhaps to increase circulating fatty acids and glucose. In pre-eclampsia, increased leptin has been reported and Anim-Nyame et al. (2000) reported significant differences from 20 weeks gestation onwards in women destined to develop pre-eclampsia, although other studies did not find this (Martinez-Abundis et al., 2000).

Measurement of placental peptides may have utility in prediction of pre-eclampsia, especially as they may reflect trophoblast function which in turn may reflect the severity of disease.

AT1 receptor autoantibodies

The presence of agonistic auto-antibodies against the angiotensin II AT1 receptor have been reported in the serum of individuals with PE (Xia *et al.*, 2003). The antibody also downregulates the AT1 receptor in a similar manner to angiotensin II but stimulates superoxide production from placental or vascular tissue (Dechend *et al.*, 2003). They also inhibit trophoblast invasion in an in vitro assay and increase trophoblast PAI-1 production (Xia *et al.*, 2002, 2003) and thus may account for two features of pre-eclampsia (reduced invasion and increased PAI-1). In cross-sectional studies these auto-antibodies are claimed to be found in the majority of patients with severe pre-eclampsia. This, however, needs to be confirmed in prospective longitudinal studies. Whether these antibodies exist prior to development of pre-eclampsia or are found in individuals with mild disease remains to be determined.

Conclusion

The majority of pre-eclampsia occurs in nulliparous individuals and yet within this group 75% occurs at term in association with relatively low maternal and fetal morbidity. Less than 1% of the nulliparous population develop pre-eclampsia at <34 weeks. Such a low incidence of clinically significant disease may preclude the use of expensive screening tests in such a low-risk population.

The greatest expenditure associated with pre-eclampsia in the developed world is in the care of premature infants delivered of women with early onset or severe pre-eclampsia. Identification of individuals who may develop the early onset/severe pre-eclampsia phenotype is then the most desirable in terms of reducing neonatal and maternal morbidity and mortality and subsequent societal expense. Screening should perhaps focus primarily on multiparous individuals with a history of pre-eclampsia and women of any parity with underlying medical disease or multifetal pregnancy, as these women account for the majority of early onset severe pre-eclampsia resulting in preterm delivery. The inclusion of risk factors such as blood pressure at initial prenatal care visit, body mass index, family history and, possibly, smoking as well as short pre-conception exposure to paternal antigens, could expand the screen to include a greater number of otherwise low-risk nulliparas destined to develop early onset pre-eclampsia (Figure 15.2). A second round of screening or surveillance could then include the use of biochemical and biophysical markers, maternal and perhaps fetal genotype to identify such phenotypes and select the group of patients felt to be at highest risk for the development of pre-eclampsia. These biochemical/biophysical tests may also provide alternative and earlier definitions

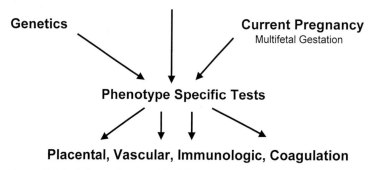

Figure 15.2 Defining patients at risk of developing pre-eclampsia.

of disease than simply hypertension/proteinuria and suggest who may benefit from different therapeutic interventions (placental/vascular), as well as ongoing pregnancy surveillance. Current treatment is limited to the administration of steroids for fetal lung maturation and seizure prophylaxis for the mother, and resolution of disease is limited to delivery of the infant and its placenta. This does not dismiss the potential of future prophylactic treatments such as antioxidants. Using such a two-step screening approach, a small percentage of nulliparas and multiparas destined to develop pre-eclampsia may be screen-negative (low risk by clinical and biochemical screen). The advantage of a two-step approach is to limit the number of individuals undergoing potentially costly screening and surveillance.

By far the majority of studies of pre-eclamptic women to date have been cross-sectional of women with mild disease at term. Although there are now more longitudinal studies emerging, they mostly still employ small patient numbers and a priori still focus on mild disease at term. What is needed are large-scale prospective studies powered to correlate predictive markers with clinically and economically significant outcomes for mother and fetus, i.e. they need to study early onset/severe pre-eclampsia

REFERENCES

Aldrich, C., Verp, M. S., Walker, M. A. and Ober, C. (2000). A null mutation in HLA-G is not associated with preeclampsia or intrauterine growth retardation. *J. Reprod. Immunol.*, **47**, 41–8.

American College of Obstetricians and Gynecologists. (1996). *Hypertension in Pregnancy*. Washington: The College. Technical Bulletin No. 219.

Anderson, G. D. and Sibai, B. M. (1986). In *Obstetrics Normal and Problem Pregnancies*, eds. S. Gabbe, J. Nieby and J. Simpson. New York: Churchill Livingstone, 845 pp.

Anim-Nyame, N., Hills, F. A., Sooranna, S. R., Steer, P. J. and Johnson, M. R. (2000). A longitudinal study of maternal plasma insulin-like growth factor binding protein-1 concentrations during normal pregnancy and pregnancies complicated by pre-eclampsia. *Hum. Reprod.*, **15**, 2215–19.

Aquilina, J., Barnett, A., Thompson, O. and Harrington, K. (1999). Second-trimester maternal serum inhibin A concentration as an early marker for preeclampsia. *Am. J. Obstet. Gynecol.*, **181**, 131–6.

Arborgast, B., Leeper, S. and Merrick, R. (1996). Plasma factors that determine endothelial cell lipid toxicity in vitro correctly identify women with preeclampsia in early and late gestation. *Hypertens. Pregn.*, **15**, 263–79.

Arngrimsson, R., Hayward, C., Nadaud, S., *et al.* (1997). Evidence for a familial pregnancy-induced hypertension locus in the eNOS-gene region. *Am. J. Hum. Genet.*, **61**, 354–62.

Bahado-Singh, R. O., Oz, U., Isozaki, T., *et al.* (1998). Midtrimester urine human chorionic gonadotropin beta-subunit core fragment levels and the subsequent development of pre-eclampsia. *Am. J. Obstet. Gynecol.*, **179**, 738–41.

Baker, P. N., Krasnow, J., Roberts, J. M. and Yeo, K. T. (1995). Elevated serum levels of vascular endothelial growth factor in patients with preeclampsia. *Obstet. Gynecol.*, **86**, 815–21.

Barden, A., Beilin, L. J., Ritchie, J., Croft, K. D., Walters, B. N. and Michael, C. A. (1996). Plasma and urinary 8-iso-prostane as an indicator of lipid peroxidation in pre-eclampsia and normal pregnancy. *Clin. Sci. (Lond.)*, **91**, 711–18.

Belgore, F. M., Blann, A. D., Li-Saw-Hee, F. L., Beevers, D. G. and Lip, G. Y. (2001). Plasma levels of vascular endothelial growth factor and its soluble receptor (SFlt-1) in essential hypertension. *Am. J. Cardiol.*, **87**, 805–7, A9.

Bower, S., Bewley, S. and Campbell, S. (1993). Improved prediction of preeclampsia by two-stage screening of uterine arteries using the early diastolic notch and color Doppler imaging. *Obstet. Gynecol.*, **82**, 78–83.

Brockelsby, J., Hayman, R., Ahmed, A., Warren, A., Johnson, I. and Baker, P. (1999). VEGF via VEGF receptor-1 (Flt-1) mimics preeclamptic plasma in inhibiting uterine blood vessel relaxation in pregnancy: implications in the pathogenesis of preeclampsia. *Lab. Invest.*, **79**, 1101–11.

Caritis, S., Sibai, B., Hauth, J., *et al.* (1998). Low-dose aspirin to prevent preeclampsia in women at high risk. National Institute of Child Health and Human Development Network of Maternal–Fetal Medicine Units. *N. Engl. J. Med.*, **338**, 701–5.

Caron, C., Goudemand, J., Marey, A., Beague, D., Ducroux, G. and Drouvin, F. (1991). Are haemostatic and fibrinolytic parameters predictors of pre-eclampsia in pregnancy-associated hypertension? *Thromb. Haemost.*, **66**, 410–14.

Chappell, L. C., Seed, P. T., Kelly, F. J., *et al.* (2002). Vitamin C and E supplementation in women at risk of preeclampsia is associated with changes in indices of oxidative stress and placental function. *Am. J. Obstet. Gynecol.*, **187**, 777–84.

Chavarria, M. E., Lara-Gonzalez, L., Gonzalez-Gleason, A., Sojo, I. and Reyes, A. (2002). Maternal plasma cellular fibronectin concentrations in normal and pre-eclamptic pregnancies: a longitudinal study for early prediction of preeclampsia. *Am. J. Obstet. Gynecol.*, **187**, 595–601.

Chesley, L. C., Annitto, J. E. and Cosgrove, R. A. (1968). The familial factor in toxemia of pregnancy. *Obstet. Gynecol.*, **32**, 303–11.

Chien, P. F., Arnott, N., Gordon, A., Owen, P. and Khan, K. S. (2000). How useful is uterine artery Doppler flow velocimetry in the prediction of pre-eclampsia, intrauterine growth retardation and perinatal death? An overview. *Br. J. Obstet. Gynaecol.*, **107**, 196–208.

Cincotta, R. B. and Brennecke, S. P. (1998). Family history of pre-eclampsia as a predictor for pre-eclampsia in primigravidas. *Int. J. Gynaecol. Obstet.*, **60**, 23–7.

Cotter, A. M., Molloy, A. M., Scott, J. M. and Daly, S. F. (2001). Elevated plasma homocysteine in early pregnancy: a risk factor for the development of severe pre-eclampsia. *Am. J. Obstet. Gynecol.*, **185**, 781–5.

Dechend, R., Viedt, C., Muller, D. N., *et al.* (2003). AT1 receptor agonistic antibodies from preeclamptic patients stimulate NADPH oxidase. *Circulation*, **107**, 1632–9.

Dekker, G. A., de Vries, J. I., Doelitzsch, P. M., *et al.* (1995). Underlying disorders associated with severe early-onset preeclampsia. *Am. J. Obstet. Gynecol.*, **173**, 1042–8.

Eskenazi, B., Fenster, L. and Sidney, S. (1991). A multivariate analysis of risk factors for preeclampsia. *J. Am. Med. Ass.*, **266**, 237–41.

Estelles, A., Gilabert, J., Espana, F., Aznar, J. and Galbis, M. (1991). Fibrinolytic parameters in normotensive pregnancy with intrauterine fetal growth retardation and in severe preeclampsia. *Am. J. Obstet. Gynecol.*, **165**, 138–42.

Fitzgerald, D. J., Entman, S. S., Mulloy, K. and FitzGerald, G. A. (1987a). Decreased prostacyclin biosynthesis preceding the clinical manifestation of pregnancy-induced hypertension. *Circulation*, **75**, 956–63.

Fitzgerald, D. J., Mayo, G., Catella, F., Entman, S. S. and FitzGerald, G. A. (1987b). Increased thromboxane biosynthesis in normal pregnancy is mainly derived from platelets. *Am. J. Obstet. Gynecol.*, **157**, 325–30.

Fleischer, A., Schulman, H., Farmakides, G., *et al.* (1986). Uterine artery Doppler velocimetry in pregnant women with hypertension. *Am. J. Obstet. Gynecol.*, **154**, 806–13.

Gratton, R. J., Asano, H. and Han, V. K. (2002). The regional expression of insulin-like growth factor II (IGF-II) and insulin-like growth factor binding protein-1 (IGFBP-1) in the placentae of women with pre-eclampsia. *Placenta*, **23**, 303–10.

Grobman, W. A. and Wang, E. Y. (2000). Serum levels of activin A and inhibin A and the subsequent development of preeclampsia. *Obstet. Gynecol.*, **96**, 390–4.

Grobman, W. A. and Kazer, R. R. (2001). Serum insulin, insulin-like growth factor-I, and insulin-like growth factor binding protein-1 in women who develop preeclampsia. *Obstet. Gynecol.*, **97**, 521–6.

Haig, D. (1993). Genetic conflicts in human pregnancy. *Q. Rev. Biol.*, **68**, 495–532.

Harrison, G. A., Humphrey, K. E., Jones, N., *et al.* (1997). A genomewide linkage study of preeclampsia/eclampsia reveals evidence for a candidate region on 4q. *Am. J. Hum. Genet.*, **60**, 1158–67.

Hietala, R., Turpeinen, U. and Laatikainen, T. (2001). Serum homocysteine at 16 weeks and subsequent preeclampsia. *Obstet. Gynecol.*, **97**, 527–9.

Hornig, C., Barleon, B., Ahmad, S., Vuorela, P., Ahmed, A. and Weich, H. A. (2000). Release and complex formation of soluble VEGFR-1 from endothelial cells and biological fluids. *Lab. Invest.*, **80**, 443–54.

Hsu, C. D., Chan, D. W., Iriye, B., Johnson, T. R., Hong, S. F. and Repke, J. T. (1994). Elevated serum human chorionic gonadotropin as evidence of secretory response in severe preeclampsia. *Am. J. Obstet. Gynecol.*, **170**, 1135–8.

Hutt, R., Ogunniyi, S. O., Sullivan, M. H. and Elder, M. G. (1994). Increased platelet volume and aggregation precede the onset of preeclampsia. *Obstet. Gynecol.*, **83**, 146–9.

Izumi, A., Minakami, H., Kuwata, T. and Sato, I. (1997). Calcium-to-creatinine ratio in spot urine samples in early pregnancy and its relation to the development of preeclampsia. *Metabolism*, **46**, 1107–8.

Key, T. J., Pike, M. C., Moore, J. W., Wang, D. Y. and Morgan, B. (1990). The relationship of free fatty acids with the binding of oestradiol to SHBG and to albumin in women. *J. Steroid Biochem.*, **35**, 35–8.

Koga, K., Osuga, Y., Yoshino, O., *et al.* (2003). Elevated serum soluble vascular endothelial growth factor receptor 1 (sVEGFR-1) levels in women with pre-eclampsia. *J. Clin. Endocrinol. Metab.*, **88**, 2348–51.

Konijnenberg, A., Stokkers, E. W., van der Post, J. A., *et al.* (1997). Extensive platelet activation in preeclampsia compared with normal pregnancy: enhanced expression of cell adhesion molecules. *Am. J. Obstet. Gynecol.*, **176**, 461–9.

Laasanen, J., Heinonen, S., Hiltunen, M., Mannermaa, A. and Laakso, M. (2002). Polymorphism in the peroxisome proliferator-activated receptor-gamma gene in women with preeclampsia. *Early Hum. Dev.*, **69**, 77–82.

Le Bouteiller, P., Pizzato, N., Barakonyi, A. and Solier, C. (2003). HLA-G, pre-eclampsia, immunity and vascular events. *J. Reprod. Immunol.*, **59**, 219–34.

Lim, K. H., Friedman, S. A., Ecker, J. L., Kao, L. and Kilpatrick, S. J. (1998). The clinical utility of serum uric acid measurements in hypertensive diseases of pregnancy. *Am. J. Obstet. Gynecol.*, **178**, 1067–71.

Lindoff, C., Ingemarsson, I., Martinsson, G., Segelmark, M., Thysell, H. and Astedt, B. (1997). Preeclampsia is associated with a reduced response to activated protein C. *Am. J. Obstet. Gynecol.*, **176**, 457–60.

Livingston, J. C., Barton, J. R., Park, V., Haddad, B., Phillips, O. and Sibai, B. M. (2001). Maternal and fetal inherited thrombophilias are not related to the development of severe preeclampsia. *Am. J. Obstet. Gynecol.*, **185**, 153–7.

Lyall, F. (2002). The human placental bed revisited. *Placenta*, **23**, 555–62.

Lyall, F., Greer, I. A., Boswell, F. and Fleming, R. (1997). Suppression of serum vascular endothelial growth factor immunoreactivity in normal pregnancy and in pre-eclampsia. *Br. J. Obstet. Gynaecol.*, **104**, 223–8.

Makkonen, N., Heinonen, S., Hiltunen, M., Helisalmi, S., Mannermaa, A. and Kirkinen, P. (2001). Apolipoprotein E alleles in women with pre-eclampsia. *J. Clin. Pathol.*, **54**, 652–4.

Martinez-Abundis, E., Gonzalez-Ortiz, M. and Pascoe-Gonzalez, S. (2000). Serum leptin levels and the severity of preeclampsia. *Arch. Gynecol. Obstet.*, **264**, 71–3.

Masuzaki, H., Ogawa, Y., Sagawa, N., *et al.* (1997). Nonadipose tissue production of leptin: leptin as a novel placenta-derived hormone in humans. *Nat. Med.*, **3**, 1029–33.

Maynard, S. E., Min, J. Y., Merchan, J., *et al.* (2003). Excess placental soluble fms-like tyrosine kinase 1 (sFlt1) may contribute to endothelial dysfunction, hypertension, and proteinuria in preeclampsia. *J. Clin. Invest.*, **111**, 649–58.

McKay, D. G. (1981). Chronic intravascular coagulation in normal pregnancy and preeclampsia. *Contrib. Nephrol.*, **25**, 108–19.

Millar, J. G., Campbell, S. K., Albano, J. D., Higgins, B. R. and Clark, A. D. (1996). Early prediction of pre-eclampsia by measurement of kallikrein and creatinine on a random urine sample. *Br. J. Obstet. Gynaecol.*, **103**, 421–6.

Missfelder-Lobos, H., Teran, E., Lees, C., Albaiges, G. and Nicolaides, K. H. (2002). Platelet changes and subsequent development of pre-eclampsia and fetal growth restriction in women with abnormal uterine artery Doppler screening. *Ultrasound Obstet. Gynecol.*, **19**, 443–8.

Moses, E. K., Lade, J. A., Guo, G., *et al.* (2000). A genome scan in families from Australia and New Zealand confirms the presence of a maternal susceptibility locus for pre-eclampsia, on chromosome 2. *Am. J. Hum. Genet.*, **67**, 1581–5.

Muttukrishna, S., Knight, P. G., Groome, N. P., Redman, C. W. and Ledger, W. L. (1997). Activin A and inhibin A as possible endocrine markers for pre-eclampsia. *Lancet*, **349**, 1285–8.

Muttukrishna, S., North, R. A., Morris, J., *et al.* (2000). Serum inhibin A and activin A are elevated prior to the onset of pre-eclampsia. *Hum. Reprod.*, **15**, 1640–5.

Myatt, L., Brewer, A. and Prada, J. (1992). In 39th Annual Meeting, *Society for Gynecologic Investigation*, San Antonio, Texas.

Myatt, L. and Miodovnik, M. (1999). Prediction of preeclampsia. *Semin. Perinatol.*, **23**, 45–57.

Myatt, L. for the NICHD MFMU Network. (2001). Do women at high risk develop preeclampsia earlier in gestation than those at low risk? *Am. J. Obstet. Gynecol.*, **184**, S81.

Myatt, L. for the NICHD MFMU Network. (2002). Differences in the time of diagnosis of mild vs severe preeclampsia between low and high risk patient groups. *Hypertens. Pregn.*, **21** (Suppl. 1), 63.

Naicker, T., Khedun, S. M., Moodley, J. and Pijnenborg, R. (2003). Quantitative analysis of trophoblast invasion in preeclampsia. *Acta Obstet. Gynecol. Scand.*, **82**, 722–9.

Nebert, D.W. (2000). Extreme discordant phenotype methodology: an intuitive approach to clinical pharma-cogenetics. *Eur. J. Pharmacol.*, **410**, 107–20.

Nevils, B. and Conrad, K. (1995). Increased circulating levels of TNFa in preeclampsia: a possible role for cytokines in the pathogenesis of the disease. *J. Soc. Gyn. Invest.*, **2**, 311.

O'Brien, M., Dausset, J., Carosella, E. D. and Moreau, P. (2000). Analysis of the role of HLA-G in preeclampsia. *Hum. Immunol.*, **61**, 1126–31.

O'Brien, T. E., Ray, J. G. and Chan, W. S. (2003). Maternal body mass index and the risk of preeclampsia: a systematic overview. *Epidemiology*, **14**, 368–74.

Ohkuchi, A., Minakami, H., Aoya, T., *et al.* (2001). Expansion of the fraction of Th1 cells in women with preeclampsia: inverse correlation between the percentage of Th1 cells and the plasma level of PAI-2. *Am. J. Reprod. Immunol.*, **46**, 252–9.

Pang, Z. J. and Xing, F. Q. (2003). Comparative study on the expression of cytokine–receptor genes in normal and preeclamptic human placentas using DNA microarrays. *J. Perinat. Med.*, **31**, 153–62.

Pearson, H. (2002). Reproductive immunology: immunity's pregnant pause. *Nature*, **420**, 265–6.

Perkins, A. V., Linton, E. A., Eben, F., Simpson, J., Wolfe, C. D. and Redman, C.W. (1995). Corticotrophin-releasing hormone and corticotrophin-releasing hormone binding protein in normal and pre-eclamptic human pregnancies. *Br. J. Obstet. Gynaecol.*, **102**, 118–22.

Petraglia, F., De Vita, D., Gallinelli, A., *et al.* (1995). Abnormal concentration of maternal serum activin-A in gestational diseases. *J. Clin. Endocrinol. Metab.*, **80**, 558–61.

Phupong, V., Dejthevaporn, T., Tanawattanacharoen, S., Manotaya, S., Tannirandorn, Y. and Charoenvidhya, D. (2003). Predicting the risk of preeclampsia and small for gestational age infants by uterine artery Doppler in low-risk women. *Arch. Gynecol. Obstet.*, **268**, 158–61.

Pijnenborg, R., Bland, J. M., Robertson, W. B. and Brosens, I. (1983). Uteroplacental arterial changes related to interstitial trophoblast migration in early human pregnancy. *Placenta*, **4**, 397–413.

Pouta, A. M., Hartikainen, A. L., Vuolteenaho, O. J., Ruokonen, A. O. and Laatikainen, T. J. (1998). Mid-trimester N-terminal proatrial natriuretic peptide, free beta hCG, and alpha-fetoprotein in predicting preeclampsia. *Obstet. Gynecol.*, **91**, 940–4.

Ranheim, T., Staff, A. C. and Henriksen, T. (2001). VEGF mRNA is unaltered in decidual and placental tissues in preeclampsia at delivery. *Acta Obstet. Gynecol. Scand.*, **80**, 93–8.

Regan, C. L., Levine, R. J., Baird, D. D., *et al.* (2001). No evidence for lipid peroxidation in severe preeclampsia. *Am. J. Obstet. Gynecol.*, **185**, 572–8.

Reimer, T., Koczan, D., Gerber, B., Richter, D., Thiesen, H. J. and Friese, K. (2002). Microarray analysis of differentially expressed genes in placental tissue of pre-eclampsia: up-regulation of obesity-related genes. *Mol. Hum. Reprod.*, **8**, 674–80.

Roberts, J. M., Taylor, R. N., Musci, T. J., Rodgers, G. M., Hubel, C. A. and McLaughlin, M. K. (1989). Pre-eclampsia: an endothelial cell disorder. *Am. J. Obstet. Gynecol.*, **161**, 1200–4.

Saito, S., Sakai, M., Sasaki, Y., Tanebe, K., Tsuda, H. and Michimata, T. (1999). Quantitative analysis of peripheral blood Th0, Th1, Th2 and the Th1:Th2 cell ratio during normal human pregnancy and preeclampsia. *Clin. Exp. Immunol.*, **117**, 550–5.

Sakai, M., Tsuda, H., Tanebe, K., Sasaki, Y. and Saito, S. (2002). Interleukin-12 secretion by peripheral blood mononuclear cells is decreased in normal pregnant subjects and increased in preeclamptic patients. *Am. J. Reprod. Immunol.*, **47**, 91–7.

Saleh, A. A., Bottoms, S. F., Farag, A. M., *et al.* (1992). Markers for endothelial injury, clotting and platelet activation in preeclampsia. *Arch. Gynecol. Obstet.*, **251**, 105–10.

Sattar, N., Ramsay, J., Crawford, L., Cheyne, H. and Greer, I. A. (2003). Classic and novel risk factor parameters in women with a history of preeclampsia. *Hypertension*, **42**, 39–42.

Savvidou, M. D., Hingorani, A. D., Tsikas, D., Frolich, J. C., Vallance, P. and Nicolaides, K. H. (2003). Endothelial dysfunction and raised plasma concentrations of asymmetric dimethylarginine in pregnant women who subsequently develop pre-eclampsia. *Lancet*, **361**, 1511–17.

Serin, I. S., Ozcelik, B., Basbug, M., *et al.* (2002). Predictive value of tumor necrosis factor alpha (TNF-alpha) in preeclampsia. *Eur. J. Obstet. Gynecol. Reprod. Biol.*, **100**, 143–5.

Sibai, B. M., el-Nazer, A. and Gonzalez-Ruiz, A. (1986). Severe preeclampsia-eclampsia in young primigravid women: subsequent pregnancy outcome and remote prognosis. *Am. J. Obstet. Gynecol.*, **155**, 1011–16.

Sibai, B. M., Caritis, S. N., Thom, E., *et al.* (1993). Prevention of preeclampsia with low-dose aspirin in healthy, nulliparous pregnant women. The National Institute of Child Health and Human Development Network of Maternal–Fetal Medicine Units. *N. Engl. J. Med.*, **329**, 1213–18.

Sibai, B. M., Gordon, T., Thom, E., *et al.* (1995). Risk factors for preeclampsia in healthy nulliparous women: a prospective multicenter study. The National Institute of Child Health and Human Development Network of Maternal–Fetal Medicine Units. *Am. J. Obstet. Gynecol.*, **172**, 642–8.

Sibai, B. M., Ewell, M., Levine, R. J., *et al.* (1997). Risk factors associated with preeclampsia in healthy nulliparous women. The Calcium for Preeclampsia Prevention (CPEP) Study Group. *Am. J. Obstet. Gynecol.*, **177**, 1003–10.

Smith, G. C., Stenhouse, E. J., Crossley, J. A., Aitken, D. A., Cameron, A. D. and Connor, J. M. (2002). Early pregnancy levels of pregnancy-associated plasma protein a and the risk of intrauterine growth restriction, premature birth, preeclampsia, and stillbirth. *J. Clin. Endocrinol. Metab.*, **87**, 1762–7.

Solomon, C. G., Graves, S. W., Greene, M. F. and Seely, E. W. (1994). Glucose intolerance as a predictor of hypertension in pregnancy *Hypertension*, **23**, 717–21.

Sowers, J. R., Saleh, A. A. and Sokol, R. J. (1995). Hyperinsulinemia and insulin resistance are associated with preeclampsia in African-Americans. *Am. J. Hypertens.*, **8**, 1–4.

Sugimoto, H., Hamano, Y., Charytan, D., *et al.* (2003). Neutralization of circulating vascular endothelial growth factor (VEGF) by anti-VEGF antibodies and soluble VEGF receptor 1 (sFlt-1) induces proteinuria. *J. Biol. Chem.*, **278**, 12,605–8.

Suhonen, L. and Teramo, K. (1993). Hypertension and pre-eclampsia in women with gestational glucose intolerance. *Acta Obstet. Gynecol. Scand.*, **72**, 269–72.

Tjoa, M. L., van Vugt, J. M., Go, A. T., Blankenstein, M. A., Oudejans, C. B. and van Wijk, I. J. (2003). Elevated C-reactive protein levels during first trimester of pregnancy are indicative of preeclampsia and intrauterine growth restriction. *J. Reprod. Immunol.*, **59**, 29–37.

Torry, D. S., Wang, H. S., Wang, T. H., Caudle, M. R. and Torry, R. J. (1998). Preeclampsia is associated with reduced serum levels of placenta growth factor. *Am. J. Obstet. Gynecol.*, **179**, 1539–44.

Vaillant, P., David, E., Constant, I., *et al.* (1996). Validity in nulliparas of increased beta-human chorionic gonadotrophin at mid-term for predicting pregnancy-induced hypertension complicated with proteinuria and intrauterine growth retardation. *Nephron*, **72**, 557–63.

Vince, G. S., Starkey, P. M., Austgulen, R., Kwiatkowski, D. and Redman, C. W. (1995). Interleukin-6, tumour necrosis factor and soluble tumour necrosis factor receptors in women with pre-eclampsia. *Br. J. Obstet. Gynaecol.*, **102**, 20–5.

Wilson, M. L., Goodwin, T. M., Pan, V. L. and Ingles, S. A. (2003). Molecular epidemiology of preeclampsia. *Obstet. Gynecol. Surv.*, **58**, 39–66.

Wolf, M., Sandler, L., Munoz, K., Hsu, K., Ecker, J. L. and Thadhani, R. (2002). First trimester insulin resistance and subsequent preeclampsia: a prospective study. *J. Clin. Endocrinol. Metab.*, **87**, 1563–8.

Xia, Y., Wen, H. Y. and Kellems, R. E. (2002). Angiotensin II inhibits human trophoblast invasion through AT1 receptor activation. *J. Biol. Chem.*, **277**, 24,601–8.

Xia, Y., Wen, H., Bobst, S., Day, M. C. and Kellems, R. E. (2003). Maternal autoantibodies from preeclamptic patients activate angiotensin receptors on human trophoblast cells. *J. Soc. Gynecol. Investig.*, **10**, 82–93.

Yamada, N., Arinami, T., Yamakawa-Kobayashi, K., *et al.* (2000). The 4G/5G polymorphism of the plasminogen activator inhibitor-1 gene is associated with severe preeclampsia. *J. Hum. Genet.*, **45**, 138–41.

Yoshimura, T., Chowdhury, F. A., Yoshimura, M. and Okamura, H. (2003). Genetic and environmental contributions to severe preeclampsia: lack of association with the endothelial nitric oxide synthase Glu298Asp variant in a developing country. *Gynecol. Obstet. Invest.*, **56**, 10–13.

Zhou, Y., McMaster, M., Woo, K., *et al.* (2002). Vascular endothelial growth factor ligands and receptors that regulate human cytotrophoblast survival are dysregulated in severe preeclampsia and hemolysis, elevated liver enzymes, and low platelets syndrome. *Am. J. Pathol.*, **160**, 1405–23.

16

Long-term implications of pre-eclampsia for maternal health

Gordon C. S. Smith

Introduction

The immediate clinical consequences and associations of pre-eclampsia are the subject of intense study and are reviewed in depth throughout this volume. It is natural for any woman who experiences a hypertensive disorder in pregnancy to enquire what implications this has, if any, for her future health. While the long-term outcome of women who experience pre-eclampsia has been the subject of research, there are still major uncertainties regarding this area due to the inherent problems of long-term longitudinal clinical studies. The aim of this chapter is to summarize the recent evidence regarding the implications of pre-eclampsia occurring during pregnancy for a woman's health in later life. Moreover, methodological issues related to addressing this research question will also be reviewed both to assist interpretation of the existing literature and to provide guidance for how future studies might be conducted.

Methodological issues in determining long-term associations with pre-eclampsia

Study design

Epidemiological studies generally aim to quantify the association between developing a given disease and some characteristic in a population. The characteristic can take many forms, such as a blood test, environmental exposure or socio-economic factor. The first step in any study is to determine whether the outcome and exposure are associated to a degree which is greater than expected by chance. Any analysis assumes that a sufficient number of individuals were studied to allow detection of an association, were any to exist. Having demonstrated an association, the next step is to determine whether the association is likely to be causal. There are multiple criteria for supporting a causal interpretation (Rothman and Greenland, 1998), these are described elsewhere and providing strong evidence for causality is often the work of multiple studies using different approaches. In a given study it is important, however, to exclude the possibility that any association between an exposure and an outcome is due to a common dependence on some other determinant (confounding).

Case control studies

The approach of a case control study is to identify a group with the condition of interest and compare the proportion who have the exposure of interest with a group of unaffected individuals (controls). This type of study is infrequently used in the long-term outcome of pre-eclampsia. Studies which examine the outcome of a group of women who experienced pre-eclampsia with a group of women who did not are frequently described by their authors as "case control studies." In fact, this is inaccurate since the groups are defined by the exposure of interest (i.e. pre-eclampsia), not the outcome of interest (e.g. chronic hypertension), as would occur in a case control study.

Matched cohort studies

Cohort studies are defined as the analysis of a group of individuals who are all drawn from some definable population and are followed up over a period of time. The follow-up may be conducted retrospectively or prospectively. Following up groups of women with pre-eclampsia and then comparing them with a group who did not are matched cohort studies. The key issue in such studies is the selection of the unexposed (control) group. Since the analysis depends on statistical comparison with the control group, it is essential that the control group is a random sample of the unexposed population. The selection of controls, as is performed in a matched cohort study, allows the possibility of bias.

Population-based cohort studies

This study design takes a defined population (e.g. all women attending a given hospital for antenatal care or all women in a given country) and compares the incidence of the outcome in relation to the exposure of interest. Since the unexposed group is unselected, there is less likelihood of bias being introduced in the comparisons. An important issue in these studies is how the event was ascertained. For example, if events were ascertained by questionnaire, were the response rates similar in relation to exposure? Alternatively, if they were ascertained by record linkage to other local data sources, was there systematic migration or lack of migration in relation to the exposure?

Prospective cohort studies

Prospective cohort studies represent the "gold standard" in determining association. In this design a group of women is identified and followed up. The incidence of events is related to the

exposure of interest. A prospective design allows definition of exposure to be performed in a standardized way for the whole cohort, which will reduce the chance of bias being introduced in definitions. The major drawback of prospective cohort studies is their expense.

Nested case control studies

A nested case control study is a variant on a cohort study. A cohort is followed up and all women experiencing events are ascertained. All the cases are compared with a random selection of controls from within the cohort. The random selection of controls allows identification of a non-biased group of controls. Confining any analysis to cases and controls considerably reduces the costs of the study, particularly if detailed investigations of cases and controls is planned.

Definition of exposure, maternal characteristics and events

A key reason why studies may differ in the nature and strength of associations described with hypertensive disorders in pregnancy is the definition of the exposure. Different study designs are likely to have different methods of definition. Generally, small studies and prospective studies will tend to have more precise definitions. Studies involving a retrospective review of case notes will depend on the degree of standardization of clinical care to allow comparison between women. The inclusion criteria for the study are also likely to determine the associations observed. If a study includes women who attend late for antenatal care, those with previously unrecognized chronic hypertension who book late in pregnancy may be wrongly diagnosed as having gestational hypertension. This would lead to an apparent but potentially spurious association between pregnancy-induced hypertension and later chronic hypertension. Another important issue is parity. The number of pregnancies women have is clearly highly variable and this can vary systematically in relation to important maternal characteristics. The risk that a woman will have any pregnancy affected by pre-eclampsia is clearly increased with the total number of pregnancies, particularly if some of these are to different partners. The potential for bias in these classifications can be overcome by relating long-term outcome to a diagnosis of pre-eclampsia in the first pregnancy which, all other things being equal, might be regarded as a standardized measure of a woman's tendency to develop the disease.

There is a general rule of epidemiological databases that the information available on each individual varies in inverse proportion to the total number in the study group. Large-scale population databases have the advantage that they include a sufficient number of women to be powered to detect rare events, such as premature death due to cerebrovascular disease. The drawback of such studies is that the exposure (e.g. pre-eclampsia), the other maternal characteristics (e.g. smoking and obesity) and the outcome (e.g. differentiation between ischemic or thrombotic stroke) are likely to be incompletely defined. In practice, groups with a documented diagnosis of pre-eclampsia in such databases are likely to include women with chronic hypertension and women who did not experience pre-eclampsia. Conversely, groups where the diagnosis is not documented are likely to include women who did experience pre-eclampsia. The effect of misclassification clearly depends on the extent of the overlap.

The issues outlined above are important in interpreting the existing literature regarding the long-term outcome following pre-eclampsia. Hypertension is a chronic condition that increases the risk of many cardiovascular events. If a diagnosis of apparent pre-eclampsia during pregnancy is simply a marker for women with first and early diagnosis of chronic hypertension, then it would be anticipated that associations would be apparent between pre-eclampsia and later hypertension and cardiovascular disease. The definition of pre-eclampsia and the clinical information available for the definition to be made

are the key determinants of the potential for misclassification. Variations in the definition and the clinical information employed are likely to account for much of the variability in the literature.

Early studies on remote prognosis of eclampsia and pre-eclampsia

The literature on this subject up to 1980 was reviewed in some depth by Leon Chesley, who is perhaps one of the key figures in much of the early work (Chesley, 1980). The majority of these studies employ cohorts of women who experienced some form of hypertensive disorder of pregnancy. Comparison was made either with matched control groups or population average incidences for the given outcome. The vast majority of these early studies focused on chronic hypertension as the outcome. The conclusion of these early studies was that eclampsia and pre-eclampsia were not associated with an increased risk of chronic hypertension in later life. Gestational hypertension was associated with an increased risk of chronic hypertension. The apparent paradox that the mildest form of the disease had the strongest association with long-term prognosis was explained by the fact that women diagnosed with "gestational hypertension" probably had first diagnosis of essential hypertension in pregnancy. Since the early work described above, more recent studies have re-examined this research question and have often employed larger cohorts of women. The following sections will describe the major findings of subsequent large scale studies.

Hypertensive disorders in pregnancy and hypertension in later life

There is more information about the risk of hypertension in later life and previous pre-eclampsia than any other long-term outcome.

This is probably because hypertension is relatively common in younger women. Relatively young women remain the focus for most of these studies for the pragmatic reason that computerized databases of pregnancy outcome are relatively recent and represent the most convenient way for initiating large-scale longitudinal studies, due to the expense of dedicated prospective observational studies.

Wilson *et al.* described the long-term outcome for a cohort of women delivering in Aberdeen, Scotland between 1951 and 1970 (Wilson *et al.*, 2003). Women were classified into normotensive, gestational hypertension (i.e. hypertension without proteinuria) and pre-eclampsia (i.e. hypertension with proteinuria). Hypertension in later life was ascertained by questionnaire and physical examination of respondents within the cohort. While this is open to recall bias and respondent bias, the cohort was also linked to computerized databases of hospital discharge data and death certificate data. There were associations between both gestational hypertension and pre-eclampsia and later hypertension both by questionnaire and physical examination of respondents and by linkage of the whole cohort to hospital discharge data. The relative risks were in the region of 2−4.

A large-scale prospective cohort study of women recruited to the control group of a matched cohort study of the oral contraceptive pill related a previous diagnosis of pre-eclampsia to the risk of later chronic hypertension. The authors described a relative risk of 2.4 (2.1−2.6). However, the criteria for diagnosis of pre-eclampsia were not defined and it is likely that this group included many women with misclassified hypertension (Hannaford *et al.*, 1997).

A matched cohort study of 273 women with well-defined hypertensive disorders of pregnancy demonstrated associations between both gestational hypertension and pre-eclampsia and later chronic hypertension. The incidence was 45% in the pregnancy-induced hypertension group and 14% in controls ($P < 0.001$) This study correctly excluded women where the data were lacking to classify the pregnancy-related hypertension, due to missing data or late booking. Interestingly, there was no association between eclampsia and later hypertension, although only 29 women were followed up who had experienced this event (Marin *et al.*, 2000).

Sibai and colleagues describe prospective follow-up of 179 women who experienced eclampsia but did not have pre-existing hypertension (Sibai *et al.*, 1992). They demonstrated that the likelihood of hypertension in later life depended on the gestational age where the index event took place: 18% if eclampsia occurred <31 weeks, 12% if eclampsia occurred between 31 and 36 weeks and 5% if eclampsia occurred at term. This trend is statistically significant ($P = 0.03$ by chi square test for trend − not reported by authors). They also found that women who had pre-eclampsia in subsequent pregnancies had a greater risk of later hypertension than women whose subsequent pregnancies were not affected by pre-eclampsia (25% versus 2%, $P < 0.0001$).

The same authors had earlier reported a matched cohort study of 406 women aged <26 years who developed severe pre-eclampsia during their first pregnancy. The diagnostic criteria employed were strict and women with unclassifiable hypertension were excluded. The incidence of chronic hypertension was 15% compared with 6% in the control group and the difference was highly statistically significant (Sibai *et al.*, 1986).

The studies described above strongly suggest that both pre-eclampsia and eclampsia are related to the risk of chronic hypertension in later life. Use of strict diagnostic criteria means that some of these studies cannot be explained by misclassification. The relationship between gestational age at the time of the eclamptic event and the risk of later hypertension does suggest heterogeneity within this group and that long-term implications of a diagnosis of pre-eclampsia or eclampsia might vary according to the gestational age at onset in the affected pregnancy.

Hypertensive disorders in pregnancy and ischemic heart disease in later life

A number of studies have demonstrated associations between a diagnosis of pre-eclampsia in pregnancy and ischemic heart disease (IHD) in later life. This association is plausible given the evidence outlined above for a relationship with hypertension, which is a well-recognized risk factor for IHD. However, IHD is relatively uncommon in young women. Consequently, the most feasible studies for addressing this question are register-based studies, since these can include a sufficient number of women to be powered to address the research question. In all but one of these studies, however, the definition of exposure is based on the coding of clinical records, which is open to misclassification.

The analysis of controls for the oral contraception cohort, reported by Hannaford and described above, reported relative risks of 1.5–2.2 for a number of different IHD conditions. The association persisted when the analysis was stratified by chronic hypertension and the analysis was adjusted for age, smoking and social class (Hannaford et al., 1997). A national retrospective cohort study of 129,920 women having first births in Scotland between 1980 and 1984 demonstrated an approximately twofold risk of death or hospital admission due to IHD in relation to a diagnosis of pre-eclampsia (Smith et al., 2001). The diagnosis of pre-eclampsia was based on coding in a maternity register and 18% of women were documented as experiencing pre-eclampsia, indicating that the diagnostic criteria were relatively broad. The association was not attenuated by adjusting for maternal age, social deprivation, height or essential hypertension. Smoking data were lacking in this cohort but it is unlikely that smoking might have explained the observed association since pre-eclampsia is less common among smokers (England et al., 2002). A national registry based study in Denmark of over 600,000 births also demonstrated an increased risk of death due to cardiovascular causes (Irgens et al., 2001). These authors demonstrated that the relative risk of death associated with a diagnosis of pre-eclampsia varied in relation to gestational age. For term births the relative risk was 1.6 and for preterm births it was 8.1. However, previous studies have shown that preterm birth is a risk factor for IHD independently of pre-eclampsia (Smith et al., 2001, 2000). Irgens et al. did not perform a formal statistical test for interaction.

Each of these large-scale studies supports the hypothesis that a diagnosis of pre-eclampsia is associated with an increased risk of later IHD. However, in all studies the accuracy of diagnosis is debatable as they are based on large-scale registers of case note data. A single large-scale study has been described with well-defined data on the diagnosis of pre-eclampsia (Wilson et al., 2003), the Aberdeen study described above. This study generated somewhat inconsistent results. There was a twofold risk of death due to IHD on the basis of record linking to death certificate data although due to small numbers this was of borderline statistical significance ($P = 0.09$). Surprisingly, there was no trend of an increased risk of hospital admission for IHD (relative risk 0.9, upper 95% CI 1.4). However, there was no association between gestational hypertension and either hospital admission or death due to IHD. In the presence of these inconsistencies, further work will be required to define the strength and nature of the association, if any, between hypertensive disorders in pregnancy and later risk of IHD.

Hypertensive disorders in pregnancy and cerebrovascular disease in later life

Hypertension is a major etiological factor in cerebrovascular disease. A number of studies have attempted to determine whether pre-eclampsia during pregnancy is associated with an increased risk of cerebrovascular disease in later life. The cohort study reported by Hannaford reported a non-significant trend toward an increased risk of cerebrovascular disease in relation to a history of pre-eclampsia. However, they did report that women who had no diagnosis of a hypertensive disorder of pregnancy had a lower risk of cerebrovascular disease in later life than nulliparous women (Hannaford *et al.*, 1997). The cohort study of 600,000 women from Denmark found a fivefold risk of stroke among women delivered preterm with a diagnosis of pre-eclampsia but no excess risk of stroke among those who experienced pre-eclampsia but delivered at term (Irgens *et al.*, 2001). These and other authors have shown that preterm birth in the absence of pre-eclampsia is associated with an increased risk of later stroke (Irgens *et al.*, 2001; Pell *et al.*, 2004). The linked Aberdeen data allowed comparison of women with gestational hypertension and those with pre-eclampsia. The association with later cerebrovascular disease was stronger among the pre-eclampsia group (relative risk 2.1 for hospital admission and 3.5 for death) than among the gestational hypertensive group (relative risk 1.4 for hospital admission and 2.9 for death) and, indeed, was only statistically significant in the former group. These data generally support the interpretation that pre-eclampsia is associated with later cerebrovascular disease. It is unknown, however, whether this association is wholly explained by the association between pre-eclampsia and chronic hypertension.

Hypertensive disorders in pregnancy and venous thromboembolism in later life

Some studies have suggested that pre-eclampsia may be more common among women with inherited and acquired thrombophilias (Kupferminc *et al.*, 2000), although the data are inconsistent (Morrison *et al.*, 2002). Furthermore, pathological examination of placentae from women with pre-eclampsia often demonstrate thrombotic changes (Sikkema *et al.*, 2002). These associations have led to studies of the possible association between pre-eclampsia and venous thromboembolism in later life. Hannaford *et al.* reported a relative

risk for venous thromboembolism of 1.6 for women with a history of pre-eclampsia (Hannaford *et al.*, 1997). When stratified by chronic hypertension, the relationship appeared stronger among women who were normotensive. A more recent analysis of almost 300,000 pregnancies from Canada demonstrated a twofold risk of venous thromboembolism among women with a pregnancy diagnosis of pre-eclampsia (van Walraven *et al.*, 2003). Both studies included both first and subsequent pregnancies, employed register bases definitions of pre-eclampsia and could not adjust for important potential confounders, such as obesity. While these data suggest a possible association between pre-eclampsia and venous thromboembolism, further studies are clearly required.

Possible mechanisms of association between pre-eclampsia and later disease

Pre-eclampsia shares common features with some determinants of disease in later life. A candidate mechanism linking the two is insulin resistance. It has been suggested that pre-eclampsia is a manifestation of the insulin resistance syndrome and the evidence supporting this is reviewed elsewhere (Solomon and Seely, 2001). Although insulin resistance in pregnancy is associated with an increased risk of pre-eclampsia, the relative risk is modest, at approximately 2. This would not be considered a strong association and is consistent with the clinical impression that the majority of women with gestational diabetes do not experience severe adverse outcomes in pregnancy. One of the problems in the clinical investigation of the causes of pre-eclampsia is the multiorgan involvement in the affected individual. Literally dozens of circulating factors have been shown to be altered among women with pre-eclampsia, but it is unclear whether these are causal or epiphenomena. It has been shown that the risk of pre-eclampsia is associated with first trimester circulating maternal concentrations of pregnancy-associated plasma protein-A (PAPP-A), a trophoblast-derived regulator of the insulin-like growth factor system (Smith *et al.*, 2002). This observation suggests the factors determining later pre-eclampsia may be evident in the very earliest weeks post-conception. The relatively weak link between factors such as insulin resistance in late pregnancy and the risk of pre-eclampsia may reflect the importance of conditions in very early pregnancy in determining the risk of disease.

Clearly, insulin resistance is just one of many possible mechanisms linking pre-eclampsia and cardiovascular disease in later life. Another is thrombophilia. There are reports that women with inherited thrombophilias are at increased risk of pregnancy complications (Gharavi *et al.*, 2001) and of IHD (Rosendaal *et al.*, 1997a, b). However, genetic epidemiology is plagued by small-scale studies and a systematic tendency of journals to publish positive results. This results in a characteristic pattern of a flurry of interest in a given mutation followed by a series of negative results (Bonnici *et al.*, 2002). Consistent with this, recent large-scale studies of inherited thrombophilias and pre-eclampsia have been negative (Morrison *et al.*, 2002). Nevertheless, both pre-eclampsia and diseases such as IHD show strong familial associations (Morgan and Ward, 1999; Slack and Evans, 1966). It is plausible, given the common features of the pathophysiology of these conditions, that there may be common genetic determinants of IHD and pregnancy complications. Consistent with this, a recent study has shown that a family history of early onset IHD is associated with an increased risk of delivering a low birthweight baby (Pell *et al.*, 2003). It is currently well recognized that development of gestational diabetes during pregnancy identifies women who are insulin resistant and at increased risk of developing type 2 diabetes in later life (Linne *et al.*, 2002). In this case pregnancy could be seen as a test of the body's predisposition toward diabetes. It is possible that the failure of the mother to adapt to placentation and fetal growth leading to obstetric complications such as pre-eclampsia, intrauterine growth restriction or preterm birth reflects

occult cardiovascular, microvascular or hemostatic dysfunction. Since these will also make her susceptible to hypertension, atherosclerosis and thrombotic disorders, a woman's reproductive history may, therefore, also become informative in assessing her future risk of cardiovascular disease. The true nature and mechanism of these associations will only be resolved by large-scale prospective studies.

Note

This review summarizes the literature to October 2003. For information on more recent studies, see Ray, J. G. (2006). *Drug Dvpt Res.*, **67**, 607–11.

REFERENCES

Bonnici, F., Keavney, B., Collins, R. and Danesh, J. (2002). Angiotensin converting enzyme insertion or deletion polymorphism and coronary restenosis: meta-analysis of 16 studies. *Br. Med. J.*, **325**, 517–20.

Chesley, L. C. (1980). Hypertension in pregnancy: definitions, familial factor, and remote prognosis. *Kidney Int.*, **18**, 234–40.

England, L. J., Levine, R. J., Qian, C., *et al.* (2002). Smoking before pregnancy and risk of gestational hypertension and preeclampsia. *Am. J. Obstet. Gynecol.*, **186**, 1035–40.

Gharavi, A. E., Pierangeli, S. S., Levy, R. A. and Harris, E. N. (2001). Mechanisms of pregnancy loss in antiphospholipid syndrome. *Clin. Obstet. Gynecol.*, **44**, 11–19.

Hannaford, P., Ferry, S. and Hirsch, S. (1997). Cardiovascular sequelae of toxaemia of pregnancy. *Heart*, **77**, 154–8.

Irgens, H. U., Reisaeter, L., Irgens, L. M. and Lie, R. T. (2001). Long term mortality of mothers and fathers after pre-eclampsia: population based cohort study 1 *Br. Med. J.*, **323**, 1213–17.

Kupferminc, M. J., Fait, G., Many, A., Gordon, D., Eldor, A. and Lessing, J. B. (2000). Severe preeclampsia and high frequency of genetic thrombophilic mutations. *Obstet. Gynecol.*, **96**, 45–9.

Linne, Y., Barkeling, B. and Rossner, S. (2002). Natural course of gestational diabetes mellitus: long term follow up of women in the SPAWN study. *Br. J. Obstet. Gynaecol.*, **109**, 1227–31.

Marin, R., Gorostidi, M., Portal, C. G., Sanchez, M., Sanchez, E. and Alvarez, J. (2000). Long-term prognosis of hypertension in pregnancy. *Hypertens. Pregn.*, **19**, 199–209.

Morgan, T. and Ward, K. (1999). New insights into the genetics of preeclampsia. *Semin. Perinatol.*, **23**, 14–23.

Morrison, E. R., Miedzybrodzka, Z. H., Campbell, D. M., *et al.* (2002). Prothrombotic genotypes are not associated with pre-eclampsia and gestational hypertension: results from a large population-based study and systematic review. *Thromb. Haemost.*, **87**, 779–85.

Pell, J. P., Smith, G. C., Dominiczak, A., *et al.* (2003). Family history of premature death from ischaemic heart disease is associated with an increased risk of delivering a low birth weight baby. *Heart*, **89**, 1249–50.

Pell, J. P., Smith G. C. S. and Walsh, D. (2004). Pregnancy complications and subsequent maternal cerebrovascular events: a retrospective cohort study of 119,668 births. *Am. J. Epidemiol.*, **159**, 336–42.

Rosendaal, F. R., Siscovick, D. S., Schwartz, S. M., *et al.* (1997a). Factor V Leiden (resistance to activated protein C) increases the risk of myocardial infarction in young women. *Blood*, **89**, 2817–21.

Rosendaal, F. R., Siscovick, D. S., Schwartz, S. M., Psaty, B. M., Raghunathan, T. E. and Vos, H. L. (1997b). A common prothrombin variant (20210 G to A) increases the risk of myocardial infarction in young women. *Blood*, **90**, 1747–50.

Rothman, K. J. and Greenland, S. (1998). *Modern Epidemiology*, 2nd edn. Philadelphia: Lippincott-Raven.

Sibai, B. M., el Nazer, A. and Gonzalez-Ruiz, A. (1986). Severe preeclampsia–eclampsia in young primigravid women: subsequent pregnancy outcome and remote prognosis. *Am. J. Obstet. Gynecol.*, **155**, 1011–16.

Sibai, B. M., Sarinoglu, C. and Mercer, B. M. (1992). Eclampsia. VII. Pregnancy outcome after eclampsia and long-term prognosis. *Am. J. Obstet. Gynecol.*, **166**, 1757–61.

Sikkema, J. M., Franx, A., Bruinse, H. W., van der Wijk, N. G., de Valk, H. W. and Nikkels, P. G. (2002). Placental pathology in early onset pre-eclampsia and intra-uterine growth restriction in women with and without thrombophilia. *Placenta*, **23**, 337–42.

Slack, J. and Evans, K. A. (1966). The increased risk of death from ischaemic heart disease in first degree relatives of 121 men and 96 women with ischaemic heart disease. *J. Med. Genet.*, 239–49.

Smith, G. C. S., Pell, J. P. and Walsh, D. (2001). Pregnancy complications and maternal risk of ischaemic heart disease: a retrospective cohort study of 129,290 births. *Lancet*, **357**, 2002–6.

Smith, G. C. S., Stenhouse, E. J., Crossley, J. A., Aitken, D. A., Cameron, A. D. and Connor, J. M. (2002). Early pregnancy levels of pregnancy-associated plasma protein A and the risk of intra-uterine growth restriction, premature birth, pre-eclampsia and stillbirth. *J. Clin. Endocrinol. Metab.*, **87**, 1762–7.

Smith, G. D., Whitley, E., Gissler, M. and Hemminki, E. (2000). Birth dimensions of offspring, premature birth, and the mortality of mothers. *Lancet*, **356**, 2066–7.

Solomon, C. G. and Seely, E. W. (2001). Brief review: hypertension in pregnancy: a manifestation of the insulin resistance syndrome? *Hypertension*, **37**, 232–9.

van Walraven, C., Mamdani, M., Cohn, A., Katib, Y., Walker, M. and Rodger, M. A. (2003). Risk of subsequent thromboembolism for patients with pre-eclampsia. *Br. Med. J.*, **326**, 791–2.

Wilson, B. J., Watson, M. S., Prescott, G. J., *et al.* (2003). Hypertensive diseases of pregnancy and risk of hypertension and stroke in later life: results from cohort study. *Br. Med. J.*, **326**, 845.

PART II

Clinical Practice

17

Classification and diagnosis of pre-eclampsia

Robyn A. North

Introduction

Pre-eclampsia is a pregnancy-specific condition characterized by placental dysfunction and a maternal response featuring systemic inflammation with activation of the endothelium and coagulation. This multifactorial disease presents as a syndrome of symptoms and signs, with associated hematological and biochemical abnormalities. Most consider hypertension and proteinuria to be the hallmarks of pre-eclampsia, but the clinical manifestations of this syndrome are very heterogeneous. Some women develop severe maternal disease requiring intensive care, whereas others remain asymptomatic with mild hypertension and proteinuria. Approximately one in six babies born to mothers with pre-eclampsia is very preterm. In contrast, two-thirds are delivered after 37 weeks, most of whom are normally grown, healthy babies. It is the very nature of the condition that creates difficulties in classifying pre-eclampsia precisely.

Over the decades a number of classifications have been promoted by different groups of experts or representative bodies (Anonymous, 1990, 2000, 2002; Brown *et al.*, 2000; Davey and MacGillivray, 1988; Helewa *et al.*, 1997; Hughes, 1972; Redman and Jefferies, 1988). This range of definitions has served to confuse clinicians and researchers as to the most appropriate definition to use (Chappell *et al.*, 1999; Harlow and Brown, 2001). The most recent classification proposals are more closely aligned, with some commonality in terminology and criteria for abnormal blood pressure and proteinuria. It is now widely accepted that

gestational hypertension is the presence of de novo hypertension (usually diastolic blood pressure >90 mmHg and/or systolic blood pressure >140 mmHg) occurring in the second half of pregnancy and pre-eclampsia is the combination of gestational hypertension with new proteinuria (Anonymous, 2000, 2002; Brown *et al.*, 2000; Helewa *et al.*, 1997). In recognition that severe disease may occur in the absence of proteinuria (Douglas and Redman, 1994), the Australasian Society of Hypertension in Pregnancy (ASSHP) has widened these criteria to include the presence of other multisystem manifestations, whether or not proteinuria is present (Brown *et al.*, 2000).

In this chapter current classifications are summarized. The objectives of defining pre-eclampsia will be discussed from the perspective of a clinician and then a researcher. We will review how the different classification systems address these issues. The inherent difficulties and pitfalls when measuring blood pressure and proteinuria will be considered. The problems diagnosing superimposed pre-eclampsia in the presence of underlying medical conditions, such as essential hypertension, renal disease or diabetes, will also be addressed. The chapter concludes with future approaches to define and diagnose this elusive disease.

Current classification systems

Gestational hypertension

Recent classifications from American (Anonymous, 2000, 2002), Canadian (Helewa *et al.*, 1997) and

Australasian (Brown *et al.*, 2000) representative bodies have defined gestational hypertension as a blood pressure ≥140/90 mmHg after 20 weeks gestation. In a general pregnant population, blood pressure greater than 140/90 mmHg is more than two standard deviations above the mean between 20 and 34 weeks gestation, and approximately two standard deviations above the mean from 35 weeks to term (Stone *et al.*, 1995). There are minor differences in the criteria for gestational hypertension between these consensus statements. The Canadian's elected to use only a diastolic blood pressure >90 mmHg in the definition, requiring confirmation on at least two occasions 4 h apart. The Australasian definition specifies a systolic blood pressure greater or equal to 140 mmHg and/or diastolic blood pressure of at least 90 mmHg, taken repeatedly over several hours and an absence of any features of multisystem disease. In the USA, the National Institutes of Health working group report on blood pressure in pregnancy, endorsed by the American College of Obstetricians and Gynecologists (ACOG), has defined gestational hypertension as a systolic blood pressure greater than 140 mm Hg or diastolic blood pressure greater than 90 mmHg after 20 weeks gestation, without reference to repeated recordings. All classification systems include women in whom the blood pressure rise is only present intrapartum, and in the USA this may comprise a substantial proportion of all pre-eclamptics (Zhang *et al.*, 2001). As gestational hypertension may progress to pre-eclampsia (Barton *et al.*, 2001; Saudan *et al.*, 1998), it is recognized that the final diagnosis of gestational hypertension can only be made postpartum (Anonymous, 2000). Resolution of the high blood pressure by 3 months postpartum is required in order to confirm the woman does not have chronic hypertension.

Pre-eclampsia

The Canadian consensus statement did not use the term "pre-eclampsia," but the more cumbersome "gestational hypertension with proteinuria,"

which was then subdivided into those with and without adverse conditions. The adverse conditions were the presence of severe hypertension, maternal multisystem complications (convulsions, thrombocytopenia, oliguria, pulmonary edema, right upper quadrant pain or elevated liver enzymes) or adverse placental/fetal outcomes (suspected abruption placentae, intrauterine growth restriction, oligohydramnios or absent or reversed-end umbilical artery end diastolic flow). This classification advanced thinking by addressing the importance of the presence or absence of severe maternal and fetal sequelae. It was, however, a retrograde step to focus the terminology on hypertension. Although development of hypertension is usually the first sign, it is only one sign amongst many in the pre-eclampsia syndrome.

Neither the terminology proposed by the Canadians nor the unwieldy terminology used in the earlier ISSHP classification has been widely applied internationally. Cumbersome language fails to address the human element in the uptake of terminology and medicine is not immune to the impact of branding. The widespread use of "HELLP syndrome" highlights this. HELLP is the acronym coined in 1982 for hemolysis, elevated liver enzymes, and low platelets (Weinstein, 1982). It is just a term for a set of multisystem complications that occur in pre-eclampsia. The simple, easy to remember name evokes the response that this is a severe medical problem, contributing to the widespread global uptake of this terminology. However, the terminology has fueled the incorrect concept that this is a separate disease to pre-eclampsia rather than part of the spectrum. Other combinations of complications, such as "ELLP" syndrome, also occur, probably even more commonly than "HELLP."

The American classification separates gestational hypertension from pre-eclampsia by the presence of proteinuria with the new onset-hypertension (Anonymous, 2000, 2002). Proteinuria is diagnosed on a 24 h urinary protein measurement ($\geq 0.3 \, \text{g} \, 24 \, \text{h}^{-1}$) or if this is not feasible, a fixed time interval collection corrected for creatinine excretion. The American classification identifies a group of mothers and babies at potential danger, and comment that the following features of severe disease increase the certainty of the diagnosis:

- blood pressure of 160 mmHg or more systolic, or 110 mmHg or more diastolic;
- proteinuria of 2.0 g or more in 24 h (2+ or 3+ on qualitative examination);
- increased serum creatinine (> 1.2 mg dl^{-1} unless known to be previously elevated);
- platelet count less than 100,000 cell mm^{-1} and/or evidence of microangiopathic hemolytic anemia (with increased lactic acid dehydrogenase);
- elevated hepatic enzymes (alanine transaminase or aspartate transaminase);
- persistent headache or other cerebral or visual disturbances;
- persistent epigastric pain;
- eclampsia (convulsions).

Recent ACOG criteria are based on the above consensus document with the following minor modifications to the list of severe features (Anonymous, 2002). Severe hypertension required the blood pressure to be $\geq 160/100$ mmHg on two or more occasions 6 h apart while the patient is on bedrest, the proteinuria cut-off was elevated to 5 g 24 h^{-1} or 3+ on two random urine samples and oliguria (defined as < 500 ml 24 h^{-1}). Pulmonary edema or cyanosis and fetal growth restriction were added to the list.

The importance of thinking about pre-eclampsia as a multisystem disease, that requires systematic assessment of each organ potentially involved, is the foundation of the Australasian (ASSHP) classification. In this definition all women with features of multisystem disease are included under the diagnosis of pre-eclampsia, whether or not they have significant proteinuria (Table 17.1) (Brown *et al.*, 2000). This contrasts with the American classification where a woman with gestational hypertension (i.e. has no proteinuria) who develops one or more severe manifestations is still considered to have gestational hypertension. It should be noted that in the Australasian definition women with gestational hypertension and proteinuria, but no other severe complications, are considered to have

Table 17.1. Australasian Society for the Study of Hypertension in Pregnancy 2000 Classification System for Pre-eclampsia

---

Gestational hypertension (de novo systolic blood pressure ≥ 140 mmHg and/or diastolic blood pressure ≥ 90 mmHg) and any of the following:
Proteinuria: ≥ 300 mg 24 h^{-1} or a spot urine protein/creatinine ratio ≥ 30 mg mmol^{-1}
Renal insufficiency: serum creatinine > 0.09 mmol l^{-1} or oliguria
Liver disease: epigastric/right upper quadrant pain and/or raised serum transaminases
Neurological problems: convulsions (eclampsia); hyperreflexia and clonus; severe headaches with hyperreflexia; persistent visual disturbance (scotomas)
Hematological disturbance: thrombocytopenia, disseminated intravascular coagulation, hemolysis
Fetal growth restriction

---

pre-eclampsia. Inclusion of fetal growth restriction, but exclusion of other feto-placental problems, such as placental abruption, is an inconsistency in the ASSHP classification. The clinical importance of severe hypertension (BP $\geq 170/110$ mmHg) is recognized, but they do not separate severe from milder hypertension within the diagnostic criteria.

Objectives when defining pre-eclampsia

Clinician's perspective

Like any diagnostic "test," the definition of pre-eclampsia ultimately classifies women as having or not having the condition. Once labeled as pre-eclampsia, a treatment threshold is crossed, triggering a series of changes in clinical management. The criteria used to classify pre-eclampsia have, therefore, significant implications for clinical care.

The objectives of defining pre-eclampsia are twofold:

1. to identify women and their babies with severe maternal or fetal complications due to pre-eclampsia; and
2. to identify women at significant risk of subsequently developing severe maternal and/or fetal

sequelae due to pre-eclampsia who require more intensive monitoring and timely delivery to prevent these problems.

Defining pre-eclampsia by the most common early manifestations of the syndrome (hypertension and proteinuria), clusters a broad range of clinical scenarios, from mild disease posing no immediate threat to maternal or fetal health through to women with eclampsia, severe liver and renal dysfunction associated with a coagulopathy and/or severe fetal compromise. For some these severe complications are present at the time of diagnosis, others develop them in the ensuing days or weeks. For many, pre-eclampsia never progress beyond the initial manifestations of mild disease. Thus the current definitions of pre-eclampsia function in dual capacity, as a diagnostic tool for severe maternal or fetal disease and as a screening test that identifies women at significant risk of subsequently developing severe sequelae of pre-eclampsia.

Like all screening tests, sensitivity and specificity are balanced around the cut-off criteria utilized. No definition is perfect, but the object is to identify all women who develop severe disease (high sensitivity) and exclude all at minimal risk of significant sequelae (high specificity). If the definition is too broad, an inclusive approach will result in the diagnosis of women with very mild disease. Classifications that included the criteria of edema (Anonymous, 1990; Hughes, 1972) or an isolated rise in blood pressure with the final blood pressure remaining less than 140/90 mmHg (Anonymous, 1990), resulted in labeling many women with pre-eclampsia who were at little risk of serious maternal or fetal morbidity. An isolated rise in blood pressure has now been shown to occur in 27–67% of pregnancies, and identifies women who have an essentially normal pregnancy outcome (North et al., 1999; Ohkoshi et al., 2003; Villar and Sibai, 1989). A further study reported no increase in important adverse outcomes among the 2% of nulliparous women with proteinuria and a 15 mmHg rise in diastolic blood pressure, but whose blood pressure remained less than

90 mmHg (Levine et al., 2000). An isolated rise in blood pressure and the presence of edema have now been dropped from recent classifications (Anonymous, 2000, 2002; Brown et al., 2000; Helewa et al., 1997).

Equally, if criteria are too stringent, then some women who are at risk of developing severe maternal disease will not be identified and appropriate management not implemented. Redman and Jefferies found that if more strict criteria for hypertension (a rise in diastolic blood pressure of at least 25 mmHg to at least 90 mmHg) were employed, this identified pregnancies with increased rates of proteinuria, lower birthweights and increased perinatal mortality (Redman and Jefferies, 1988). These criteria for hypertension were shown to be associated with a higher rate of small for gestational age babies than if an absolute BP cut-off was utilized (Perry and Beevers, 1994). Redman's criteria have been used in major clinical trials (CLASP, 1994) but have not been widely accepted in clinical practice. The reason for this includes the requirement of an early blood pressure to make the diagnosis. This is not available in a significant number of pregnancies, especially in certain sectors where women often present late in pregnancy. This definition also excludes women with proteinuria combined with a diastolic blood pressure greater than 90 mmHg, but whose increase in blood pressure is less than 25 mmHg. Amongst these women, the precise number who would develop severe maternal or fetal complications is unknown. As several million pregnancies are complicated by pre-eclampsia annually, failure to recognize even a small percentage translates into large numbers of women potentially placed at risk globally.

The current classifications of gestational hypertension and pre-eclampsia do identify two groups of women with very different risk profiles (Figure 17.1) (Brown and Buddle, 1995a; North et al., 1999). US-based studies also report fewer major adverse maternal or fetal in gestational hypertension compared with pre-eclampsia (Barton et al., 2001; Hauth et al., 2000). It should be

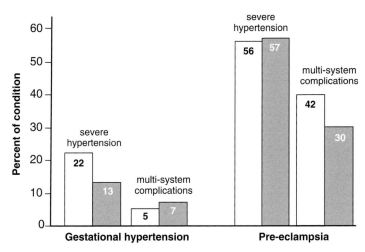

Figure 17.1 Among women with gestational hypertension and pre-eclampsia, the proportion who develop severe hypertension or multi-system complications. Multi-system complications included renal insufficiency, thrombocytopenia, liver dysfunction, imminent eclampsia, eclampsia and pulmonary edema. □, North *et al.* (1999); ■, Brown and Buddle (1995a).

recognized that within the gestational hypertension group, there are small subgroups of women at relatively greater risk of morbidity. These include those with severe hypertension (Hauth *et al.*, 2000) and those with early-onset disease (Barton *et al.*, 2001; Saudan *et al.*, 1998).

The Australasian definition, with its emphasis on a systematic approach to determine if the woman has multisystem involvement or if her baby's health is adversely affected, can be readily applied to clinical practice (Figure 17.2). After determining whether a woman has gestational hypertension, a systematic review should be undertaken for symptoms and signs, with supportive evidence from laboratory investigations or ultrasound scan, of maternal multisystem disease and adverse fetal/ placental outcomes. According to the ASSHP classification, if these are present, the woman has pre-eclampsia and if they are absent she has gestational hypertension. This approach can also be applied in the daily assessment of women with pre-eclampsia who are being conservatively managed in an attempt to increase gestational age at birth.

Research perspective

In contrast to clinical obstetrics where the classification needs to be inclusive, for most research it is preferable that only women with definite disease are studied. This applies particularly to basic research into the pathogenesis of the condition. It remains contentious as to whether the researcher should insist on proteinuria to make the diagnosis of pre-eclampsia (Anonymous, 2002) or whether women with gestational hypertension and no proteinuria but other manifestations of multisystem disease are included (Brown *et al.*, 2000). This decision remains with the researcher.

Recent studies have highlighted the variable often poor quality definitions used in studies on pre-eclampsia (Chappell *et al.*, 1999; Harlow and Brown, 2001). In particular, almost a third of studies provided no definition and up to a fifth of papers relied on urinary dipstick to determine proteinuria. The sine qua non is that the definition of the condition be provided when performing research on pre-eclampsia. Given the limitations of urinary dipstick to determine proteinuria, as described

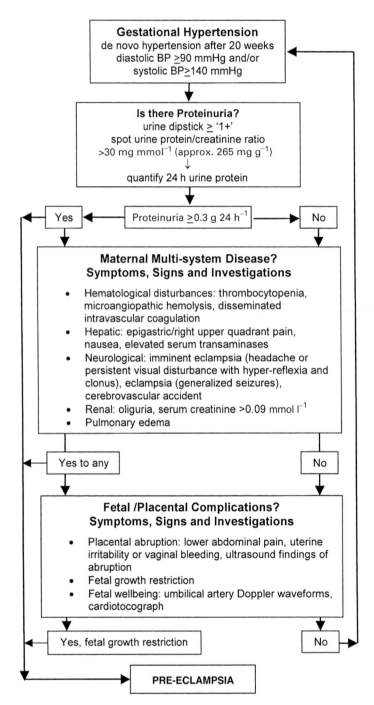

Figure 17.2 Approach to diagnosis of gestational hypertension and pre-eclampsia, using modified ASSHP classification (Brown *et al.*, 2000).

below, more accurate methods of measuring the vital signs are required in studies. It has been recommended that normal blood pressure should be documented before 12 weeks gestation or after 12 weeks postpartum (Anonymous, 2000). This is relevant for some research, but could reduce the applicability of certain clinical studies to general obstetric populations where this information is not available for many women. It is also often proposed that only nulliparous women be studied, as a significant number of multiparous women with pre-eclampsia have underlying disease. However, 30–40% of women with pre-eclampsia are multiparous and these women often have important morbidity. The research question should determine whether or not multiparous women are included.

There is increasing interest in studying phenotypic subgroups of pre-eclampsia, such as early-onset versus late-onset disease or pre-eclampsia with and without fetal growth restriction (von Dadelszen et al., 2003). At present, there is no recommended standard method of defining these subtypes. Often the definition utilized is determined by logistics and power issues, rather than the underlying research hypothesis. In the future this needs to be addressed if we are to advance understanding of this spectrum of conditions currently included under the label of pre-eclampsia.

Inherent difficulties and pitfalls when measuring blood pressure

Blood pressure falls with pregnancy, and is significantly lower by the end of the first trimester, reaching a nadir between 20 and 24 weeks' gestation, increasing back to nonpregnant values by term. Blood pressure constantly fluctuates in response to numerous physiological variables. Posture (increased diastolic with standing), exercise, smoking (5–10 mmHg increase within minutes), coffee, cold weather and stress increase blood pressure. White coat hypertension (sustained hypertension in clinic, but normal blood pressures

Table 17.2. Recommendations for recording blood pressure in pregnancy*

Measure blood pressure in both arms at first visit, thereafter the right arm. In labor, if a left lateral position is used, use the left arm.

The pregnant woman should be seated, feet supported, for 2–3 min.

Appropriate sized cuff (large if arm circumference >33 cm).

The cuff should be at the level of the heart.

Systolic blood pressure should be palpated at brachial artery and cuff inflated to 20 mmHg above this level.

Deflate cuff slowly, at approximately 2 mmHg per second.

Record systolic and diastolic blood pressure.

Use Korotkoff V (disappearance of sound) for diastolic blood pressure, and only use phase IV (muffling) if phase V is not present.

*Based on ASSHP recommendations (Brown et al., 2000).

at home) occurs in fewer than 5% of pregnant women (Brown et al., 1999). Neither white coat hypertension nor the white coat effect (a >20 mmHg difference between clinic and home blood pressures) is associated with adverse pregnancy outcomes (Brown et al., 1999). Blood pressure normally decreases with sleep, resulting in a circadian rhythm (Taylor et al., 2001). Nocturnal hypertension is particularly common in women with pre-eclampsia compared to other causes of hypertension in pregnancy (Brown et al., 2001).

As the diagnosis of pre-eclampsia is based on blood pressure measurement, it should be performed accurately. Measurement of blood pressure is subject to equipment, technique and observer errors. Traditionally mercury sphygmomanometers are used to measure blood pressure in pregnancy. Recommendations for taking blood pressure are summarized in Table 17.2. Device errors include inability to see mercury meniscus, meniscus not returning to zero and perished rubber or a faulty valve that prevents slow and controlled release of cuff inflation (Shennan and Halligan, 1999). Technique errors include incorrect position of patient (e.g. lying supine), incorrect cuff size leading to overestimation (5–10 mmHg diastolic and 7–13 mmHg systolic) if the cuff is too small and underestimation of blood pressure (3–5 mmHg) if the cuff is too large (Maxwell *et al.*, 1982), failure to have the cuff at the level of the heart, digit preference and rounding to the nearest 5 or 10 mmHg (Stone *et al.*, 1995). Interobserver variability is greater with the use of Korotkoff IV (muffling) rather than Korotkoff V (disappearance) to measure the diastolic blood pressure (Shennan *et al.*, 1996a). A small randomized trial found use of Korotkoff V instead of IV was safe (Brown *et al.*, 1998), and the current recommendation is to use Korotkoff V (Anonymous, 2002; Brown *et al.*, 2000). Aneroid sphygmomanometers in pregnant women are also widely used in the community, despite limited validation in pregnant women. Aneroids become less accurate over time and require regular calibration (usually six-monthly).

Recognition of the inherent errors of mercury measurements and the wish to remove mercury containing equipment from many hospitals has fueled considerable interest in automated blood pressure devices (Halligan *et al.*, 1995). Before introduction into clinical care, electronic or ambulatory blood pressure devices require validation according to the British Hypertension Society (BHS) (O'Brien *et al.*, 1993b) or the American Association for the Advancement of Medical Instrumentation (AAMI). The hemodynamic changes with pregnancy have usually not been accounted for in the algorithms used to calculate blood pressure in automated monitors. Although several monitors performed satisfactorily through a range of normal blood pressures in pregnancy (Clarke *et al.*, 1991; Gupta *et al.*, 1997; O'Brien *et al.*, 1993a; Penny *et al.*, 2001; Reinders *et al.*, 2003; Shennan *et al.*, 1993), only the Microlife 3BTO-A monitor has been validated for use in pre-eclampsia (Golara *et al.*, 2002; Gupta *et al.*, 1997; Natarajan *et al.*, 1999; Quinn, 1994; Reinders *et al.*, 2003, 2005; Shennan *et al.*, 1996b). Use of non-validated electronic monitors can result in clinically important inaccuracies in blood pressure measurement

(Lo *et al.*, 2002). Automated monitors used in theatres and high-dependency units, such as the Dinamap®, may also be inaccurate in pre-eclampsia (Franx *et al.*, 1994).

Inherent difficulties and pitfalls when determining proteinuria

Urinary protein excretion increases in normal pregnancy, with the upper 95% confidence limit of total protein excretion being 200–260 mg 24 h^{-1} and urinary albumin excretion of 29 mg 24 h^{-1} (Higby *et al.*, 1994; Kuo *et al.*, 1992). The gold standard for determining proteinuria remains the 24 h urinary protein excretion.

In the setting of gestational hypertension and pre-eclampsia there is a clinical need for a quick and accurate test to determine the presence of proteinuria. Women with gestational hypertension are usually managed as outpatients and the presence of proteinuria changes their diagnosis to pre-eclampsia, consequently modifying their care. As pre-eclamptic women are at significantly greater risk of developing severe maternal and fetal complications (Brown and Buddle, 1995a; Hauth *et al.*, 2000; North *et al.*, 1999), they are usually managed as inpatients, allowing more intensive observation and investigation. Therefore a positive test for proteinuria in a woman with gestational hypertension commonly leads to hospitalization. A rapid test for proteinuria is also required as part of the armamentarium when assessing acutely ill women with probable severe pre-eclampsia, as delivery may supervene before a 24 h urinary collection is complete. The urinary dipstick has been the primary method of rapidly measuring proteinuria, but it is fraught with incorrect results.

Dipstick urinalysis to determine proteinuria

The dipstick test for urinary protein is simple and easy to perform. It is, however, subject to

Table 17.3. False negative and false positive rates for urinary dipstick measurements in pregnancy

Incorrect dipstick result	Proteinuria on dipstick			
	"−" or trace	"+" or $0.3\,\mathrm{g\,l^{-1}}$	"++" or $1\,\mathrm{g\,l^{-1}}$	"3+−4+" or $3\text{–}5\,\mathrm{g\,l^{-1}}$
False negatives*	$8\text{–}66\%^{\dagger}$			
False positives**		$17\text{–}83\%^{\gamma}$	$6\text{–}18\%^{\delta}$	$0\text{–}8\%^{\delta}$

*Dipstick is negative, but the 24 h protein $\geq 0.3\,\mathrm{g\,24\,h^{-1}}$.
**Dipstick is positive, but the 24 h protein is $< 0.3\,\mathrm{g}$.
†Brown and Buddle (1995b), Kuo *et al.* (1992), Meyer *et al.* (1994), Waugh *et al.* (2001).
γBrown and Buddle (1995b), Meyer *et al.* (1994), Saudan *et al.* (1997).
δBrown and Buddle (1995b), Meyer *et al.* (1994).

physiological factors, as well as genuine errors, that result in a significant number of false positive and false negative results. Urinary protein excretion varies throughout the day, with physiological modification occurring in response to variables such as posture and exercise (Douma *et al.*, 1995; Halligan *et al.*, 1999).

A urinary dipstick value is a concentration measurement, and therefore subject to changes in urine dilution. The effect of testing the more concentrated early-morning specimen, rather than a urine specimen collected later in the day, is an improvement in sensitivity to detect significant proteinuria, but this is at the expense of more false positives. The order of effect is, however, small with sensitivity of $\geq$"1+" reducing from 86% in an early morning specimen to 82% in a random urine specimen, with the positive predictive values increasing from 38% to 46%, respectively (Brown and Buddle, 1995b). Urinary dipstick of "1+" is equivalent to $0.3\text{–}0.5\,\mathrm{g\,l^{-1}}$ on most available brands. Given the average daily urine volume is 1.5 l (Halligan *et al.*, 1999), this equates to a 24 h urinary protein of 0.45–0.75 g. Therefore when the 24 h urinary protein is just abnormal $(0.3\text{–}0.5\,\mathrm{g\,24\,h^{-1}})$, it follows there will be false negatives on urinary dipstick testing.

Amongst women with hypertensive problems, there are high rates of incorrect urinary dipstick results (Table 17.3). Of concern, up to 66% of hypertensive women with a negative urinary dipstick were found to have significant proteinuria (Meyer *et al.*, 1994). In another study, 40% of 66 hospital staff tested a protein solution at $380\,\mathrm{mg\,l^{-1}}$ (i.e. equivalent to $>0.3\,\mathrm{g\,24\,h^{-1}}$ urinary protein excretion) as negative, and 8% still called a $1.0\,\mathrm{g\,l^{-1}}$ solution negative (Kuo *et al.*, 1992). Studies report markedly different sensitivity [22% (Waugh *et al.*, 2001), 67% (Meyer *et al.*, 1994) and 86% (Brown and Buddle, 1995b)] of urinary dipstick $\geq$"1+" to detect significant proteinuria $(>0.3\,\mathrm{g\,24\,h^{-1}})$ in hypertensive women. The performance of a urinary dipstick changes with the type of dipstick employed (Higby *et al.*, 1995) and the method of quantifying protein in the 24 h urine (Waugh *et al.*, 2001). Of interest, two studies that reported very different sensitivity (22% and 86%), used the same method to measure 24 h urinary protein (benzethonium chloride assay), but different brands of urinary dipstick (Brown and Buddle, 1995b; Waugh *et al.*, 2001). The center with high sensitivity also reported a high false positive rate at "1+" (67%), indicating staff may have been trained to have a low threshold to read a test as positive. Further, the dipstick cannot be used to accurately quantify proteinuria at levels greater than $0.3\,\mathrm{g\,24\,h^{-1}}$ (Kuo *et al.*, 1992; Meyer *et al.*, 1994).

Observer error when reading urinary dipsticks is a well-recognized problem. Training staff reduces observer error (Bell *et al.*, 1999). To remove observer variation, there are automated dipstick readers that can be used in a clinic setting and these have been shown to improve the performance of urinary dipstick compared to the gold standard, 24 h urine protein excretion (Saudan *et al.*, 1997). Automated dipstick readers are, therefore, the preferred option with trained staff the second choice, but asking patients to test their own urine is inappropriate.

The clinicians' interpretation of the significance of the false positive and false negative rates with urinary dipsticks determines their management response. The clinician may dismiss the "1+" urinary dipstick as probably a false positive. On balance, most studies report more true positives than false positives. In the presence of gestational hypertension the prudent approach is to assume the woman has significant proteinuria, and therefore pre-eclampsia, and to arrange a random urine protein : creatinine ratio and/or a 24 h urinary protein to confirm or refute the dipstick result. A midstream urine may be performed at the same time to exclude a urinary tract infection. Equally important is the clinician's response to the false negative result in women with gestational hypertension. Failure to detect proteinuria on dipstick should not offer unqualified reassurance that this rules out pre-eclampsia, especially if there are other features of the pre-eclamptic syndrome. Overall 26–46% of women with gestational hypertension progress to pre-eclampsia (Barton *et al.*, 2001; Saudan *et al.*, 1998). The gestation at presentation modifies the rate of disease progression, with progression occurring in 42% of women with gestational hypertension presenting before 30 weeks, falling to 7% among those presenting after 37 weeks' gestation (Saudan *et al.*, 1998). Appreciation of the false negative rate on urinary dipstick enables the clinician to factor this in when planning follow-up of women with gestational hypertension.

24 h urinary protein excretion

Although the gold standard, the 24 h urinary protein is subject to inaccuracies due to incomplete collection of the specimen or the effects of dehydration. Variation in the 24 h urinary protein measurement due to such factors could be minimized if a 24 h protein creatinine ratio was used rather than the absolute 24 h protein excretion. Further research is necessary to determine the threshold value for an abnormal 24 h protein creatinine ratio in pregnancy. There is no international agreement on the optimal laboratory method to measure urinary protein, and a range of methods (e.g. turbidometric methods such as the benzethonium chloride method, Coomassie brilliant blue dye-binding) are widely used. The lack of a universal method to estimate urinary proteins, alters the range of proteins that are measured and consequently the levels reported (Waugh *et al.*, 2001). This inevitably limits comparison of values between different centers, a fact not widely appreciated.

Protein : creatinine ratio

To circumvent the practical difficulties of collecting 24 h urine specimens and the limitations of urinary dipstick measurements, researchers have investigated the use of the protein : creatinine ratio on a spot urine specimen. This should not be confused with an albumin (measured by immunoassay) : creatinine ratio which has not been shown to be of value in testing for proteinuria associated with hypertensive disorders of pregnancy.

Most (Jaschevatzky *et al.*, 1990; Neithardt *et al.*, 2002; Ramos *et al.*, 1999; Robert *et al.*, 1997; Saudan *et al.*, 1997), but not all (Durnwald and Mercer, 2003; Rodriguez-Thompson and Lieberman, 2001), studies have reported a good correlation ($r = 0.92–0.94$) between a spot protein : creatinine ratio and the 24 h urinary protein. However, only a few studies are appropriately designed to evaluate the usefulness of a protein : creatinine ratio as a screening/diagnostic test for significant proteinuria (24 h protein ≥ 0.3 g) in hypertensive disorders of pregnancy and both are relatively underpowered (Durnwald and Mercer, 2003; Saudan *et al.*, 1997). In the first study of a hundred women seen because of hypertensive problems in pregnancy, a spot urinary protein:creatinine ratio was compared with 24 h urinary protein (abnormal $>0.3\,g\,24\,h^{-1}$) (Saudan *et al.*, 1997). Using a cut-off value of $30\,mg\,mmol^{-1}$ for an abnormal protein:creatinine ratio, sensitivity was 93%, specificity 95%, and positive predictive value 95% with a negative predictive value of 90%. None of the false negatives had a 24 h urinary protein greater than 0.4 g. The conclusion from this study was this method could be used to rapidly screen hypertensive pregnant women for proteinuria. A recent study of 220 women evaluated for suspected pre-eclampsia has found the ratio did not perform as well as this, although they used a different method to measure proteinuria (biuret reaction rather than the benzethonium chloride turbidometric method used by Saudan and co-workers) (Durnwald and Mercer, 2003). Using a cut-off of $300\,mg\,g^{-1}$ (equivalent to approximately $34\,mg\,mmol^{-1}$) to define an abnormal protein:creatinine ratio, they reported a sensitivity of 81%, specificity 56%, positive predictive value of 86% and a negative predictive value of 48%. In other words, 19% of women with significant proteinuria on a 24 h urine were not detected by a protein:creatinine ratio, the majority of women with a positive test do have significant proteinuria but half the women with a negative protein:creatinine ratio result had significant proteinuria. Overall the protein:creatinine ratio with a $300\,mg\,g^{-1}$ cut-off correctly categorized 75% of women with respect to proteinuria being present or absent. From the ROC analysis data, if a lower cut-off ($200\,mg\,g^{-1}$) was used then sensitivity increased to 91%, specificity remained low at 48% and 39% of women with a normal protein:creatinine ratio had significant proteinuria on a 24 h urine. At this lower cut-off value, overall 80% of women were correctly categorized as having or not having proteinuria.

In summary, a protein:creatinine ratio is probably a more accurate method to screen for proteinuria than urinary dipstick, particularly at "1+", and possibly "2+" on dipstick. In the setting of gestational hypertension with either a negative, trace or "1+" on dipstick, then a spot 24 h urine protein:creatinine ratio may be a helpful screening test to identify those women with and without proteinuria. If proteinuria is "≥3+" on dipstick, the rate of false positive tests is so low that the protein:creatinine adds little as a screening test and protein excretion should be quantified directly on a 24 h specimen. The protein : creatinine ratio has not been found to be an accurate method of quantifying protein excretion and should not be used to track progression of proteinuria in pre-eclampsia. Centers will need to evaluate local performance of the protein:creatinine ratio, as performance may be influenced by their patient population and the method of measuring protein. Further research is required to refine the role of a protein:creatinine ratio in the management of women with gestational hypertension and pre-eclampsia. At present it should not replace the 24 h urinary protein as the definitive test to determine whether a woman has significant proteinuria.

Diagnosis of superimposed pre-eclampsia in chronic hypertension, renal disease and diabetes

In contrast to gestational hypertension and pre-eclampsia that occur in the second half of pregnancy, hypertension that is evident before 20 weeks' gestation is diagnosed as chronic hypertension. The Australasian and American classifications are consistent in their definitions of chronic hypertension, blood pressure ≥140 mmHg systolic and/or ≥90 mmHg diastolic pre-conception or in the first half of pregnancy (Anonymous, 2000; Brown *et al.*, 2000). Rare exceptions include hydatidiform molar pregnancies, severe renal disease or antiphospholid syndrome and occasional chromosomal anomalies, where true pre-eclampsia can occur before 20 weeks. For women presenting with hypertension for the first time in early pregnancy, it is necessary to confirm that their blood pressure remains elevated at least

3 months after delivery. Chronic hypertension is subdivided into essential and secondary due to underlying causes such as renal disease (e.g. glomerulonephritis, reflux nephropathy, adult polycystic kidney disease), systemic disease with renal complications (e.g. systemic lupus erythematosus, diabetes), renal artery stenosis or endocrine disorders (e.g. cushings, phaeochromocytoma) (Brown *et al.*, 2000).

The diagnosis of superimposed pre-eclampsia in the context of chronic hypertension, renal disease or diabetes is difficult. The signs (hypertension and proteinuria) used to make the diagnosis may already be present. Further, new or worsening hypertension or proteinuria can occur alone in these conditions, and do not indicate pre-eclampsia per se. As a consequence of these inherent difficulties, recent definitions do not offer very precise criteria for the diagnosis of superimposed pre-eclampsia (Anonymous, 2000; Brown *et al.*, 2000). Superimposed pre-eclampsia is likely when there is a significant increase in blood pressure ($>30/15$ mmHg) in the second half of pregnancy associated with either the development of new proteinuria >0.3 g 24 h^{-1} or a sudden increase (doubling) in prior proteinuria. Other supportive features of multisystem and fetal manifestations (see Table 17.1) are necessary to be secure that this is pre-eclampsia, not just pregnancy-induced aggravation of signs present because of the underlying medical condition (Brown *et al.*, 2000). Given the difficulties diagnosing superimposed pre-eclampsia, and the progressive nature of pre-eclampsia toward severe maternal and fetal morbidity, surveillance should be increased in cases of suspected superimposed pre-eclampsia.

Future

In the last two decades there have been significant advances in understanding pre-eclampsia and with this, better diagnostic classifications. The diagnosis of pre-eclampsia is currently still based on a collection of symptoms, signs and a few laboratory tests. Many of the measures used are imprecise, inaccurate and subject to significant operator variability. The need for large prospective clinical trials to properly evaluate current criteria used to define pre-eclampsia, and to identify subgroups at particular risk of severe sequelae, have been highlighted (Anonymous, 2000). In addition, internationally agreed upon diagnostic criteria for disease subsets, such as early-onset pre-eclampsia or those with a growth restricted fetus, need to be developed (von Dadelszen *et al.*, 2003).

The lack of reliable, objective methods to define and diagnose pre-eclampsia has created the clinical need for a diagnostic test that accurately identifies women with pre-eclampsia, especially those with rapidly progressive disease. Technological advances, such as in proteomics, have created the opportunity to develop such novel diagnostic tests for the syndrome. The objectives of novel diagnostic tests should be clear. Amongst women with pre-eclampsia will the aim be to detect all with hypertension and proteinuria in the second half of pregnancy, or those with multisystem disease or perhaps those who will develop multisystem disease in the near future? In addition, there is a need for a diagnostic test that recognizes superimposed pre-eclampsia when there is underlying maternal disease.

In the future, it is likely that there will be more objective methods of diagnosing and risk-classifying women with pregnancy-induced hypertensive complications. Improved diagnostic/screening criteria for pre-eclampsia would advance obstetric care, with the potential to decrease severe maternal morbidity through timely delivery and to reduce infant morbidity and mortality through unnecessary iatrogenic delivery of the very preterm infant.

REFERENCES

Anonymous. (1990). National High Blood Pressure Education Program Working Group report on ambulatory blood pressure monitoring. *Arch. Int. Med.*, **150**, 2270–80.

Anonymous. (2000). National High Blood Pressure Education Program Working Group report on high blood pressure in pregnancy. NIH Publication No. 00-3029.

Anonymous. (2002). American College of Obstetricians and Gynecologists. Diagnosis and management of preeclampsia and eclampsia. ACOG Practice Bulletin No. 33. *Obstet. Gynecol.*, **99**, 159–67.

Barton, J. R., O'Brien J. M., Bergauer, N. K., Jacques, D. L. and Sibai, B. M. (2001). Mild gestational hypertension remote from term: progression and outcome. *Am. J. Obstet. Gynecol.*, **184**, 979–83.

Bell, S., Halligan, A., Martin, A., *et al.* (1999). The role of observer error in antenatal dipstick proteinuria analysis. *Br. J. Obstet. Gynaecol.*, **106**, 1177–80.

Brown, M. and Buddle, M. (1995a). The importance of nonproteinuric hypertension in pregnancy. *Hypertens. Preg.*, **14**, 57–65.

Brown, M. and Buddle, M. (1995b). Inadequacy of dipstick proteinuria in hypertensive pregnancy. *Aust. N. Z. J. Obstet. Gynaecol.*, **35**, 366–9.

Brown, M., Buddle, M., Farrell, T., Davis, G. and Jones, M. (1998). Randomised trial of management of hypertensive pregnancies by Korotkoff phase IV or phase V. *Lancet*, **352**, 777–81.

Brown, M. A., Robinson, A. and Jones, M. (1999). The white coat effect in hypertensive pregnancy: much ado about nothing? *Br. J. Obstet. Gynaecol.*, **106**, 474–80.

Brown, M. A., Hague, W. M., Higgins, J., *et al.* (2000). The detection, investigation and management of hypertension in pregnancy: full consensus statement. *Aust. N. Z. J. Obstet. Gynaecol.*, **40**, 139–55.

Brown, M. A., Davis, G. K. and McHugh, L. (2001). The prevalence and clinical significance of nocturnal hypertension in pregnancy. *J. Hypertens.*, **19**, 1437–44.

Chappell, L., Poulton, L., Halligan, A. and Shennan, A. H. (1999). Lack of consistency in research papers over the definition of pre-eclampsia. *Br. J. Obstet. Gynaecol.*, **106**, 983–5.

Clarke, S., Hofmeyr, G. J., Coats, A. J. and Redman, C. W. G. (1991). Ambulatory blood pressure monitoring in pregnancy: validation of the TM-2420 monitor. *Obstet. Gynecol.*, **77**, 152–5.

CLASP. (1994). Collaborative Low-dose Aspirin Study in Pregnancy: a randomised trial of low-dose aspirin for the prevention and treatment of pre-eclampsia among 9364 pregnant women. *Lancet*, **343**, 619–29.

Davey, D. A. and MacGillivray, I. (1988). The classification and definition of the hypertensive disorders of pregnancy. *Am. J. Obstet. Gynecol.*, **158**, 892–8.

Douglas, K. A. and Redman, C. W. (1994). Eclampsia in the United Kingdom. *Br. Med. J.*, **309**, 1395–400.

Douma, C. E., van der Post, J. A., van Acker, B. A. C., Boer, K. and Koopman, M. G. (1995). Circadian variation of urinary albumin excretion in pregnancy. *Br. J. Obstet. Gynaecol.*, **102**, 107–10.

Durnwald, C. and Mercer, B. (2003). A prospective comparison of total protein/creatinine ratio versus 24-hour urine protein in women with suspected pre-eclampsia. *Am. J. Obstet. Gynecol.*, **189**, 848–52.

Franx, A., van der Post, J., Elfering, I., *et al.* (1994). Validation of automated blood pressure recording in pregnancy. *Br. J. Obstet. Gynaecol.*, **101**, 66–9.

Golara, M., Benedict, A., Jones, C., Randhawa, M., Poston, L. and Shennan, A. H. (2002). Inflationary oscillometry provides accurate measurement of blood pressure in pre-eclampsia. *Br. J. Obstet. Gynaecol.*, **109**, 1143–7.

Gupta, M., Shennan, A. H., Halligan, A., Taylor, D. J. and de Swiet, M. (1997). Accuracy of oscillometric blood pressure monitoring in pregnancy and pre-eclampsia. *Br. J. Obstet. Gynaecol.*, **104**, 350–5.

Halligan, A., Bell, S. and Taylor, D. (1999). Dipstick proteinuria: caveat emptor. *Br. J. Obstet. Gynaecol.*, **106**, 1113–15.

Halligan, A., Shennan, A., Thurston, H., de Swiet, M. and Taylor, D. (1995). Ambulatory blood pressure measurement in pregnancy: the current state of the art. *Hypertens. Preg.*, **14**, 1–16.

Harlow, F. H. and Brown, M. A. (2001). The diversity of diagnoses of preeclampsia. *Hypertens. Preg.*, **20**, 57–67.

Hauth, J. C., Ewell, M. G., Levine, R. J., *et al.* (2000). Pregnancy outcomes in healthy nulliparas who developed hypertension. *Obstet. Gynecol.*, **95**, 24–8.

Helewa, M., Burrows, R., Smith, J., Williams, K., Brain, P. and Rabkin, S. (1997). Report of the Canadian Hypertension Society consensus conference: 1. Definitions, evaluation and classification of hypertensive disorders in pregnancy. *Can. Med. Assoc. J.*, **157**, 715–25.

Higby, K., Suiter, C. R., Phelps, J. Y., Siler-Khoder, T. and Langer, O. (1994). Normal values of urinary albumin and total protein excretion during pregnancy. *Am. J. Obstet. Gynecol.*, **171**, 984–9.

Higby, K., Suiter, C. R. and Siler-Khoder, T. (1995). A comparison between two screening methods for detection of microproteinuria. *Am. J. Obstet. Gynecol.*, **173**, 1111–14.

Hughes, E. ed. (1972). *Obstetric–Gynecologic Terminology*. Philadelphia: Davis, pp. 422–3.

Jaschevatzky, O. E., Rosenberg, R. P., Shalit, A., Zonder, H. B. and Grunstein, S. (1990). Protein/creatinine ratio in random urine specimens for quantitation of protein-uria in preeclampsia. *Obstet. Gynecol.*, **75**, 604–6.

Kuo, V., Koumantakis, G. and Gallery, E. (1992). Protein-uria and its assessment in normal and hypertensive pregnancy. *Am. J. Obstet. Gynecol.*, **167**, 723–8.

Levine, R. J., Ewell, M. G., Hauth, J. C., *et al.* (2000). Should the definition of preeclampsia include a rise in diastolic blood pressure of >/=15 mmHg to a level <90 mmHg in association with proteinuria? *Am. J. Obstet. Gynecol.*, **183**, 787–92.

Lo, C., Taylor, R. S., Gamble, G., McCowan, L. and North, R. A. (2002). Use of automated home blood pressure monitoring in pregnancy: is it safe? *Am. J. Obstet. Gynecol.*, **187**, 1321–8.

Maxwell, M. H., Waks, A. U., Schroth, P. C., Karam, M. and Dornfield, L. P. (1982). Error in blood pressure measure-ment due to incorrect cuff size in obese patients. *Lancet*, **ii**, 33–6.

Meyer, N., Mercer, B., Friedman, S. and Sibai, B. (1994). Urinary dipstick protein: a poor predictor of absent or severe proteinuria. *Am. J. Obstet. Gynecol.*, **170**, 137–41.

Natarajan, P., Shennan, A. H., Penny, J., Halligan, A. W., de Swiet, M. and Anthony, J. (1999). Comparison of auscultatory and oscillometric automated blood pres-sure monitors in the setting of preeclampsia. *Am. J. Obstet. Gynecol.*, **181**, 1203–10.

Neithardt, A. B., Dooley, S. L. and Borensztajn, J. (2002). Prediction of 24-hour protein excretion in pregnancy with a single voided urine protein-to-creatinine ratio. *Am. J. Obstet. Gynecol.*, **186**, 883–6.

North, R. A., Taylor, R. S. and Schellenberg, J. C. (1999). Evaluation of a definition of pre-eclampsia. *Br. J. Obstet. Gynaecol.*, **106**, 767–73.

O'Brien, E., Mee, F., Atkins, N., Halligan, A. and O'Malley, K. (1993a). Accuracy of the SpaceLabs 90207 ambulatory blood pressure measuring system in nor-motensive pregnant women determined by the British Hypertension Society protocol. *J. Hypertens.*, **11**, S282–3.

O'Brien, E., Petrie, J., Littler, W., *et al.* (1993b). The British Hypertension Society protocol for the evaluation of blood pressure measuring devices. *J. Hypertens.*, **11**, S43–62.

Ohkoshi, A., Iwasaki, R., Ojima, T., *et al.* (2003). Increase in systolic blood pressure of ≥30 mmHg and/or diastolic blood pressure of ≥15 mmHg during pregnancy: is it pathologic? *Hypertens. Preg.*, **22**, 275–86.

Penny, J., Shennan, A., Rushbrook, J., Halligan, A., Taylor, D. J. and De Swiet, M. (2001). Validation of the Welch Allyn QuietTrak ambulatory blood pressure monitor in pregnancy. *Hypertens. Preg.*, **15**, 313–21.

Perry, I. J. and Beevers, D. G. (1994). The definition of pre-eclampsia. *Br. J. Obstet. Gynaecol.*, **101**, 587–91.

Quinn, M. (1994). Automated blood pressure measure-ment devices: a potential source of morbidity in preeclampsia? *Am. J. Obstet. Gynecol.*, **170**, 1303–7.

Ramos, J. G. L., Martins-Costa, S. H., Mathias, M. M., Guerin, Y. L. S. and Barros, E. G. (1999). Urinary protein/creatinine ratio in hypertensive pregnant women. *Hypertens. Preg.*, **18**, 209–18.

Redman, C. W. and Jefferies, M. (1988). Revised definition of pre-eclampsia. *Lancet*, **1**, 809–12.

Reinders, A., Cuckson, A. C., Jones, C. R., Poet, R., O'Sullivan, G. and Shennan, A. (2003). Validation of the Welch Allyn 'Vital Signs' blood pressure measure-ment device in pregnancy and pre-eclampsia. *Br. J. Obstet. Gynaecol.*, **110**, 134–8.

Reinders, A., Cuckson, A. C., Lee, J. T. M. and Shennan, A. H. (2005). An accurate automated pressure device for use in pregnancy and pre-eclampsia: the Microlife 3BTO-A. *Br. J. Obstet. Gynaecol.*, **112**, 915–20.

Robert, M., Sepandj, F., Liston, R. M. and Dooley, K. C. (1997). Random protein–creatinine ratio for the quan-titation of proteinuria in pregnancy. *Obstet. Gynecol.*, **90**, 893–5.

Rodriguez-Thompson, D. and Lieberman, E. S. (2001). Use of a random urinary protein-to-creatinine ratio for the diagnosis of significant proteinuria during pregnancy. *Am. J. Obstet. Gynecol.*, **185**, 808–11.

Saudan, P., Brown, M., Buddle, M. and Jones, M. (1998). Does gestational hypertension become pre-eclampsia? *Br. J. Obstet. Gynaecol.*, **105**, 1177–84.

Saudan, P., Brown, M., Farrell, T. and Shaw, L. (1997). Improved methods of assessing proteinuria in hyper-tensive pregnancy. *Br. J. Obstet. Gynaecol.*, **104**, 1159–64.

Shennan, A., Gupta, M., Halligan, A., Taylor, D. and de Swiet, M. (1996a). Lack of reproducibility in preg-nancy of Korotkoff phase IV as measured by mercury sphygmomanometry. *Lancet*, **347**, 139–42.

Shennan, A., Halligan, A., Gupta, M., Taylor, D. and de Swiet, M. (1996b). Oscillometric blood pressure measurements in severe pre-eclampsia: validation of the SpaceLabs 90207. *Br. J. Obstet. Gynaecol.*, **103**, 171–3.

Shennan, A.H. and Halligan, W.F. (1999). Measuring blood pressure in normal and hypertensive pregnancy. *Baill. Clin. Obstet. Gynaecol.*, **13**, 1–26.

Shennan, A.H., Kissane, J. and de Swiet, M. (1993). Validation of the SpaceLabs 90207 ambulatory blood pressure monitor for use in pregnancy. *Br. J. Obstet. Gynaecol.*, **100**, 904–8.

Stone, P., Cook, D., Hutton, J., Purdie, G., Murray, H. and Harcourt, L. (1995). Measurements of blood pressure, oedema and proteinuria in a pregnant population of New Zealand. *Aust. N.Z. J. Obstet. Gynaecol.*, **35**, 32–7.

Taylor, R.S., Gamble, G., McCowan, L. and North, R.A. (2001). Sleep effects on ambulatory blood pressure measurements in pregnant women. *Am. J. Hypertens.*, **14**, 38–43.

Villar, M.A. and Sibai, B.M. (1989). Clinical significance of elevated mean arterial blood pressure in second trimester and threshold increase in systolic or diastolic blood pressure during third trimester. *Am. J. Obstet. Gynecol.*, **160**, 419–23.

von Dadelszen, P., Magee, L. and Roberts, J.M. (2003). Subclassification of preeclampsia. *Hypertens. Preg.*, **22**, 143–8.

Waugh, J., Bell, S.C., Kilby, M., Lambert, P., Shennan, A. and Halligan, A. (2001). Effect of concentration and biochemical assay on the accuracy of urine dipsticks in hypertensive pregnancies. *Hypertens. Preg.*, **20**, 205–17.

Weinstein, L. (1982). Syndrome of hemolysis, elevated liver enzymes, and low platelet count: a severe consequence of hypertension in pregnancy. *Am. J. Obstet. Gynecol.*, **142**, 159–67.

Zhang, J., Klebanoff, M.A. and Roberts, J.M. (2001). Prediction of adverse outcomes by common definitions of hypertension in pregnancy. *Obstet. Gynecol.*, **97**, 261–7.

18

Measuring blood pressure in pregnancy and pre-eclampsia

Andrew H. Shennan and Annemarie De Greeff

Introduction

Blood pressure is measured routinely during the antenatal period. Accurate blood pressure measurement is essential to the diagnosis and management of hypertension in pregnancy. The gold standard for measuring indirect blood pressure is the mercury sphygmomanometer, although it is widely acknowledged that it has associated errors and that alternatives are not dependent on the skill of the observer, which can have significant advantages.

One such alternative is automated equipment. However, the inherent inaccuracies of most automated devices are confounded by the altered hemodynamic state of pregnancy and especially pre-eclampsia. Evidence already points to significant inaccuracies in women with pre-eclampsia. However, as most of these devices are intended for home monitoring they have the potential to reduce inpatient monitoring whilst improving surveillance. The role of this type of monitoring is yet to be to established.

It is of critical importance that these devices are evaluated according to a recognized protocol, i.e. the British Hypertension Society, the European Society of Hypertension or the Association for the Advancement of Medical Instrumentation, before their accuracy in clinical practice, and especially an obstetric population, can be assumed.

Accurate and precise technique and the use of properly calibrated and well-maintained equipment is vital.

The importance of blood pressure in pregnancy

The importance of blood pressure measurement during pregnancy has been recognized for more than a century (Seligman, 1987) and is a fundamental part of antenatal care. For many women their pregnancy will be the first point of medical contact and they may have been unaware of any pre-existing hypertension up to this point.

Early diagnosis of hypertension has important implications for the management and prognosis of both the mother and the fetus. It is dependent on the accurate measurement of blood pressure, as hypertension is often the only early sign of impending pre-eclampsia. It is not, however, necessarily indicative of pre-eclampsia or indeed eclampsia.

A survey of eclamptic women in the United Kingdom in 1992 demonstrated that a significant proportion of women did not have a blood pressure measurement that adequately distinguished them from the general antenatal population and fits occurred in hospital without severe hypertension (Douglas and Redman, 1994). There is also evidence of an increased perinatal mortality rate associated with blood pressures recorded below 140/90 mmHg (Browne and Dodds, 1942; Chesley, 1976; Rippmann, 1968).

If eclampsia occurs at normal pressures, it may be that blood pressure measurement will become much less significant in identifying women prone to eclampsia. Currently clinicians rely mainly on blood pressure to identify, diagnose and manage these women and an increasing proportion of women will be "missed" according to current blood pressure criteria. It is uncertain to what degree the current errors associated with mercury sphygmomanometery as well as automated devices could contribute to the failure of current screening methods.

Women with chronic hypertension are usually essentially hypertensive and sometimes have underlying renal disease. They are at an increased risk (Ferrazzani et al., 1990; Mabie et al., 1986; Rey and Couturier, 1994; Sibai and Anderson, 1986; Sibai et al., 1983), regardless of whether they present with superimposed pre-eclampsia or not. Compared to normotensive pregnancies, women with chronic hypertension have an increased risk of fetal loss (McCowan et al., 1996). However, they have lower associated fetal and maternal morbidity compared to pre-eclamptic women (Ferrazzani et al., 1990; Mabie et al., 1986; Rey and Couturier, 1994; Sibai and Anderson, 1986; Sibai et al., 1983). Maternal mortality in women who have pre-eclampsia is mainly contributed to intracerebral hemorrhage (CEMD, 2004; HMSO, 1996). This direct arterial injury commonly occurs as a result of severe hypertension, when the limits of the auto regulation of the brain circulation have been exceeded (Strandgaard et al., 1973). An association between abruptio placentae and hypertension in pregnancy has been shown (Brosens and Renaer, 1972) and if severe hypertension is noted before 20 weeks gestation, it could result in adverse effects in the fetus.

Indirect determinants of blood pressure, whether it be Korotkoff sounds or oscillations, are dependent on the hemodynamics of the circulation. Blood pressure is a function of peripheral vascular resistance and cardiac output, both of which change during pregnancy and even more dramatically in pre-eclampsia. These changes will result in a change in blood pressure and have the potential to influence the characteristics of arterial oscillations that are generated during a blood pressure measurement cycle. As the vast majority of automated blood pressure devices rely on oscillometry to determine blood pressure, their accuracy in the

chronic hypertensive or normotensive state cannot be assumed to be equivalent in pre-eclampsia.

Pre-eclampsia

Pre-eclampsia is a multisystem disease that affects the maternal neurological, cardiovascular, renal, coagulation and hepatic systems to variable degrees. Later manifestations of the disease include symptoms of headache, epigastric pain and visual disturbance. The measurement of blood pressure is only a surrogate indicator of end organ involvement of the cardiovascular system. This partly explains the relatively poor relationship between blood pressure and outcome in this condition, although it defines the disease.

Widespread vascular endothelial damage goes some way in explaining the multisystem nature of the disease (Roberts and Redman, 1993) and it is presumed that differential effects of this pathological process explain the varied presentation of the disease and why hypertension may not be the first indication of the syndrome. Processes such as deported placental syncytiotrophoblasts (Smarason et al., 1993) and abnormal lipid profiles, thought to originate from the placenta (Branch et al., 1994; Lorentzen et al., 1995; Wang et al., 1991) are being linked to the pathophysiology of pre-eclampsia. Increased sympathetic vasoconstrictor activity to skeletal muscle, which reverts to normal after delivery, has been described (Howell and Brush, 1901).

In normal pregnancy, cardiac output increases by about 40% to compensate for the profound vasodilatation. This is achieved by an increase in stroke volume and heart rate. Increased cardiac output ensures that the blood pressure is maintained and adequate oxygen is supplied to the uterus and the fetus. It also supports the increased metabolic rate of the mother. Blood volume increases to a peak at 32 weeks gestation. In pre-eclampsia the cardiac output is often reduced, with increased blood pressure and therefore a profound increase in peripheral vascular resistance. There is

Table 18.1. Summary of the hemodynamic changes in pregnancy

	Change	Amount
Cardiac output	Increased (40%)	4.5–6.0 l min^{-1}
Stroke volume	Increased	65–70 ml
Heart rate	Increased	70–85 ml
Systemic vascular resistance	Reduced	1700–980 dynes s^{-1} cm^{-5}
Blood pressure	Reduced	5–10 mmHg
Blood volume	Increased	2600–3800 ml

associated reduced vascular volume and often surrounding tissue edema. It is important to bear in mind that the circulatory pathophysiology of a woman with pre-eclampsia may be different from that of a woman who has an underlying condition unrelated to the pregnancy which causes the equivalent level of blood pressure.

Table 18.2 summarizes the normal hemodynamic changes that occur in pregnancy.

Diagnosis of pre-eclampsia is currently dependent on clinical markers of "end-organ" damage, primarily blood pressure and proteinurea. Although pre-eclampsia is multisystem in nature, there is a clear association between both proteinurea and blood pressure and increasing perinatal mortality and morbidity (Butler and Bonham, 1963; Chua and Redman, 1992; Ferrazzani *et al.*, 1990; Moore and Redman, 1983; Naeye and Friedman, 1979).

Blood pressure and defining pre-eclampsia

Approximately 1 in 5 women will have a raised blood pressure recorded in the latter half of pregnancy (Redman, 1995) and a large proportion of these women will not be at any increased risk. A number of definitions have been developed over the years in an attempt to more accurately identify women at risk more accurately. They are primarily based on the level of blood pressure

and/or rise thereof from the baseline pressure measured in the first half of pregnancy (ACOG, 1986; Davey and MacGillivray, 1988; Redman and Jefferies, 1988).

Pregnancy-induced hypertension is defined as hypertension without proteinurea (Greer, 1992). It has been argued that this diagnosis can only be made retrospectively, however, as the hypertension is not always due to the pregnancy (Davey and MacGillivray, 1988).

The International Society for the Study of Hypertension in Pregnancy (ISSHP) has suggested the term "gestational hypertension" to be used for all hypertensive pregnant women (i.e. with/without proteinurea) who have not previously been hypertensive or proteinuric. Women who are gestationally hypertensive and then go on to develop proteinurea are then assumed to be pre-eclamptic until proven otherwise. This definition is adopted from that of Davey and MacGillivray.

The National High Blood Pressure Education Program Working Group Report on High Blood Pressure in Pregnancy defines pre-eclampsia as reaching a given blood pressure threshold (140/90 mmHg; Korotkoff phase 5 diastolic).

Redman and Jefferies, on the other hand, have suggested a diagnosis of pre-eclampsia when a threshold of blood pressure (diastolic of 90 mmHg; Korotkoff phase 4) and an incremental rise from the baseline (>25 mmHg) in the first half of pregnancy is reached.

All these definitions are confounded by the fact that they rely on blood pressure which is inherently variable, i.e. no single reading can be taken as representative of an individual's true blood pressure and readings are often taken using conventional mercury sphygmomanometry with its associated errors. A single raised reading can have substantial consequences for the individual and will invariably result in more frequent hospital visits and increased anxiety about the pregnancy. Toward the end of pregnancy it may even result in induction or delivery. Accurate characterization of blood pressure cannot be obtained from a single or a few readings.

In one study a comparison was made between the Redman and Jefferies definition and the classification suggested by Davey and MacGillivray (ISSHP definition) (Perry and Beevers, 1994). The outcome of 692 nulliparous women was evaluated. Eleven of the 12 women who developed proteinuric hypertension (as defined by the ISSHP) were identified by Redman and Jefferies' definition of using blood pressure parameters alone. In contrast, 33 of the 55 women who were classified as having gestational hypertension by the ISSHP definition fulfilled the Redman/Jefferies criteria. When comparing the ponderal index of these 33 babies with the babies of the 22 gestational hypertensives who were "missed" by Redman/Jefferies, there was a significant difference (22 vs. 24.9, $p<0.01$). The study concludes that the Redman/Jefferies definition (which incorporates an incremental rise in blood pressure) has advantages over the ISSHP definition, as it selects important features such as women who have proteinurea and poor outcome while also making a distinction between non-proteinuric pre-eclampsia and other causes of gestational hypertension. However, the authors also stress that a distinction should be made between proteinuric and non-proteinuric hypertension.

Systolic vs. diastolic pressure

There is some evidence to suggest that systolic pressure has a better relationship to outcome than diastolic pressure (Chesley and Annito, 1947; Fisher, 1985; Tervila et al., 1973), despite diastolic pressure being favored by most definitions described above.

In a recent study including more than 4000 hypertensive pregnant women, systolic pressure had a better correlation with perinatal mortality, low Apgar scores (<7), birth weight under 2500 g, and small for gestational age babies as compared with the diastolic pressure (Tervila et al., 1973). This study showed that the diastolic pressure could

be excluded without significant disadvantage in predicting outcome.

Systolic pressure is also more readily reproduced (Shennan et al., 1996a). Recommendations adopted by the WHO and the ISSHP (Davey and MacGillivray, 1988) state that systolic pressure is more variable than diastolic pressure and that it does not make any contribution toward the diagnostic or prognostic significance of the hypertensive disorders of pregnancy. There is little evidence to support this.

Incremental rise from baseline

The current thresholds for systolic and diastolic pressures (140/90 mmHg) are a compromise between clinical safety and over-diagnosis. It is dependent on gestation, i.e. a diastolic of 90 mmHg corresponds to 3 standard deviations (SD) above the mean for mid pregnancy, 2 SD at 34 weeks, and 1.5 SD at term (Greer, 1992). Other suggested thresholds vary from 125/75 mmHg (Chesley, 1976) to 135/85 mmHg (Rippmann, 1968).

Low thresholds are not clinically useful due to the large number of "false positives," i.e. women with high readings, but normal outcome. The higher thresholds obliterate this problem, but will inevitably miss some individuals who are at risk of an adverse outcome.

Pregnant women with pre-existing disease have different risks associated with their pregnancy than those without, and therefore thresholds to define chronic hypertension in pregnancy may be different from conventional definitions. Definitions that rely on a threshold alone may fail to distinguish these women which could be due to their increased risk of developing pre-eclampsia (Ferrazzani et al., 1990; Mabie et al., 1986; McCowan et al., 1996; Rey and Couturier, 1994; Sibai et al., 1983).

The American College of Gynecologists suggested that the baseline blood pressure should be taken as the average of values obtained before 20 weeks gestation. If these values were not available a threshold of 140/90 mmHg would be sufficient. A rise in blood pressure of 30 mmHg for systolic pressure and 15 mmHg for diastolic pressure is taken as a sign of hypertensive complication. This was met with criticism as the normal rise of diastolic pressure in the second half of pregnancy is usually greater than 10 mmHg (Chesley, 1976; MacGillivray et al., 1969). More recently this incremental rise has been recognized as inappropriate and is no longer recommended.

An increment of 25 mmHg was suggested following a retrospective study looking at the difference between blood pressure at the antenatal booking visit and the highest blood pressure recorded (Redman and Jefferies, 1988). This increment was associated with a significant reduction in birth weight, which was assumed to be an indication of intrauterine growth restriction and therefore a feature of pre-eclampsia. However, it is likely that the blood pressures studied were single readings predisposing it to the errors associated with single blood pressure readings, e.g. white coat hypertension. Therefore, the definition might not be valid in the case of repeated measurements being taken over time.

In summary, thresholds of blood pressure are being used increasingly in favor of incremental rises, but the astute clinician must be aware of the basic physiology that influences blood pressure change and therefore must be aware of possible pathology even if a threshold is not crossed.

History of blood pressure measurement

The first blood pressure recording was done in 1733 by the Reverend Stephen Hales (1677–1761). He inserted a brass tube into the crural artery of a restrained mare and observed the column of blood that rose in the tube.

Pioseuille used the first mercury sphygmomanometer in 1828 when he measured direct arterial pressure in a dog. Using mercury considerably reduced the height of the pressure column required (by a factor of 13.6). This study was the origin of the units for measuring blood pressure, i.e. millimeters of mercury (mmHg).

In 1847 Carl Ludwig fitted a floating pen onto the mercury sphygmomanometer, thus obtaining a graphical record of intra-arterial pressure and removing the observer error of having to estimate the maximum and minimum levels of the mercury column.

Thirty years later, Ritter von Basch applied a water-filled bag over a superficial artery which was backed by bone. By palpating an artery more distal whilst applying force to the bag, the pressure which resulted in occlusion could be read from a fluid-filled column attached to the bag. He was therefore able to measure blood pressure indirectly (i.e. without breaking the skin) for the first time.

Around the same time, E. J. Marey, a French physiologist, described enclosing the bare arm in a water-filled cylinder connected to a reservoir that could be raised. This in turn was connected to a mercury manometer. Marey described pulsatile oscillations which increased, then decreased, when the reservoir was raised until the arm blanched. A number of authors used variations on this technique, including air-filled systems (e.g. Potain in 1902).

The main principle of indirect blood pressure measurement had therefore been established, i.e. detecting the passage of a pulse wave once an occluding pressure is relieved. The four basic methods were palpatory, flush, oscillometric and auscultatory: all gave an acceptable technique for identifying systolic blood pressure, but at that time only the auscultatory method could identify diastolic pressure with any accuracy.

In 1896 the Italian physician Scipione Riva Rocci described an indirect method of measuring blood pressure using an air-inflating arm-occluding cuff (Riva Rocci, 1896; Zanchetti and Mancia, 1996). Systolic blood pressure could be determined by palpating a distal artery. Hill and Barnard, working in England at the same time, also described the use of an air-inflated cuff (Hill and Barnard, 1897). Half a decade later, it was suggested by Henrich von Recklinghausen to use a 12-cm wide cuff. He argued that the 5-cm wide cuff used by Riva Rocci gave erroneously high systolic pressures which could be corrected by using the larger cuff (von Recklinghausen, 1901).

Blood pressure variability

Blood pressure varies continually throughout the day, making a single or even a few readings unrepresentative, either through the circumstance of the individual or through errors obtained in the measurement of the blood pressure. An accurate baseline pressure is often difficult to obtain due to presence of various stimuli.

Variations in blood pressure can be contributed to race, age, sex, time of day, activity, emotion, posture, etc. (MacGillivray et al., 1969). Within-patient variation can be due to systemic variation, e.g. women have a lower blood pressure than men after the age of 45 (Kannel, 1974); circadian rhythm – blood pressure will be lower during sleep than wakefulness, especially during the first two hours of sleep (Coccagna et al., 1971) [attenuation and reversal of the diurnal variation have been described in pre-eclampsia (Dame et al., 1977; Halligan et al., 1996; Murnaghan et al., 1980; Redman et al., 1976; Sawyer et al., 1981; Seligman, 1971)]; diastolic pressure will increase on standing; dynamic exercise increases the systolic pressure while cessation of prolonged exercise will cause a decrease (Kenney and Seals, 1993), etc. Smoking (Cellina et al., 1975; Mann et al., 1991) or drinking coffee (Jeong and Dimsdale, 1990; Smits et al., 1985) will also cause a rise in blood pressure and many daily activities such as micturition, defecation, eating and drinking can have significant effects on the blood pressure. These random variations of blood pressure will most likely result in sampling errors.

Gestational effects on blood pressure

A decrease during the first half of pregnancy is commonly described (Gallery et al., 1977; Moutquin et al., 1985; Page and Christianson, 1976), with a return to pre-pregnancy levels by the third trimester. Large changes have been reported even in early pregnancy (between 6 and 10 weeks gestation) (Redman, 1995). However, this study only included 10 women due to the difficulty of obtaining longitudinal data preconceptually. It is therefore evident that the gestation at which women present for their booking visit will influence the "baseline" pressure recorded. Hypertensive women may present as "normotensive" in the early second trimester.

White coat hypertension

The anxiety caused by the measurement itself or the environment in which it is taken can influence blood pressure by what is known as a defense reaction (Mancia et al., 1983, 1987). When the blood pressure of the patient is constantly higher when measured in the clinical environment than at home, it is known as white coat hypertension, i.e. patients who have white coat hypertension have a blood pressure that is within the normal range outside the clinic setting (Pickering et al., 2002). This phenomenon was first described more than 60 years ago (Ayman and Golshine, 1940).

The mechanism of white coat hypertension is still being investigated. It is thought that it may be due to an exaggerated learning or orientating response to stressful stimuli. However, studies have failed to demonstrate an increase in laboratory stressors when comparing individuals with white coat and sustained hypertension (Floras et al., 1981; Siegel et al., 1990). There is also no difference in the variability of blood pressure between hypertensive and normotensive adults (Siegel et al., 1990; White and Baker, 1986). It is possible that this defense reaction could be a learned or conditioned response, i.e. the patient associates the clinic with an unpleasant experience and the normal habituation does not occur. One study showed that in a group of young men, those who received a letter stating that they were hypertensive (prior to their appointment) had a significantly higher blood pressure (by 16/10 mmHg) than those who were sent a neutral letter. White coat hypertension may also be dependent on the interaction between subject and observer based on gender (Millar and Accioloy, 1996).

Its prevalence in a non-pregnant population is between 20 and 40% and there is some evidence that it is more commonly found in women (Hoegholm *et al.*, 1992; Khoury *et al.*, 1992; Krakoff *et al.*, 1988). It is unlikely to be a benign condition in non-pregnant individuals, as the risk appears to fall somewhere in between those who are normotensive and those with sustained hypertension (Julius *et al.*, 1990).

Its significance in an obstetric population has not been determined. Rayburn *et al.* (1984) showed that in the vast majority of cases where clinic blood pressures differed significantly from home readings, the readings taken at home were lower. More recent studies have shown that the presence of white coat hypertension may be more clinically significant in early pregnancy (Broughton Pipkin *et al.*, 1998) rather than late pregnancy (Brown *et al.*, 1999). There are no comparisons between pregnant and non-pregnant individuals as to the degree that this defense reaction causes blood pressure to change. It seems likely though that the influence of stress and anxiety is greater in the pregnant patient (e.g. admission to hospital, delivery, etc.).

Korotkoff sounds

Nicolai Sergei Korotkoff described the auscultatory method for measuring blood pressure in the early

Table 18.2. Korotkoff sounds in pregnancy

Phase I:	"A loud clear-cut snapping tone."
Phase II:	"A succession of murmurs."
Phase III:	"The disappearance of the murmurs and the appearance of a tone resembling to a degree the first phase but less well marked."
Phase IV:	(The tone) "becomes less clear in quality or dull."
Phase V:	"The disappearance of all sounds."

1900s (Segall, 1987). It relies on the auscultation of Korotkoff sounds heard over the brachial artery, distal to a deflating cuff. In 1907 Ettinger described the "muffling" in the sequence of vascular sounds and in 1911 Goodman and Howell described five distinct phases, still being used today, as shown in Table 18.2.

The origin of the Korotkoff sounds are not fully understood but it is generally accepted that they are related to either pressure-induced movements of the arterial wall or turbulent flow through a compressed arterial lumen or both (Dock, 1980; London and London, 1967). A study using Doppler ultrasound during a cuff deflation in pregnancy demonstrated that phase I was consistently identified at the onset of flow distal to the cuff, while phase IV was associated with the onset of continuous flow. Phase V occurred when there was an increase in the diastolic component of the arterial waveform (Quinn, 1995).

An auscultatory gap (where no sounds may be heard) can sometimes occur between phases II and III (Cook and Taussig, 1917) and subsequent work has shown this phenomenon to be related to venous congestion. Variation in blood pressure measuring techniques are not uncommon (Perry *et al.*, 1990) and are known to differ widely from the recommended guidelines (Petrie *et al.*, 1986).

Accurate determination of diastolic pressure is still largely dependent on the auscultation of Korotkoff sounds. Various controversies exist around which Korotkoff phase should be used

Table 18.3. Suggested recommendations for blood pressure measurement in pregnancy

	Recommendation
Instrument	Mercury, aneroid or electronic sphygmomanometer for auscultation or validated oscillometric automated device
Setting	Relaxed, quiet environment, preferably after rest
Position	Lying or sitting (cuff at heart level)
Arm	Either arm – right is preferred (higher value if difference >10 mmHg). Dependent upon arm if in a lateral position
Korotkoff sounds	First (systolic) and fifth (diastolic); if diastolic persistently <40 mmHg use muffling/fourth sound and make a note

to identify diastolic pressure: the muffling sound known as Korotkoff phase 4 (K4) or the "disappearance of sound" (K5). In non-pregnant individuals, phase 5 is universally recognized to be the diastolic identification point (Kirkendall *et al.*, 1981; Petrie *et al.*, 1986). In pregnancy, hemodynamic changes may cause a number of women to have sounds approaching (or at) zero cuff pressure (MacGillivray *et al.*, 1969). This could be as a result of the diaphragm of the stethoscope being applied with too great pressure (Brown and Whitworth, 1991; Perry *et al.*, 1990; Rubin, 1996).

As K5 is invariably heard and therefore more reproducible than the muffling sounds of K4 (Rubin, 1996; Shennan *et al.*, 1996a), it is our view that K5 should be used in pregnancy. In randomized controlled trials the abandonment of K4 appears to be safe and even beneficial (Brown *et al.*, 1998).

Mercury sphygmomanometry

Despite recognized shortcomings, mercury sphygmomanometry remains the gold standard for blood pressure measurement since being introduced by Riva Rocci. Various inherent errors can be attributed to the observer, the instrument itself or the stethoscope. The error is further confounded by the variability of blood pressure and the number of measurements taken. In pregnancy alone, the associated hemodynamic changes relating to peripheral vascular resistance, cardiac output and the use of antihypertensive/fluid therapy has the potential to influence the characteristics of arterial oscillations and blood flow at a given mean arterial pressure. Subsequently, it can also influence the accuracy of indirect measurement using automated oscillometric devices.

Recommendations for measurement in pregnancy are shown in Table 18.3.

Common errors experienced with the mercury sphygmomanometer include oxidized mercury in the glass tubing that obscures clear visualization, incorrect calibration, i.e. the meniscus does not settle at zero before inflation and cracked tubing.

Inappropriate cuff dimensions can also lead to errors in measurement. It is recommended that the length of the cuff should be at least 80% and the width 40% of the circumference measured around the middle of the upper arm (Petrie *et al.*, 1986). Using a cuff that is smaller than this recommendation will result in overestimation of blood pressure by between 5 and 10 mmHg for diastolic and 7–13 mmHg for systolic pressures (Maxwell *et al.*, 1982). If the opposite occurs, i.e. using a cuff that is too large for the patient, diastolic pressure will be underestimated by 3–5 mmHg. It is clear from these examples that "under-cuffing" is more of a problem than "over-cuffing." The upper arm should be measured at the approximate mid-point to establish the correct size to use and the arm should be supported at heart level.

The cuff should be inflated rapidly over 3–5 s. The device must be able to reach 200 mmHg or 40 mmHg above the estimated systolic blood pressure. Sometimes a period of silence is observed between the systolic and diastolic points. This is known as an auscultatory gap. If the cuff is not sufficiently inflated the returning sounds following this gap might be mistaken for the systolic point resulting in underestimation of systolic blood pressure. It is therefore important to initially inflate the cuff while palpating the distal (radial) pulse to determine the approximate systolic pressure prior to auscultation.

A smooth deflation rate of 2–3 mmHg per second or pulse (using the control release valve) should be maintained. Too slow deflation may cause sufficient discomfort to the patient to increase the blood pressure (Petrie *et al.*, 1986) and too rapid or jerky deflation will cause under- and over-estimation of the systolic and diastolic blood pressure, respectively.

The stethoscope can also contribute to error in measurement by influencing the quality of sound available to the observer. As the length of the tubing increases, the sound transmission will diminish.

During measurement the observer can be subject to "digit preference," i.e. rounding the reading to the nearest 5 or 10 mmHg. It is recommended that blood pressure be measured to the nearest 2 mmHg (Petrie *et al.*, 1986). The observer may also choose to ignore blood pressure measurements that would require any action. This is known as threshold avoidance. Other factors that can influence his/her ability to obtain an accurate measurement include concentration, reaction time, hearing and visual acuity.

In pregnancy, posture can play a particularly important role in accurate blood pressure measurement. Measurements are frequently taken with the woman lying in the left lateral position. This is due to the fact that during advanced gestation, lying supine will cause compression of the inferior vena cava by the gravid uterus. Blood pressure seems to be lowest when measured in the left lateral position, using the uppermost arm, and it increases on sitting or standing (Wichman *et al.*, 1984).

When the inherent inaccuracies of indirect blood pressure measurement compared with true intra-arterial pressure are considered and are added to the worst observer practices (measuring blood pressure to the nearest 10 mmHg), a diastolic measurement of 90 mmHg may be as high as 128 mmHg or as low as 74 mmHg (de Swiet, 1991). Management based on the extremes of this range would be entirely different.

The debate surrounding the abandonment of mercury in the clinical setting is ongoing. It is a bio-accumulable substance and is toxic to the environment. However, the quantity of mercury contained in sphygmomanometers around the world is not nearly equivalent to that used in the industry and crematoriums, for example. Nevertheless, there is a notion to eliminate its use from the clinical setting.

Aneroid and random-zero sphygmomanometers

In an attempt to obliterate observer bias associated with mercury sphygmomanometery, the Hawksley random-zero sphygmomanometer was introduced. However, evidence suggests that it underestimates blood pressure (O'Brien *et al.*, 1990) and therefore is not a suitable replacement for the mercury sphygmomanometer.

Aneroid devices were also suggested as a mercury-free alternative and are popular for use in the community, as it is easily portable. They are reported to become less accurate over time (Coleman *et al.*, 2005; Waugh *et al.*, 2002) and with extended use. Modern aneroids may use better materials but there are few data assessing them longitudinally. It therefore remains a recommendation to do regular calibration checks to reduce possible error in measurement.

Automated blood pressure measuring devices

In 1890, Roy and Adami demonstrated arterial oscillations at different pressures by applying a tight-fitting water chamber to the wrist. The mean arterial pressure was represented at the point of maximum oscillation (Hill and Barnard, 1897) and changes in the amplitude of these oscillations could be used to detect systolic and diastolic pressures (Howell and Brush, 1901).

Initially it was thought that an increase in the amplitude of the oscillations corresponded to the systolic pressure, while the diastolic pressure was represented by the lowest point of the maximum oscillations (Erlanger, 1903). Subsequent studies showed that diastolic pressure was in fact below the maximum oscillations.

Most automated devices available today use oscillometry to determine the blood pressure. Their accuracy and suitability as a replacement for the mercury sphygmomanometer have been the subject of research and discussion for more than two decades. Although they address some of the errors associated with mercury sphygmomanometry, their accuracy cannot be assumed without evaluation against mercury sphygmomanometry.

The need for a standardized protocol became apparent in the late 1980s after the widespread introduction of automated devices to the market. Various protocols have since been published with the aim of establishing a minimum standard of accuracy. The Association for the Advancement of Medical Instrumentation (1993), the British Hypertension Society (O'Brien et al., 1993a) and the European Society for Hypertension (O'Brien et al., 2002) all published protocols and both Germany and Australia have unpublished recommended national standards.

The need to evaluate devices in an obstetric population specifically is well-documented. Various devices deemed accurate in adults have been shown to underestimate blood pressure in a hypertensive pregnant population by clinically significant amounts (Franx et al., 1997; Gupta et al., 1996; Hehenkamp et al., 2002; Natarajan et al., 1999; Quinn, 1994; Reinders et al., 2003). Revised protocols of the AAMI and BHS now make specific provision for the evaluation of automated devices in pregnancy, although it does not address pre-eclamptic women in particular.

Device accuracy also varies depending on whether it is compared to mercury sphygmomanometry or intra-arterial readings. Automated auscultatory devices have shown decreased accuracy in pre-eclampsia despite passing the protocol in a pregnant population (Nataranjan et al., 1998; Penny et al., 1996) and the same has been found for oscillometric devices (Gupta et al., 1996; Penny et al., 1997).

It is thought that the accuracy of automated devices might be influenced by the altered compliance in pre-eclampsia. Care should be taken when interpreting blood pressure measurements taken with automated devices in women with pre-eclampsia.

Self-initiated and ambulatory monitoring

Ambulatory monitoring allows some normality with regard to daily activity. The device is worn for 24 h and programmed to take blood pressure measurements at a set time interval. Most devices will give some warning, e.g. a beeping sound, that the cuff is about to inflate. This is an indication to the patient to stop any activity and to keep their arm still. Home monitors are designed to be initiated manually.

Whether self-initiated blood pressures are different from those initiated by the clinician, is not known. It is, however, quite likely as even the gender of the investigator performing the measurement can influence the reading (Millar and Accioly, 1996).

In the non-pregnant population, ambulatory blood pressure measurements correlate better with target organ damage (Asmar et al., 1988; Bianchi et al., 1994; Devereux et al., 1983;

Table 18.4. Meta-analysis of 10 validation studies in pregnant women with and without pre-eclampsia

	Mercury		Intra-arterial	
	Pregnancy	PET	Pregnancy	PET
Subjects (n)	597	176	8	30
Systolic*	−1.13 (5.80)	−4.60 (8.04)	4.11 (10.95)	−17.76 (10.12)
Diastolic*	−1.20 (6.03)	−5.16 (7.19)	3.00 (8.00)	−8.17 (6.59)

*Mean pressure difference and standard deviation (SD) mmHg.

Shimada *et al.*, 1992) and direct cardiovascular morbidity (Perloff *et al.*, 1983, 1989, 1991) than casual blood pressure measurements. Its use in a hypertensive adult population is quite extensive.

It was first used in pregnancy in the late 1980s (O'Brien *et al.*, 1991) and soon thereafter in hypertensive pregnancy (Rath *et al.*, 1990). Normal values of 24-h ambulatory blood pressure measurement have been determined (Contard *et al.*, 1993; Ferguson *et al.*, 1994; Halligan *et al.*, 1993) and it is known that women with pre-eclampsia have an attenuated nocturnal fall in blood pressure.

It was thought that ambulatory monitoring could have a predictive value related to the absence of a nocturnal fall (>12 mmHg) in women destined to become pre-eclamptic (Halligan *et al.*, 1993; Moutquin *et al.*, 1992). Other studies have shown that significantly higher systolic and mean arterial pressures occur at 18 and 28 weeks gestation in those women who subsequently develop pre-eclampsia (Kyle *et al.*, 1993). The predictive capability of ambulatory monitoring is limited by the need to screen a large number of women with relatively intensive monitoring. It does, however, appear to be useful in evaluating hypertensive pregnancies. It is a better predictor of adverse obstetric outcome than conventional mercury sphygmomanometry (Peek *et al.*, 1996; Penny *et al.*, 1998) with regard to severe hypertension. Disappointingly, it remains a weak predictor of subsequent proteinurea, i.e. pre-eclampsia.

Validated devices in pre-eclampsia

In the latest UK Confidential Enquiry into Maternal Deaths (CEMD, 2004), it was highlighted that automated devices can systematically underestimate the blood pressure in pre-eclampsia to a serious degree. Accurate measurement and avoidance of inaccurate devices was a key recommendation. An increasing number of studies are being published in an attempt to address this problem.

Not many devices have been validated in pregnancy. To date only 16 studies have been identified (Brown *et al.*, 1995; Franx *et al.*, 1994, 1997; Golara *et al.*, 2002; Gupta *et al.*, 1996; Kwek *et al.*, 1998; Modesti *et al.*, 1996; Nataranjan *et al.*, 1999; O'Brien *et al.*, 1993b; Penny *et al.*, 1996, 1997; Quinn, 1994; Reinders *et al.*, 2003, 2005; Shennan *et al.*, 1993, 1996b). In most cases, the devices were evaluated against mercury sphygmomanometry, but in two studies intra-arterial evaluation was performed. Nine studies included data from pre-eclamptic women. From these, 10 devices were identified with sufficient data to perform a meta-analysis (Table 18.4).

It is clear from the data that devices have a tendency to underestimate the blood pressure, especially in pre-eclampsia. The degree of error does not preclude their use in clinical practice, but it is worth noting that some machines do have a large unacceptable error. The recommendation remains that each device intended for use in an obstetric population should be evaluated accordingly.

Doppler ultrasound

This method of blood pressure measurement is particularly useful in noisy environments when the Korotkoff sounds are quiet (below 200 Hz), e.g. in children or shocked patients. A piezoelectric crystal generates an ultrasonic wave of about 8 megahertz, which is directed at the brachial artery beneath an occluding cuff. Reflected waves are detected by a second crystal, and the distortions created by the oscillating artery will cause a shift in frequency (the Doppler effect) (Stegall *et al.*, 1968). This shift is either amplified or electronically displayed. The accuracy of these measurements have not been extensively evaluated, particularly in pregnancy.

Summary and recommendations

Pre-eclampsia has huge implications for health service resources. Obstetric day-care units are inundated by referrals for the monitoring of blood pressure and other clinical signs of pre-eclampsia (Anthony, 1992) and up to a quarter of all antenatal admissions are for the monitoring or management of women with hypertension (Rosenberg and Twaddle, 1990).

The fundamental importance of blood pressure measurement during pregnancy is well recognized. Our clinical knowledge is derived from mercury sphygmomanometry and when used properly it remains the best indirect determinant of blood pressure.

New technology in blood pressure measurement should be evaluated against mercury sphygmomanometry for accuracy, especially in a pre-eclamptic population where significant underestimation of blood pressure has been shown. If an oscillometric, automated device is to be used the mean arterial value (MAP) is more likely to be accurate than the systolic or diastolic pressure (Penny *et al.*, 1997). If in doubt, it is advisable to confirm readings obtained by automated devices with mercury sphygmomanometry or intra-arterial lines.

Measurements should be taken in a quiet, relaxed environment, after a period of rest. It should be ensured that the cuff is at heart level. Whether the patient is lying or sitting is not critical, but it should be ensured that women do not lie flat on their backs, as this will cause supine hypotension. In hypertensive women blood pressure should be measured in both the right and the left arm. If the difference between the arms is consistent and more than 10 mmHg, the higher reading should be adopted from then on. High readings should be confirmed after a period of rest.

During measurement we recommend that Korotkoff phase 5 be used to identify the diastolic pressure, except in rare cases where sounds continue to be heard through to 0 mmHg (then use Korotkoff phase 4). Multiple/repeated readings will give a better risk assessment than single readings and an average of the readings is advised. Care should be taken to ensure the correct deflation rate and measurement should be to the nearest 2 mmHg.

Blood pressure is a convenient, cheap and easy-to-use screening method. Many other tests, far more involved than measuring blood pressure, have been suggested as predictors of pre-eclampsia (Dekker and Sibai, 1991). None of these perform well at identifying women at risk of an adverse outcome. The correct measurement of blood pressure remains a fundamental and crucial skill in the management of pregnancy, and there is ample evidence it is not performed well.

REFERENCES

Anthony, J. (1992). Improving antenatal care. The role of the antenatal assessment unit. *Health Trends*, **24**, 123–5.

Asmar, R. G., Brunel, P. C., Pannier, B. M., Lacolley, P. J. and Safar, M. E. (1988). Arterial distensibility and ambulatory blood pressure monitoring in essential hypertension. *Am. J. Cardiol.*, **61**(13), 1066–70.

Association for the Advancement of Medical Instrumentation. (1993). *American National Standard*. Electronic or automated sphygmomanometers. Arlington, VA: AAMI.

American College of Obstetricians and Gynecologists. (1986). *Management of Preeclampsia*. 91.

Ayman, D. and Golshine, A. D. (1940). Blood pressure determinations by patients with essential hypertension: the difference between clinic and home readings before treatment. *Am. J. Med. Sci.*, **200**, 465–75.

Bianchi, S., Bigazzi, R., Baldari, G., Sgherri, G. and Campese, V. M. (1994). Diurnal variations of blood pressure and microalbuminuria in essential hypertension. *Am. J. Hypertens.*, **7**(1), 23–9.

Branch, D. W., Mitchell, M. D., Miller, E., Palinski, W. and Witztum, J. L. (1994). Pre-eclampsia and serum antibodies to oxidised low-density lipoprotein. *Lancet*, **343**(8898), 645–6.

Brosens, I. and Renaer, M. (1972). On the pathogenesis of placental infarcts in pre-eclampsia. *J. Obstet. Gynaecol. Br. Cwlth*, **79**(9), 794–9.

Broughton Pipkin, F., Sharif, J. and Lal, S. (1998). Predicting high blood pressure in pregnancy: a multivariate approach. *J. Hypertens.*, **16**, 221–9.

Brown, M. A. and Whitworth, J. A. (1991). Recording diastolic blood pressure in pregnancy. *Br. Med. J.*, **303**(6794), 120–1.

Brown, M. A., Buddle, M. L., Farrell, T., Davis, G. and Jones, M. (1998). Randomised trial of management of hypertensive pregnancies by Korotkoff phase IV or phase V. *Lancet*, **352**, 777–81.

Brown, M. A., Buddle, M. L., Bennett, M., Smith, B., Morris, R. and Whitworth, J. A. (1995). Ambulatory blood pressure in pregnancy: comparison of the SpaceLabs 90207 and Accutracker II monitors with intraarterial recordings. *Am. J. Obstet. Gynecol.*, **173**(1), 218–23.

Brown, M. A., Robinson, A. and Jones, M. (1999). The white coat effect in hypertensive pregnancy: much ado about nothing? *Br. J. Obstet. Gynaecol.*, **106**, 474–80.

Browne, F. J. and Dodds, G. H. (1942). Pregnancy in the patient with chronic hypertension. *J. Obstet. Gynaecol. Br. Empire*, **49**, 1–17.

Butler, N. R. and Bonham, D. G. (1963). Toxaemia in pregnancy. In: *Perinatal Mortality*. Edinburgh: E and S Livingstone, pp. 86–100.

Cellina, G. U., Honour, A. J. and Littler, W. A. (1975). Direct arterial pressure, heart rate, and electrocardiogram during cigarette smoking in unrestricted patients. *Am. Heart J.*, **89**, 18–25.

CEMD. The sixth report of the Confidential Enquiries into Maternal Deaths in the United Kingdom. (2004). *Why mothers die 2000–2002*. London: CEMD (www.cemd.org.uk).

Chesley, L. C. (1976). Blood pressure, edema and proteinuria in pregnancy. 1. Historical developments. *Prog. Clin. Biol. Res.*, **7**, 19–66.

Chesley, L. C. and Annitto, J. E. (1947). Pregnancy in the patient with hypertensive disease. *Am. J. Obstet. Gynecol.*, **53**, 372–81.

Chua, S. and Redman, C. W. (1992). Prognosis for pre-eclampsia complicated by 5 g or more of proteinuria in 24 hours. *Eur. J. Obstet. Gynecol. Reprod. Biol.*, **43**, 9–12.

Coccagna, G., Mantovani, M., Brignani, F., Manzini, A. and Lugaresi, E. (1971). Laboratory note. Arterial pressure changes during spontaneous sleep in man. *Electroencephalogr. Clin. Neurophysiol.*, **31**, 277–81.

Coleman, A. J., Steel, S. D., Ashworth, M., Vowler, S. L. and Shennan, A. (2005). Accuracy of the pressure scale of sphygmomanometers in clinical use within primary care. *Blood Press. Monit.*, **10**(4), 181–8.

Contard, S., Chanudet, X., Coisne, D., *et al.* (1993). Ambulatory monitoring of blood pressure in normal pregnancy. *Am. J. Hyperten.*, **6**(10), 880–4.

Cook, J. E. and Taussig, A. E. (1917). Auscultatory blood pressure determination. *J. Am. Med. Ass.*, **68**, 1088.

Dame, W. R., Bachour, G., Bottcher, H. D., Beller, F. K. (1977). Continuous monitoring of direct intra-arterial blood pressure in normal and preeclamptic pregnancies (author's transl.) *Geburtshilfe Frauenheilkd*, **37**(8), 708–14.

Davey, D. A. and MacGillivray, I. (1988). The classification and definition of the hypertensive disorders of pregnancy. *Am. J. Obstet. Gynecol.*, **158**, 892–8.

de Swiet, M. (1991). Blood pressure measurement in pregnancy. *Br. J. Obstet. Gynaecol.*, **98**, 239–40.

Dekker, G.A. and Sibai, B.M. (1991). Early detection of preeclampsia. *Am. J. Obstet. Gynecol.*, **165**(1), 160–72.

Devereux, R.B., Pickering, T.G., Harshfield, G.A., *et al.* (1983). Left ventricular hypertrophy in patients with hypertension: importance of blood pressure response to regularly recurring stress. *Circulation*, **68**(3), 470–6.

Dock, W. (1980). Occasional notes. Korotkoff's sounds. *N. Engl. J. Med.*, **302**, 1264–7.

Douglas, K. and Redman, C. (1994). Eclampsia in the United Kingdom. *Br. Med. J.*, **309**(6966), 1395–400.

Erlanger, J. (1903). A new instrument for determining the minimum and maximum blood-pressures in man. *Johns Hopkins Hosp. Rep.*, **12**, 53–110.

Ettinger, W. (1907). Auskultatorische Methode der Blutdruckbestimmung und ihr praktischer Wert. *Wein klinische Wochenschrift*, **LVIII**, 243.

Ferguson, J.H., Neubauer, B.L. and Shaar, C.J. (1994). Ambulatory blood pressure monitoring during pregnancy. Establishment of standards of normalcy. *Am. J. Hypertens.*, **7**(9, Pt. 1), 838–43.

Ferrazzani, S., Caruso, A., De Carolis, S., Martino, I.V. and Mancuso, S. (1990). Proteinuria and outcome of 444 pregnancies complicated by hypertension. *Am. J. Obstet. Gynecol.*, **162**, 366–71.

Fisher, C.M. (1985). The ascendancy of diastolic blood pressure over systolic. *Lancet*, **2**, 1349–50.

Floras, J.S., Jones, J.V., Hassan, M.O., Osikowska, B., Sever, P.S. and Sleight, P. (1981). Cuff and ambulatory blood pressure in subjects with essential hypertension. *Lancet*, **2**, 107–9.

Franx, A., Van der Post, J.A.M., van Montfrans, G.A. and Bruinse, H.W. (1997). Comparison of an auscultatory versus an oscillometric ambulatory blood pressure monitor in normotensive, hypertensive and pre-eclamptic pregnancy. *Hypertens. Pregn.*, **16**, 187–202.

Franx, A., Elfering, I.M., Merkus, H.M.W.M. and van Montfrans, G.A. (1994). Validation of automated blood pressure recording in pregnancy. *Br. J. Obstet. Gynaecol.*, **101**, 66–9.

Gallery, E.D., Hunyor, S.N., Ross, M. and Gyory, A.Z. (1977). Predicting the development of pregnancy-associated hypertension. The place of standardised blood-pressure measurement. *Lancet*, **1**(8025), 1273–5.

Golara, M., Benedict, A., Jones, C., Randhawa, M., Poston, L. and Shennan, A.H. (2002). Inflationary oscillometry provides accurate measurement of blood pressure in pre-eclampsia. *Br. J. Obstet. Gynaecol.*, **109**(10), 1143–7.

Goodman, E.H. and Howell, A.A. (1911). Further clinical studies in the auscultatory method of determining blood pressure. *Am. J. Med. Sci.*, **142**, 334–52.

Greer, I.A. (1992). Hypertension. In: *High-risk Pregnancy*. Oxford: Butterworth Heinemann, pp. 31–93.

Gupta, M., Shennan, A.H., Halligan, A.W., Taylor, D.J. and de Swiet, M. (1996). Accuracy of oscillometric blood pressure monitoring in pregnancy and pre-eclampsia. *Br. J. Obstet. Gynaecol.*, **104**, 350–5.

Halligan, A., O'Brien, E., O'Malley, K., *et al.* (1993). Twenty-four-hour ambulatory blood pressure measurement in a primigravid population. *J. Hypertens.*, **11**, 869–73.

Halligan, A., Shennan, A., Lambert, P.C., de Swiet, M. and Taylor, D.J. (1996). Diurnal blood pressure difference in the assessment of preeclampsia. *Obstet. Gynecol.*, **87**(2), 205–8.

Hehenkamp, W.J., Rang, S., van Goudoever, J., Box, W.J., Wolf, H. and van der Post, J.A. (2002). Comparison of Portapres with standard sphygmo-manometery in pregnancy. *Hypertens. Preg.*, **21**(1), 65–76.

Hill, L. and Barnard, H. (1897). A simple and accurate form of sphygmometer or arterial pressure gauge contrived for clinical use. *Br. Med. J.*, **2**, 904.

HMSO. (1996). Department of Health and Social Security, editor. *Report on Confidential Enquiries into Maternal Deaths in the United Kingdom 1991–1993*. London: HMSO.

Hoegholm, A., Kristensen, K.S., Madsen, N.H. and Svendsen, T.L. (1992). White coat hypertension diagnosed by 24-h ambulatory monitoring. Examination of 159 newly diagnosed hypertensive patients. *Am. J. Hypertens.*, **5**(2), 64–70.

Howell, W.H. and Brush, C.E. (1901). A critical note upon clinical methods of measuring blood pressure. *Boston Med. Surg. J.*, **145**, 146–51.

Jeong, D.U. and Dimsdale, J.E. (1990). The effects of caffeine on blood pressure in the work environment. *Am. J. Hypertens.*, **3**, 749–53.

Julius, S., Mejia, A., Jones, K., *et al.* (1990). "White coat" versus "sustained" borderline hypertension in Tecumseh, Michigan. *Hypertension*, **16**, 617–23.

Kannel, W.B. (1974). Role of blood pressure in cardiovascular morbidity and mortality. *Progr. Cardiovasc. Dis.*, **17**, 5–24.

Kenney, M. J. and Seals, D. R. (1993). Postexercise hypotension. Key features, mechanisms, and clinical significance. *Hypertension*, **22**, 653–64.

Khoury, S., Yarows, S. A., O'Brien, T. K. and Sowers, J. R. (1992). Ambulatory blood pressure monitoring in a nonacademic setting. Effects of age and sex. *Am. J. Hypertens.*, **5**(9), 616–23.

Kirkendall, W. M., Feinleib, M., Freis, E. D. and Mark, A. L. (1981). Recommendations for human blood pressure determination by sphygmomanometers. Subcommittee of the AHA Postgraduate Education Committee. *Stroke*, **12**(4), 555A–64A.

Krakoff, L. R., Eison, H., Phillips, R. H., Leiman, S. J. and Lev, S. (1988). Effect of ambulatory blood pressure monitoring on the diagnosis and cost of treatment for mild hypertension. *Am. Heart J.*, **116**(4), 1152–4.

Kwek, K., Chan, Y. G., Tan, K. H. and Yeo, G. S. (1998). Validation of an oscillometric electronic sphygmomanometer in an obstetric population. *Am. Heart J.*, **11**, 978–82.

Kyle, P. M., Clark, S. J., Buckley, D., *et al.* (1993). Second trimester ambulatory blood pressure in nulliparous pregnancy: a useful screening test for pre-eclampsia? *Br. J. Obstet. Gynaecol.*, **100**(10), 914–19.

Lewis, G. and Drife, J., eds. (2001). *Why Mothers Die 1997–1999. The Fifth Report of the Confidential Enquiries into Maternal Deaths in the United Kingdom.* London: RCOG Press.

Littler, W. A., Honour, A. J., Carter, R. D. and Sleight, P. (1975). Sleep and blood pressure. *Br. Med. J.*, **3**(5979), 346–8.

London, S. B. and London, R. E. (1967). Critique of indirect diastolic end point. "Muffling" vs "Last" Sound. *Arch. Int. Med.*, **119**, 39–49.

Lorentzen, B., Drevon, C. A., Endresen, M. J. and Henriksen, T. (1995). Fatty acid pattern of esterified and free fatty acids in sera of women with normal and pre-eclamptic pregnancy. *Br. J. Obstet. Gynaecol.*, **102**(7), 530–7.

Mabie, W. C., Pernoll, M. L. and Biswas, M. K. (1986). Chronic hypertension in pregnancy. *Obstet. Gynecol.*, **67**, 197–205.

MacGillivray, I., Rose, G. A. and Rowe, B. (1969). Blood pressure survey in pregnancy. *Clin. Sci.*, **37**, 395–407.

Mancia, G., Bertinieri, G., Grassi, G., *et al.* (1983). Effects of blood-pressure measurement by the doctor on patient's blood pressure and heart rate. *Lancet*, **2**, 695–8.

Mancia, G., Parati, G., Pomidossi, G., Grassi, G., Casadei, R. and Zanchetti, A. (1987). Alerting reaction and rise in blood pressure during measurement by physician and nurse. *Hypertension*, **9**, 209–15.

Mann, S. J., James, G. D., Wang, R. S. and Pickering, T. G. (1991). Elevation of ambulatory systolic blood pressure in hypertensive smokers. A case-control study. *J. Am. Med. Ass.*, **265**, 2226–8.

Maxwell, M. H., Waks, A. U., Schroth, P. C., Karam, M. and Dornfeld, L. P. (1982). Error in blood-pressure measurement due to incorrect cuff size in obese patients. *Lancet*, **2**, 33–6.

McCowan, L. M., Buist, R. G., North, R. A. and Gamble, G. (1996). Perinatal morbidity in chronic hypertension. *Br. J. Obstet. Gynaecol.*, **103**, 123–9.

Millar, J. A. and Accioly, J. M. (1996). Measurement of blood pressure may be affected by an interaction between subject and observer based on gender. *J. Hum. Hypertens.*, **10**, 449–53.

Modesti, P. A., Costoli, A., Cecioni, I., Toccafondi, S., Carnemolla, A. and Serneri, G. G. N. (1996). Clinical evaluation of the QuietTrak blood pressure recorder according to the protocol of the British Hypertension Society. *Blood Press. Monit.*, **1**, 63–8.

Moore, M. P. and Redman, C. W. (1983). Case-control study of severe pre-eclampsia of early onset. *Br. Med. J.*, **287**, 580–3.

Moutquin, J. M., Rainville, C., Giroux, L., *et al.* (1985). A prospective study of blood pressure in pregnancy: prediction of preeclampsia. *Am. J. Obstet. Gynecol.*, **151**(2), 191–6.

Moutquin, J. M., Desmarais, L., Bastide, A., *et al.* (1992). Prediction of pre-eclampsia: ambulatory arterial hypertension. *J. Gynecol. Obstet. Biol. Reprod.*, **21**(3), 313–15.

Murnaghan, G. A., Mitchell, R. H., Ruff, S., Bonnar, J., MacGillivray, I., Symonds, E. M., eds. (1980). *Pregnancy Hypertension*. Lancaster, England: MTP Press, pp. 107–12.

Naeye, R. L. and Friedman, E. A. (1979). Causes of perinatal death associated with gestational hypertension and proteinuria. *Am. J. Obstet. Gynecol.*, **133**, 8–10.

Nataranjan, P., Shennan A. H., Penny, J., Halligan, A. and de Swiet, M. (1998). Auscultatory versus oscillometric blood pressure measurement in pre-eclampsia. *Proceedings of the International Society for the Study of Hypertension in Pregnancy*, Oxford.

Natarajan, P., Shennan, A. H., Penny, J., Halligan, A. W., de Swiet, M. and Anthony, J. (1999). Comparison of auscultatory and oscillometric automated blood pressure monitors in the setting of pre-eclampsia. *Am. J. Obstet. Gynecol.*, **181**, 1203–10.

National High Blood Pressure Education Program Working Group Report on High Blood Pressure in Pregnancy. (1990). *Am. J. Obstet. Gynecol.*, **163**(5, Pt. 1), 1691–712.

O'Brien, E., Mee, F., Atkins, N. and O'Malley, K. (1990). Inaccuracy of the Hawksley random zero sphygmomanometer. *Lancet*, **336**, 1465–8.

O'Brien, E., Mee, F., Atkins, N. and O'Malley, K. (1991). Accuracy of the Del Mar Avionics Pressurometer IV determined by the British Hypertension Society protocol. *J. Hypertens.*, **9**(6), 567–8.

O'Brien, E., Petrie, J., Littler, W., *et al.* (1993a). The British Hypertension Society protocol for the evaluation of blood pressure measuring devices. *J. Hypertens.*, **11**(Suppl. 2), S43–62.

O'Brien, E., Mee, F., Atkins, N., Halligan, A. and O'Malley, K. (1993b). Accuracy of the SpaceLabs 90207 ambulatory blood pressure measuring system in normotensive pregnant women determined by the British Hypertension Society protocol. *J. Hypertens.*, **11**(Suppl. 5), S282–3.

O'Brien, E., Pickering, T., Asmar, R., *et al.* (2002). Working Group on Blood Pressure Monitoring of the European Society of Hypertension International protocol for validation of blood pressure measuring devices in adults. *Blood Press. Monit.*, **7**, 3–17.

Page, E. W. and Christianson, R. (1976). Influence of blood pressure changes with and without proteinuria upon outcome of pregnancy. *Am. J. Obstet. Gynecol.*, **126**(7), 821–33.

Peek, M., Shennan, A., Halligan, A., Lambert, P. C., Taylor, D. J. and de Swiet, M. (1996). Hypertension in pregnancy: which method of blood pressure measurement is most predictive of outcome? *Obstet. Gynecol.*, **88**(6), 1030–3.

Penny, J. A., Shennan, A. H., Rushbrook, J., Halligan, A. W., Taylor, D. J. and de Swiet, M. (1996). Validation of the QuietTrak ambulatory blood pressure monitor for use in pregnancy. *Hypertens. Pregn.*, **15**(3), 313–21.

Penny, J. A., Shennan, A. H., Halligan, A. W., Taylor, D. J., de Swiet, M. and Anthony, J. (1997). Blood pressure measurement in severe pre-eclampsia. Letter. *Lancet*, **349**, 1518.

Penny, J., Halligan, A. W., Shennan, A. H., *et al.* (1998). Automated, Ambulatory or Conventional measurement in pregnancy: which is the better predictor of severe hypertension? *Am. J. Obstet. Gynecol.*, **178**, 521–6.

Perloff, D., Sokolow, M. and Cowan, R. (1983). The prognostic value of ambulatory blood pressures. *J. Am. Med. Ass.*, **249**(20), 2792–8.

Perloff, D., Sokolow, M., Cowan, R. M. and Juster, R. P. (1989). Prognostic value of ambulatory blood pressure measurements: further analyses. *J. Hypertens.*, **7**(3), S3–10.

Perloff, D., Sokolow, M., Cowan, R. M., Juster, R. P. and Cowan, R. (1991). Prognostic value of ambulatory blood pressure measurements: further analyses. The prognostic value of ambulatory blood pressure monitoring in treated hypertensive patients. *J. Hypertens.*, **9**(1), S33–9.

Perry, I. J. and Beevers, D. G. (1994). The definition of pre-eclampsia. *Br. J. Obstet. Gynaecol.*, **101**, 587–91.

Perry, I. J., Stewart, B. A., Brockwell, J., *et al.* (1990). Recording diastolic blood pressure in pregnancy. *Br. Med. J.*, **301**(6762), 1198.

Petrie, J. C., O'Brien, E. T., Littler, W. A. and de Swiet, M. (1986). Recommendations on blood pressure measurement. *Br. Med. J.*, **293**, 611–15.

Pickering, T. G., Gerin, W. and Schwartz, A. R. (2002). What is the white coat effect and how should it be measured? *Blood Press. Monit.*, **7**, 293–300.

Quinn, M. (1994). Automated blood pressure measurement devices: a potential source of morbidity and pre-eclampsia. *Am. J. Obstet. Gynecol.*, **170**(5), 1303–7.

Quinn, M. (1995). Korotkoff's sounds in pregnancy. Ultrasound. *Obstet. Gynecol.*, **6**, 58–61.

Rath, W., Schrader, J., Guhlke, U., *et al.* (1990). 24-hour blood pressure measurement in normal pregnancy in hypertensive pregnant patients. *Klin. Wochenschr.*, **68**(15), 768–73.

Rayburn, W. F., Zuspan, F. P. and Piehl, E. J. (1984). Self-monitoring of blood pressure during pregnancy. *Am. J. Obstet. Gynecol.*, **148**(2), 159–62.

Redman, C. W. (1995). Hypertension in pregnancy. In: de Swiet, ed., *Medical Disorders in Obstetric Practice*, 2nd edn. Oxford: Blackwell Science, pp. 182–225.

Redman, C. W. and Jefferies, M. (1988). Revised definition of pre-eclampsia. *Lancet*, **1**, 809–12.

Redman, C. W., Beilin, L. J. and Bonnar, J. (1976). Reversed diurnal blood pressure rhythm in hypertensive pregnancies. *Clin. Sci. Mol. Med.*, **51**, 687–9.

Reinders, A., Cuckson, A. C., Jones, C. R., Poet, R., O'Sullivan, G. and Shennan, A. H. (2003). Validation of the Welch Allyn 'Vital Signs' blood pressure measurement device in pregnancy and pre-eclampsia. *Br. J. Obstet. Gynaecol.,* **110**, 134–8.

Reinders, A., Cuckson, A. C., Lee, J. and Shennan, A. H. (2005). An accurate automated blood pressure device for use in pregnancy and pre-eclampsia: the Microlife 3BTO-A. *Br. J. Obstet. Gynaecol.,* **112**(7), 915–20.

Rey, E. and Couturier, A. (1994). The prognosis of pregnancy in women with chronic hypertension. *Am. J. Obstet. Gynecol.,* **171**, 410–16.

Rippmann, E. T. (1968). Gestosis of late pregnancy. Nomenclature and scoring. *Gynaecologia,* **165**, 12–20.

Riva Rocci, S. (1896) Un nuovo sfigmomanometro. *Gazz. Med. Torino,* **50**, 981–96.

Roberts, J. M. and Redman, C. W. (1993). Pre-eclampsia: more than pregnancy-induced hypertension. *Lancet,* **341**(8858), 1447–51. Published erratum appears in *Lancet,* 1993, **342**(8869), 504.

Rosenberg, K. and Twaddle, S. (1990). Screening and surveillance of pregnancy hypertension – an economic approach to the use of daycare. *Baill. Clin. Obstet. Gynaecol.,* **4**(1), 89–107.

Roy, C. S. and Adami, J. G. (1890). Heart-beat and pulse-wave. *Practitioner,* **45**, 20–33.

Rubin, P. (1996). Measuring diastolic blood pressure in pregnancy. *Br. Med. J.,* **313**, 4–5.

Sawyer, M. M., Lipshitz, J., Anderson, G. D., Dilts, P. V. Jr. and Halperin, L. (1981). Diurnal and short-term variation of blood pressure: comparison of preeclamptic, chronic hypertensive, and normotensive patients. *Obstet. Gynecol.,* **58**(3), 291–6.

Segall, H. N. (1987). To the question of methods of determining the blood pressure (from the clinic of Professor C. P. Federov) by N. S. Korotkoff. In: *Classic Papers in Hypertension. Blood Pressure and Renin,* ed. J. D. Swales. London: Science Press Ltd, pp. 152–7.

Seligman, S. (1987). Which blood pressure? *Br. J. Obstet. Gynaecol.,* **94**, 497–8.

Seligman, S. A. (1971). Diurnal blood-pressure variation in pregnancy. *J. Obstet. Gynaecol. Br. Cwlth,* **78**(5), 417–22.

Shennan, A. H., Kissane, J. and de Swiet, M. (1993). Validation of the SpaceLabs 90207 ambulatory blood pressure monitor for use in pregnancy. *Br. J. Obstet. Gynaecol.,* **100**, 904–8.

Shennan, A. H., Gupta, M., Halligan, A., Taylor, D. J. and de Swiet, M. (1996a). Lack of reproducibility in pregnancy of Korotkoff phase IV as measured by mercury sphygmomanometry. *Lancet,* **347**(i), 139–42.

Shennan, A. H., Halligan, A., Gupta, M., Taylor, D. and de Swiet, M. (1996b). Oscillometric blood pressure measurement in severe pre-eclampsia: validation of the SpaceLabs 90207. *Br. J. Obstet. Gynaecol.,* **103**, 171–3.

Shimada, K., Kawamoto, A., Matsubayashi, K., Nishinaga, M., Kimura, S. and Ozawa, T. (1992). Diurnal blood pressure variations and silent cerebrovascular damage in elderly patients with hypertension. *J. Hypertens.,* **10**(8), 875–8.

Sibai, B. M. and Anderson, G. D. (1986). Pregnancy outcome of intensive therapy in severe hypertension in first trimester. *Obstet. Gynecol.,* **67**, 517–22.

Sibai, B. M., Abdella, T. N. and Anderson, G. D. (1983). Pregnancy outcome in 211 patients with mild chronic hypertension. *Obstet. Gynecol.,* **61**, 571–6.

Siegel, W. C., Blumenthal, J. A. and Divine, G. W. (1990). Physiological, psychological, and behavioral factors and white coat hypertension. *Hypertension,* **16**, 140–6.

Smarason, A. K., Sargent, I. L., Starkey, P. M. and Redman, C. W. (1993). The effect of placental syncytiotrophoblast microvillous membranes from normal and pre-eclamptic women on the growth of endothelial cells in vitro. *Br. J. Obstet. Gynaecol.,* **100**(10), 943–9.

Smits, P., Thien, T. and van't Laar, A. (1985). Circulatory effects of coffee in relation to the pharmacokinetics of caffeine. *Am. J. Cardiol.,* **56**, 958–63.

Stegall, H. F., Kardon, M. B. and Kemmerer, W. T. (1968). Indirect measurement of arterial blood pressure by Doppler ultrasonic sphygmomanometry. *J. Appl. Physiol.,* **25**(6), 793–8.

Strandgaard, S., Olesen, J., Skinhoj, E. and Lassen, N. (1973). Autoregulation of brain circulation in severe arterial hypertension. *Br. Med. J.,* **1**(852), 507–10.

Tervila, L., Goecke, C. and Timonen, S. (1973). Estimation of gestosis of pregnancy (EPH-gestosis). *Acta Obstet. Gynecol. Scand.,* **52**, 235–43.

von Recklinghausen, H. (1901). Uber Blutdruckmessung beim Menschen. *Exp. Pathol. Pharmacol.,* **XLVI**, 78.

Wang, Y. P., Walsh, S. W., Guo, J. D. and Zhang, J. Y. (1991). The imbalance between thromboxane and prostacyclin in preeclampsia is associated with an imbalance between lipid peroxides and vitamin E in maternal blood. *Am. J. Obstet. Gynaecol.,* **165**(6, Pt. 1), 1695–700.

Waugh, J., Halligan, A., Rushbrook, J. and Shennan, A. H. (2002). Validation of the hidden errors of aneroid sphygmomanometers. *Blood Press. Monit.,* **7**, 309–12.

White, W. B. and Baker, L. H. (1986). Episodic hypertension secondary to panic disorder. *Arch. Int. Med.*, **146**, 1129–30.

Wichman, K., Ryden, G. and Wichman, M. (1984). The influence of different positions and Korotkoff sounds on the blood pressure measurements in pregnancy. *Acta Obstet. Gynecol. Scand.*, **118**, 25–8.

Zanchetti, A. and Mancia, G. (1996). The centenary of blood pressure measurement: a tribute to Scipione Riva Rocci. *J. Hypertens.*, **14**, 1–12.

19

Immune maladaptation in the etiology of pre-eclampsia; an updated epidemiological perspective

Gus Dekker and Pierre Yves Robillard

Introduction

Shallow, endovascular cytotrophoblast invasion in the spiral arteries and endothelial cell dysfunction are two key features in the pathophysiology of pre-eclampsia (Roberts and Redman, 1993). However, the cause of pre-eclampsia remains unknown. In humans, organ transplants will be rejected if there are differences between donor and recipient with respect to histocompatibility complex genes, i.e. human leukocyte antigens. The feto-placental unit contains paternal antigens that are foreign to its maternal host. The concept that pre-eclampsia may be an immunologic disorder dates back to the beginning of the century (McQuarrrie, 1923; Medawar, 1953; Scott and Beer, 1976; Veit, 1902). In the early 1950s, Medawar (1953) proposed the concept of the "fetus as an allograft." Since then it has been assumed that implantation of the fetal placenta would be controlled by a maternal immune response mediated by T cells recognizing paternally derived allo-antigens expressed by the placenta. Ongoing research in the last decade has shown that implantation might predominantly involve a novel allogenetic recognition system based on natural killer cells rather than T cells. Dr. Ashley Moffett's chapter provides a detailed overview of our current understanding on the immune biology and immune pathology of placentation as it relates to pre-eclampsia, with a focus on the important role of NK-cells.

In this chapter we aim to provide an up-to-date review on epidemiologic studies corroborating or refuting the hypothesis that maladaptation between the maternal immune system and the feto-placental allograft is involved in the etiology of pre-eclampsia.

Primipaternity versus the birth interval hypothesis

Genuine pre-eclampsia is a disease of first pregnancies (Roberts and Redman 1993). A previous normal pregnancy is associated with a markedly lowered incidence of pre-eclampsia, even a previous abortion provides some protection in this respect (Strickland et al., 1986). The protective effect of multiparity is, however, lost with change of partner. Need (1975) was the first to describe that in a patient's first pregnancy without pre-eclampsia, the response of maternal lymphocytes, in a mixed lymphocyte culture, against lymphocytes of the first father was much less than against the different father of the subsequent pregnancy which was complicated by severe pre-eclampsia. Feeney and Scott (Feeny, 1980; Feeney and Scott, 1980) in a retrospective survey of 34,000 multigravida deliveries, found 47 patients with pre-eclampsia occurring after previous normal pregnancies. In 13 (28%) of these patients the affected pregnancy was by a new father, as compared with only 4.3% in the large control group. In Nigeria, Ikedife found that 34 out of

46 (74%) multiparous eclamptic patients had a new partner for the affected pregnancy, as compared to 5–10% in multiparous women with normal pregnancies (Ikedife, 1980).

The term primipaternity was introduced by Robillard *et al.* (1993) exploring the relationship between severe pre-eclampsia and changes in paternity patterns among multigravidas in Guadeloupe (French West Indies). Multiparous patients with severe pre-eclampsia and/or eclampsia and controls were examined. Information concerning paternity for the index and previous pregnancies was collected from three groups: women with pre-eclampsia; women with chronic hypertension; and a control group consisting of women without hypertension during pregnancy. In 21/34 (61.7%) of the mothers with pre-eclampsia, the father of the current pregnancy was different than that of the former, compared to 4/40 (10%) among chronic hypertensive women and 10/60 (16.6%) in the control group ($P < 0.0001$). Because the patterns of changing paternity were significantly correlated with pre-eclampsia in multiparae but not with chronic hypertension and controls, the authors proposed that pre-eclampsia might be a problem of primipaternity rather than primigravidity. Because concerns related to definitions used by Robillard *et al.* (1993) were expressed, Amsterdam researchers (Tubbergen *et al.*, 1999), using very strict diagnostic criteria, studied 333 multiparous patients with pre-eclampsia and/or HELLP syndrome. The control group consisted of 182 multiparous women without pre-eclampsia. The prevalence of new paternity was significantly higher ($P<0.0001$) both for pre-eclamptic and HELLP patients in comparison with the controls with an odds ratio of 8.6 (95% CI: 3.1–23.5) and 10.9 (95% CI: 3.7–32.3), respectively. In the discussion paragraph Tubbergen *et al.* (1999) stress that every multiparous woman ought to be asked if her pregnancy originates from the same partner. According to the primipaternity concept, multiparous women with a new partner should have the same antenatal care approach as primigravidas. Using a cohort approach, Trupin *et al.* (1996)

studied 5068 nulliparas and 5800 multiparas, 573 of whom had new partners. The pre-eclampsia incidence in nulliparas (3.2%) and multiparas with changed paternity (3%) was found to be similar, as compared to the significantly lower pre-eclampsia incidence (1.9%) in multiparas with no change in partners.

The primipaternity concept was recently challenged by Skjaerven *et al.* (2002). These investigators used data from the Medical Birth Registry of Norway, a population-based registry that includes births that occurred between 1967 and 1998. They studied 551,478 women who had two or more singleton deliveries, and 209,423 women who had three or more singleton deliveries. Pre-eclampsia occurred during 3.9% of first pregnancies, 1.7% of second pregnancies and 1.8% of third pregnancies when the woman had the same partner. The risk in a second or third pregnancy was directly related to the time that had elapsed since the preceding delivery and, when the interbirth interval was 10 years or more, the risk approximated that among nulliparous women. A change of paternity for the second pregnancy was associated with a reduced risk of pre-eclampsia after controlling for the time since first delivery (OR 0.80, 95% CI: 0.72–0.90), but the interaction between change in paternity and time between deliveries was significant only for women with no previous pre-eclampsia. The interaction between history of pre-eclampsia and time interval between the two deliveries was highly significant and, for women with no previous pre-eclampsia, the risk of pre-eclampsia in second pregnancy increased with increasing time interval. For intervals longer than 15 years, the OR was 2.11 (95% CI: 1.75–2.53). For women with previous pre-eclampsia, the risk tended to decrease with increasing time interval between deliveries. Skjaerven *et al.* (2002) concluded that the protective impact of a new father for the second pregnancy challenges the hypothesis of primipaternity, and implies that the increase in pre-eclampsia risk ascribed to a new father by others is due to insufficient control for interbirth interval.

It should be noted that other investigators had previously described the birth interval effect. Mostello *et al.* (2002) conducted a population-based, case-control study using birth certificate data from Missouri. Data from women delivered of their first two singleton pregnancies between 1989 and 1997 (2332 cases with pre-eclampsia in the second pregnancy, and 2370 control cases) were analyzed. Significant risk factors for pre-eclampsia in a second pregnancy included longer birth interval, previous preterm delivery, previous small-for-gestational-age newborn, renal disease, chronic hypertension, diabetes mellitus, obesity, black race and inadequate prenatal care. Importantly, in contrast to the Norwegian study, same paternity was found to be *protective*.

Basso *et al.* (2001) studied the outcome of the second birth in a cohort of Danish women with pre-eclampsia in the previous birth (8401 women) and in all women with pre-eclampsia in the second (but not first) birth together with a sample of women with two births (26,596 women). A long interbirth interval was associated with a higher risk of pre-eclampsia in women with no previous pre-eclampsia when the father was the same. Similar to the Norwegian investigators, they found that partner change was associated with an increased risk of pre-eclampsia in women with no history of pre-eclampsia; this effect disappeared after adjustment for the interbirth interval. The investigators mentioned that they saw different results when stratified on the length of the interbirth interval.

Conde-Agudelo and Belizan (2000), studying the impact of interbirth interval on maternal morbidity and mortality, reported the first truly large study on the effect of prolonged birth interval as a risk factor for pre-eclampsia. These investigators, using the Perinatal Information System database of the Latin American Center for Perinatology and Human Development in Montevideo, studied 456,889 parous women delivering singleton infants. They showed that short (<6 months) and long (> 59 months) interbirth intervals were observed for 2.8 and 19.5% of

women, respectively. After adjustment for major confounding factors, compared with those conceiving at 18−23 months after a previous birth, women with interbirth intervals of 5 months or less had higher risks for maternal death (OR = 2.54; 95% CI: 1.22−5.38), third trimester bleeding (1.73; 1.42−2.24), premature rupture of membranes (1.72; 1.53−1.93), puerperal endometritis (1.33; 1.22−1.45) and anemia (1.30; 1.18−1.43). Compared with women with interbirth intervals of 18−23 months, women with interbirth intervals longer than 59 months had significantly increased risks of pre-eclampsia (1.83; 1.72−1.94) and eclampsia (1.80; 1.38−2.32).

We strongly feel that there is a different interpretation to the Norwegian data that does not necessarily disagree with the primipaternity hypothesis. First of all, the Norwegian study has several important weaknesses. Birth registries do not contain the details necessary for adequate investigation of paternity in humans. Besides a 12% rate of missing data on paternities reported in the study of Skjaerven *et al.* (2002), it is known that there is a significant rate (1−30%) of false claimed paternities in stable couples in developed countries (Lucassen and Parker, 2001). Those, nevertheless, fall in the "same father" group in the present study. Thus, conclusions concerning the association between paternity and pre-eclampsia based on birth registry alone should be avoided; they are a crude indication of the real paternities and do not contain the necessary information on sexual cohabitation, which is fundamental to scholarly advance of these continued discussions. Skjaerven *et al.* (2002) also suggest that the diagnosis of pre-eclampsia in their study included the presence of 0.3 g of protein per 24 h. The Norwegian authors have not addressed the fact that most Western countries, and we do not know of any reason to assume that Norway behaved differently, only started to use 24-h urine analysis during the 1980s. Thus the diagnosis of proteinuria in at least 60% of their "pre-eclamptic" patients may be in question. This is a very relevant concern, since the index of patients of interest in the Norwegian study are multiparous women often of relatively advanced age; it is notoriously difficult to come to a reliable diagnosis of pre-eclampsia in this category of women.

Second, there appears to be a significant degree of biologic inconsistency in the paper. Skjaerven *et al.* (2002) fail to discuss the findings of a study published by Li and Wi (2000), who reported a cohort study based on 140,147 women with two consecutive births during 1989–1991 identified through linking of annual California birth certificate data. Among women without pre-eclampsia/eclampsia in the first birth, changing partners resulted in a 30% increase in the risk of pre-eclampsia/eclampsia in the subsequent pregnancy compared with those who did not change partners (95% CI: 1.1–1.6). On the other hand, among women with pre-eclampsia/eclampsia in the first birth, changing partners resulted in a 30% reduction in the risk of pre-eclampsia/eclampsia in the subsequent pregnancy (95% CI: 0.4–1.2). Even more interestingly, the same group of Norwegian authors (Lie *et al.*, 1998), in a previous report, also found that the risk of developing pre-eclampsia in mothers who had had pre-eclampsia in their first pregnancy was 13.1% if she had her second pregnancy with the same partner. This risk dropped to 11.8% if she changed the partner. If anything, one would assume a longer birth interval after experiencing a traumatic life event such as a pregnancy complicated by pre-eclampsia in combination with the time required to find a new partner. As such, their own previously published data (Lie *et al.*, 1998), as well as the data of Li and Wi (2000), appear to contradict the "birth interval hypothesis." It should also be noted that, in a publication in the *International Journal of Epidemiology* (Trogstad *et al.*, 2001) preceding the *New England Journal of Medicine* publication (on the same population cohort, with different authors), it is specifically emphasized that birth interval is not a risk factor in women with previous pre-eclampsia with same or new paternity pregnancies. Again, these findings make the birth interval hypothesis implausible.

It is hard to conceive of any risk factor (environmental, infection, stress, BMI, etc.) that would increase the risk in women with previously normal pregnancies and, at the same time, decrease the risk in women with previous pre-eclamptic pregnancies.

Be this as it may, considering the combined Norwegian and Latin American data, let us assume that a prolonged pregnancy interval is an important risk factor for future pre-eclampsia in multiparous women, independent of maternal age. What are the possible alternative explanations?

1. Both the Norwegian study and the Latin American study confirm common knowledge that the majority (>80%) of couples normally have an interval of <5 years between their offspring. Because of this, one has to rethink the most common possible reasons why some couples (less than 20%) would apparently "opt" to have prolonged intervals between their offspring. So far, all of the studies mentioned earlier have studied subsequent pregnancy outcome in multiparous women but, in reality, pregnancy outcome only included pregnancies after 16 (Norway) or 19 (Latin America) weeks' gestation. In other words, all miscarriages were ignored. The occurrence of one or more miscarriages, a very common event for many women in Western societies, may explain a significant proportion of the couples apparently "opting" for a prolonged birth interval. Women with recurrent miscarriages are known to have a higher incidence of adverse pregnancy outcome in subsequent ongoing pregnancies (Jivraj *et al.*, 2001).

2. Diminished fertility could also account for the long birth interval of >5 years in less than 20% of couples. The most common causes of diminished fertility include Polycystic Ovarian (PCO) syndrome and obesity, both having clear associations with pre-eclampsia in subsequent pregnancies (Dekker, 1999; de Vries *et al.*, 1998). However, even unexplained infertility has a clear association with pre-eclampsia. In 1983, Moore and Redman described, in a case control study of

24 patients with severe pre-eclampsia diagnosed before 34 weeks' gestation, and 48 randomly selected controls matched for age and parity, that a history of infertility is a significant risk factor for pre-eclampsia. Pandian *et al.* (2001) examined outcome of singleton pregnancies in couples with unexplained infertility and explored the impact of fertility treatment. The authors studied women with unexplained infertility identified in the Aberdeen Fertility Clinic, and they used the general obstetric population as a control group. Women with unexplained infertility were significantly older (30.8 versus 27.9 years) and more likely to be primiparous (59 versus 40%, 95% CI = +1.3 to +1.9). After adjusting for age and parity, the women with a history of infertility had a higher incidence of pre-eclampsia and placental abruption. The authors concluded that women with unexplained infertility are at higher risk for obstetrical complications including pre-eclampsia. Interestingly, another Scandinavian group (Basso *et al.*, 2003) recently examined the association between subfecundity and pre-eclampsia. By using interview data collected during the second trimester of pregnancy (1998–2001) from women participating in the Danish National Birth Cohort, they identified 20,034 and 24,698 singleton live births to primiparous and multiparous women, respectively, for whom pre-eclampsia information was available from hospital birth records. Among women with no known hypertension, the authors estimated a higher risk of pre-eclampsia in those with longer times to pregnancy after adjustment for maternal age, pre-pregnancy body mass index, and smoking. Compared with primiparas who became pregnant right away (referent category), the risk of pre-eclampsia increased with increasing interval to conception and then stabilized for women taking 6 months or longer to conceive – in which women the risk of pre-eclampsia increased by 50%. Multiparas also had an increased risk, but only those reporting a time-to-pregnancy longer than

12 months (odds ratio = 2.47, 95% CI: 1.30, 4.69). The authors found that a long time-to-pregnancy was associated with pre-eclampsia, supporting the hypothesis that some factors delaying clinically recognized conception might also participate in a causal pathway for pre-eclampsia.

3. The third explanation is more hypothetical. In Western societies, the percentage of marriages ending in divorce is gradually increasing to more than 40%. As such, the number of relationships facing a near crisis is even higher. Two mechanisms may be operational in these relationships: many such women may have secret extramarital relationships, sometimes resulting in unplanned pregnancies. These women have two options. They may divorce and start a new life with a new partner (which would be counted as new paternity) or stay with their husband and, for obvious reasons, never acknowledge the change in paternity. The true frequency of non-paternity is not known but, as mentioned earlier, published reports suggest an incidence from as low as 1% per generation up to about 30% in Western populations (Lucassen and Parker, 2001). This mechanism may be relevant (at least partially) in explaining the Norwegian study findings. Women with very prolonged pregnancy intervals often have their first pregnancies as teenagers or in their early 20s; such women are known to have a higher risk for future marital infidelity and divorce (Atkins *et al.*, 2001). In some married couples with children, sex drive decreases to a lower level because of marital stress and/or extramarital affairs. This may result in minimal sperm exposure over prolonged periods of time (and less chance of pregnancy). Some of these couples may decide to have another baby in order to save/revive their marriage. It might be that these emotional decisions are accompanied by a sudden reactivation of sexuality and a resulting short interval between "the decision" and the subsequent pregnancy. If ongoing sperm exposure is required to boost

the active process of NK-related partner-specific immune tolerance, one would expect a high incidence of pre-eclampsia in these "save the relationship" pregnancies (Dekker, 2002).

Eskenazia and Harleyb (2001) also reviewed the evidence for and against the primipaternity hypothesis versus the birth interval hypothesis, and stressed that, while neither Lie *et al.* (1998) nor Li and Wi (2000) report odds ratios controlling for the time interval between deliveries, both groups reported that time interval was examined and was not a confounder. Furthermore, time between deliveries is unlikely to be a confounder in the Li and Wi (2000) study given that the authors restricted their population to births that were between 1 and 3 years apart.

A very important study strongly supporting the primipaternity concept was recently published by Saftlas *et al.* (2003). These authors studied nulliparous women previously recruited in the Calcium for Pre-eclampsia Prevention Trial, 1992–1995. They specifically examined whether nulliparous women with a prior abortion who then change partner lose the protective effect of the prior pregnancy. Their data show that women with a history of abortion who conceived again with the same partner had nearly half the risk of pre-eclampsia (adjusted odds ratio = 0.54, 95% CI: 0.31, 0.97) as women without a history of abortion. In contrast, women with an abortion history who conceived with a new partner had the same risk of pre-eclampsia as women without a history of abortion (adjusted odds ratio = 1.03, 95% CI: 0.72, 1.47). Thus, the protective effect of a prior abortion operated only among women who conceived again with the same partner. According to these investigators their data strongly support an immune-based etiologic mechanism, whereby prolonged exposure to fetal antigens from a previous pregnancy protects against pre-eclampsia in a subsequent pregnancy with the same father. In their discussion, Saftlas *et al.* (2003) also emphasize that the Scandinavian investigators (Skjaerven *et al.*, 2002) ignored the effect of

history of abortions, particularly induced abortions. They state "Because induced abortions protect against preeclampsia and are obtained more frequently by unmarried, separated, or divorced women than by women in stable unions, failure to account for termination of pregnancies conceived between registered births would result in erroneously long interbirth intervals attributed to women who change partners. Moreover, adjustment for induced abortions would decrease the relative risk associated with interbirth interval and increase the relative risk associated with changing partners." Although the inter-pregnancy interval was not ascertained directly in the CPEP Trial, which enrolled only nulliparous women (median age, 19.7 years), the average inter-pregnancy interval approximated 1 year, given that the average age of primigravidas was 1 year less than that for women who had one previous pregnancy. Saftlas *et al.* (2003) stress that confounding by inter-pregnancy interval is also unlikely because the odds ratios for women above or below the median age were virtually identical, despite the fact that the interpregnancy interval was, of necessity, shorter for women below than above the median age. In addition, the average age of women who changed partners was only about a month more than that of women who remained with the same partner.

In summary, the primipaternity hypothesis continues to stand strong. However, we should not be blind to the fact that there may be an additional effect associated with prolonged birth intervals. Khong *et al.* (2003) recently demonstrated that structural changes of the spiral arteries needed for the pregnancy do not completely resolve following parturition, and that the degree of anatomical changes are related to the number of previous pregnancies; duplication and fragmentation of the internal elastic lamina, and the proportion of non-muscular tissue increased with increasing parity. It would be very important to know whether or not these changes regress with prolonged birth intervals.

Sperm exposure

Marti and Herrmann (1977) were the first to recognize that repeated sperm exposure might prevent pre-eclampsia. They studied 83 primigravidas, 28 with pre-eclampsia, and 55 with an uncomplicated pregnancy. The pre-eclamptics had an average of 59.5 physiologic exposures to semen while the non-pre-eclamptic control group had 191.6 exposures. In addition, the number of women using oral contraceptives (allowing sperm exposure) and the total period of oral contraceptive use was significantly lower in the pre-eclamptic women. The authors stated that their findings might provide an explanation for the high incidence of pre-eclampsia in teenage pregnant girls. One possible flaw in this study was introduced by the fact that pre-eclampsia was defined by a gestosis index score (Goecke and Schwabe, 1965). The gestosis index (Goecke and Schwabe, 1965) combines systolic and diastolic blood pressure, proteinuria and edema to classify patients as having mild, moderate or severe Edema–Proteinuria–Hypertension (EPH) gestosis. Thus, the presence of physiologic edema is enough to classify a normotensive pregnant woman as having mild EPH gestosis. Using more contemporary definitions to define pregnancy-induced hypertensive disorders, the issue of sperm exposure protecting against pre-eclampsia was reassessed by Klonoff et al. (1989). A case-control study was conducted comparing the contraceptive and reproductive histories of 110 primiparous women with pre-eclampsia to 115 pregnant women without pre-eclampsia. Controls were frequency matched to cases by age, race, and distance from the hospital. Unconditional logistic regression analysis indicated a 2.37-fold (95% CI: 1.01–5.58) increased risk of pre-eclampsia for users of contraceptives that prevent exposure to sperm, e.g. condoms, diaphragms, spermicides, and withdrawal. A dose–response gradient was observed, with increasing risk of pre-eclampsia for those with fewer episodes of sperm exposure. According to Klonoff et al. (1989), barrier methods may

contribute to as much as 60% of pre-eclamptic cases. Mills et al. (1991) could not confirm these "adverse" effects of barrier contraceptives. After the publication of Klonoff et al. (1989), they analyzed, post hoc, data from two prospective pregnancy studies (the "Kaiser Permanente Birth Defects Study" and the "Vaginal Infection and Prematurity Study"), primarily consisting of women who were delivered in the mid-seventies, to examine the relationship between contraceptive use before conception, and pre-eclampsia. The pre-eclampsia rates among women using barrier contraceptives were not significantly higher than the rates in women using non-barrier contraceptives or those not using any contraceptives in either study. However, the Mills et al. (1991) study had not been specifically designed to explore the relationship between contraceptive use and pre-eclampsia, and it should be noted that only contraceptive use in the year before the study pregnancy was evaluated. It is possible that women who had used barrier methods during the study period could have used non-barrier methods prior to this time. Women often stop taking oral contraceptives some time before actually trying to get pregnant, because of a concern about the baby being exposed to "pill" hormones, or a worry that their ovulatory function is no longer intact after many years of oral contraceptives (Mosher and Pratt, 1990; Serfaty, 1992). Also, although it is stated (Mills et al., 1991) that contemporary criteria were used to diagnose pregnancy-induced hypertensive disorders, the reported incidences of pregnancy-induced hypertensive disorders in this study was substantially higher than reported by most authorities. In the "Kaiser Permanente Birth Defects Study," 6.1% of primigravida developed pre-eclampsia, which is consistent with studies in the literature. However, looking at their multiparae, one is struck by a 5.4% incidence of pre-eclampsia, which is very high. In the "Vaginal Infection and Prematurity Study," the pre-eclampsia incidence in nulliparae was 16.4%, and 13.3% in multiparous women. These data raise serious concerns about the validity of the conclusions made by Mills *et al.* (1991).

Several studies in other countries have since confirmed the increased risk of pre-eclampsia associated with barrier contraceptives (Cepicky and Podrouzek, 1990; Hernandez-Valencia *et al.*, 2000). Quite recently, Einarsson *et al.* (2003) published data supporting the risks associated with barrier contraceptives. These Texan authors used a case-control design in which women with pre-eclampsia (cases) were matched with two women without pre-eclampsia (controls) by age and parity. A total of 113 cases were compared with 226 controls. Women with a short period of cohabitation (<4 months) using barrier methods for contraception had a substantially elevated risk for development of pre-eclampsia compared with women with more than 12 months of cohabitation before conception (odds ratio 17.1, $P = 0.004$).

Robillard *et al.* (1994) were the first to perform a prospective study on the relationship between sperm exposure and pre-eclampsia. They studied the duration of sexual cohabitation with the father prior to conception and the incidence of pregnancy-induced hypertension. During a five-month period, 1011 consecutive women delivering in one obstetric unit were interviewed about paternity and duration of sexual cohabitation before conception. Obstetric charts were abstracted to identify three groups: those with pregnancy-induced hypertension, chronic hypertension, and normal blood pressure. The incidence of pregnancy-induced hypertension was 11.9% among primigravidae, 4.7% among same-paternity multigravidas, and 24.0% among new-paternity multigravidas. For both primigravidae and multigravidas, length of sexual cohabitation before conception was inversely related to the incidence of pregnancy-induced hypertension ($P < 0.0001$). Similar results were observed after control for race, education, maternal age, marital status, and number of pregnancies. Taking women cohabitating for more than 12 months as a reference, the adjusted odds ratio (OR) for developing pre-eclampsia when the cohabitation period was 0–4 months

was 11.6 (95% CI: 6.4–20.9), for a period of 5–8 months it was 5.9 (95% CI: 2.9–12.5), and for a period of 9–12 months it was 4.2 (95% CI: 1.7–10.4). In this prospective study, Robillard *et al.* (1994) demonstrated that multigravidas with a pregnancy-induced hypertensive disorder had a new partner in 66.7% of cases as compared to 24.1% in normotensive multigravidas ($P = 0.0001$). The very high incidence (24.0%) of pregnancy-induced hypertension among new-paternity multigravidas was shown to be related to a remarkably short period of sperm exposure preceding conception. Robillard *et al.* (1994) concluded that pregnancy-induced hypertensive disorders is a problem of primipaternity rather than primigravidity, and that an extended duration of sexual cohabitation before conception protects against pregnancy-induced hypertensive disorders. In this study 21 patients developed proteinuric pregnancy-induced hypertension (pre-eclampsia), while the other 81 patients developed pregnancy-induced hypertension. In the analysis, these patients were counted together as pregnancy-induced hypertension. Thus, although this prospective study has provided very convincing data, further studies are necessary in order to assess if sperm exposure provides protection against genuine pre-eclampsia, and especially pre-eclampsia associated with adverse perinatal outcome. In a relatively small case-control study, Verwoerd *et al.* (2002) found that multigravidae, but not primigravidae, with a period of unprotected sexual cohabitation of >6 months, had a decreased risk of pre-eclampsia. In contrast to Robillard's study, Morcos *et al.* (2000) found in a recent retrospective case-control study of 68 women of mixed parity with pregnancy-induced hypertension, that in primiparous women a shorter duration of sexual cohabitation was associated with only a small and non-significant reduction in the risk of pregnancy-induced hypertension. For multiparous women, a longer interval between conception and ceasing the use of barrier contraceptives was associated with a greater risk of pregnancy-induced hypertension. However, the study of Morcos *et al.* (2000) has some major problems: (a) a relatively high percentage (20–40% of cases) had a history of a previous abortion, and (b) both cases and controls had some significant fertility limiting factors. The mean number of months of sexual activity without any birth control was 13.2 and 10.9 months, respectively, in the primiparous hypertensive cases and controls, and 49.4 and 27.1 months, respectively, in the multiparous hypertensive cases and controls.

Alternative mucosal sperm exposure

Oral administration of myelin and collagen has a significant beneficial effect in patients with multiple sclerosis and rheumatoid arthritis, respectively. This effect (oral tolerization) is probably related to the specific way in which the antigen is processed by the digestive tract immune system. Oral tolerance is a long-recognized method of inducing immune tolerance. Interestingly, antigens that stimulate the gut-associated lymphoid tissue (GALT) preferentially generate a Th2 type response (Weiner *et al.*, 1994). In 1986, two distinct and mutually inhibitory types of T-helper cells were described (Mossman *et al.*, 1986). The first type of cell, termed Th1, secretes IL-2, IFN-γ, and lymphotoxin. This contrasts with Th2 cells, which secrete IL-4, IL-6, and IL-10 (Mossman and Moore, 1991). Th1 cytokines are associated with cell-mediated immunity and delayed hypersensitivity reactions, while Th2 cytokines foster antibody responses and allergic reactions. Because Th1 cytokines are considered harmful to pregnancy, and Th2 cytokines such as IL-10 can downregulate production of Th1 cytokines, it was proposed by Wegman in the early 1990s that successful pregnancy is a Th2 phenomenon (Marzi *et al.*, 1996; Wegmann *et al.*, 1993). Nowadays we know that this paradigm is clearly an oversimplification. However, based on the concept of mucosal tolerance, and the type 1 versus type 2 paradigm, Koelman *et al.* (2000) evaluated whether oral sex is associated with a lower incidence of pre-eclampsia; 41 primiparous women with a history

of pre-eclampsia, strictly defined by the combined presence of pregnancy-induced hypertension, proteinuria and hyperuricemia, and a control group of 44 women with a normal pregnancy were asked if they had oral sex (intraoral ejaculation) with their partner before the index pregnancy. In the 41 pre-eclamptic women 18 (44%) had oral sex with their partner before the index pregnancy versus 36 out of 44 (82%) in the control group ($P=0.0003$). In addition, 7 of the 41 (17%) pre-eclamptic patients versus 21 out of the 44 control patients (48%) confirmed that they had swallowed the sperm ($P=0.003$). Thus, oral sex before the first pregnancy appears to be associated with a significantly decreased incidence of pre-eclampsia. The authors admitted that further studies are needed to assess whether these findings reflect oral tolerization to paternal antigens or if oral sex is associated with increased genital tract exposure to sperm.

Where is the critical paternal antigen and how is the female organism exposed to the paternal HLA message?

The exact way by which the female organism is exposed to the paternal HLA message is uncertain.

Koelman *et al.* (2000) demonstrated the presence of soluble class I HLA molecules in seminal plasma representing a potentially straightforward way of endometrial exposure. Interestingly, soluble HLA molecules have also been demonstrated to induce apoptosis in human cytotoxic T cells (Zavazava and Kronke, 1996), and induction of apoptosis may be a mechanism for inducing specific tolerance against a partner's HLA cell membrane molecules. An alternative model, proposed by Clark (1993, 1994), states that the genital tract has unusual T cells with $\gamma\delta$ rather than $\alpha\beta$ type receptors for antigen. He suggested that these T cells respond to antigens in the vagina and uterus without the usual requirement for simultaneous binding to an HLA-A, -B, -C, or -D type antigen on the antigen-presenting cells (APC). Such a mechanism would pave the way for recognition of human trophoblast lacking classical HLA surface antigens.

However, based on his study of pregnancies after intra-uterine insemination, Smith *et al.* (1997) suggested that the protective factor is on the spermatozoa themselves and not in the seminal fluid. This was strongly supported by a subsequent study by Wang *et al.* (2002). They used a very elegant model to confirm the protective effect of previous sperm exposure and to analyse whether or not this protection is conveyed by sperm cells or seminal plasma. These authors looked at outcomes in pregnancies following Intra-Cytoplasmatic Sperm Injection (ICSI), where fertilization is achieved by injecting the sperm into the oocyte plasma. ICSI is used initially in cases where there are severe semen defects, including azoospermia. In some patients it is necessary to obtain sperm surgically. Couples in which the male partner has azoospermia and where sperm cells are obtained surgically provide an ideal "model" to test the protective partner-specific immune-tolerance conveyed by sperm cells. The model allows independent analysis of what may be present in seminal fluid, since in these couples there is no exposure of the female genital tract to sperm cells during intercourse, while exposure to seminal fluid is unaffected. Altogether, 1621 deliveries conceived after standard IVF, ICSI using sperm cells obtained by masturbation, and ICSI using surgically obtained sperm cells were analyzed; 195 (12.0%) had gestational hypertension, and 67 of them (4.1%) had pre-eclampsia. The risk of gestational hypertension was doubled, while the risk of pre-eclampsia was tripled in ICSI using surgically obtained sperm compared with standard IVF and ICSI using sperm obtained by masturbation. This study clearly confirms that previous exposure to the actual sperm cells must convey a major part of the protection, since women in the ICSI group using sperm cells obtained by transcutaneous surgical methods had not experienced any previous contact with their partner's sperm cells – and it was only in this subset of patients with longstanding infertility that the increased

incidence of both pre-eclampsia and gestational hypertension was seen.

Hall *et al.* (2001) came to different conclusions. These investigators examined the outcomes of pregnancies of women who conceived by donor insemination, as compared with women who conceived after IVF with their partner's spermatozoa. This was a retrospective cohort study of 218 women attending an IVF clinic, 45 of whom conceived with donor insemination and 173 of whom conceived with their partner's spermatozoa. Cases were identified from the IVF unit and data were extracted from patients' notes by blinded observers. Analysis showed no difference between the groups, with 22% of women who conceived with donor spermatozoa and 24% who conceived with partner spermatozoa developing some form of hypertensive disease of pregnancy. Insemination with their partner's spermatozoa was not associated with a reduction of hypertensive disease, and neither was donor spermatozoa insemination associated with an increased incidence. It should be noted that (a) this is a very small study, and (b) the incidence of pregnancy-induced hypertensive disorders is very high in both groups. We feel, however, that Hall *et al.* (2001) made one significant error that can explain their contrasting findings. The group of women requiring IVF using their partner's sperm cells almost certainly had additional fertility limiting factors when compared with the group who conceived with donor sperm. As mentioned earlier, Basso *et al.* (2003) found that some factors delaying clinically recognized conception might also be in a causal pathway for pre-eclampsia.

In summary, sperm exposure does provide some protection against developing pre-eclampsia. Actual exposure to the sperm cells appears to be the important factor. Deposition of semen in the female genital tract provokes a cascade of cellular and molecular events that resemble a classic inflammatory response. The critical factor appears to be seminal vesicle-derived transforming growth factor β (TGFβ). Seminal vesicle-derived TGFβ is secreted predominantly in a latent form.

Seminal plasmin and uterine factors transform the latent form into bioactive TGFβ (Tremellen *et al.*, 1998). Intra-uterine insemination of TGFβ in vivo results in an increase in granulocyte–monocyte colony stimulating factor (GM-CSF) production that is sufficient to initiate an endometrial leukocytosis comparable with that seen following mating (Robertson, 2002). The introduction of TGFβ into the uterus, in combination with paternal ejaculate antigens, favors the growth and survival of the semi-allogenic fetus, as evidenced by a significant increase in fetal and placental weight in animal studies. This is believed to be facilitated in two ways. First, by initiating a post-mating inflammatory reaction, TGFβ increases the ability to sample and process paternal antigens contained within the ejaculate. Another important role of TGFβ and the subsequent post-coital inflammatory response, is the initiation of a strong type 2 immune deviation. The processing of an antigen by antigen-presenting cells in an environment containing TGFβ is likely to initiate a Th2 phenotype within these responding T-cells (Robertson, 2002). By initiating a type 2 immune response toward paternal ejaculate antigens, seminal TGFβ may inhibit the induction of type 1 responses to the semi-allogenic conceptus that are thought to be responsible for poor placental and fetal development. Decidual macrophages, present in an immune-suppressive phenotype from the moment of implantation, may inhibit NK cell lytic activity through the release of molecules such as TGF, interleukin-10 (IL-10) and prostaglandin-E2 (PGE2). Under the influence of the local cytokine environment, antigen-presenting cells (such as macrophages and dendritic cells) may take up, process and present ejaculate antigens (sperm, somatic cells, and soluble antigens) to T cells in the draining lymph nodes (Tremellen *et al.*, 1998). In mice, uptake of sperm mRNA encoding for paternal HLA by decidual antigen-presenting cells has been shown to occur. There is subsequent translation of this sperm mRNA encoding paternal MHC class I within these maternal antigen-presenting cells. These antigen-presenting cells

traffic from the uterus to the draining lymph nodes during the post-coital inflammatory response. It is unknown whether or not this fascinating mechanism is operative in humans. HLA-G is certainly not involved here, since human sperm cells do not have mRNA for HLA-G (Hiby *et al.*, 1999; Watson *et al.*, 1983). Since HLA-G is monomorphic it would also be a very unlikely candidate to represent the paternal HLA specificity. Classic HLA-A and HLA-B are also very unlikely since these are not expressed by trophoblast.

Donor insemination and oocyte donation

Analogous to short periods of sperm exposure, artificial donor insemination has been reported by several investigators to result in a substantial increase in the incidence of pre-eclampsia (Schenker and Ezra, 1994). Concerning artificial donor insemination, the first major study was reported by Need *et al.* in 1983. They reported on 584 pregnancies following artificial donor insemination (ADI) in programs throughout Australia. The overall incidence of pre-eclampsia (proteinuric pregnancy-induced hypertension) was high (9.3%) compared with the expected incidence of 0.5–5%. The incidence was increased in both multigravid and primigravid women. The expected pre-eclampsia incidence in Australian primigravid women was 5%, while it was 10.1% in primigravid women pregnant after ADI. This increase in the incidence of pre-eclampsia in primigravid women after ADI supports the findings of Robillard *et al.* (1994), who demonstrated the protective effects of a prolonged period of sperm exposure. The expected pre-eclampsia incidence was 0.9% in multigravid patients, while it was 7.8% in the multigravid ADI patients. Thus, the expected protective effect of a previous pregnancy was not seen, and in fact there was a 47-fold increase in pre-eclampsia (observed versus expected) in ADI pregnancies after a previous full-term pregnancy, and a 15-fold increase after a pregnancy of shorter duration. The data from the multigravid patients who had ADI also tend to support the concept of primipaternity described by several independent groups of investigators (Feeney, 1980; Feeney and Scott 1980; Ikedife, 1980; Robillard *et al.*, 1993; Trupin *et al.*, 1996; Tubbergen *et al.*, 1999). Grefenstette *et al.* (1990) described the outcome of 487 pregnancies conceived after ADI with frozen semen, and found a significantly increased incidence of pregnancy-induced hypertension when compared both with their control group, and with control group from the national study conducted by INSERM in France in 1981.

The first report concerning the effect of oocyte donation on the incidence of pregnancy-induced hypertensive disorders was by Serhal and Craft (1987). They reported that 5 of their first 10 pregnant patients with oocyte donation, all of whom were normotensive prior to pregnancy, developed proteinuric hypertension. Two years later, they published a series of 61 pregnancies following oocyte donation; the incidence of pre-eclampsia was 38% (Serhal and Craft, 1989). A similar incidence (32%) has been reported by Pados *et al.* (1994), and by Soderstrom-Anttila and Hovatta (1995) (41%). However, the impact of oocyte donation/ADI on the incidence of pre-eclampsia has not been consistently reported by others. Perkins (1993) followed a small series of 44 AID initiated pregnancies. The incidence of hypertensive complications in this group, 36 of whom were nulliparous, did not differ from the rate for all pregnancies at their institution. Friedman *et al.* (1996) compared perinatal outcomes in a small series of 22 consecutive ovum donor pregnancies. They were matched for age, parity and order of gestation with a control group of 22 women who underwent standard IVF embryo transfer during the same period. Both groups showed a similar rate of hypertensive disorders. Antinori *et al.* (1995) reporting on 44 pregnancies achieved after oocyte donation, found an incidence of pregnancy-induced hypertensive disorders of 13%, which is increased only modestly as compared to that in the literature, especially considering the relatively

higher age of the women in this study. Hendler *et al.* (1997) compared pregnancy outcomes in 35 singleton pregnancies of at least 24 weeks duration conceived following oocyte donation at one reproductive center, with 95 singleton pregnancies conceived after IVF in women of similar maternal age who delivered during the same period (1988–1996). The incidence of pregnancy-induced hypertensive disorders was 25.7% in the oocyte donation group, versus 4.2% in the control group ($P < 0.01$). The comparable maternal age in the oocyte-donation women as compared to the regular IVF patients is an important feature of this study. This is because most studies reporting a high incidence of hypertensive complications in pregnancies following oocyte donation are confounded by the increased age of the patients, which in and of itself is associated with an increased risk of developing hypertension (Michalas *et al.*, 1996). Salha *et al.* (1999) compared the effects of different types of donated gametes. In this retrospective cohort study, a total of 144 women were studied. Of these, 72 were infertility patients who had conceived as a result of sperm, ovum or embryo donation. The other 72 women were age- and parity-matched control patients who became pregnant with their own gametes, either spontaneously or following intrauterine insemination with their partner's spermatozoa. Study patients were divided into three groups depending on the origin of the donated gametes. Group 1 consisted of pregnancies achieved by intrauterine insemination with washed donor spermatozoa ($n = 33$). Group 2 comprised women who conceived using donated oocytes ($n = 27$), and group 3 consisted of women who conceived as a result of embryo donation ($n = 12$). The incidence of pregnancy-induced hypertension in the donated gametes study group was 12.5% (9/72) compared with 2.8% (2/72) in the control group. In addition, pre-eclampsia was diagnosed in 18.1% (13/72) of the donated gametes study group compared to 1.4% (1/72) in the age- and parity-matched controls.

In summary, in line with the immune maladaptation hypothesis, pregnancies conceived with donated gametes, and more specifically donor embryo pregnancies, are clearly at an increased risk of pre-eclampsia. With the likelihood of increased use of these reproductive techniques in the foreseeable future, clinical obstetricians need to adapt their antenatal care for these higher-risk pregnancies.

"Dangerous" partner

There are data that provide evidence for the existence of the so-called "dangerous" father. Lie *et al.* (1998) published a Norwegian population study (1967–1992; about 60,000 births per year) in which they identified 363,758 pairs of first and second pregnancies where the two children had the same mother and father; 14,266 pairs of pregnancies where the children had the same mother but different fathers; and 26,152 pairs where the children had the same father but different mothers. One of the major findings of this study was that men who fathered one pre-eclamptic pregnancy were nearly twice as likely to father a pre-eclamptic pregnancy in a different woman (1.8; 95% CI: 1.2–2.6; after adjustment for parity), regardless of whether that woman had already had a pre-eclamptic pregnancy or not. Thus mothers had a substantially increased risk in their second pregnancy (2.9%) if they became pregnant by a man who had previously fathered a pre-eclamptic first pregnancy in another woman. This risk was nearly as high as the average risk amongst first pregnancies. Whether or nor being a "dangerous" man relates to his specific HLA, seminal factors (e.g. lower TGFβ) or other factors is yet to be determined.

There is a well-recognized inherited maternal predisposition to pre-eclampsia. Whether there is a paternally inherited component, however, is not certain, but Esplin *et al.* (2001) used records from the Utah Population Database to identify 298 men and 237 women born in Utah between 1947 and 1957 whose mothers had had pre-eclampsia during their pregnancy. For each man and woman in the study group, they identified two matched, unrelated control subjects who were not the products of pregnancies complicated by pre-eclampsia. They then identified 947 children of the 298 male study subjects and 830 children of the 237 female study subjects who had been born between 1970 and 1992. These children were matched to offspring of the control subjects (1950 offspring of the male control group and 1658 offspring of the female control group). After adjustment for the offspring's year of birth, maternal parity, and the offspring's gestational age at delivery, the odds ratio of an adult whose mother had had pre-eclampsia of having a child who was itself the product of a pregnancy complicated by pre-eclampsia was 2.1 (95% CI: 1.0–4.3; $P = 0.04$) in the male study group and 3.3 (95% CI: 1.5–7.5; $P = 0.004$) in the female study group. The authors concluded that both men and women who were the product of a pregnancy complicated by pre-eclampsia were significantly more likely than control men and women to have a child who was the product of a pregnancy complicated by pre-eclampsia.

Perspectives

The studies, mostly epidemiologic, reviewed in this chapter strongly suggest that immune maladaptation is involved in the etiology of pre-eclampsia. Exposure to sperm provides at least partial protection against the development of pre-eclampsia. Immune maladaptation may cause the characteristic shallow endovascular trophoblast invasion of pre-eclampsia, and lead to placental ischemia and endothelial cell dysfunction, a theory in line with the placenta ischemia hypothesis (Smarason *et al.*, 1993). Alternatively, immune maladaptation may cause the release of toxic cytokines, radical species and proteolytic enzymes from the decidua, which may then cause damage and/or disturb the normal function of the trophoblast and the maternal endothelium (Dekker and Sibai, 1998). The immune maladaptation hypothesis does not contradict studies showing the involvement of genetic factors in the etiology of pre-eclampsia. As early as 1985, Beer and Need hypothesized that a female who is a genetically poor responder, challenged by a male who by genetic design is a poor stimulator, would definitely lead to a poor or inadequate maternal immune response. Westendorp et al. (1997) demonstrated the relation between genetic factors and cytokine production. These investigators found that a certain innate anti-inflammatory cytokine profile (low TNF and high IL-10 levels) may contribute to fatal meningococcal disease. In theory, similar genetic factors, if controlling the Th1/Th2 balance, may affect the maternal response against foreign fetal (paternal) antigens. Chen et al. (1996) demonstrated the presence of an increased TNF-α mRNA expression in leucocytes from pre-eclamptic women as compared with normal pregnant and non-pregnant women. This high expression of TNF-α may be associated with the TNF1 allele, whose frequency was found to be markedly increased in pre-eclampsia (Chen et al., 1996). However, in a recent larger study, Lachmeijer et al. (2001) failed to find any association between nine polymorphisms in the TNF region and pre-eclampsia or HELLP syndrome. In accordance with Hefler et al. (2001), these authors also found that polymorphisms in the IL-1 and interleukin-1 receptor antagonist (IL1ra) gene and pre-eclampsia or HELLP syndrome did not show any association.

The conclusions derived from the studies we have reviewed in this chapter may have practical consequences for practising physicians, even if the exact etiology of pre-eclampsia remains unresolved:

1. According to the primipaternity concept, a multiparous woman with a new partner should be approached as having the same risk of pre-eclampsia as a primigravid woman.
2. Artificial donor insemination, oocyte donation, and especially embryo donation are associated with an increased risk of developing pregnancy-induced hypertensive disorders.

3. A prolonged period of sperm exposure provides partial protection against pregnancy-induced hypertensive disorders. In this day and age, all women with multiple partners are strongly advised to use condoms in order to prevent sexually transmitted diseases. However, a certain period of sperm exposure within a stable relationship, when pregnancy intended, may be associated with at least partial protection against pre-eclampsia.

The observation of an inverse relationship between the duration of sexual cohabitation and the incidence of pre-eclampsia suggests that long-term sperm exposure may be important for the human implantation success (Robertson et al., 2003). This makes physiological sense since the human female is one of the few mammals exposed to her partner's semen on multiple occasions prior to conception. From an evolutionary perspective, it can be argued that induction of paternal antigen tolerance through repeated sperm exposure may have reproductive advantages. This may be by promoting implantation and survival of embryos conceived in a long-term relationship where it could be argued that the male parent may be more committed to the well-being of the resultant child. In terms of evolution, the relatively high incidence of pre-eclampsia represents a significant reproductive disadvantage in humans as compared with other mammals. Eclampsia is still a complicating factor in up to 1% of births in developing countries, and was present in a similar proportion of births in the developed countries until the 1950s (Robillard et al., 2002). Many authors think that this disease might hide an adaptive advantage somewhere. This may be true for the increase in blood pressure per se, since the increased maternal systemic blood pressure will increase perfusion pressure (Dadelszen et al., 2000). However, overall the clinical syndrome of pre-eclampsia–eclampsia has forced womankind to adapt to a tremendous reproductive burden.

The major difference between the human embryo and their mammal counterparts is the size of its brain which requires about 60% of total fetal nutritional needs during brain development in the second and third trimester of pregnancy (Martin, 1996). Robillard *et al.* (2002) recently proposed the hypothesis that the large size of the human fetal brain requires deep endovascular trophoblast invasion. According to this hypothesis, such deep endovascular trophoblast invasion can only occur if there are major immunogenetic compromises in terms of maternal–paternal tissue tolerance. These authors proposed that the low fecundability rate and loss of estrus represent the price mankind had to pay for a large brain, the necessary deep endovascular trophoblast invasion, and an acceptably low incidence of pre-eclampsia.

The human female has a very low fecundability rate, 25% at the age of maximum fecundity. In mathematical models on populations, demographers use a mean interval of 7–8 months after constitution of couples (without contraception). Being very fertile in a first pregnancy may be considered a disadvantage with respect to the high associated pre-eclampsia risk. According to Robillard *et al.* (2002, 2003), a fecundability rate of 25%, as observed in the human species, is the best compromise between the risk of pre-eclampsia and multiparity with the same partner, without threatening fertility for subsequent pregnancies.

Conclusion

Recently, in the understanding of the etiology of pre-eclampsia, clinical (epidemiological) studies have been found to be fundamental in order to reorient the debate toward the potential for immunological mechanisms. The term "primipaternity" (Robillard *et al.*, 1993) has been chosen to challenge the dogma that "pre-eclampsia is a disease of primigravidas" promulgated in most of the last century's obstetrical textbooks. Nevertheless, this term "primipaternity" carries some ambiguity. Fortunately for the human species, the great majority of multiparae who change partners do not present with pre-eclampsia (and neither do the great majority of primigravidae).

The Guadeloupean prospective cohort (Robillard *et al.*, 1994) study on primiparae (as well as multiparae who reported changing partners) confirmed the results of Marti and Herrmann (1977): there was a 40–45% chance of hypertensive disorders of pregnancy in a minority of women where conception occurred within the first 4 months of sexual cohabitation. Therefore, "changing paternity" should be considered only as one of many risk factors for pre-eclampsia. Collectively, these studies arrive at the same logical conclusion, which is that the duration of sexual cohabitation, and the first conception of a couple, are not independent risk factors, and that the biological explanation of this might well be the need for sperm exposure before conception. For this reason Robillard, Dekker and Hulsey proposed the alternative "primipaternity" model in 1999 (Robillard *et al.*, 1999). In this model pre-eclampsia is associated with "couples conceiving rapidly after their constitution."

A critical review of the major epidemiological reports published during the twentieth century, and in particular the landmark books of Dieckmann (1952), Chesley (1978) and MacGillivray (1983) reveals a number of inconsistencies that may now be explained. For example, pre-eclampsia was reported by these authors to be much more prevalent in teenage or unmarried primigravidae. This finding was difficult to explain on the basis of pre-eclampsia only being a disease of primigravidae. With the primipaternity model, however, it now becomes reasonable. We have also made two predictions based on the primipaternity model: (1) that fertilization with anonymous donor sperm should increase the incidence of pre-eclampsia; and (2) that the protective effect of a prior termination of pregnancy or miscarriage should only be present in cases where the subsequent pregnancy is with the same male partner. This last prediction has recently been confirmed by Saftlas *et al.* (2003).

REFERENCES

Antinori, S., Versaci, C., Panci, C., Caffa, B. and Gholami, G. H. (1995). Fetal and maternal morbidity and mortality in menopausal women aged 45–63 years. *Hum. Reprod.*, **10**, 464–9.

Atkins, D. C., Baucom, D. H. and Jacobson, N. S. (2001). Understanding infidelity: correlates in a national random sample. *J. Fam. Psychol.*, **15**, 735–49.

Basso, O., Christensen, K. and Olsen, J. (2001). Higher risk of pre-eclampsia after change of partner. An effect of longer interpregnancy intervals. *Epidemiology*, **12**, 624–9.

Basso, O., Weinberg, C. R., Baird, D. D., Wilcox, A. J. and Olsen, J. (2003). Danish National Birth Cohort. Subfecundity as a correlate of preeclampsia: a study within the Danish National Birth Cohort. *Am. J. Epidemiol.*, **157**, 195–202.

Beer, A. E. and Need, J. A. (1985). Immunological aspects of preeclampsia/eclampsia. In *Birth Defects: Original Article Series*, ed. B.K. Young, chapter 21, New York, March of Dimes Birth Defects, pp. 131–54.

Cepicky, P. and Podrouzek, P. (1990). Barrier contraception increases the risk of pre-eclampsia. *Cesk. Gynekol.*, **55**, 620–1 (Czech).

Chen, G., Wilson, R., Wang, S. H., Zheng, H. Z., Walker, J. J. and McKillop, J. H. (1996). Tumour necrosis factor-alpha (TNF-α) gene polymorphism and expression in preeclampsia. *Clin. Exp. Immunol.*, **104**, 154–9.

Chesley, L. C. (1978). *Hypertensive Disorders in Pregnancy*. New York, Appleton-Century Crofts.

Clark, D. A. (1993). Cytokines, decidua, and early pregnancy. *Oxf. Rev. Reprod.*, **15**, 83–111.

Clark, D. A. (1994). Does immunological intercourse prevent preeclampsia. *Lancet*, **344**, 969–70.

Conde-Agudelo, A. and Belizan, J. M. (2000). Maternal morbidity and mortality associated with interpregnancy interval: cross sectional study. *Br. Med. J.*, **321**, 1255–9.

Dadelszen, von P., Ornstein, M. P., Bull, S. B., Logan, A. G., Koren, G. and Magee, L. A. (2000). Fall in mean arterial pressure and fetal growth restriction in pregnancy hypertension: a meta-analysis. *Lancet*, **355**, 87–92.

Dekker, G. A. (1999). Risk factors for preeclampsia. *Clin. Obstet. Gynecol.*, **42**, 422–35.

Dekker, G. A. (2002). The partner's role in the etiology of preeclampsia. *J. Reprod. Immunol.*, **57**, 203–15.

Dekker, G. A. and Sibai, B. M. (1998). Etiology and pathogenesis of preeclampsia; current concepts. *Am. J. Obstet. Gynecol.*, **179**, 1359–75.

Diekmann, W. J. (1952). *The Toxemias of Pregnancy* (2nd edn). St Louis, C. V. Mosby.

Einarsson, J. I., Sangi-Haghpeykar, H. and Gardner, M. O. (2003). Sperm exposure and development of preeclampsia. *Am. J. Obstet. Gynecol.*, **188**, 1241–3.

Eskenazia, B. and Harleyb, K. (2001). Perinatal epidemiology. Commentary: revisiting the primipaternity theory of pre-eclampsia. *Int. J. Epidemiol.*, **30**, 1323–4.

Esplin, M. S., Fausett, M. B., Fraser, A., *et al.* (2001). Paternal and maternal components of the predisposition to preeclampsia. *N. Engl. J. Med.*, **344**, 867–72.

Feeney, J. G. (1980). Pre-eclampsia and changing paternity. In *Proceedings of the First Congress of the International Society for the Study of Hypertension in Pregnancy*, ed. J. Bonnar, I. MacGillivray and M. Symonds. London: MTP Press Ltd, pp. 41–4.

Feeney, J. G. and Scott, J. S. (1980). Pre-eclampsia and changed paternity. *Eur. J. Obstet. Gynecol. Reprod. Biol.*, **11**, 35–8.

Friedman, F. Jr., Copperman, A. B., Brodman, M. L., Shah, D., Sandler, B. and Grunfeld, L. (1996). Perinatal outcome after embryo transfer in ovum recipients: a comparison with standard in vitro fertilization. *J. Reprod. Med. Obstet. Gynecol.*, **41**, 640–4.

Goecke, C. and Schwabe, G. (1965). Vorschlag einer Stadien-Einteilung der Gestose. *Zentralbl. Gynaekol.*, **87**, 1439.

Grefenstette, I., Royere, D., Barthelemy, C. I., Tharanne, M. J. and Lansac, J. (1990). The outcome of 470 pregnancies obtained using AID with frozen semen. *J. Gynecol. Obstet. Biol. Reprod.*, **19**, 737–44.

Hall, G., Noble, W., Lindow, S. and Masson, E. (2001). Long-term sexual co-habitation offers no protection from hypertensive disease of pregnancy. *Hum. Reprod.*, **16**, 349–52.

Hefler, L. A., Tempfer, C. B. and Gregg, A. R. (2001). Polymorphisms within the interleukin-1 beta gene cluster and preeclampsia. *Obstet. Gynecol.*, **97**, 664–8.

Hendler, I., Dulitzky, M., Soriano, D., *et al.* (1997). Pregnancy outcome after oocyte donation. *Am. J. Obstet. Gynecol.*, **176**, S133.

Hernandez-Valencia, M., Saldana Quezada, L., Alvarez Munoz, M. and Valdez Martinez, E. (2000). Barrier family planning methods as risk factor which predisposes to preeclampsia. *Ginecol. Obstet. Mex.*, **68**, 333–8 (in Spanish).

Hiby, S. E., King, A., Sharkey, A. and Loke, Y. W. (1999). Molecular studies of trophoblast HLA-G: polymorphisms, isoforms, imprinting and expression in preimplantation embryo. *Tissue Antigens*, **53**, 1–13.

Ikedife, D. (1980). Eclampsia in multiparae. *Br. Med. J.*, **280**, 985–6.

Jivraj, S., Anstie, B., Cheong, Y. C., Fairlie, F. M., Laird, S. M. and Li, T. C. (2001). Obstetric and neonatal outcome in women with a history of recurrent miscarriage: a cohort study. *Hum. Reprod.*, **16**, 102–6.

Koelman, C. A., Coumans, A. B., Nijman, H. W., Doxiadis, I. I. N., Dekker, G. A. and Claas, F. H. J. (2000). Correlation between oral sex and a low incidence of preeclampsia: a role for soluble HLA in seminal fluid? (Hypothesis.) *J. Reprod. Med.*, **46**, 155–66.

Khong, T. Y., Adema, E. D. and Erwich, J. J. (2003). On an anatomical basis for the increase in birth weight in second and subsequent born children. *Placenta*, **24**, 348–53.

Klonoff Cohen, H. S., Savitz, D. A., Cefalo, R. C. and McCann, M. F. (1989). An epidemiologic study of contraception and preeclampsia. *J. Am. Med. Assoc.*, **262**, 3143–7.

Lachmeijer, A. M., Crusius, J. B., Pals, G., Dekker, G. A., Arngrímsson, R. and ten Kate, L. P. (2001). Polymorphisms in the tumor necrosis factor and lymphotoxin-alpha gene region and preeclampsia. *Obstet. Gynecol.*, **98**, 612–19.

Li, D. K. and Wi, S. (2000). Changing paternity and the risk of preeclampsia/eclampsia in the subsequent pregnancy. *Am. J. Epidemiol.*, **151**, 57–62.

Lie, R. T., Rasmussen, S., Brunborg, H., Gjessing, H. K., Lie-Nielsen, E. and Irgens, L. M. (1998). Fetal and maternal contributions to risk of pre-eclampsia: a population based study. *Br. Med. J.*, **316**, 1343–7.

Lucassen, A. and Parker, M. (2001). Revealing false paternity: some ethical considerations. *Lancet*, **357**, 1033–5.

Marti, J. J. and Herrmann, U. (1977). Immunogestosis: a new etiologic concept of "essential" EPH gestosis, with special consideration of the primigravid patient. *Am. J. Obstet. Gynecol.*, **128**, 489–93.

Martin, R. D. (1996). Scaling of the mammalian brain: the maternal energy hypothesis. *News Physiol. Sci.*, **11**, 149–56.

Marzi, M., Vigano, A., Trabattoni, D., *et al.* (1996). Characterization of type 1 and type 2 cytokine production profile in physiologic and pathologic human pregnancy. *Clin. Exp. Immunol.*, **106**, 127–33.

McQuarrie, I. (1923). Isoagglutination in the new born infants and their mother: a possible relationship between interagglutination and the toxemias of pregnancy. *Johns Hopkins Hosp. Bull.*, **34**, 51–4.

MacGillivray, I. (1983). *Pre-Eclampsia: The Hypertensive Disease of Pregnancy.* London, Saunders.

Medawar, P. B. (1953). Some immunological and endocrinological problems raised by the evolution of viviparity in vertebrates. In: *Evolution 7. Society for Experimental Biology.* New York: Academic Press, pp. 320–38.

Michalas, S., Loutradis, D., Drakakis, P., *et al.* (1996). Oocyte donation to women over 40 years of age: pregnancy complications. *Eur. J. Obstet. Gynecol. Reprod. Biol.*, **64**, 175–8.

Mills, J. L., Klebanoff, M. A., Graubard, B. I., Carey, J. C. and Berendes, H. W. (1991). Barrier contraceptive methods and preeclampsia. *J. Am. Med. Assoc.*, **265**, 70–3.

Moore, M. P. and Redman, C. W. (1983). Case-control study of severe pre-eclampsia of early onset. *Br. Med. J. (Clin. Res. Ed.)*, **287**, 580–3.

Morcos, C. C., Bourguet, P. S. G., Prabcharan, O., *et al.* (2000). Pregnancy-induced hypertension and duration of sexual cohabitation. *J. Reprod. Med.*, **45**, 207–12.

Mosher, W. D. and Pratt, W. F. (1990). Contraceptive use in the United States, 1973–1988. *Adv. Data*, **182**, 1–10.

Mosmann, T. R., Cherwinski, H. and Bond, M. W. (1986). Two types of murine helper T cell clone. I. Definition according to profiles of lymphokine activities and secreted proteins. *J. Immunol.*, **136**, 2348–57.

Mosmann, T. R. and Moore, K. W. (1991). The role of Il-10 in cross-regulation of TH1 and TH2 responses. *Immunol. Today*, **12**, 49.

Mostello, D., Catlin, T. K., Roman, L., Holcomb Jr., W. L. and Leet, T. (2002). Preeclampsia in the parous woman: who is at risk. *Am. J. Obstet. Gynecol.*, **187**, 425–9.

Need, J. A. (1975). Pre-eclampsia in pregnancies by different fathers. *Br. Med. J.*, **ii**, 548–9.

Need, J. A., Bell, B., Meffin, E. and Jones, W. R. (1983). Pre-eclampsia in pregnancies from donor inseminations. *J. Reprod. Immunol.*, **5**, 329–38.

Pados, G., Camus, M., Van Steirteghem, A., Bonduelle, M. and Devroey, P. (1994). The evolution and outcome of pregnancies from oocyte donation. *Hum. Reprod.*, **9**, 538–42.

Pandian, Z., Bhattacharya, S. and Templeton, A. (2001). Review of unexplained infertility and obstetric outcome: a 10 year review. *Hum. Reprod.*, **16**, 2593–7.

Perkins, R. P. (1993). Pregnancy following donor insemination: implications for preeclampsia. *J. Matern. Fetal. Med.*, **2**, 52–4.

Roberts, J. M. and Redman, C. W. G. (1993). Pre-eclampsia: more than pregnancy-induced hypertension. *Lancet*, **341**, 1447–51.

Robertson, S. A. (2002). Transforming growth factor beta – a mediator of immune deviation in seminal plasma. *J. Reprod. Immunol.*, **57**, 109–28.

Robertson, S. A., Bromfield, J. J. and Tremellen, K. P. (2003). Seminal 'priming' for protection from preeclampsia – a unifying hypothesis. *J. Reprod. Immunol.*, **59**, 253–65.

Robillard, P. Y., Hulsey, T. C., Alexander, G. R., Keenan, A., de Caunes, F. and Papiernik, E. (1993). Paternity patterns and risk of preeclampsia in the last pregnancy in multiparae. *J. Reprod. Immunol.*, **24**, 1–12.

Robillard, P. Y., Hulsey, T. C., Perianin, J., Janky, E., Miri, E. H. and Papiernik, E. (1994). Association of pregnancy-induced hypertension with duration of sexual cohabitation before conception. *Lancet*, **344**, 973–5.

Robillard, P. Y., Dekker, G. A. and Hulsey, T. C. (1999). Revisiting the epidemiological standard of preeclampsia: primigravidity or primipaternity? *Eur. J. Obstet. Gynecol. Reprod. Biol.*, **84**, 37–41.

Robillard, P. Y., Dekker, G. A. and Hulsey, T. C. (2002). Evolutionary adaptations to pre-eclampsia/eclampsia in humans: low fecundability rate, loss of oestrus, prohibitions of incest and systematic polyandry. *Am. J. Reprod. Immunol.*, **47**, 104–11.

Robillard, P. Y., Hulsey, T. C., Dekker, G. A. and Chaouat, G. (2003). Preeclampsia and human reproduction. An essay of a long term reflection. *J. Reprod. Immunol.*, **59**, 93–100.

Saftlas, A. F., Levine, R. J., Klebanoff, M. A., et al. (2003). Abortion, changed paternity, and risk of preeclampsia in nulliparous women. *Am. J. Epidemiol.*, **157**, 1108–14.

Salha, O., Sharma, V., Dada, T., et al. (1999). The influence of donated gametes on the incidence of hypertensive disorders of pregnancy. *Hum. Reprod.*, **14**, 2268–73.

Schenker, J. G. and Ezra, Y. (1994). Complications of assisted reproductive techniques. *Fertil. Steril.*, **61**, 411–22.

Scott, J. R. and Beer, A. A. (1976). Immunologic aspects of pre-eclampsia. *Am. J. Obstet. Gynecol.*, **125**, 418–27.

Serfaty, D. (1992). Medical aspects of oral contraceptive discontinuation. *Adv. Contracept.*, **8**, 21–33.

Serhal, P. F. and Craft, I. (1987). Immune basis for pre-eclampsia: evidence from oocyte recipients. *Lancet*, **ii**, 744.

Serhal, P. F. and Craft, I. L. (1989). Oocyte donation in 61 patients. *Lancet*, **I**, 1185–7.

Skjaerven, R., Wilcox, A. J. and Lie, R. T. (2002). The interval between pregnancies and the risk of pre-eclampsia. *New. Engl. J. Med.*, **346**, 33–8.

Smarason, A. K., Sargent, I. L., Starkey, P. M. and Redman, C. W. G. (1993). The effect of placental syncytiotrophoblast microvillous membranes from normal and pre-eclamptic women on the growth of endothelial cells in vivo. *Br. J. Obstet. Gynaecol.*, **100**, 943–9.

Smith, G. N., Walker, M., Tessier, J. L. and Millar, K. G. (1997). Increased incidence of preeclampsia in women conceiving by intrauterine insemination with donor versus partner sperm for treatment of primary infertility. *Am. J. Obstet. Gynecol.*, **177**, 455–8.

Soderstrom Anttila, V. and Hovatta, O. (1995). An oocyte donation program with goserelin down-regulation of voluntary donors. *Acta Obstet. Gynecol. Scand.*, **74**, 288–92.

Strickland, D. M., Guzick, D. S., Cox, K., et al. (1986). The relationship between abortion in the first pregnancy and development of pregnancy-induced hypertension in the subsequent pregnancy. *Am. J. Obstet. Gynecol.*, **154**, 146–8.

Tremellen, K. P., Seamark, R. F. and Robertson, S. A. (1998). Seminal transforming growth factor 1 stimulates granulocyte–macrophage colony-stimulating factor production and inflammatory cell recruitment in the murine uterus. *Biol. Reprod.*, **58**, 1217–25.

Trogstad, L. I., Eskild, A., Magnus, P., Samuelsen, S. O. and Nesheim, B. I. (2001). Changing paternity and time since last pregnancy; the impact on pre-eclampsia risk. A study of 547238 women with and without previous pre-eclampsia. *Int. J. Epidemiol.*, **30**, 1317–22.

Trupin, L. S., Simon, L. P. and Eskenazi, B. (1996). Change in paternity: a risk factor for preeclampsia in multiparas. *Epidemiology*, **7**, 240–4.

Tubbergen, A. M., Lachmeijer, S. M., Althuisius, M. E., Vlak, H. P., van Geijn H. and Dekker, G. A. (1999). Change in paternity: a risk factor for preeclampsia in multiparous women? *J. Reprod. Immunol.*, **45**, 81–8.

Veit, J. (1902). Über Albuminurie in der Schwangerschaft. Ein Beitrag zur Physiologie der Schwangerschaft. *Berliner Klin. Wchschr.*, **3**, 513–16.

Verwoerd, G. R., Hall, D. R., Grove, D., Maritz, J. S. and Odendaal, H. J. (2002). Primipaternity and duration of exposure to sperm antigens as risk factors for pre-eclampsia. *Int. J. Gynaecol. Obstet.*, **78**, 121–6.

Vries de, M. J., Dekker, G. A. and Schoemaker, J. (1998). Higher risk of preeclampsia in the polycystic ovary syndrome. A case control study. *Eur. J. Obstet. Gynecol. Reprod. Biol.*, **76**, 91–5.

Wang, J. X., Knottnerus, A. M., Schuit, G., Norman, R. J., Chan, A. and Dekker, G. A. (2002). Surgically obtained sperm, and risk of gestational hypertension and pre-eclampsia. *Lancet*, **359**, 673–4.

Watson, J. G., Carroll, J. and Chaykin, S. (1983). Reproduction in mice: the fate of spermatozoa not involved in fertilization. *Gamete Res.*, **7**, 75–84.

Wegmann, T. G., Lin, H., Guilbert, L. and Mosmann, T. R. (1993). Bidirectional cytokine interactions in the maternal–fetal relationship: is successful pregnancy a Th2 phenomenon? *Immunol. Today*, **15**, 353–6.

Weiner H. L., Friedman A., Miller A., *et al.* (1994). Oral tolerance: immunologic mechanisms and treatment of animal and human-organ specific autoimmune diseases by oral administration of autoantigens. *Ann. Rev. Immunol.*, **12**, 809–37.

Westendorp, R. G. J., Langermans, J. A. M., Huizinga, T. W. J., *et al.* (1997). Genetic influence on cytokine production and fatal meningococcal disease. *Lancet*, **349**, 170–3.

Zavazava, N. and Kronke, M. (1996). sHLA class I molecules induce apoptosis in alloreactive cytotoxic T cells. *Nat. Med.*, **2**, 1005–11.

20

Genetics of pre-eclampsia and counseling the patient who developed pre-eclampsia

Kenneth Ward

Introduction

Pre-eclampsia runs in families. Analysis of affected families provides compelling evidence that pre-eclampsia is a polygenic, multifactorial disease. It is unlikely that any particular genotype is necessary for the disease to occur; rather, "pre-eclampsia genes" act as susceptibility loci (along with environmental influences) to lower a woman's threshold for developing pre-eclampsia. The available data suggest that some pre-eclampsia-associated mutations are relatively common, and present in a large percentage of women. Other alleles will be "private" mutations, affecting one woman or only a handful of women in an extended family. However, any mutation identified that can dramatically affect even one woman's risk may give us new insights into the pathophysiologic cascade which leads to pre-eclampsia.

Recognizing that a condition is genetic enables the use of gene discovery techniques such as linkage disequilibrium and haplotype mapping to find the genes and the molecular pathways responsible for the illness. Gene mapping techniques have been applied in every field of medicine to uncover the molecular underpinnings of complex human diseases. Undoubtedly, discoveries of pre-eclampsia-related genes will lead to improved means of classification and diagnosis. A major lesson of modern genetics is that syndromes defined on the basis of clustering of clinical symptoms often reveal marked heterogeneity once they are understood at a molecular level. In this respect, the boundaries around pre-eclampsia, gestational hypertension, and HELLP syndrome are likely to be redrawn when genetic determinants can be examined directly. Proceeding from genes to biological or clinical manifestations or "phenotypes" constitutes a radical alternative in the logic of scientific inference.

One potential outcome from genetic studies of pre-eclampsia would be the discovery of a gene that has a critical role and that is common in the population. Correlation of genotypes with clinical phenotypes could allow specific diagnostic and novel predictive insights. Better predictions will allow targeting of the women most at-risk for preventative therapies. Given the inconsistent efficacy of "preventative therapies" such as low-dose aspirin or calcium supplementation in different populations, it is entirely possible that these treatments do work in certain genetic subsets, but not all. Once the molecular pathophysiology and the population genetics of pre-eclampsia are known, investigators may be able to propose other existing agents as rational prevention therapy. Novel treatments with fewer side effects, better techniques for monitoring the disease progression, even a redesign of prenatal care are likely because of future discoveries.

Unfortunately, despite hundreds of studies regarding the genetics of pre-eclampsia, we are still at an early stage of our understanding. Pre-eclampsia is an extremely complex disease to study using genetic methods; the tools are only now becoming available to meet this challenge. This chapter will review the progress to date in understanding the genetics of pre-eclampsia. It will discuss the limited circumstances in which genetic testing should be considered in patients who had pre-eclampsia. Finally, it will propose a postpartum evaluation that helps to categorize patients into clinical subsets that may allow improved counseling for the woman who has pre-eclampsia.

Family reports

Numerous early reports of familial clustering of pre-eclampsia/eclampsia were summarized by Chesley et al. in 1968. They found that Elliott was the first to report familial incidence of eclampsia in 1873, when he reported a woman who died of eclampsia during her fifth pregnancy. Three of her four daughters subsequently died of eclampsia as well. The older reports focus on eclampsia, since "pre-" eclampsia could not be recognized until roughly 150 years ago when it became possible to check for proteinuria. Clinical blood pressure measurements have only been possible for the last 100 years. The recognition that proteinuric, pregnancy-induced hypertension is pre-eclampsia came in the early 1900s. At about the same time, physicians reported that like eclampsia, pre-eclampsia is also familial.

Chesley also conducted many of the landmark studies on the genetics of pre-eclampsia (Chesley and Cosgrove, 1955; Chesley et al., 1962, 1968, 1976; Cooper et al., 1988). He studied 240 eclamptic women who had delivered at one hospital in New Jersey, and he collected outcome data on the subsequent generations (who delivered at hospitals throughout the United States). Remarkably persistent in this effort, Chesley was able to find information on 96% of all the daughters of his index cases, greatly reducing the possibility of ascertainment bias. The quality of the available obstetrics records varied, so it is not certain that all of the patients he called pre-eclamptic had proteinuric hypertension. Chesley and his collaborators found elevated rates of pre-eclampsia in the mothers, sisters, daughters, and granddaughters of probands with eclampsia. Pre-eclampsia was not more prevalent in the in-laws of the eclamptic probands, suggesting that maternal rather than fetal genes are critical. Chesley's group suggested that pre-eclampsia might be due to a single recessive gene carried by one out of every four women.

There have been more than 20 other family studies over the past few decades (recently summarized in Lachmeijer et al., 2002). Studies in a variety of populations (USA, United Kingdom, Scotland, Iceland, etc.) agree that first-degree relatives of women previously diagnosed with pre-eclampsia are 3–4 times more likely to develop pre-eclampsia than matched controls.

Most of these family studies also attempt to fit the recurrence risk data to a genetic model. Pre-eclampsia would be considered a dominant trait if the risk occurs even when only one chromosome of a pair has a defect, or recessive if the risk is only expressed when mutations exist on both alleles for a locus. For most genetic diseases, penetrance is less than 100%. For highly penetrant, autosomal dominant conditions, the gene is expressed in each generation (i.e. vertical transmission). New mutations are relatively common for most dominant traits. Dominant phenotypes can be extremely variable. Autosomal recessive conditions are only expressed when both versions (i.e. alleles) of the involved gene are abnormal. Carrier rates are high if the recessive disease is common in the population. Conclusions regarding the inheritance of pre-eclampsia have varied: some authors favor a recessive hypothesis, others suggest there is a maternal and fetal genotype interaction, while the most recent analysis suggests that pre-eclampsia is a polygenic trait with a strong maternal factor. Taken together, these segregation analyses suggest a "major gene" effect. All models suggest that mutations conferring susceptibility to pre-eclampsia are relatively common.

Whether every family has the same gene involved, or a private mutation, is impossible to determine from the published segregation analyses. Some families with a high occurrence of pre-eclampsia show simple Mendelian patterns of inheritance. In such families, the pre-eclampsia predisposition is likely to be due to mutation(s) at a single genetic locus. It is possible that there are only a few pre-eclampsia-causing alleles which are common in the population. Alternatively, frequent new mutations may be creating thousands of disease-associated alleles in the dozens of critical genes involved in the pathophysiologic cascade. Unfortunately, none of the published models has adequately included the very high new mutation rate that would be expected for pre-eclampsia. History shows that mortality from eclampsia was high until the last few generations. Usually the only way a lethal gene will stay common in the population is if there are frequent new mutations or if the gene is positively selected for on some other basis. Both mechanisms remain possibilities in pre-eclampsia.

Dominance and recessiveness are empiric terms that depend entirely upon the clinical definition used for the disease; they are attributes describing the phenotype, not attributes of the gene or allele. For instance, the retinoblastoma gene is a recessive tumor suppressor gene at the cellular level, but abnormalities in the gene are responsible for the autosomal dominant tendency for children to develop retinoblastomas. As we learn more about the tremendous variation that occurs at every genetic locus, the distinctions between dominant and recessive conditions have become blurred. Even in the classic, "single-gene" Mendelian disorders, there can be tremendous quantitative and qualitative differences in the phenotype among persons who have the same allele or the same genetic mutation. This variability can be evident as non-penetrance of certain features (or the entire phenotype) and as differences in the severity of features, the frequency of cyclic or episodic events, or the age of onset of the first clinical sign of the disorder. The genetic background of the affected person can also cause genetic variability. The phenotype may be further influenced by maternal factors such as cytoplasmic

inheritance, the intrauterine environment, or imprinting. Furthermore, each genotype undergoes subtle changes over time through somatic mutation, gene amplification, or transpositions and positional effects.

Most pre-eclampsia families show a polygenic multifactorial pattern of inheritance in affected families. Polygenic multifactorial inheritance usually operates according to a threshold model. Several genetic and environmental factors must collaborate for the disease to develop. Only after these factors reach a critical point (threshold) is the phenotypic effect seen. The intrinsic heritability of the condition is frequently the most important factor to affect the observed recurrence risk. In disorders with a relatively high heritability, the recurrence risk of the disorder approximates the square root of the population incidence. Different ethnic groups will vary in their population frequency of different disorders. The recurrence risk is higher for common disorders or within populations with a high incidence of the disorder. The number of affected individuals in a family affects the recurrence risk. The greater the number of family members who have been affected with a multifactorial condition, the more likely it is that the genetic background is favorable for expression of the condition. Consanguinity increases the risk of recurrence because of the greater likelihood of deleterious genes being shared. In some instances (i.e. Hirschsprung disease) the severity of the disorder predicts the recurrence risk, while in others (i.e. neural tube defects) it does not.

There have been several reports of a paternal or fetal genetic effect on the occurrence of pre-eclampsia (Astin et al., 1981; Feeney and Scott, 1980; Need, 1975). For example, Astin et al. (1981) at the University of Utah reported a man who lost two consecutive wives to eclampsia. His third wife was also affected with severe pre-eclampsia. The observation that pre-eclampsia is extremely common in a molar pregnancy (in which all the fetal chromosomes are derived from the father) is considered further evidence of the role of paternal genes. Cooper et al. found an increased rate of pre-eclampsia if the proband's own mother was eclamptic during the pregnancy in which she delivered the proband (Cooper *et al.*, 1988). Arngrimsson *et al.* found a small increase in the incidence of pre-eclampsia in the daughter-in-laws of women who had pregnancy-induced hypertension (Arngrimsson *et al.*, 1990). Esplin *et al.* (2001) used a population database to identify 298 men and 237 women whose mothers had had pre-eclampsia during their pregnancy. They examined birth certificate data for the children of these men and women to see whether they were the product of a pregnancy complicated by pre-eclampsia. The odds ratio was 2.1 (95% confidence interval [CI], 1.0–4.3; $P = 0.04$) in the males and 3.3 (95% CI, 1.5–7.5; $P = 0.004$) in the female study group, again suggesting both a maternal and a paternal genetic predisposition.

Twin studies

Twin studies can be used to measure the heritability of a condition (the proportion of the occurrence which is due to genetic factors as opposed to environmental factors). Only a handful of twin studies have been published concerning pre-eclampsia or eclampsia (Lachmeijer *et al.*, 1998; O'Shaughnessy *et al.*, 2000; Thompson *et al.*, 1981; Thornton and Macdonald, 1999; Thornton and Onwude, 1991; Treloar *et al.*, 2001). The early studies suffered from small numbers and they lacked DNA zygosity tests to prove whether the twins were monozygotic. In most of these studies it is uncertain whether both twins had the same opportunity to develop pre-eclampsia. In 1998, Lachmeijer *et al.* reported three sets of monozygotic twins concordant for pre-eclampsia. O'Shaughnessy *et al.* (2000) identified four sets of monozygous twins and a monozygous triplet gestation; all with zygosity confirmed using DNA testing. Two of the twin pairs were concordant for pre-eclampsia and two of the triplets had pregnancy-induced hypertension, although only one of the triplets had proteinuria. More recently,

Treloar *et al.* (2001) looked at two large cohorts of Australian female twin pairs and they made a retrospective diagnosis of pre-eclampsia from medical and hospital records. Using strict diagnostic criteria, they found no concordant female twin pairs for severe pre-eclampsia or eclampsia. The study indicates that maternal genes do not play a major role in Australian patients. These data are inconsistent with the segregation data summarized above.

Consanguinity studies

Another approach to estimating heritability is to examine consanguineous families. Unfortunately, the few consanguinity studies in the literature all suffer from problems with methodology. Stevenson and coworkers conducted a 1976 study in Turkey, where a fifth of all the deliveries are consanguineous. Using clinical definitions that are probably too inclusive, they found that the incidence of "toxemia" was decreased when the couple was consanguineous (Stevenson *et al.*, 1976). George *et al.* (1992) studied pregnancy outcomes in 814 primigravida in South India. Of these pregnancies, 26% were felt to be consanguineous. They studied pregnancy-induced hypertension rather than proteinuric pre-eclampsia specifically. Most of the marriages were either cousin–cousin or uncle–niece. They found the odds of pre-eclampsia were 1.12 in consanguineous couples compared to non-consanguineous couples (with a confidence interval of 0.72–1.75).

Genetic association studies

Regardless of the genetic theory invoked, it is perhaps obvious that genes should play a role in the pathophysiology of pre-eclampsia. Mutant genes in any of dozens of pathways discussed in the other chapters in this book could affect a woman's risk of developing pre-eclampsia. There are many challenges when applying gene mapping and discovery techniques to common diseases (Botstein *et al.*, 2003; Broeckel *et al.*, 2003; Clark, 2003; Phillips and Belknap, 2002) (Table 20.1). Pre-eclampsia is an extremely complex disease with unique issues which are present in the study

Table 20.1. Common errors in genetic association studies

Inadequate sample size
Non-specific diagnoses
Subgroup analysis without corrections for multiple testing
Poorly matched control group
Hidden ethnic biases
Failure to replicate findings in a second population
Inappropriate conversion of quantitative traits to
  categories
Positive publication bias
Casual inferences from limited association data
Failure to consider linkage disequilibrium with
  neighboring loci
Failure to consider known gene–gene and
  gene–environment interactions
Random error

of other diseases (Table 20.2) (Bernard and Giguere, 2003).

Over a hundred genetic association studies concerning pre-eclampsia have now been published [recently reviewed in Lachmeijer *et al.* (2001), Wilson *et al.* (2003)]. Genetic association studies using a case control format are relatively easy to perform. Polymorphisms or, preferably, functional variants of the "candidate gene" are assayed in both populations and chi-square contingency tests are applied. Unfortunately, these simple studies often lead to false conclusions, as spurious associations can arise due to hidden biases (Table 20.3). Association studies cannot prove biologic causation, but if they are performed carefully, they can uncover a predisposing or causative gene that had not been suspected, or a marker linked to the chromosomal region of the disease gene (linkage disequilibrium).

Any genetic hypothesis of pre-eclampsia must explain the first pregnancy effect. It is widely known that most women will not have pre-eclampsia with future pregnancies unless another

Table 20.2. Special problems with the study of pre-eclampsia genes

- Gender-limited trait
- Pregnancy-limited expression
- Age of onset of the condition is delayed until the reproductive years
- Specificity of the diagnosis
- Phenocopies are common – does the patient have a primary or secondary disease?
- Heterogeneity
- The blood pressure and proteinuria criteria in common use depend upon arbitrary cut-offs along a continuous distribution of values
- Hypertension and proteinuria are not the pathologic features of the pre-eclampsia syndrome
- The normal reference ranges for blood pressure and proteinuria also vary with respect to measurement protocols, gestational age, and ethnic background
- Expanded versus narrow definition of pre-eclampsia (should we use proteinuric hypertension, gestational hypertension, or a placental phenotype such as reduced placental invasion, or a renal phenotype such as glomerular endotheliosis, etc.)
- Full expression of the disease gene can be interrupted by appropriate medical care or early delivery
- Alleles must be extremely common with spouses bringing the gene into pedigrees frequently, and there is probably genetic heterogeneity
- Large percentage of cases likely to be due to new mutations
- No convincing animal model of pre-eclampsia exists
- Is it the genotype of the mother, the fetus, or an interaction between the two?
- Lack of genetically well-characterized populations

Table 20.3. Published linkage studies on pre-eclampsia

Author	Year	Model	Type	Results
Wilton	1990, 1991	AR	Cand	HLA region excluded
Cooper	1991	AR	Cand	1q32, 14q32-3 excluded
Haywood	1992	AR	General	25% of genome excluded
Arngrimssom	1993	NP	Cand	Linkage with AGT
Harrison	1997	Various	General	Linkage with 4q
Arngrimssom	1997	Various	Cand	Linkage with 7q36
Arngrimssom	1999	NP	General	Significant linkage 2p13
Moses	2000	NP	General	Several suggestive locations
Lachmeijer	2001	NP	General	Several suggestive locations

condition exists (twins, diabetes). This has suggested an immunogenetic mechanism to many investigators, but other explanations are feasible. For instance, certain enzymes in pregnancy are permanently induced and never go back to baseline levels after delivery (Brown, 1995).

The "candidate" genes that have been tested to date code for proteins involved in maternal adaptation, trophoblast invasion, placentation, hemodynamic factors/blood pressure regulation, placental perfusion, oxidative stress, thrombosis, cytokines and other inflammatory mediators. Unfortunately, most of the published studies lack rigor or they are underpowered. Results are often inconsistent across populations. Inconsistent findings may indicate that the positive associations are spurious, or they may actually support the hypothesized candidate gene if the population genetics of the candidate gene(s) are different in the study populations. Unfortunately, we often lack critical data to differentiate these opposite conclusions.

In our own work, we observed significant association of pre-eclampsia with the T235 variant of the angiotensinogen gene (Ward et al., 1993). We studied women with carefully defined pre-eclampsia (excluding HELLP syndrome) and ethnically matched controls. Primigravidae and parous women were analyzed separately. The T235 association has been corroborated by several studies and refuted by others. We cannot resolve these different conclusions using allelic association

alone. To do so would require greater knowledge of the frequency of T235 in all populations, the frequencies of all other angiotensinogen alleles, and all the alleles of linked genes, the allelic variants in all genes involved in all the known and unknown pathways of angiotensinogen action, etc.

Once an association is observed and replicated in other studies, investigations must shift toward understanding the biology behind the statistics. With respect to angiotensinogen, we now know that there is a promoter mutation that alters expression of the gene which is "marked" by the T235 variant (Inoue et al., 1997). We have described how angiotensinogen is expressed in remodeling vessels in the first trimester uterus (Morgan et al., 1998) and that the T235 allele is expressed at higher levels than the M235 allele in heterozygous women (Morgan et al., 1997). We have also shown that the T235 allele correlates with first-trimester vascular pathology (Morgan et al., 1999) and with the activities of a renal angiotensinogen mechanism for regulating blood volume (Lalouel et al., 2001).

Linkage analyses

Several investigators are now studying the genetics of pre-eclampsia using linkage analysis in affected families and affected sibling pairs (see Table 20.3) (Arngrimsson et al., 1993, 1999; Harrison et al., 1997; Hayward et al., 1992; Moses et al., 2000; Tabor et al., 2002; Wilton et al., 1990). Polymorphic

DNA markers mapped to locations that describe regular intervals in the human genome are tested in family or affected sibling pairs. The analysis detects any violations of Mendel's second law, which states that independent traits segregate independently. Whenever two independent traits are closely located on the same chromosome, Mendel's second law is violated. Thus linkage between pre-eclampsia and these reference markers can be used to map the chromosomal location of a disease gene. Linkage studies require an accurate diagnosis of the disease under study (which can be difficult with pre-eclampsia, and precise histories of family relationships among the study participants). Furthermore, linkage analysis of large pedigrees requires that the appropriate genetic model be used in the LOD score analysis.

Counseling the woman who has pre-eclampsia

Unfortunately, few if any of the molecular genetic observations regarding pre-eclampsia are ready for use in predictive, diagnostic, or prognostic protocols (Khoury and Wagener, 1995).

For instance, even though angiotensinogen T235 is associated with a several-fold increased risk of pre-eclampsia in the Utah population, and even though most patients with pre-eclampsia are homozygous or heterozygous for T235, over 60% of the obstetric population has T235 and only 5–8% will develop pre-eclampsia. Thus, even with a postulated key role and a statistically high attributable risk, the T235 genetic marker has a low positive predictive value.

Eventually a panel of laboratory tests analyzed with clinical factors (such as parity, age, body mass index, and family history) will be incorporated into a clinically useful test. The test will be similar to the maternal serum screening tests used currently to predict the risk of Down's syndrome. Until these tests are available, genetic counseling of close relatives will depend upon the published

empiric risks and upon identification of patients with underlying diseases related to pre-eclampsia.

The traditional six-week postpartum visit provides an opportunity to assure that the maternal recovery from pre-eclampsia is complete, and to screen for underlying conditions (Walker, 1996). In an uncomplicated pregnancy, most of the physiologic changes brought on by pregnancy have returned to baseline (although this is often a new baseline when compared to the patient's physiology before her first pregnancy). The primary exception is the dilation of the maternal renal pelves, calyces, and ureters which may persist for 8–12 weeks postpartum. Functionally, the increased renal plasma flow, glomerular filtration rate, and creatinine clearance rate associated with pregnancy return to normal by 6 weeks after delivery.

At the six-week visit, it is important to recheck the patient's blood pressure to be certain that she does not have chronic hypertension. Hypertension due to pre-eclampsia usually decreases to baseline within 2 weeks of delivery; when it does take longer, the maternal blood pressure almost always returns to normal by 12 weeks postpartum. Other changes in the cardiovascular system caused by pregnancy (i.e. increase in heart rate, cardiac output, and blood volume) generally return to baseline by 6 weeks postpartum.

A careful history and physical should be performed to rule out cardiomyopathy, to look for signs of an autoimmune disease flare, to confirm that the patient has recovered completely from pre-eclampsia. It is prudent to test for Factor V Leiden and other thrombophilias if the patient has a positive family history of thromboembolism, if there were prominent placental infarcts, or if the patient plans to use hormonal contraceptives. If oliguria or severe proteinuria were present peripartum, it is reasonable to check a 24 h urine collection for protein and creatinine clearance and a complete urinalysis. I also have a low threshold for ordering an ANA, sedimentation rate, rheumatoid factor, and anti-phospholipid antibodies in patients with a family history of autoimmune disease or if the patient has symptoms consistent with an autoimmune syndrome. Finally, given the association of pre-eclampsia and insulin resistance, most patients who had severe disease should have a glucose tolerance test, and a fasting lipid profile particularly if the patient is morbidly obese or if she also had gestational diabetes.

Whenever possible, I try to see any pre-eclamptic patients for another visit 12–16 weeks after delivery. This extra visit provides an opportunity to do a complete review of systems, to recheck the blood pressure, and to perform a brief physical exam targeted by the patient's symptoms. This provides a more optimal setting to discuss laboratory results from the hospital or the six-week visit, to go over the placental pathology, to follow up any prior medical consultations, to discuss recurrence risks, and to make appropriate referrals.

If the patient had typical pre-eclampsia, has normal laboratory values, a low body mass index, and none of the following risk factors:

1. onset before 30 weeks gestation;
2. black race;
3. different father than prior gestation;
4. recurrent pre-eclampsia in a multiparous patient;
5. HELLP syndrome,

she can be counseled that she faces a slightly higher risk of pre-eclampsia than other multiparous women, but that over 90% will not have recurrent disease with subsequent pregnancies. Close monitoring for developing pre-eclampsia is advised throughout future gestations. Recent large randomized trials utilizing potential preventive therapies (calcium, low-dose aspirin) have, overall, produced disappointing results. Thus, no clear treatment or preventive therapies are available presently. Many clinicians continue to use low-dose aspirin in women with thrombophilia-like or "collagen vascular" syndromes. Calcium supplementation is safe for most patients and it can be considered in patients with hypercalciuria.

The risks of isolated pre-eclampsia with respect to long-term health have been studied by many authors. Bryans (1966) reviewed 53 papers reporting follow-up on 2637 women, and he found that 13% of patients developed hypertension. Chesley (1980) was able to report 33 years average follow-up on 270 eclamptics from 1931 to 1951; he found no excess hypertension or CV mortality in primiparas, but more hypertension was observed in multiparas with eclampsia. Fisher *et al.* (1981) reported that primiparas with renal biopsy-proven pre-eclampsia had only a 10% rate of hypertension, and that this was the same as age- and race-matched controls from the National Health Survey. It appears that the more secure the diagnosis of pre-eclampsia/eclampsia, the lower the rate of ultimate hypertension. Other forms of pregnancy-induced hypertension such as gestational hypertension have a higher recurrence rate and a greater risk for remote cardiovascular disease.

Conclusions

Pre-eclampsia is a familial disorder and one or more major predisposing genes are likely to be characterized in the next several years. Multicenter efforts with precise clinical definitions are needed to assure adequate power and to properly define pathologic subsets. The search for a pre-eclampsia gene could lead to the development of simple tests for susceptibility to pre-eclampsia, a greater understanding of its primary physiology, and the development of rational treatment or preventative strategies.

At present, the woman who had typical pre-eclampsia in her first pregnancy should be advised that her first-degree relatives do have an increased risk of pre-eclampsia in their first pregnancies. Since pregnancy-associated hypertension is often secondary to another underlying disease, a careful postpartum evaluation should be performed. Unless there is some other risk factor, extensive DNA testing cannot be recommended.

REFERENCES

Arngrimsson, R., Bjornsson, S., Geirsson, R.T., Bjornsson, H., Walker, J.J. and Snaedal, G. (1990). Genetic and familial predisposition to eclampsia and pre-eclampsia in a defined population. *Br. J. Obstet. Gynaecol.*, **97**(9), 762–9.

Arngrimsson, R., Purandare, S., Connor, M., *et al.* (1993). Angiotensinogen: a candidate gene involved in preeclampsia? *Nat. Genet.*, **4**(2), 114–15.

Arngrimsson, R., Sigurard ttir, S., Frigge, M.L., *et al.* (1999). A genome-wide scan reveals a maternal susceptibility locus for pre-eclampsia on chromosome 2p13. *Hum. Mol. Genet.*, **8**(9), 1799–805.

Astin, M., Scott, J.R. and Worley, R.J. (1981). Pre-eclampsia/eclampsia: a fatal father factor. *Lancet*, **2**(8245), 533.

Bernard, N. and Giguere, Y. (2003). Genetics of pre-eclampsia: what are the challenges? *J. Obstet. Gynaecol. Can.*, **25**(7), 578–85.

Botstein, D. and Risch, N. (2003). Discovering genotypes underlying human phenotypes: past successes for Mendelian disease, future approaches for complex disease. *Nat. Genet.*, **33** (Suppl.), 228–37.

Broeckel, U. and Schork, N.J. (2004). Identifying genes and genetic variation underlying human diseases and complex phenotypes via recombination mapping. *J. Physiol.*, **554**(pt. 1), 40–5.

Brown, M.A. (1995). The physiology of pre-eclampsia. *Clin. Exp. Pharmacol. Physiol.*, **22**(11), 781–91.

Bryans, C.I., Jr. (1966). The remote prognosis in toxemia of pregnancy. *Clin. Obstet. Gynecol.*, **9**(4), 973–90.

Chesley, L.C. (1980). Hypertension in pregnancy: definitions, familial factor, and remote prognosis. *Kidney Int.*, **18**(2), 234–40.

Chesley, L.C. and Cosgrove, R.A. (1955). A continuing follow-up study of eclamptic women. *Obstet. Gynecol.*, **5**(5), 697–714.

Chesley, L.C., Cosgrove, R.A. and Annitto, J.E. (1962). Pregnancies in the sisters and daughters of eclamptic women. *Obstet. Gynecol.*, **20**, 39–46.

Chesley, L.C., Annitto, J.E. and Cosgrove, R.A. (1968). The familial factor in toxemia of pregnancy. *Obstet. Gynecol.*, **32**(3), 303–11.

Chesley, L.C., Annitto, J.E. and Cosgrove, R.A. (2000). *American Journal of Obstetrics and Gynecology*, Volume 124, 1976: The remote prognosis of eclamptic women. Sixth periodic report. *Am. J. Obstet. Gynecol.*, **182**(1, Pt. 1), 247; discussion, 248.

Clark, A.G. (2003). Finding genes underlying risk of complex disease by linkage disequilibrium mapping. *Curr. Opin. Genet. Dev.*, **13**(3), 296–302.

Cooper, D.W., Hill, J.A., Chesley, L.C. and Bryans, C.I. (1988). Genetic control of susceptibility to eclampsia and miscarriage. *Br. J. Obstet. Gynaecol.*, **95**(7), 644–53.

Esplin, M.S., Fausett, M.B., Fraser, A., *et al.* (2001). Paternal and maternal components of the predisposition to preeclampsia. *N. Engl. J. Med.*, **344**(12), 867–72.

Feeney, J.G. and Scott, J.S. (1980). Pre-eclampsia and changed paternity. *Eur. J. Obstet. Gynecol. Reprod. Biol.*, **11**(1), 35–8.

Fisher, K.A., Luger, A., Spargo, B.H. and Lindheimer, M.D. (1981). Hypertension in pregnancy: clinical–pathological correlations and remote prognosis. *Medicine (Baltimore)*, **60**(4), 267–76.

George, K., Vedamony, J., Idikulla, J. and Rao, P.S. (1992). The effect of consanguinity on pregnancy-induced hypertension. *Aust. N.Z. J. Obstet. Gynaecol.*, **32**(3), 231–2.

Harrison, G.A., Humphrey, K.E., Jones, N., *et al.* (1997). A genomewide linkage study of preeclampsia/eclampsia reveals evidence for a candidate region on 4q. *Am. J. Hum. Genet.*, **60**(5), 1158–67.

Hayward, C., Livingstone, J., Holloway, S., Liston, W.A. and Brock, D.J. (1992). An exclusion map for pre-eclampsia: assuming autosomal recessive inheritance. *Am. J. Hum. Genet.*, **50**(4), 749–57.

Inoue, I., Nakajima, T., Williams, C.S., *et al.* (1997). A nucleotide substitution in the promoter of human angiotensinogen is associated with essential hypertension and affects basal transcription in vitro. *J. Clin. Invest.*, **99**(7), 1786–97.

Khoury, M.J. and Wagener, D.K. (1995). Epidemiological evaluation of the use of genetics to improve the predictive value of disease risk factors. *Am. J. Hum. Genet.*, **56**(4), 835–44.

Lachmeijer, A.M., Aarnoudse, J.G., ten Kate, L.P., Pals, G. and Dekker, G.A. (1998). Concordance for pre-eclampsia in monozygous twins. *Br. J. Obstet. Gynaecol.*, **105**(12), 1315–17.

Lachmeijer, A.M., Dekker, G.A., Pals, G., Aarnoudse, J.G., ten Kate, L.P. and Arngrimsson, R. (2002). Searching for preeclampsia genes: the current position. *Eur. J. Obstet. Gynecol. Reprod. Biol.*, **105**(2), 94–113.

Lalouel, J.M., Rohrwasser, A., Terreros, D., Morgan, T. and Ward, K. (2001). Angiotensinogen in essential hypertension: from genetics to nephrology. *J. Am. Soc. Nephrol.*, **12**(3), 606–15.

Morgan, T., Craven, C., Nelson, L., Lalouel, J. M. and Ward, K. (1997). Angiotensinogen T235 expression is elevated in decidual spiral arteries. *J. Clin. Invest.*, **100**(6), 1406–15.

Morgan, T., Craven, C. and Ward, K. (1998). Human spiral artery renin-angiotensin system. *Hypertension*, **32**(4), 683–7.

Morgan, T., Craven, C., Lalouel, J. M. and Ward, K. (1999). Angiotensinogen Thr235 variant is associated with abnormal physiologic change of the uterine spiral arteries in first-trimester decidua. *Am. J. Obstet. Gynecol.*, **180**(1, Pt. 1), 95–102.

Moses, E. K., Lade, J. A., Guo, G., *et al.* (2000). A genome scan in families from Australia and New Zealand confirms the presence of a maternal susceptibility locus for pre-eclampsia, on chromosome 2. *Am. J. Hum. Genet.*, **67**(6), 1581–5.

Need, J. A. (1975). Pre-eclampsia in pregnancies by different fathers: immunological studies. *Br. Med. J.*, **1**(5957), 548–9.

O'Shaughnessy, K. M., Ferraro, F., Fu, B., Downing, S. and Morris, N. H. (2000). Identification of monozygotic twins that are concordant for preeclampsia. *Am. J. Obstet. Gynecol.*, **182**(5), 1156–7.

Phillips, T. J. and Belknap, J. K. (2002). Complex-trait genetics: emergence of multivariate strategies. *Nat. Rev. Neurosci.*, **3**(6), 478–85.

Stevenson, A. C., Say, B., Ustaoglu, S. and Durmus, Z. (1976). Aspects of pre-eclamptic toxaemia of pregnancy, consanguinity, twinning in Ankara. *J. Med. Genet.*, **13**(1), 1–8.

Tabor, H. K., Risch, N. J. and Myers, R. M. (2002). Opinion: candidate-gene approaches for studying complex genetic traits: practical considerations. *Nat. Rev. Genet.*, **3**(5), 391–7.

Thompson, B., Sauve, B., MacGillivray, I. and Campbell, D. (1981). Reproductive performance in twin sisters. *Prog. Clin. Biol. Res.*, **69A**, 169–73.

Thornton, J. G. and Macdonald, A. M. (1999). Twin mothers, pregnancy hypertension and pre-eclampsia. *Br. J. Obstet. Gynaecol.*, **106**(6), 570–5.

Thornton, J. G. and Onwude, J. L. (1991). Pre-eclampsia: discordance among identical twins. *Br. Med. J.*, **303**(6812), 1241–2.

Treloar, S. A., Cooper, D. W., Brennecke, S. P., Grehan, M. M. and Martin, N. G. (2001). An Australian twin study of the genetic basis of preeclampsia and eclampsia. *Am. J. Obstet. Gynecol.*, **184**(3), 374–81.

Walker, J. J. (1996). Care of the patient with severe pregnancy induced hypertension. *Eur. J. Obstet. Gynecol. Reprod. Biol.*, **65**(1), 127–35.

Ward, K., Hata, A., Jeunemaitre, X., *et al.* (1993). A molecular variant of angiotensinogen associated with preeclampsia. *Nat. Genet.*, **4**(1), 59–61.

Wilson, M. L., Goodwin, T. M., Pan, V. L. and Ingles, S. A. (2003). Molecular epidemiology of preeclampsia. *Obstet. Gynecol. Surv.*, **58**(1), 39–66.

Wilton, A. N., Cooper, D. W., Brennecke, S. P., Bishop, S. M. and Marshall, P. (1990). Absence of close linkage between maternal genes for susceptibility to pre-eclampsia/eclampsia and HLA DR beta. *Lancet*, **336**(8716), 653–7.

21

Thrombophilias and pre-eclampsia

Isobel D. Walker

Introduction

Pre-eclampsia remains a leading cause of maternal and fetal morbidity and mortality. It is a pregnancy-specific multisystem disorder, occurring most commonly in primigravidae and characterized by the development of hypertension and proteinuria in the second half of pregnancy. The incidence in a second pregnancy is less than 1% in women who have had a normotensive first pregnancy, but is increased in women who have had pre-eclampsia in their first pregnancy, particularly in women whose first pregnancy was complicated by severe pre-eclampsia (Campbell *et al.*, 1985). This issue is more completely discussed in the chapter by Dekker and Robillard in this book. The pathogenesis of pre-eclampsia is not fully understood but it is believed that genetic predisposition and immune maladaptation lead to placental ischemia and perturbation of the maternal vascular endothelium. Coagulation activation is an important feature and hypercoagulable states, including both inherited and acquired thrombophilias, have been associated not only with pregnancy thromboembolism but also with other adverse pregnancy events.

Normal hemostasis

The primary initiator of coagulation is tissue factor. Tissue factor (TF) is expressed by epithelial, stromal and perivascular cells throughout the body but not normally by cells in contact with the circulation. Following vascular damage, membrane-bound TF complexes with factor VII (FVII). Cleavage of FVII results in the formation of activated FVIIa. Thereafter TF–FVIIa complex can directly activate factor X (FX). TF–FVIIa complex may also activate FX indirectly via activation of factor IX (FIX). Factor IXa, in complex with activated Factor VIII (FVIIIa) on the platelet surface (tenase), activates FX.

Thrombin has multiple functions within hemostasis, including the cleavage of fibrinogen to form fibrin, platelet activation, activation of factor XIII (FXIII) and the feedback activation of clotting factors V (FV) and VIII (FVIII). It is produced by activation of prothrombin by prothrombinase, a phospholipid-bound complex of activated Factor X (FXa) and its cofactor activated Factor V (FVa). Factor V is activated by FXa and thrombin. Cleavage of prothrombin by FXa results in the release of prothrombin fragment 1+2 (F1+2).

Natural anticoagulant mechanisms regulate thrombin by inhibition of the activity of formed thrombin by antithrombin and by downregulating thrombin production by the protein C/protein S system. Excess thrombin is rapidly inhibited by serine protease inhibitors (serpins) including antithrombin and heparin co-factor II. Thrombin is also inactivated on the endothelial cell surface by thrombomodulin. Prior to activation by thrombin to activated protein C (APC), protein C circulates as a two-chain zymogen (Esmon *et al.*, 1982, 1983; Esmon and Owen, 1981a). The activation process is enhanced approximately 20,000-fold when thrombin is bound to thrombomodulin

(Esmon and Owen, 1981b). Formation of the thrombin–thrombomodulin complex at the endothelial surface accelerates activation of protein C by thrombin. Formation of this complex blocks the ability of thrombin to catalyze fibrin formation, Factor XIII activation, platelet activation and feedback activation of coagulation cofactors. Thus thrombomodulin plays a key role in the conversion of thrombin from a procoagulant to an anticoagulant.

Once APC is generated it binds to protein S on the surface of activated cells and this complex then inactivates FVa and FVIIIa, downregulating thrombin generation. Approximately 60% of plasma protein S is bound to the β chain of C4b-binding protein and is inactive. The remaining 40%, designated free protein S, is uncomplexed and is the active moiety. Free protein S increases the affinity of APC for negatively charged phospholipid surfaces on platelets or the endothelium, enhancing complex formation of APC with FVa and FVIIIa. In addition, protein S has an independent anticoagulant effect on the free form of FIXa–FVIIIa–phospholipid complex (tenase) and the FVa–FXa–phospholipid complex (prothrombinase).

The principal inhibitor of the FVII–tissue factor pathway is the tissue factor pathway inhibitor (TFPI) which binds and inhibits FXa and forming a larger quaternary complex with TF–FVIIa and calcium. This greatly reduces the functional duration of the TF–FVIIa complex.

The fibrinolytic system provides a further level of regulation of fibrin clot propagation. Tissue-type plasminogen activator (t-PA) binds to fibrin to generate plasmin. Plasminogen activator inhibitors (PAI-1 and PAI-2) inactivate plasminogen activators.

Hemostasis in normal pregnancy

Pregnancy is associated with a progressive increase in the concentrations of many clotting factors including fibrinogen, FVIIC, FVIIIC,

von Willebrand antigen and ristocetin cofactor, FXC and FXIIC (Clark, 2003; Clark et al., 1998).

There is no significant effect of gestation on antithrombin activity or antigen levels. Results from a number of longitudinal and cross-sectional studies have demonstrated no consistent significant effect of gestation on protein C activity or antigen levels. Pregnancy does, however, result in a significant decrease in plasma levels of both total and free protein S (Clark, 2003; Clark et al., 1998). Levels less than those observed in nonpregnant subjects have been recorded throughout first-trimester pregnancy (Fernandez et al., 1989; Malm et al., 1988).

Thrombomodulin is found on maternal vascular endothelial cells and on the trophoblastic surface of the placenta (Maruyama et al., 1985). Thrombomodulin levels increase continuously throughout pregnancy. Increasing gestational age is associated with an increase in the activation of protein C and an increase in thrombin-mediated antithrombotic activity. Resistance to activated protein C increases throughout pregnancy (Clark et al., 1998; Cumming et al., 1995; Mathonnet et al., 1996). Plasma levels of TFPI increase in response to heparin, during the third trimester, and during labor (Bombeli et al., 1997; Novotny et al., 1991).

A significant positive relationship exists between gestational stage and the level of prothrombin fragment F1+2 (Cadroy et al., 1993; Comeglio et al., 1996; Kjellberg et al., 1999). Elevated levels of thrombin antithrombin (TAT) complex are found in about 50% of pregnant women during their first trimester, and in 100% during the second and third trimesters (Bremme et al., 1992), indicating that pregnancy is associated with increased thrombin generation. A higher level of fibrinopeptide A (a fragment released after the activation of fibrinogen) is also a feature of pregnancy and indicates an increase in fibrin generation.

Plasminogen activity and plasminogen activator inhibitor (PAI-1 and PAI-2) levels increase throughout pregnancy. The pregnant uterine decidua is a rich source of PAI-1 and the placenta produces PAI-2. There is also believed to be an increase in tissue plasminogen activator antigen release, but a reduction in tissue plasminogen activator activity (Clark, 2003).

The overall balance of the prothrombotic and antithrombotic thrombin effects in pregnancy are not known, but the net effect appears to be a shift toward hypercoagulability with increased levels of procoagulants and reduced anticoagulant activity.

Placental development

Establishment of the placenta requires that fetal cytotrophoblast stem cells invade the decidua and penetrate into the maternal spiral arteries. Trophoblasts replace maternal endothelium as far as the inner third of the myometrium transforming their phenotype and adopting characteristics such as the presence of von Willebrand factor, CD31 markers, adhesion molecules and coagulation components so as to resemble the endothelium they replace. The invasion of syncytiotrophoblasts into the spiral arteries results in widening of these arteries increasing the blood flow available to the developing placenta and fetus.

The special structure of the placenta demands efficient mechanisms for ensuring fast activation and localized regulation of hemostasis. The presence of both procoagulant and anticoagulant components on the placental endothelial cells and syncytiotrophoblast is essential. Tissue factor pathway inhibitor is primarily found in the endothelial cells and a variant, tissue factor pathway inhibitor 2, purified from placentae, has been localized in the syncytiotrophoblast lining the villi. Thrombomodulin is localized in endothelial cells and apical membranes of syncytiotrophoblast. Annexin V, an anticoagulant that binds to negative membrane phospholipids, is abundant in normal placental syncytiotrophoblasts.

In pre-eclampsia, the cytotrophoblast infiltrates the decidual portion of the spiral arteries but fails to penetrate the myometrial portion – possibly as a result of an abnormal maternal immune response to paternally derived antigens on the trophoblasts. Instead of the normal development of large tortuous vascular channels, the vessels remain narrow (Knight *et al.*, 1998; Meekins *et al.*, 1994). The resultant placental hypoperfusion causes increased placental apoptosis with the release of syncytiotrophoblast fragments into the maternal circulation leading to endothelial cell damage. Widespread cytokine-mediated oxidative stress and inflammation cause further maternal endothelial dysfunction (Knight *et al.*, 1998; Redman and Sargent, 2000). Significant differences exist in gene expression in cytotrophoblast isolated from pre-eclamptic and normal placenta.

Fetal blood circulation is confined to the blood vessels transversing the villi. There is no direct contact between maternal and fetal circulations and all exchange processes are performed through the outer layer of syncytiotrophoblast. Maternal blood, carrying oxygen, flows through the decidual spiral arteries, bathing the intervillous spaces and syncytiotrophoblasts lining the villi. Systemic (plasmatic) factors are of maternal origin, but the cellular regulatory mechanisms such as tissue factor, thrombomodulin and annexin V are fetal. Some components such as tissue factor pathway inhibitor and tissue plasminogen activator are derived from both sources. It is plausible that disorders of maternal hemostasis which result in the generation of increased amounts of thrombin may cause thrombosis in the intervillous spaces on the maternal side of the placenta. This would impair placental perfusion and further impede the normal transformation of the spiral arteries.

Thrombophilia

In Europe the term thrombophilia has a laboratory basis and is used to describe disorders of hemostasis which appear to predispose to venous thrombosis. In North America the term thrombophilia is used clinically to describe individuals who develop venous thrombosis either spontaneously or who have a first event at a young age. A definition which encompasses laboratory and clinical aspects is lacking, but clinicians investigating and managing patients should remain aware that both the clinical history and the laboratory findings are relevant. Thrombophilia may be inherited, acquired or complex – the result of environmental influences such as diet or other lifestyle factors interacting with genetic background.

Heritable thrombophilias

Currently a limited number of genetic abnormalities are accepted as independent risk factors for venous thromboembolism. These defects include those due to reduction in anticoagulant function – deficiency of the natural anticoagulants antithrombin, protein C or protein S – and those which are associated with increased (gain of function) procoagulant activity, Factor V Leiden (FV Leiden) and the G20210A prothrombin polymorphism (FII G20210A). The natural anticoagulant deficiencies are the result of a large number of potential gene defects. FV Leiden and the FII G20210A polymorphism are the result of single nucleotide polymorphisms. It is likely that there are other as yet unidentified heritable abnormalities of hemostasis associated with an increased risk of thrombosis. Some additional candidates such as dysplasminogenemia, thrombomodulin variants, tissue factor pathway inhibitor deficiency, protein Z deficiency and heparin co-factor II deficiency have been studied. However, none has been demonstrated conclusively to contribute to heritable thrombophilia.

Natural anticoagulant deficiencies

Two major phenotypes of heritable antithrombin deficiency are recognized. Type I defects are characterized by quantitative reduction of qualitatively normal protein, and type II deficiency is due to the production of a qualitatively abnormal antithrombin protein. Heritable antithrombin deficiency is uncommon, the prevalences of heterozygous type I and type II mutations being, respectively, 0.021 and 0.145% (Tait et al., 1994). Family studies suggest that antithrombin deficiency is a more severe defect than deficiencies of protein C or protein S.

The prevalence of heterozygous protein C deficiency in the general population is approximately 0.3% (Tait et al., 1995). The prevalence of protein S deficiency in the general population is not firmly established but it has been suggested that it may be around 0.03–0.13% (Dykes et al., 2001). Other studies have, however, suggested that the prevalence may be considerably higher (Faioni et al., 1997). Because of the lack of clear information about the prevalence of protein S deficiency it has not been possible to calculate accurately the "size" of the risk associated with protein S deficiency.

Gain of function defects

Activated protein C (APC) resistance is defined as an impaired plasma anticoagulant response to APC added in vitro. This phenomenon has been observed in the plasma of about 5% of the general population and over 20% of unselected consecutive patients with venous thrombosis. In 1993 Dahlback et al. reported that increased APC resistance cosegregated with thrombosis in families with familial venous thromboembolism. The majority of patients with familial APC resistance have the same point mutation in the gene for FV, a guanine to adenine transition at nucleotide position 1691, the factor V Leiden mutation (FV Leiden) (Bertina et al., 1994). This mutation causes a substitution of glutamine for arginine at position 506, one of the major sites at which APC cleaves factor Va. It is much more common than any other heritable thrombophilia in Caucasian populations, having a reported prevalence of between 2 and 15% (Rees et al., 1995). It is more prevalent in individuals of Northern European extraction than in those from Southern Europe (Ridker et al., 1997;

Rosendaal *et al.*, 1995). Homozygous FV Leiden has a prevalence of 0.06–0.25% and is reported to increase the risk of venous thrombosis approximately 80-fold (Rosendaal *et al.*, 1995). It has been suggested that carriage of the FV Leiden mutation may have a species benefit in so far as it may be associated with a reduced blood loss intrapartum (Lindqvist *et al.*, 1998).

The most recently described heritable thrombophilic defect is a single nucleotide change of guanine to adenine at position 20210 in the 3′ untranslated region of the prothrombin gene (FII G20210A) (Poort *et al.*, 1996). This polymorphism is associated with increased plasma prothrombin levels and an increased risk of venous thromboembolism. The prevalence of this polymorphism in Northern European populations is around 2% (Poort *et al.*, 1996). Higher prevalences have been reported in Southern Europe where FII G20210A is the most prevalent heritable thrombophilic defect (Souto *et al.*, 1998)

Dysfibrinogenemia

The majority of individuals with dysfibrinogenemia remain asymptomatic and are identified co-incidentally. However, in about 20% there is an increased tendency to arteriovenous thromboembolism (Haverkate and Samama, 1995). Dysfibrinogenemia has been found in only 0.8% of patients with a history of venous thromboembolism (Haverkate and Samama, 1995), but a high incidence of postpartum thrombosis and an increased risk of pregnancy loss have been reported in women with thrombophilic fibrinogen variants.

Combinations of heritable defects

Combinations of deficiencies of natural anticoagulants – antithrombin, protein C and protein S – are rare because of the low allelic frequencies of each of these defects, but FV Leiden and the FII G20210A polymorphism are common and combinations of these defects with each other,

with a natural anticoagulant deficiency or with an acquired or complex thrombophilia, are frequently found.

Acquired thrombophilic defects

Antiphospholipids

Antiphospholipids are a heterogeneous collection of IgG and IgM (and less frequently IgA) immunoglobulins. Lupus inhibitors are detected on functional testing where they cause prolongation of phospholipid-dependent coagulation reactions. Anticardiolipins react with anionic phospholipids in solid phase immunoassays. Historically it was believed that antiphospholipids react with negatively charged phospholipids. Recently, however, it has been shown that they react not with phospholipids but with plasma proteins bound to suitable (not necessarily phospholipid) surfaces such as β_2 glycoprotein 1(β_2GP1), human prothrombin, annexin V and proteins C and S.

Antiphospholipids (APLs) may occur in association with a wide variety of conditions including connective tissue disorders, infections, and exposure to certain drugs (Greaves *et al.*, 2000) and sometimes with no evident underlying pathology or drug exposure (Love and Santoro, 1990). The persisting presence of APLs (persisting in at least two samples collected at least 6 weeks apart) is associated with an increased risk of both venous and arterial thrombosis (Long *et al.*, 1991; Love and Santoro, 1990), and for many years has been known to increase the risk of recurrent fetal loss (Ginsberg *et al.*, 1992). The clinical criteria for the antiphospholipid syndrome also include one or more premature births of a morphologically normal neonate at or beyond 34 weeks of gestation because of severe pre-eclampsia or eclampsia.

The frequency of APLs in the general population is poorly documented but has been estimated to be between 1 and 2% (Creagh *et al.*, 1991; Rosendaal, 1999a, 1999b). The thrombotic risk associated with incidental APL positivity appears to be relatively low (Finazzi *et al.*, 1996). Among patients with venous thromboembolism the frequency of APLs is reported to be between 5 and 15% (Ginsberg *et al.*, 1992; Mateo *et al.*, 1997; Simioni *et al.*, 1996).

Acquired APC resistance

Resistance to activated protein C may be acquired in patients with increased plasma levels of FVIII or with antiphospholipids. There is evidence that APC resistance correlates with increased venous thrombosis risk irrespective of whether or not FV Leiden is present and there is an inverse relationship between the degree of the response to APC and thrombosis risk (De Visser *et al.*, 1999).

Mixed thrombophilic defects

Homocysteine and methylene tetrahydrofolate reductase

Plasma homocysteine levels are increased in individuals with reduced levels of folate, cobalamin or pyridoxine due to dietary deficiency, drugs or underlying disease. Hyperhomocysteinemia may also be caused by genetic abnormalities affecting the trans-sulphuration or remethylation pathways of homocysteine metabolism. A common mutation in the gene encoding methylene tetrahydrofolate reductase (MTHFR) in which a cytidine residue at position 677 (C677T) in the gene is replaced by thymidine has been described. The resultant variant is thermolabile and, in its homozygous form, is associated with an approximately 50% reduction of the enzyme activity. In the presence of folate deficiency, homozygosity for this mutation results in elevated plasma homocysteine levels and a slightly increased risk of venous thrombosis. Of white populations, 10–15% are homozygous (677TT) for this variant. The mechanisms whereby hyperhomocysteinemia promote thrombosis are not clear but seem to involve endothelial injury through oxidative stress, increased expression of

tissue factor, impaired endogenous anticoagulant activity (protein C, thrombomodulin) and reduced fibrinolysis.

Elevated FVIII activity

FVIII levels are in part genetically regulated and partly a response to environmental factors such as stress, estrogen use or pregnancy. An elevated plasma concentration of FVIII, but not of von Willebrand factor, is an independent risk factor for venous thromboembolism (Koster *et al.*, 1995). To date no specific genetic abnormality has been identified (Kraaijenhagen *et al.*, 2000). The risk of venous thrombosis increases steadily with increasing FVIII levels.

Thrombophilia and pre-eclampsia: the evidence

Over the past few years there have been numerous reports postulating associations between abnormalities of hemostasis and vascular complications of pregnancy. It has been suggested that women with thrombophilia are at increased risk, not only of pregnancy-associated thromboembolism, but also of other adverse pregnancy outcomes including pre-eclampsia and fetal loss. Studies of pre-eclampsia have been bedevilled by varying definitions and diagnostic criteria. Some have included women with pregnancy-induced hypertension without proteinuria and others have included women with chronic hypertension. Some studies have included only primigravidae (De Groot *et al.*, 1999) and some have included both primigravidae and multigravidae. Some studies have included women with recurrent pre-eclampsia.

Most studies searching for a link between thrombophilias and pre-eclampsia have examined only white patients. Few studies have included African Americans, in whom the prevalences of heritable thrombophilias are different from those in white populations (Livingston *et al.*, 2001). Most are observational or case-control studies, many of which lack any or adequate control groups. Vitamin supplementation policies during pregnancy vary from country to country. Supplementation with folate may decrease maternal homocysteine levels and may be a significant confounder. Some studies have reported activated protein C resistance without clarifying whether this is acquired APC resistance or associated with the FV Leiden mutation.

Heritable and mixed thrombophilias and pre-eclampsia

The evidence to support a role for heritable thrombophilias in the pathogenesis of pre-eclampsia is conflicting. Studies reported by Dekker *et al.* (1995), Kupferminc *et al.* (2000a), Dizon-Townson *et al.* (1996), van Pampus *et al.* (1999), Grandone *et al.* (1997, 1999), Lindoff *et al.* (1997) and others have demonstrated that patients with a history of pre-eclampsia were more likely to have evidence of a heritable thrombophilia than the normal population or normotensive gravidae. In contrast, numerous studies including those reported by Lindquvist *et al.* (1999), Livingston *et al.* (2001), de Groot *et al.* (1999), Young *et al.* (2001), O'Shaughnessy *et al.* (1999), Murphy *et al.* (2000) and Morrison (Morrison *et al.* 2002) have failed to find any significant relationship between heritable thrombophilias and pre-eclampsia risk.

Only studies which have recruited patients with both hypertension (≥140/90 mmHg or an increase in systolic blood pressure (SBP) ≥30 mmHg and/or an increase in diastolic blood pressure (DBP) ≥15 mmHg above baseline on at least two occasions at least 4 h apart) and proteinuria (≥300 mg 24 h or ++) have been included in the tables in this review. The degree of each, however, varies from study to study.

APC resistance and factor V Leiden

Because increased APC resistance and FV Leiden are the most prevalent thrombophilias in Caucasian populations, much attention has been directed toward studying the association, if any, of these defects with pre-eclampsia. In an early study, 8 of 50 women with a history of severe, early pre-eclampsia were found to have increased APC resistance (Dekker *et al.*, 1995). No controls were included, but in a further study the same group later reported that FV Leiden was more common in women with a history of early onset severe pre-eclampsia (6%: 32/284) than in normotensive controls (1.5%: 1/67). Although the authors reported an association between FV Leiden and pre-eclampsia (odds ratio 4.20), the confidence interval was very wide (0.55–32.15) and the association not statistically significant (Van Pampus *et al.*, 1999). Other studies have similarly failed to find a statistically significant association between FV Leiden carriage and pre-eclampsia (Table 21.1) (De Groot *et al.*, 1999; Grandone *et al.*, 1999; Lindoff *et al.*, 1997; Livingston *et al.*, 2001; Morrison *et al.*, 2002; Murphy *et al.*, 2000; O'Shaughnessy *et al.*, 1999; Young *et al.*, 2001). In a study from Japan, none of the cases or controls were found to carry FV Leiden (Kobashi *et al.*, 1999).

The study reported by de Groot *et al.* (1999) is interesting. One hundred and sixty-three women with a history of pre-eclampsia and controls matched for age and delivery date were tested for FV Leiden, FII G20210A, protein C, protein S, and antithrombin deficiency. The prevalence of these genetic risk factors was similar in the patient group (12.9%) and the control group (12.9%). There was, however, an unexplained high prevalence of FV Leiden in the control group (9.2%) and the odds ratio of 1.07 was not significant (95% CI 0.51–2.25). When the prevalence of FV Leiden in the patients was compared with the prevalence of FV Leiden in the background population previously reported by the authors, the prevalence in the patients was noted to be significantly greater.

Studies which have adopted stringent criteria and recruited only patients with severe pre-eclampsia have noted a significantly increased prevalence of FV Leiden (usually about 2.5–5-fold)

Table 21.1. FV Leiden and pre-eclampsia

Author	Recruitment	Case definition	Controls	Cases/ controls	Odds ratio (95% CI)
Dizon Townson et al., 1996	Recruited at labor	SBP > 160 mmHg or DBP > 110 mmHg on ≥2 occasions and proteinuria > 500 mg 24 h or +++/++++	Normotensive nonpregnant	158/403	2.21 (1.06–4.59)
Lindoff et al., 1997	Consecutive primigravidae	BP > 140/90 mmHg at least twice in 24 h and proteinuria > 300 mg 24 h	Healthy pregnant same population	50/50	1.98 (0.61–6.38)
Grandone et al., 1997	Primigravidae in labor	SBP > 140 mmHg and DBP > 90 mmHg on two occasions and proteinuria > 300 mg 24 h	Healthy pregnant same population	96/128	4.9 (1.3–18.3)
Nagy et al., 1998	Consecutive women with severe pre-eclampsia	SBP > 160 mmHg and DBP > 90 mmHg and proteinuria ≥1000 mg 24 h	Healthy pregnant	68/71	3.06 (1.03–9.13)
Grandone et al., 1999	Recruited in labor	SBP > 140 mmHg and DBP > 90 mmHg on two occasions and proteinuria > 300 mg 24 h	Healthy pregnant same population	70/216	3.2 (0.78–13.14)
Mimuro et al., 1998	Prospective	SBP > 135 mmHg and/or DBP > 90 mmHg on two occasions and proteinuria > 300 mg 24 h or ++	Normal pregnant and nonpregnant	50/200	12.96 (1.41–118.8)
O'Shaughnessy et al., 1999	Prospective Mainly primigravid	SBP > 160 mmHg or DBP > 110 mmHg and proteinuria > 300 mg 24 h	Normotensive pregnant	110/97	0.88 (0.33–2.33)
De Groot et al., 1999	Retrospective population-based case control	↑ SBP > 30 mmHg or ↑DBP > 15 mmHg or late pregnancy BP > 140/90 mmHg and proteinuria ++	Normal pregnancy	163/163	1.07 (0.51–2.25)
Van Pampus et al., 1999	Prospective; severe pre-eclampsia	DBP > 110 mmHg and proteinuria > 500 mg 24 h and delivery <36 weeks or HELLP	Healthy primigravidae	345/67	4.20 (0.55–32.15)
Kupferminc et al., 1999	Consecutive women with pregnancy complications including pre-eclampsia	BP > 160/110 mmHg and proteinuria > 500 mg 24 h or platelets <100,000 mm^{-3} or HELLP	Matched normal pregnancies	110/110	5.3 (1.80–15.60)

Reference	Study	Criteria	Comparison group	n	Odds ratio (95% CI)
Kuperminc et al., 2000a	Consecutive women with pre-eclampsia	BP >160/110 mmHg and proteinuria >500 mg 24 h or platelets <100,000 mm⁻³ or HELLP	Matched normal pregnancies	63/126	4.61 (1.83–11.58)
Rigo et al., 2000	High-risk obstetric patients	SBP >160 mmHg or DBP >110 mmHg on ≥2 occasions and proteinuria >300 mg 24 h or +++	Matched normal pregnancies	120/101	0.33 (2.13–25.30)
Murphy 2000 (Murphy, Donoghue, Nallen, D'Mello, Regan, Whitehead, & Fitzgerald 2000)	Prospective. All primi-gravidae booking	SBP >140 mmHg or DBP >110 mmHg or DBP >90 mmHg on 2 occasions and proteinuria +	Normotensive pregnant; no IUGR history	12/540	Not given
Von Tempelhof 2000 (Von Tempelhoff, Heilmann, Spanuth, Kunzmann, & Hommel 2000)	Prospective; women with history of pre-eclampsia	BP >160/110 mmHg and proteinuria >500 mg 24 h	Normal primiparae	29/61	5.0 (1.4–18.5)
Young et al., 2001	Pre-eclampsia in previous pregnancy	SBP >140 mmHg or DBP >90 mmHg and proteinuria >300 mg 24 h or +	≥2 normal pregnancies	282/361	1.28 (0.59–2.80)
Livingston et al., 2001	Prospective cross-sectional	SBP >160 mmHg or DBP >110 mmHg and proteinuria >300 mg 24 h	Normal pregnant	110/97	1.8 (0.44–7.34)
Morrison et al., 2002	Retrospective population-based case control	DBP >110 mmHg or DBP >90 mmHg on two occasions and proteinuria >300 mg 24 h	Previous normal pregnancy	404/164	0.87 (0.37–2.07)

SBP = systolic blood pressure; DBP = diastolic blood pressure; ↑ = increase in.

in the patients compared with the controls (Dizon-Townson *et al.*, 1996; Grandone *et al.*, 1997; Kupferminc *et al.*, 1999, 2000a; Nagy *et al.*, 1998; Rigo *et al.*, 2002; Von Tempelhoff *et al.*, 2000). The confidence intervals are, however, frequently extremely wide, and the results must be interpreted with caution.

Fetal as well as maternal carriage of FV Leiden may influence the risk of pregnancy complication. In one study placentae with a greater than 10% placental infarction have been associated with a tenfold increased fetal carrier rate for FV Leiden (Dizon-Townson *et al.*, 1997). In another, no association between fetal carriage of FV Leiden and pre-eclampsia was demonstrated (Livingston *et al.*, 2001).

Prothrombin G20210A

A limited number of studies have sought an association between the FIIG20210A polymorphism and pre-eclampsia (Table 21.2). One study – a case-control study from Italy – suggested that there may be an increased prevalence of FII G20210A in women with pre-eclampsia (Grandone *et al.*, 1999). Similarly, investigators in Israel found that the FII G20210A polymorphism was statistically significantly associated with vascular complications of pregnancy including severe pre-eclampsia, but they did not have the power to demonstrate an association with pre-eclampsia alone (Kupferminc *et al.*, 1999, 2000b). In a further study, the same group reported a statistically significant association with severe pre-eclampsia after adjusting for other covariates (Kupferminc *et al.*, 2000a). Other reported studies have failed to find an association (De Groot *et al.*, 1999; Higgins *et al.*, 2000; Livingston *et al.*, 2001; Morrison *et al.*, 2002). However, the study by Higgins *et al.*, 2000) was powered to find a threefold increase in risk, and a lesser risk may have been undetected, and the power to detect an association in the study reported by Livingston *et al.*, may have been compromised by the restricted number of Caucasians recruited (Livingston *et al.*, 2001).

Methylene tetrahydrofolate reductase 677TT

Hyperhomocysteinemia has been reported in pre-eclamptic patients (Dekker *et al.*, 1995). Homozygosity for the common thermolabile MTHFR C677T variant causes mild hyperhomocysteinemia in folate-deficient patients and has been implicated in vascular damage and increased arterial and venous thrombotic risk. It has therefore been targeted as a possible susceptibility gene for pre-eclampsia and numerous reports have been published (Table 21.3). Most studies have failed to confirm an association (Kaiser *et al.*, 2000, 2001; Kobashi *et al.*, 2000; Lachmeijer *et al.*, 2001; Laivuori *et al.*, 2000; Livingston *et al.*, 2001; Morrison *et al.*, 2002; Murphy *et al.*, 2000; O'Shaughnessy *et al.*, 1999; Powers *et al.*, 1999; Rigo Jr. *et al.*, 2000; Young *et al.*, 2001; Zusterzeel *et al.*, 2000) but a small case-control study from Japan (Sohda *et al.*, 1997), an Italian case-control study (Grandone *et al.*, 1997, 1999) and a study of Israeli Jewish women (Kupferminc *et al.*, 1999, 2000a) reported an approximately 2–3-fold increased prevalence of homozygosity for the 677TT MTHFR polymorphism in women with pre-eclampsia.

Folate supplementation reduces plasma homocysteine levels irrespective of MTHFR genotype. This is therefore an important confounding variable. Folate supplementation is more common in the USA than in other countries, and policies with respect to folate administration in pregnancy vary from country to country.

Other heritable abnormalities

Natural anticoagulant deficiencies are rare or uncommon. Although early studies suggested protein S deficiency may be associated with an increased risk of pregnancy vascular complication including pre-eclampsia, no large studies including carefully characterized patients confirming these findings have been reported.

In a case-control study of 404 women with a history of pre-eclampsia, 303 with a history of gestational hypertension and 164 control women,

Table 21.2. FII G20210A and pre-eclampsia

Author	Recruitment	Case definition	Controls	Cases/controls	Odds ratio (95% CI)
Grandone et al., 1999	Recruited in labor	SBP >140 mmHg and DBP >90 mmHg on two occasions and proteinuria >300 mg 24 h	Healthy pregnant same population	70/216	3.83 (1.49–9.87)
O'Shaughnessy et al., 1999	Prospective Mainly primigravid	SBP >160 mmHg or DBP >110 mmHg and proteinuria >300 mg 24 h	Normotensive pregnant	110/97	0.88 (0.33–2.33)
De Groot et al., 1999	Retrospective population-based case control	↑ SBP >30 mmHg or ↑DBP >15 mmHg or late pregnancy BP >140/90 mmHg and proteinuria ++	Healthy same population non pre-eclamptic	163/163	0.83 (0.25–2.77)
Kupferminc et al., 1999	Consecutive women with pregnancy complications including pre-eclampsia	BP >160/110 mmHg and proteinuria >500 mg 24 h or platelets <100,000 mm^{-3} or HELLP	Matched women with normal pregnancies	110/110	0.2 (0.4–13.9)
Kupferminc et al., 2000a	Consecutive women with pre-eclampsia	BP >160/110 mmHg and proteinuria >500 mg 24 h or platelets <100,000 mm^{-3} or HELLP	Matched women with normal pregnancies	63/126	2.63 (0.68–10.16)
Kupferminc et al., 2000b	Consecutive women with pre-eclampsia	BP >160/110 mmHg and proteinuria >500 mg 24 h or platelets <100,000 mm^{-3} or HELLP	Matched women with normal pregnancies	80/156	2.9 (0.89–9.44)
Higgins et al., 2000	History of pre-eclampsia	↑ SBP >25 mmHg and/or ↑DBP >15 mmHg or SBP >140 and/or DBP >90 mmHg on ≥2 occasions and proteinuria >300 mg 24 h or ++	Normotensive pregnant women	189/119	1.53 (0.33–7.01)
Livingston et al., 2001	Prospective cross-sectional. Mainly primigravid	SBP >160 mmHg or DBP >110 mmHg and proteinuria >300 mg 24 h	Normotensive pregnant	110/97	No FIIG20210A cases
Morrison et al., 2002	Retrospective population-based case control	DBP >110 mmHg or DBP >90 mmHg on two occasions and proteinuria >300 mg 24 h	Previous normotensive pregnancy	404/164	4/0 FIIG20210A cases/controls

SBP = systolic blood pressure; DBP = diastolic blood pressure; ↑ = increase in.

Table 21.3. Methylene tetrahydrofolate reductase 677T and pre-eclampsia

Author	Recruitment	Case definition	Controls	Cases/controls	Odds ratio (95% CI)
Sohda et al., 1997	Not specified	SBP > 160 mmHg or DBP > 110 mmHg on two occasions and/or proteinuria > 500 mg 24 h or +++	Healthy pregnant and nonpregnant adults	67/358	2.5 (1.3–48)
Grandone et al., 1997	Primigravidae in labor	SBP > 140 mmHg and DBP > 90 mmHg on two occasions and proteinuria > 300 mg 24 h	Healthy pregnant same population	96/128	1.8 (1.0–3.5)
Grandone et al., 1999	Recruited in labor	SBP > 140 mmHg and DBP > 90 mmHg on two occasions and proteinuria > 300 mg 24 h	Healthy pregnant same population	70/216	0.0 (1.06–3.76)
O'Shaughnessy et al., 1999	Prospective Mainly primigravid	SBP > 160 mmHg or DBP > 110 mmHg and proteinuria > 300 mg 24 h	Normotensive pregnant	110/97	0.9 (0.44–1.83)
Powers et al., 1999	Recruited in labor	↑SBP > 30 mmHg and/or ↑DBP > 15 mmHg or BP > 140/90 mmHg and/or proteinuria > 500 mg 24 h or ++	Normal pregnant women	99/114	1.28 (0.58–2.79)
Kupferminc et al., 1999	Consecutive women with pregnancy complications including pre-eclampsia	BP > 160/110 mmHg and proteinuria > 500 mg 24 h or platelets <100,000 mm^{-3} or HELLP	Matched women with normal pregnancies	110/110	2.9 (1.0–8.5)
Kupferminc et al., 2000a	Consecutive women with pre-eclampsia	BP > 160/110 mmHg and proteinuria > 500 mg 24 h or platelets <100,000 mm^{-3} or HELLP	Matched women with normal pregnancies	63/126	2.97 (1.29–6.81)
Zusterzeel et al., 2000	Retrospective; history of pre-eclampsia	DBP > 90 mmHg on two occasions and proteinuria > 300 mg 24 h	General population	81/403	1.38 (0.78–2.44)
Kobashi et al., 2000	Singleton pregnancies	↑SBP > 30 mmHg and/or ↑DBP > 15 mmHg or BP > 140/90 mmHg and/or proteinuria > 300 mg 24 h or +	Normal pregnant women	73/215	0.68 (0.30–1.55)

Study	Study type/population	Definition of pre-eclampsia	Control group	n/n	OR (95% CI)
Laivuori et al., 2000	Retrospective; pre-eclamptic primigravidae	BP >140/90 mmHg on two occasions and proteinuria >300 mg 24 h	>1 normal pregnancy	113/103	0.50 (0.14–1.77)
Kaiser et al., 2000	Primigravidae	↑SBP >25 mmHg and/or ↑DBP >15 mm or BP >140/90 mmHg and/or proteinuria >300 mg 24 h or ++ or eclampsia	Nulliparae with normotensive pregnancy	147/109	0.71 (0.33–1.57)
Rigo et al., 2000	High risk obstetric patients	SBP >160 mmHg or DBP >110 mmHg on ≥2 occasions and proteinuria >300 mg 24 h or +++	Matched women with normal pregnancies	120/101	1.13 (0.38–3.37)
Lachmeijer et al., 2001	Retrospective: history of pre-eclampsia	DBP >90 mmHg with ↑DBP >20 mmHg on ≥2 occasions and proteinuria >300 mg 24 h	Blood donors	47/120	0.92 (0.28–3.1)
Kaiser et al., 2001	Primigravidae	↑SBP >25 mmHg and/or ↑DBP >15 mmHg or BP >140/90 mmHg and/or proteinuria >300 mg 24 h or ++ or eclampsia	Matched women with normal pregnancies	156/79	0.86 (0.39–1.90)
Young et al., 2001	Pre-eclampsia in previous pregnancy	SBP >140 mmHg or DBP >90 mmHg and proteinuria >300 mg 24 h or +	≥2 previous pregnancies; non-pre-eclamptic	282/361	1.03 (0.64–1.69)
Livingston et al., 2001	Prospective cross sectional. Primigravidae	SBP >160 mmHg or DBP >110 mmHg and proteinuria >300 mg 24 h	Normotensive pregnant	110/97	1.3 (0.46–3.44)
Morrison et al., 2002	Retrospective population based case control	DBP >110 mmHg or DBP >90 mmHg on two occasions and proteinuria >300 mg 24 h	Previous normotensive pregnancy	404/164	1.01 (0.55–1.82)

SBP = systolic blood pressure; DBP = diastolic blood pressure; ↑ = increase in.

Morrison *et al.* (2002) studied the associations of five prothrombotic gene polymorphisms (FV Leiden, FII G20210A, MTHFR C677T, plasminogen activator inhibitor-1 4G/5G and the silent dimorphism 807 cytosine to thymine within the platelet collagen receptor) with these pregnancy complications. The frequency of genotypes did not differ significantly between patients and controls for any of the polymorphisms.

There have been isolated reports suggesting that thrombomodulin variants may be associated with an increased risk of pre-eclampsia (Nakabayashi *et al.*, 1999) but other workers have failed to confirm an association (Borg *et al.*, 2002; Hira *et al.*, 2003).

Acquired thrombophilias and pre-eclampsia

Antiphospholipids

Antiphospholipids are associated with placental vascular thrombosis, decidual vasculopathy, intervillous fibrin deposition and placental infarction (Infante-Rivard *et al.*, 1991; Rand *et al.*, 1997). Up to 20% of women with recurrent fetal loss may be shown to have antiphospholipids (Branch *et al.*, 1997; Out *et al.*, 1991; Parazzini *et al.*, 1991). A number of studies have also demonstrated an association between antiphospholipids and pre-eclampsia.

In a small study of 43 women who presented with severe pre-eclampsia prior to 34 weeks' gestation, 16% had significant levels of antiphospholipid antibodies. None of the normotensive controls of similar gestational age had antiphospholipid antibodies (Branch *et al.*, 1989). In a prospective study, 60 of 830 (7%) pregnant women were found to have elevated anticardiolipins. The rate of pre-eclampsia (11.7%) in the anticardiolipin-positive group was significantly higher than in the negative group (1.9%) (Yasuda *et al.*, 1995). Of 95 patients with a history of severe early-onset pre-eclampsia, 29.4% had detectable anticardiolipins (Dekker *et al.*, 1995). In an extension of this study, anticardiolipin antibodies were observed in 20.9% of 345 patients with a history of severe pre-eclampsia but in only 7.5% of the 67 healthy controls with a history of uncomplicated pregnancies (Van Pampus *et al.*, 1999).

Other authors have failed to find any association between antiphospholipids and pre-eclampsia. No significant difference in anticardiolipin antibody levels were found between a group of 33 black women with severe pre-eclampsia and 32 normotensive women in the third trimester of pregnancy (Rajah *et al.*, 1990). In another study, 113 pregnancies in women with systemic lupus erythematosus (59 in women with detectable antiphospholipids and 54 in women without detectable antiphospholipids) were examined. No relationships were seen between antiphospholipid antibodies and pregnancy-induced hypertension or pre-eclampsia. (Out *et al.*, 1992). In a prospective cohort study 389 low-risk, nulliparous pregnant women who came to the obstetrics clinic before 25 weeks gestation had blood drawn at the first prenatal visit, 239 of whom gave a further sample at delivery. The detection of antiphospholipids in neither the booking nor the delivery samples was associated with maternal complications of pregnancy (Lynch *et al.*, 1994).

Acquired APC resistance

In a study of FV Leiden-negative subjects the degree of resistance in the first trimester of pregnancy related to the risk of development of pre-eclampsia in the index pregnancy (Clark *et al.*, 2001). A sevenfold risk of pre-eclampsia was observed for those in the highest quartile when compared with those in the lowest. In this study, regression for those factors that confounded the relationship (smoking and booking blood pressure) revealed a persisting relationship between APC resistance and the risk of subsequent pre-eclampsia.

Thrombophilia and pre-eclampsia: unresolved questions

It remains controversial whether thrombophilias are involved in the etiology and/or pathogenesis of pre-eclampsia. The incidence of pre-eclampsia is increased in the mothers, sisters, daughters and granddaughters of probands with pre-eclampsia, suggesting that genetic factors may be important in its pathogenesis. Pre-eclampsia occurs significantly more frequently in blacks than in whites. Thus different populations may be predisposed to pre-eclampsia via different mechanisms. Extremes of age have been postulated as a risk factor for pre-eclampsia. The pathogenesis of severe and/or recurrent pre-eclampsia may not necessarily be the same as the pathogenesis of milder forms of the disorder.

Four main factors are postulated to contribute to the risk of pre-eclampsia: (1) immune maladaptation, (2) placental ischemia, (3) oxidative stress, and (4) genetic susceptibility. These mechanisms are not mutually exclusive and it is likely that in many cases the etiology is a combination of all four. Placental infarctions and intervillous thrombosis are commonly observed in pre-eclampsia, suggesting that thrombophilia, genetic or acquired, may play a role in the susceptibility to and pathogenesis of pre-eclampsia. The hypothesis that increased thrombin generation may increase the risk or severity of pre-eclampsia in some women is attractive.

The weight of evidence currently available would appear to support the conclusion that the more common types of thrombophilia (FV Leiden, FII G20210A or MTHFR 677TT) are not independent risk factors for pre-eclampsia. It may be that the currently identifiable thrombophilias are not major risk factors for pre-eclampsia unless additional inherited or acquired predisposing risk factors are present. In a study reported by Pabinger et al. (2001), the prevalence of pre-eclampsia was higher in women with a history of venous thromboembolism than in women with no thrombotic history. They reported that the tendency to an increased risk was not linked to any specific thrombophilic defect and was independent of the presence of all of the analyzed variables. The authors suggested that as yet unknown thrombotic risk factors may be important contributors to the risk of pre-eclampsia. Hypercoagulability, whether due to an identifiable thrombophilia or not, may characterize a subpopulation of women in whom the risk of pre-eclampsia is elevated or in whom the clinical presentation may be more severe. In particular, there is evidence that carriage of FV Leiden may increase the risk of severe pre-eclampsia in women who are susceptible to pre-eclampsia.

The question of the role of anticoagulation in the prevention or amelioration of pre-eclampsia in some women has been raised. At present, there is general agreement that there is no place for routine screening of all women attending antenatal clinics in an attempt to prevent pre-eclampsia; however, several authors have suggested that screening for thrombophilic defects may be appropriate in women who have a previous history of pre-eclampsia (Dekker et al., 1995; Dizon-Townson et al., 1996; Kupferminc et al., 1999; Lindoff et al., 1997; Van Pampus et al., 1999). In poor or undernourished women folate supplementation would seem appropriate – whether or not they are homozygous for the thermolabile MTHFR variant (677TT).

Further adequately powered studies are required to examine potential associations between thrombophilia and the risk of developing pre-eclampsia and of the potential benefits and risks of intervention with pharmacological anticoagulation.

REFERENCES

Bertina, R. M., Koeleman, B. P. C., Koster, T., et al. (1994). Mutation in blood coagulation factor V associated with resistance to activated protein C. *Nature*, **369**(6475), 64–7.

Bombeli, T., Mueller, M. and Haeberli, A. (1997). Anticoagulant properties of the vascular endothelium. *Thromb. Haem.*, **77**(3), 408–23.

Borg, A. J., Higgins, J. R., Brennecke, S. P. and Moses, E. K. (2002). Thrombomodulin Ala455Val dimorphism is not associated with pre-eclampsia in Australian and New Zealand women. *Gynecol. Obstet. Invest.*, **54**(1), 43–5.

Branch, D. W., Andres, R., Digre, K. B., Rote, N. S. and Scott, J. R. (1989). The association of antiphospholipid antibodies with severe preeclampsia. *Obstet. Gynecol.*, **73**(4), 541–5.

Branch, D. W., Silver, R., Pierangeli, S., Van, L., and Harris, E. N. (1997). Antiphospholipid antibodies other than lupus anticoagulant and anticardiolipin antibodies in women with recurrent pregnancy loss, fertile controls, and antiphospholipid syndrome. *Obstet. Gynecol.*, **89**(4), 549–55.

Bremme, K., Ostlund, E., Almqvist, I., Heinonen, K. and Blomback, M. (1992). Enhanced thrombin generation and fibrinolytic activity in normal pregnancy and the puerperium. *Obstet. Gynecol.*, **80**(1), 132–7.

Cadroy, Y., Grandjean, H., Pichon, J., *et al.* (1993). Evaluation of six markers of haemostatic system in normal pregnancy and pregnancy complicated by hypertension or pre-eclampsia. *Br. J. Obstet. Gynaecol.*, **100**(5), 416–20.

Campbell, D. M., MacGillivray, I. and Carr-Hill, R. (1985). Pre-eclampsia in second pregnancy. *Br. J. Obstet. Gynaecol.*, **92**(2), 131–40.

Clark, P. (2003). Changes of haemostasis variables during pregnancy. *Semi. Vasc. Med.*, **3**, 13–24.

Clark, P., Brennand, J., Conkie, J. A., McCall, F., Greer, I. A. and Walker, I. D. (1998). Activated protein C sensitivity, protein C, protein S and coagulation in normal pregnancy. *Thromb. Haem.*, **79**(6), 166–70.

Clark, P., Sattar, N., Walker, I. D. and Greer, I. A. (2001). The Glasgow Outcome, APCR and Lipid (GOAL) pregnancy study: significance of pregnancy associated activated protein C resistance. *Thromb. Haem.*, **85**(1), 30–5.

Comeglio, P., Fedi, S., Liotta, A. A., *et al.* (1996). Blood clotting activation during normal pregnancy. *Thromb. Res.*, **84**(3), 199–202.

Creagh, M. D., Malia, R. G., Cooper, S. M., Smith, A. R., Duncan, S. L. B. and Greaves, M. (1991). Screening for lupus anticoagulant and anticardiolipin antibodies in women with fetal loss. *J. Clin. Pathol.*, **44**(1), 45–7.

Cumming, A. M., Tait, R. C., Fildes, S., Yoong, A., Keeney, S. and Hay, C. R. M. (1995). Development of resistance to activated protein C during pregnancy. *Br. J. Haematol.*, **90**(3), 725–7.

Dahlback, B., Carlsson, M. and Svensson, P. J. (1993). Familial thrombophilia due to a previously unrecognized mechanism characterized by poor anticoagulant response to activated protein C: prediction of a cofactor to activated protein C. *Proc. Natl Acad. Sci. USA*, **90**(3), 1004–8.

De Groot, C. J. M., Bloemenkamp, K. W. M., Duvekot, E. J., *et al.* (1999). Preeclampsia and genetic risk factors for thrombosis: a case-control study. *Am. J. Obstet. Gynecol.*, **181**(4), 975–80.

Dekker, G. A., De Vries, J. I. P., Doelitzsch, P. M., *et al.* (1995). Underlying disorders associated with severe early-onset preeclampsia. *Am. J. Obstet. Gynecol.*, **173**(4), 1042–8.

De Visser, M. C. H., Rosendaal, F. R. and Bertina, R. M. (1999). A reduced sensitivity for activated protein C in the absence of factor V Leiden increases the risk of venous thrombosis. *Blood*, **93**(4), 1271–6.

Dizon-Townson, D. S., Meline, L., Nelson, L. M., Varner, M. and Ward, K. (1997). Fetal carriers of the factor V Leiden mutation are prone to miscarriage and placental infarction. *Am. J. Obstet. Gynecol.*, **177**(2), 402–5.

Dizon-Townson, D. S., Nelson, L. M., Easton, K. and Ward, K. (1996). The factor V Leiden mutation may predispose women to severe preeclampsia. *Am. J. Obstet. Gynecol.*, **175**(4), 902–5.

Dykes, A. C., Walker, I. D., McMahon, A. D., Islam, S. I. A. M. and Tait, R. C. (2001). A study of Protein S antigen levels in 3788 healthy volunteers: influence of age, sex and hormone use, and estimate for prevalence of deficiency state. *Br. J. Haematol.*, **113**(3), 636–41.

Esmon, C. T., Esmon, N. L. and Harris, K. W. (1982). Complex formation between thrombin and thrombomodulin inhibits both thrombin-catalyzed fibrin formation and factor V activation. *J. Biol. Chem.*, **257**(14), 7944–7.

Esmon, C. T. and Owen, W. G. (1981b). Identification of an endothelial cell cofactor for thrombin-catalyzed activation of protein C. *Proc. Natl Acad. Sci. USA*, **78**(4), 2249–52.

Esmon, C. T. and Owen, W. G. (1981a). Identification of an endothelial cell cofactor for thrombin-catalyzed activation of protein C. *Proc. Natl Acad. Sci. USA*, **78**(4), 2249–52.

Esmon, N. L., Carroll, R. C. and Esmon, C. T. (1983). Thrombomodulin blocks the ability of thrombin to activate platelets. *J. Biol. Chem.*, **258**(20), 12,238–42.

Faioni, E.M., Valsecchi, C., Palla, A., Taioli, E., Razzari, C. and Mannucci, P.M. (1997). Free protein S deficiency is a risk factor for venous thrombosis. *Thromb. Haem.*, **78**(5), 1343–6.

Fernandez, J.A., Estelles, A., Gilabert, J., Espana, F. and Aznar, J. (1989). Functional and immunologic protein S in normal pregnant women and in full-term newborns. *Thromb. Haem.*, **61**(3), 474–8.

Finazzi, G., Brancaccio, V., Moia, M., *et al.* (1996). Natural history and risk factors for thrombosis in 360 patients with antiphospholipid antibodies: a four-year prospective study from the Italian registry. *Am. J. Med.*, **100**(5), 530–6.

Ginsberg, J.S., Brill-Edwards, P., Johnston, M., *et al.* (1992). Relationship of antiphospholipid antibodies to pregnancy loss in patients with systemic lupus erythematosus: a cross-sectional study. *Blood*, **80**(4), 975–80.

Grandone, E., Margaglione, M., Colaizzo, D., *et al.* (1997). Factor V leiden, C > T MTHFR polymorphism and genetic susceptibility to preeclampsia. *Thromb. Haem.*, **77**(6), 1052–4.

Grandone, E., Margaglione, M., Colaizzo, D., *et al.* (1999). Prothrombotic genetic risk factors and the occurrence of gestational hypertension with or without proteinuria. *Thromb. Haem.*, **81**(3), 349–52.

Greaves, M., Cohen, H., Machin, S.J. and Mackie, I. (2000). Guidelines on the investigation and management of the antiphospholipid syndrome. *Br. J. Haematol.*, **109**(4), 704–15.

Haverkate, F. and Samama, M. (1995). Familial dysfibrinogenemia and thrombophilia – report on a study of the SSC subcommittee on fibrinogen. *Thromb. Haem.*, **73**(1), 151–61.

Higgins, J.R., Kaiser, T., Moses, E.K., North, R. and Brennecke, S.P. (2000). Prothrombin G20210A mutation: is it associated with pre-eclampsia? *Gynecol. Obstet. Invest.*, **50**(4), 254–7.

Hira, B., Pegoraro, R.J., Rom, L. and Moodley, J. (2003). Absence of Factor V Leiden, thrombomodulin and prothrombin gene variants in Black South African women with pre-eclampsia and eclampsia. *Br. J. Obstet. Gynaecol.*, **110**(3), 327–8.

Infante-Rivard, C., David, M., Gauthier, R. and Rivard, G.-E. (1991). Lupus anticoagulants, anticardiolipin antibodies, and fetal loss: a case-control study. *N. Engl. J. Med.*, **325**(15), 1063–6.

Kaiser, T., Brennecke, S.P. and Moses, E.K. (2000). Methylenetetrahydrofolate reductase polymorphisms are not a risk factor for pre-eclampsia/eclampsia in Australian women. *Gynecol. Obstet. Invest.*, **50**(2), 100–2.

Kaiser, T., Brennecke, S.P. and Moses, E.K. (2001). C677T methylenetetrahydrofolate reductase polymorphism is not a risk factor for pre-eclampsia/eclampsia among Australian women. *Hum. Hered.*, **51**(1–2), 20–2.

Kjellberg, U., Andersson, N.-E., Rosen, S., Tengborn, L. and Hellgren, M. (1999). APC resistance and other haemostatic variables during pregnancy and puerperium. *Thromb. Haem.*, **81**(4), 527–31.

Knight, M., Redman, C.W.G., Linton, E.A. and Sargent, I.L. (1998). Shedding of syncytiotrophoblast microvilli into the maternal circulation in pre-eclamptic pregnancies. *Br. J. Obstet. Gynaecol.*, **105**(6), 632–40.

Kobashi, G., Yamada, H., Asano, T., *et al.* (1999). The factor V Leiden mutation is not a common cause of pregnancy induced hypertension in Japan. *Semin. Thromb. Hem.*, **25**, 487–9.

Kobashi, G., Yamada, H., Asano, T., *et al.* (2000). Absence of association between a common mutation in the methylenetetrahydrofolate reductase gene and pre-eclampsia in Japanese women. *Am. J. Med. Genetics*, **93**(2), 122–5.

Koster, T., Blann, A.D., Briet, E., Vandenbroucke, J.P. and Rosendaal, F.R. (1995). Role of clotting factor VIII in effect of von Willebrand factor on occurrence of deep-vein thrombosis. *Lancet*, **345**(8943), 152–5.

Kraaijenhagen, R.A., In't Anker, P.S., Koopman, M.M.W., *et al.* (2000). High plasma concentration of factor VIIIc is a major risk factor for venous thromboembolism. *Thromb. Haem.*, **83**(1), 5–9.

Kupferminc, M.J., Eldor, A., Steinman, N., *et al.* (1999). Increased frequency of genetic thrombophilia in women with complications of pregnancy. *N. Engl. J. Med.*, **340**(1), 9–13.

Kupferminc, M.J., Fait, G., Many, A., Gordon, D., Eldor, A. and Lessing, J.B. (2000a). Severe preeclampsia and high frequency of genetic thrombophilic mutations. *Obstet. Gynecol.*, **96**(1), 45–9.

Kupferminc, M.J., Peri, H., Zwang, E., Yaron, Y., Wolman, I. and Eldor, A. (2000b). High prevalence of the prothrombin gene mutation in women with intrauterine growth retardation, abruptio placentae and second trimester loss. *Acta Obstet. Gynecol. Scand.*, **79**(11), 963–7.

Lachmeijer, A.M.A., Arngrimsson, R., Bastiaans, E.J., *et al.* (2001). Mutations in the gene for methylenetetrahydrofolate reductase, homocysteine levels, and vitamin status in women with a history of preeclampsia. *Am. J. Obstet. Gynecol.*, **184**(3), 394–402.

Laivuori, H., Kaaja, R., Ylikorkala, O., Hiltunen, T. and Kontula, K. (2000). 677 C right arrow T polymorphism of the methylenetetrahydrofolate reductase gene and preeclampsia. *Obstet. Gynecol.*, **96**(2), 277–80.

Lindoff, C., Ingemarsson, I., Martinsson, G., Segelmark, M., Thysell, H. and Astedt, B. (1997). Preeclampsia is associated with a reduced response to activated protein C. *Am. J. Obstet. Gynecol.*, **176**(2), 457–60.

Lindqvist, P. G., Svensson, P. J., Dahlback, B. and Marsal, K. (1998). Factor V Q506 mutation (activated protein C resistance) associated with reduced intrapartum blood loss – a possible evolutionary selection mechanism. *Thromb. Haem.*, **79**(1), 69–73.

Lindqvist, P. G., Svensson, P. J., Marsal, K., Grennert, L., Luterkor, M., and Dahlback, B. (1999). Activated protein C resistance (FV:Q506) and pregnancy. *Thromb. Haem.*, **81**(4), 532–7.

Livingston, J. C., Barton, J. R., Park, V., Haddad, B., Phillips, O. and Sibai, B. M. (2001). Maternal and fetal inherited thrombophilias are not related to the development of severe preeclampsia. *Am. J. Obstet. Gynecol.*, **185**(1), 153–7.

Long, A. A., Ginsberg, J. S., Brill-Edwards, P., *et al.* (1991). The relationship of antiphospholipid antibodies to thromboembolic disease in systemic lupus erythematosus: a cross-sectional study. *Thromb. Haem.*, **66**(5), 520–4.

Love, P. E. and Santoro, S. A. (1990). Antiphospholipid antibodies: anticardiolipin and the lupus anticoagulant in systemic lupus erythematosus (SLE) and in non-SLE disorders. Prevalence and clinical significance. *Ann. Int. Med.*, **112**(9), 682–98.

Lynch, A., Marlar, R., Murphy, J., *et al.* (1994). Antiphospholipid antibodies in predicting adverse pregnancy outcome: a prospective study. *Ann. Int. Med.*, **120**(6), 470–5.

Malm, J., Laurell, M. and Dahlback, B. (1988). Changes in the plasma levels of vitamin K-dependent proteins C and S and of C4b-binding protein during pregnancy and oral contraception. *Br. J. Haematol.*, **68**(4), 437–43.

Maruyama, I., Bell, C. E. and Majerus, P. W. (1985). Thrombomodulin is found on endothelium of arteries, veins, capillaries, and lymphatics, and on syncytiotrophoblast of human placenta. *J. Cell Biol.*, **101**(2), 363–71.

Mateo, J., Oliver, A., Borrell, M., Sala, N. and Fontcuberta, J. (1997). Laboratory evaluation and clinical characteristics of 2,132 consecutive unselected patients with venous thromboembolism – results of the Spanish multicentric study on thrombophilia (EMET-Study). *Thromb. Haem.*, **77**(3), 444–51.

Mathonnet, F., De Mazancourt, P., Bastenaire, B., *et al.* (1996). Activated protein C sensitivity ratio in pregnant women at delivery. *Br. J. Haematol.*, **92**(1), 244–6.

Meekins, J. W., Pijnenborg, R., Hanssens, M., McFadyen, I. R. and Van Asshe, A. (1994). A study of placental bed spiral arteries and trophoblast invasion in normal and severe pre-eclamptic pregnancies. *Br. J. Obstet. Gynaecol.*, **101**(8), 669–74.

Mimuro, S., Lahoud, R., Beutler, L. and Trudinger, B. (1998). Changes of resistance to activated protein C in the course of pregnancy and prevalence of factor V mutation. *Austr. N. Z. J. Obstet. Gynaecol.*, **38**(2), 200–4.

Morrison, E. R., Miedzybrodzka, Z. H., Campbell, D. M., *et al.* (2002). Prothrombotic genotypes are not associated with pre-eclampsia and gestational hypertension: results from a large population-based study and systematic review. *Thromb. Haem.*, **87**(5), 779–85.

Murphy, R. P., Donoghue, C., Nallen, R. J., D'Mello, M., Regan, C., Whitehead, A. S. and Fitzgerald, D. J. (2000). Prospective evaluation of the risk conferred by factor V Leiden and thermolabile methylenetetrahydrofolate reductase polymorphisms in pregnancy. *Arterioscler. Thromb. Vasc. Biol.*, **20**(1), 266–70.

Nagy, B., Toth, T., Rigo, J. Jr., Karadi, I., Romics, L. and Papp, Z. (1998). Detection of factor V Leiden mutation in severe pre-eclamptic Hungarian women. *Clin. Genet.*, **53**(6), 478–81.

Nakabayashi, M., Yamamoto, S. and Suzuki, K. (1999). Analysis of thrombomodulin gene polymorphism in women with severe early-onset preeclampsia. *Semin. Thromb. Hem.*, **25**(5), 473–9.

Novotny, W. F., Brown, S. G., Miletich, J. P., Rader, D. J., and Broze, G. J. Jr. (1991). Plasma antigen levels of the lipoprotein-associated coagulation inhibitor in patient samples. *Blood*, **78**(2), 387–93.

O'Shaughnessy, K. M., Fu, B., Ferraro, F., Lewis, I., Downing, S. and Morris, N. H. (1999). Factor V Leiden and thermolabile methylenetetrahydrofolate reductase gene variants in an East Anglian preeclampsia cohort. *Hypertension*, **33**(6), 1338–41.

Out, H. J., Bruinse, H. W., Christiaens, G. C. M. L., *et al.* (1992). A prospective, controlled multicenter study on the obstetric risks of pregnant women with antiphospholipid antibodies. *Am. J. Obstet. Gynecol.*, **167**(1), 26–32.

Out, H. J., Bruinse, H. W., Christiaens, G. C. M. L., *et al.* (1991). Prevalence of antiphospholipid antibodies in patients wih fetal loss. *Ann. Rheum. Dis.*, **50**(8), 553–7.

Pabinger, I., Grafenhofer, H., Kaider, A., *et al.* (2001). Preeclampsia and fetal loss in women with a history of venous thromboembolism. *Arterioscler. Thromb. Vasc. Biol.*, **21**(5), 874–9.

Parazzini, F., Acaia, B., Faden, D., Lovotti, M., Marelli, G. and Cortelazzo, S. (1991). Antiphospholipid antibodies and recurrent abortion. *Obstet. Gynecol.*, **77**(6), 854–8.

Poort, S. R., Rosendaal, F. R., Reitsma, P. H. and Bertina, R. M. (1996). A common genetic variation in the 3′-untranslated region of the prothrombin gene is associated with elevated plasma prothrombin levels and an increase in venous thrombosis. *Blood*, **88**(10), 3698–703.

Powers, R. W., Minich, L. A., Lykins, D. L., *et al.* (1999). Methylenetetrahydrofolate reductase polymorphism, folate, and susceptibility to preeclampsia. *J. Soc. Gynecol. Invest.*, **6**(2), 74–9.

Rajah, S. B., Moodley, J., Pudifin, D. and Duursma, J. (1990). Anticardiolipin antibodies in hypertensive emergencies in pregnancy. *Clin. Exp. Hypertens. Part B, Hypertens. Pregn.*, **9**(3), 267–71.

Rand, J. H., Wu, X.-X., Andree, H. A. M., *et al.* (1997). Pregnancy loss in the antiphospholipid-antibody syndrome – a possible thrombogenic mechanism. *N. Engl. J. Med.*, **337**(3), 154–60.

Redman, C. W. G. and Sargent, I. L. (2000). Placental debris, oxidative stress and pre-eclampsia. *Placenta*, **21**(7), 597–602.

Rees, D. C., Cox, M. and Clegg, J. B. (1995). World distribution of factor V Leiden. *Lancet*, **346**(8983), 1133–4.

Ridker, P. M., Miletich, J. P., Hennekens, C. H. and Buring, J. E. (1997). Ethnic distribution of factor V Leiden in 4047 men and women: implications for venous thromboembolism screening. *J. Am. Med. Ass.*, **277**(16), 1305–7.

Rigo, J. Jr., Nagy, B., Fintor, L., Tanyi, J., Beke, A., Karadi, I. and Papp, Z. (2000). Maternal and neonatal outcome of preeclamptic pregnancies: the potential roles of Factor V Leiden mutation and 5,10 methylenetetrahydrofolate reductase. *Hypertens. Pregn.*, **19**(2), 163–72.

Rigo, J. J., Nagy, B., Fintor, L., *et al.* (2002). Factor V Leiden mutation and preeclampsia 6 (multiple letters). *Am. J. Obstet. Gynecol.*, **186**(4), 853–4.

Rosendaal, F. R. (1999a). Risk factors for venous thrombotic disease. *Thromb. Haem.*, **82**(2), 610–19.

Rosendaal, F. R. (1999b). Venous thrombosis: a multicausal disease. *Lancet*, **353**(9159), 1167–73.

Rosendaal, F. R., Koster, T., Vandenbroucke, J. P. and Reitsma, P. H. (1995). High risk of thrombosis in patients homozygous for factor V Leiden (activated protein C resistance). *Blood*, **85**(6), 1504–8.

Simioni, P., Prandoni, P., Zanon, E., *et al.* (1996). Deep venous thrombosis and lupus anticoagulant. A case-control study. *Thromb. Haem.*, **76**(2), 187–9.

Sohda, S., Arinami, T., Hamada, H., Yamada, N., Hamaguchi, H. and Kubo, T. (1997). Methylenetetrahydrofolate reductase polymorphism and preeclampsia. *J. Med. Genet.*, **34**(6), 525–6.

Souto, J. C., Coll, I., Llobet, D., *et al.* (1998). The prothrombin 20210A allele is the most prevalent genetic risk factor for venous thromboembolism in the Spanish population. *Thromb. Haem.*, **80**(3), 366–9.

Tait, R. C., Walker, I. D., Perry, D. J., *et al.* (1994). Prevalence of antithrombin deficiency in the healthy population. *Br. J. Haematol.*, **87**(1), 106–12.

Tait, R. C., Walker, I. D., Reitsma, P. H., *et al.* (1995). Prevalence of protein C deficiency in the healthy population. *Thromb. Haem.*, **73**(1), 87–93.

Van Pampus, M. G., Dekker, G. A., Wolf, H., *et al.* (1999). High prevalence of hemostatic abnormalities in women with a history of severe preeclampsia. *Am. J. Obstet. Gynecol.*, **180**(5), 1146–50.

Von Tempelhoff, G.-F., Heilmann, L., Spanuth, E., Kunzmann, E. and Hommel, G. (2000). Incidence of the Factor V Leiden-mutation, coagulation inhibitor deficiency, and elevated antiphospholipid-antibodies in patients with preeclampsia or HELLP-Syndrome. *Thromb. Res.*, **100**(4), 363–5.

Yasuda, M., Takakuwa, K., Tokunaga, A. and Tanaka, K. (1995). Prospective studies of the association between anticardiolipin antibody and outcome of pregnancy. *Obstet. Gynecol.*, **86**(4), 555–9.

Young, J. K., Williamson, R. A., Murray, J. C., *et al.* (2001). Genetic susceptibility to preeclampsia: roles of cytosine-to-thymine substitution at nucleotide 677 of the gene for methylenetetrahydrofolate reductase, 68-base pair insertion at nucleotide 844 of the gene for cystathionine beta-synthase, and factor V Leiden mutation. *Am. J. Obstet. Gynecol.*, **184**(6), 1211–17.

Zusterzeel, P. L. M., Visser, W., Blom, H. J., Peters, W. H. M., Heil, S. G. and Steegers, E. A. P. (2000). Methylenetetrahydrofolate reductase polymorphisms in preeclampsia and the HELLP syndrome. *Hypertens. Pregn.*, **19**(3), 299–307.

22

Medical illness and the risk of pre-eclampsia

Catherine Nelson-Piercy

Introduction

Many different medical illnesses predispose women to pre-eclampsia. Some of these are logical, well known, and accepted, such as pre-existing hypertension or diabetes. Others are less well known or more controversial, such as migraine and asthma. Correct identification of women at increased risk for pre-eclampsia allows appropriate channeling of antenatal care and allocation of resources to maximize the chances of early diagnosis and appropriate management. In addition, strategies to screen for and prevent pre-eclampsia are often more effective in high-risk women. It is important that women with medical diseases associated with an increased risk of pre-eclampsia and the related complications of intrauterine growth restriction and prematurity are appropriately counseled, ideally prior to pregnancy. In many cases appropriate and optimal pre-conception control of the medical illness may reduce the risk of pre-eclampsia.

The risk factors for pre-eclampsia are listed in Table 22.1. This chapter will cover the general, obstetric and medical risk factors. These general and obstetric risk factors are discussed since, although not representing medical illness themselves, they may often complicate or coexist with medical illness. They may therefore add to the already elevated risk of pre-eclampsia associated with the medical illness, e.g. obese women who are more likely to be hypertensive. Medical illness may affect fertility resulting in a delay before child bearing or longer interbirth interval, e.g. women

with renal failure who have reduced fertility. It is the individualized cumulative risk of these various factors that is important for clinical practice. Thus, an obese 40-year-old woman with hypertension in her first pregnancy is at higher risk for superimposed pre-eclampsia than a multiparous hypertensive woman aged 24 and with a normal body mass index.

General risk factors

Age

The risk of pre-eclampsia is increased at the extremes of reproductive ages. Many retrospective cohort studies in different populations have demonstrated an increased risk of pre-eclampsia in older women. In a New York population Bianco and colleagues (1996) compared pregnancy outcomes in 1404 women aged 40 years or older to those of 6978 control women aged 20–29 years. They found a significant increase in the incidence of pre-eclampsia in both nulliparous [odds ratio = 1.8 (95% CI, 1.3–2.6)] and multiparous women [odds ratio 1.9 (95% CI, 1.2–2.9)]. In a group of 183 women of mixed parity aged 40 years or over at delivery the risk of developing pre-eclampsia was increased [odds ratio 1.59 (95% CI, 1.13–2.23)] compared to the general obstetric population (Lehmann and Chism, 1987).

In an Asian population of 29,375 women from Taiwan, in whom the incidence of pre-eclampsia was 1.4%, age over 34 years was associated with

Table 22.1. Risk factors for pre-eclampsia

General
Age <20 years, >35 years
Obesity
Genetic
Mother 20–25%
Sister 35–40%
Obstetric
Previous pre-eclampsia
Primiparity
Long birth interval
Multiple pregnancy
Hydatidiform mole
Hydrops/triploidy
IVF using surgically obtained sperm or donor eggs
Medical
Hypertension
Diabetes
(Type I/Insulin dependent diabetes [IDDM], Type
    II/Non-insulin dependent diabetes [NIDDM], and
    Gestational diabetes [GDM])
Renal disease
Systemic lupus erythematosus (SLE)/Antiphospholipid
    syndrome (APS)
Heritable thrombophilia (see Chapter 20)
Asthma
Migraine

a significantly increased risk [odds ratio 1.8 (95% CI, 1.4–2.4)] of pre-eclampsia (Lee *et al.*, 2000). A retrospective cross-sectional study in Latin American and Caribbean women (Conde-Agudelo and Belizan, 2000a) found an increased risk of pre-eclampsia in women aged 35 or older (RR = 1.67 (95% CI, 1.58–1.77)). A study of 9556 pregnancies demonstrated that multiparous women aged 35 or older were at two and a half times the risk [RR = 2.58 (95% CI, 1.97–3.38)] of pre-eclampsia compared to multiparous women aged 20–29 years (Bobrowski and Bottoms, 1995).

A systematic review (Duckitt and Harrington, 2005) concludes that a maternal age over 40 roughly doubles the risk of pre-eclampsia in both primiparous [RR = 1.88 (95% CI, 1.42–2.5)] and multiparous [RR = 2.0 (95% CI, 1.45–2.75)] women.

This is one of the many powerful arguments justifying the labeling of women aged 40 years or over as "high risk." It also contributes to the rationale for discouraging the delay in child bearing that so often accompanies a professional career and the changing role of women in society.

The relative risk is lower for those aged 19 or under compared to those older than 19 [RR = 1.31 95% CI, 1.15–1.49] (Duckitt and Harrington, 2005).

Obesity

Obesity is often associated with other conditions that predispose to pre-eclampsia including type II (non-insulin-dependent, maturity onset) diabetes, gestational diabetes and hypertension (see below). Few studies have been performed to clarify whether obesity acts as an independent risk factor for pre-eclampsia when it coexists with these medical conditions.

High body mass index and obesity is one of the few modifiable risk factors for pre-eclampsia. Using the Swedish Medical Birth Register, an analysis of 10,666 nulliparous women aged under 35 years revealed an incidence of pre-eclampsia of 5.2% (Ros *et al.*, 1998). The risk of pre-eclampsia was significantly increased in obese women with a body mass index (BMI) greater than 29 compared to underweight women (BMI less than 19.8) [odds ratio = 5.19 (95% CI, 2.35–11.48)] and compared to those with a normal BMI (19–26) [RR = 2.84 (95% CI, 1.75–4.59)]. The relative risk was lower, but still significant, for overweight women (pre-pregnancy BMI 26–29) compared to those with normal BMI (19–26) [RR = 2.01 (95% CI, 1.25–3.26)].

A retrospective cohort study comparing 613 morbidly obese women (BMI >35) with 11,313 non-obese women (BMI 19–27) found an over fourfold increase in the risk of pre-eclampsia in the obese women [odds ratio = 4.39 (95% CI, 3.52–5.49)] (Bianco *et al.*, 1998). A retrospective cohort study in Asian women demonstrated an odds ratio of 2.4 (95% CI, 1.8–3.1) for women with a pre-pregnancy BMI >24.2. (Lee *et al.*, 2000). In Latin American and Caribbean women

(Conde-Agudelo and Belizan, 2000a) both obese (pre-pregnancy BMI >29) and overweight (pre-pregnancy BMI 26.1−29) women had an increased risk [RR = 2.81 95% CI, 2.69−2.94; RR = 1.57 95% CI, 1.49−1.64, respectively] compared to those women with a normal pre-pregnancy BMI (19.8−26).

In 4314 healthy nulliparous women from the United States, of whom 7.6% developed pre-eclampsia, the risk of pre-eclampsia increased significantly ($P < 0.0001$) with increased BMI. When women with an initial prenatal care visit (booking visit) BMI greater than 35 were compared with controls (BMI 20−26) the odds ratio for pre-eclampsia was 2.12 (95% CI, 1.56−2.88). The relative risk was less if all overweight women (booking BMI 26−35) were compared with controls [RR = 1.46 (95% CI, 1.15−1.84)] (Sibai et al., 1997).

It has been shown that waist circumference in early pregnancy, a measure of central obesity and associated with insulin resistance, is directly associated with the risk of pre-eclampsia (Sattar et al., 2001).

Management

Obese and overweight women should be advised to eat healthily and loose weight before embarking on a pregnancy. This is particularly important for those with other risk factors for cardiovascular mortality, and for those with previous pre-eclampsia or gestational diabetes. The benefits for long-term health and pregnancy outcome should be explained. Recent studies have highlighted the subsequent risk of ischemic heart disease (Smith et al., 2001), stroke (Irgens et al., 2001) and death (Wilson et al., 2003) following a history of pre-eclampsia. Smith and colleagues found that BW < 20th percentile, preterm delivery and pre-eclampsia all approximately doubled the risk of ischemic heart disease or death in the mother after 15−19 year follow-up. The risks were additive, so if all were present there was a sevenfold increase in adverse events in the mother. This study is consistent with the Norwegian study of Irgens and coworkers (Irgens et al., 2001) showing an eightfold

risk of cardiovascular death in women who had pre-eclampsia and a preterm delivery. Wilson and colleagues (2003) have demonstrated a significant association between pre-eclampsia and death from stroke (RR 3.59, 95% CI 1.04−12.4). Irgens et al. (2001) hypothesize that genetic factors increasing the risk of cardiovascular disease may also increase the risk of pre-eclampsia. Equally there may be some common clinical risk factor, and obesity is a strong candidate.

Obstetric risk factors

Previous pre-eclampsia

This is one of the best predictors of pre-eclampsia. In a study of almost 30,000 Asian women a history of pre-eclampsia gave an odds ratio of 6.3 (95% CI, 4.4−9.2) for developing pre-eclampsia in a subsequent pregnancy (Lee et al., 2000). Systematic review revealed that if a woman had pre-eclampsia in her first pregnancy, the risk of pre-eclampsia in a second pregnancy is increased sevenfold (OR = 7.02, 95% CI 5.65−8.73) compared with women who did not have previous pre-eclampsia (Duckitt and Harrington, 2005).

The recurrence risks for pre-eclampsia are higher in women with other underlying risk factors such as pre-existing hypertension, and also in those women who suffer severe early onset pre-eclampsia. In one study of mostly African American women with previous HELLP syndrome (Sibai et al., 1993), the recurrence risk of pre-eclampsia was 75% in women with hypertension that predated the pregnancy complicated by HELLP syndrome.

Management

Pre-conceptual counseling may be helpful to women who have previously had a pregnancy complicated by pre-eclampsia. In practice this often takes place soon after the pre-eclamptic pregnancy, especially if that pregnancy was also complicated by fetal or neonatal morbidity/mortality or severe maternal morbidity. It is important to search for possible underlying risk factors for pre-eclampsia in such women, since these may require further investigation or treatment, and their presence will increase the recurrence risk of pre-eclampsia. In most women with pre-eclampsia, the hypertension and proteinuria resolve within 6 months postpartum. If either persists beyond this time further investigation is warranted, and pre-existing (or newly developed) hypertension or renal disease is likely. Similarly, mild derangement of renal function is common in pre-eclampsia and therefore a raised serum creatinine postpartum may be wrongly attributed to the pre-eclampsia. If this persists, or is out of proportion to the other clinical features of pre-eclampsia, a search for confirmation of underlying renal impairment is warranted.

Women with previous severe or early onset pre-eclampsia should be offered screening for antiphospholipid syndrome, an acquired thrombophilia (see below). The issue of screening for inherited thrombophilias is more controversial (Nelson-Piercy, 1999; Powers et al., 1999; O'Shaughnessy et al., 1999). Postnatal screening for maternal thrombophilias in 102 women with severe pre-eclampsia and other complications in a UK population did not reveal a higher prevalence than in controls (Alfirevic et al., 2001). A systematic review (Alfirevic et al., 2002) found that thrombophilias were associated with adverse pregnancy outcomes, including pre-eclampsia, but the odds ratios were small. For example, the odds ratio for heterozygous Factor V Leiden was 1.6 (95% CI 1.2–2.1) and the authors concluded that the studies published so far are too small to adequately assess the true size of this association. Furthermore, they opined that screening for thrombophilia should not become standard practice. A more recent meta-analysis by Rey and colleagues (2003) concluded that the magnitude of the association between thrombophilia and fetal loss (an outcome frequently associated with severe pre-eclampsia) varies according not only to the type of thrombophilia but also the type of fetal loss (Rey et al., 2003). For example, Factor V Leiden was

associated with late recurrent fetal loss (RR 7.83, 95% CI 2.83–21.67) but MTHFR mutation, protein C deficiency and antithrombin deficiency were not.

Those women whose previous pregnancy was complicated by pre-eclampsia are understandably anxious about recurrence and may have been inappropriately reassured that pre-eclampsia is unlikely to recur. Their relative and absolute risk is at least as high as a nulliparous woman. Much anxiety can be allayed with the knowledge that they will be closely followed up in any subsequent pregnancy to maximize the chances of early diagnosis and appropriate management. A prospective management plan should be agreed upon with the woman and carefully documented in the notes and in a letter sent to the patient and the general practitioner/primary care physician.

Parity

A retrospective cross-sectional study of Latin American and Caribbean women using a perinatal database from Uruguay (Conde-Agudelo and Belizan, 2000a) found an incidence of pre-eclampsia of 4.8%. The relative risk for pre-eclampsia in nulliparous women was 2.38 (95% CI, 2.28–2.49). In a study of Asian women from Taiwan (Lee et al., 2000), the relative risk in nulliparous women was lower (RR = 1.3, 95% CI, 1.2–1.5).

In a systematic review of 15 studies, nulliparity more than doubled the risk for pre-eclampsia (Duckitt and Harrington, 2005): RR = 2.6 (95% CI, 1.16–5.86).

However, many studies have demonstrated that although at lower risk, it is the multiparous women who often develop severe disease, and relative to their risk of pre-eclampsia, they have a higher risk of severe morbidity and mortality. Of the 15 women dying from pre-eclampsia in the UK between 1997 and 1999, over a third were multiparous (Department of Health, 2001) and in 2000–2 half of the maternal deaths from pre-eclampsia occurred in multiparous women (CEMACH, 2004). In the British Eclampsia Survey (Douglas and Redman, 1994), 18% of women with eclampsia were multiparous and did not have a history of pre-eclampsia in a previous pregnancy. Of a cohort of 89 women with renal failure complicating pre-eclampsia in Cape Town, South Africa, 57% were multiparous (Drakeley *et al.*, 2002). In a study of 37 pre-eclamptic women developing pulmonary edema, 62% were multiparous (Sibai *et al.*, 1987). Although often overlooked, the greatest age-related increases in risk for pre-eclampsia (and other adverse outcomes) occur in multiparous women (Bobrowski and Bottoms, 1995).

Long interbirth interval

In a recent retrospective study of over 500,000 women over a period of 30 years, Skjaeren and colleagues (2002) demonstrated that the risk of pre-eclampsia in a second or third pregnancy was directly related to time elapsed since the previous delivery. After controlling for change of partner, maternal age and year of delivery there was an approximately 12% increase in the risk of pre-eclampsia for each year between pregnancies [RR per year = 1.12 (95% CI, 1.11–1.13)]. The risk of pre-eclampsia in multiparous women returns to the levels seen in primiparous women (3.9%) if more than 10 years have elapsed since the last pregnancy, even if the woman has not changed partner. The authors conclude that one of the main reasons that a change of partner is associated with an increased risk of pre-eclampsia is because this is often associated with a long interbirth interval. A retrospective cross-sectional study using a perinatal database from Uruguay (Conde-Agudelo and Belizan, 2000b) found that the relative risk for pre-eclampsia in women with an inter-pregnancy interval of longer than 59 months was almost twice as high as in those with an interval of 18–23 months (RR 1.83, 95% CI 1.72–1.94). These conclusions have been challenged by others, and the findings of the Skjaerven paper (Skjaerven *et al.*, 2002) in particular are more completely discussed in the chapter by Dekker and Robillard in this book.

Multiple pregnancy

The risk of pre-eclampsia is increased in twins and higher-order multiple births. In a Swedish study of 10,666 nulliparous women aged under 35 years, twin pregnancy was associated with a quadrupling (RR = 4.17, 95% CI, 2.3–7.55) in the risk of pre-eclampsia (Ros *et al.*, 1998). A retrospective cohort study in Asian women demonstrated an odds ratio of 3.6 (95% CI, 2.4–5.5) for women with multiple pregnancies (Lee *et al.*, 2000). In Latin American and Caribbean women (Conde-Agudelo and Belizan, 2000a) the relative risk for pre-eclampsia in multiple pregnancies was 2.1 (95% CI, 1.9–2.32).

A systematic review of eight studies has shown that the risk of pre-eclampsia is more than doubled in twin compared to singleton pregnancy (Duckitt and Harrington, 2005): RR = 2.38 (95% CI, 1.71–3.32). This risk was not influenced by either chorionicity or zygosity. In the Confidential Enquiry into Maternal Deaths 1997–99 (Department of Health, 2001), 20% of those dying from pre-eclampsia had multiple pregnancies, and the report included a recommendation that this risk should be heeded and antenatal care modified accordingly.

Therefore, women with medical illnesses who are undergoing assisted reproduction, and who are often at increased risk of pre-eclampsia for other reasons, need very careful counseling regarding the added risk of pre-eclampsia related to multiple pregnancy. Indeed, in those undergoing in vitro fertilization (IVF) in whom the baseline risk is high, some would argue that only one embryo should be replaced.

Assisted reproduction

Gamete donation increases the risk of pre-eclampsia. In a study from Leeds, the rate of pre-eclampsia was increased (18.1%) in women with pregnancies conceived as the result of donated sperm, donated oocytes or donated embryos compared to controls (1.4%) with pregnancies conceived with their own gametes either spontaneously or using intrauterine insemination with their partner's sperm (Salha *et al.*, 1999). Furthermore, if surgically obtained sperm is used for intra-cytoplasmic sperm injection (ICSI) the risk of pre-eclampsia in an ensuing pregnancy is increased (11%) compared to pregnancies resulting from in vitro fertilization or ICSI using ejaculated sperm (4%), suggesting a protective effect of semen exposure (Wang *et al.*, 2002). Readers interested in a more in-depth discussion of this subject are referred to the chapter on immune maladaptation in pre-eclampsia by Dekker and Robillard in this book.

Because of the effect of certain medical conditions (for example, renal disease) or their treatments (for example, cyclophosphamide for systemic lupus erythematosus) on fertility, these issues related to assisted reproduction are extremely pertinent. Regrettably, however, the desire of women to have children tempers the assimilation of possible risks associated with assisted reproduction. It is the responsibility of the providers of assisted conception techniques to ensure that women and their partners understand these associated risks before embarking on fertility treatment.

Medical conditions predisposing to pre-eclampsia

Several medical conditions increase the risk of pre-eclampsia. The commonest are hypertension and diabetes. For most of these conditions, the risk of pre-eclampsia is higher if the underlying medical disease is more severe. Conversely the risk is less if the illness is less severe, and may be reduced by optimal control of the medical condition prior to pregnancy. The management of women with medical illness in pregnancy provides particular challenges to the clinician not just because of their higher risk of pre-eclampsia.

Pre-existing/chronic hypertension

Women with pre-existing hypertension have an increased risk of superimposed pre-eclampsia.

A Canadian study found an incidence of pre-eclampsia of 21.2% in 337 women with chronic hypertension compared to an incidence of 2.3% in the control population ($P < 0.01$) (Rey and Couturier, 1994). In a study of 169 pregnancies in 156 women with chronic hypertension 34.3% developed superimposed pre-eclampsia (Mabie *et al.*, 1986). More recent studies have confirmed these observations. A large cross-sectional study from South America found that chronic hypertension was associated with a doubling of the risk of pre-eclampsia [RR = 1.99 (95% CI 1.78–2.22)] (Conde-Agudelo and Belizan, 2000a).

This increased risk of pre-eclampsia is related to the degree of hypertension. In a study of 211 women with mild hypertension (diastolic blood pressure 90–110 mmHg) the incidence of super-imposed pre-eclampsia was 10% (Sibai *et al.*, 1983). In those women with severe hypertension, defined as a diastolic blood pressure of 110 mmHg or higher before 20 weeks gestation, a study from New Zealand of 155 hypertensive women demonstrated a risk of superimposed pre-eclampsia of 46% compared to 14% for women with mild hypertension [odds ratio 5.2 (95% confidence interval 1.5–17.2)] (McCowan *et al.*, 1996). Both diastolic and systolic hypertension increase the risk of super-imposed pre-eclampsia. In an analysis of risk factors for pre-eclampsia in nulliparous women (Sibai *et al.*, 1997) the odds ratio for a systolic blood pressure in early pregnancy of 120 mmHg or more compared with < 101 mmHg was 2.66. Similarly the odds ratio for a diastolic blood pressure of greater than 60 mmHg compared with less than 60 mmHg was 1.72 (Sibai *et al.*, 1997).

Management

Since severe hypertension carries a higher risk of super-imposed pre-eclampsia than mild hypertension (McCowan *et al.*, 1996), the blood pressure should be optimally controlled prior to pregnancy. A Cochrane review of 19 trials in 2402 women (Abalos *et al.*, 2003) showed that antihypertensive therapy given in pregnancy does not prevent super-imposed pre-eclampsia [RR = 0.99 (95% CI 0.84–1.18)], but it halves the risk of severe hypertension [RR = 0.52 (95% CI 0.41–0.64)] and therefore reduces the risk of dangerous complications such as maternal cerebral hemorrhage.

Traditionally, the drug of choice to treat pre-existing hypertension in pregnancy has been methyldopa. However, beta-blockers are becoming more popular, especially in the USA, as a first choice agent in pregnant women with chronic hypertension. Labetalol, in particular, a combined alpha- and beta-blocker, is recommended by the American College of Obstetricians and Gynecologists as a first line therapy for women with pre-existing chronic hypertension (ACOG Practice Bulletin #29, July 2001, Chronic Hypertension in Pregnancy). Beta-blockers have fewer maternal side effects than methyldopa, but their safety in the fetus is not as well established as with methyldopa. There is some concern that beta-blockers may inhibit fetal growth when used long-term (and started in the first trimester) throughout pregnancy, but claims of neonatal hypotension and hypoglycemia have not been substantiated in the randomized controlled trials performed. There is no evidence for the superiority of any one beta-blocker over the others. Beta-blockers should not be given to women with a history of asthma (Magee et al., 1999).

Second-line drugs for the treatment of hypertension in pregnancy include calcium antagonists (e.g. slow-release nifedipine), and hydralazine. These may be used in conjunction with first-line therapy in those women resistant to monotherapy. Side effects of vasodilators include headache, facial flushing and edema, and may necessitate withdrawal in some patients. Alpha-adrenergic blockers are also safe and can be used as second- or third-line therapy. Diuretics should only be used in pregnancy for the treatment of heart failure and pulmonary edema. They are relatively contraindicated in pre-eclampsia because they cause further depletion of an already reduced intravascular volume. The angiotensin-converting enzyme (ACE) inhibitors (e.g. ramipril, enalapril) should not be used in pregnancy because they may cause oligohydramnios, renal failure and hypotension in the fetus. Their use has been associated with decreased skull ossification, hypocalvaria and renal tubular dysgenesis, and there is also a risk of intrauterine death. Any woman on maintenance therapy with an ACE inhibitor should discontinue this (and if necessary switch to methyldopa or labetalol) before pregnancy. The use of these drugs in the first trimester is associated with structural malformations (Cooper et al., 2006). There are few data concerning the newer angiotensin II-receptor blockers agents (e.g. losartan) in pregnancy, but they are similar to the ACE inhibitors and therefore should be avoided (Nelson-Piercy, 2006).

It is acceptable for women to conceive while continuing to take their usual antihypertensive medication, except ACE inhibitors (Cooper et al., 2006). Once pregnancy is confirmed, this can be discontinued. If a woman only requires one antihypertensive agent to control her blood pressure outside of pregnancy, and the blood pressure is < 140/90 mmHg when first seen in pregnancy, it is usually possible to delay the introduction of antihypertensive medication because of the physiological decrease in blood pressure that occurs in early pregnancy. Women with severe hypertension (>170/110) and those requiring more than one agent should be converted directly to one of the first-line drugs.

If hypertension is noted for the first time in the first trimester or early second trimester, it is likely that it is a chronic, pre-existing problem, since pregnancy-induced hypertension (including pre-eclampsia) usually, but not invariably, appears in the second half of pregnancy. Hypertension in any young person should not be attributed to essential hypertension (particularly in the absence of a family history) before secondary causes such as renal or cardiac disease (coarctation of the aorta), and rarely Cushing's syndrome, Conn's syndrome (and other causes of hyperaldosteronism) or phaeochromocytoma have been excluded. Of these, the commonest secondary cause encountered is renal disease, including particularly in women of child-bearing age reflux nephropathy, glomerulonephritis and renal artery stenosis. Therefore, women presenting with hypertension for the first time in early pregnancy should be examined for clues to a possible secondary cause. This should include urinalysis for protein and blood, examination of the femoral pulses (looking for radiofemoral delay suggesting coarctation of the aorta) and a search for renal bruits (possible renal artery stenosis). A simple screen with serum creatinine, urea (to exclude renal impairment), and electrolytes (to exclude hypokalemia which may suggest hyperaldosteronism) should be performed. Urinary catecholamines should be measured in cases suggestive of phaeochromocytoma (Nelson-Piercy, 2006).

Diabetes

Diabetes roughly doubles the risk of pre-eclampsia (Garner *et al.*, 1990). A Canadian study of 334 diabetic pregnancies found an incidence of pre-eclampsia of 9.9% in the diabetic women compared with 4.3% in the non-diabetic controls (Garner *et al.*, 1990). Women with pre-existing diabetes (both type I and type II) have a higher risk than those with gestational diabetes. In a Swedish cohort study (Ros *et al.*, 1998) the relative risk of pre-eclampsia was higher for type I diabetes [RR = 5.58 (95% CI, 2.72−11.43)] than for gestational diabetes [RR = 3.11 (95% CI, 1.61−6.0)]. This increased risk in type I diabetes is remarkably similar to that found in a Finnish study where the odds ratio for pre-eclampsia was 5.2 (95% CI 3.3−8.4) (Hiilesmaa *et al.*, 2000).

Among women with type I diabetes the risk of pre-eclampsia varies from 12.8% (Hiilesmaa *et al.*, 2000), to 14% (Garner *et al.*, 1990) to 21.3% (Ros *et al.*, 1998) and systematic review demonstrates a fourfold increased risk for pre-existing diabetes (Duckitt and Harrington, 2005).

The risk of pre-eclampsia relates to the severity of the underlying diabetes. Women without microvascular complications of diabetes are at lower risk than those with renal or retinal complications (Sibai, 2000). The Finnish study, for example, where the incidence of pre-eclampsia was 12.8%, specifically excluded women with nephropathy (Hiilesmaa *et al.*, 2000). In a literature review, Sibai (2000) demonstrated that the rates of pre-eclampsia for women with type 1 diabetes without nephropathy ranged from 9 to 17%, but that for those with diabetic nephropathy the rates were 35−66%.

A Danish study of 240 Caucasian women with pre-existing type I diabetes found an increasing incidence of pre-eclampsia with worsening nephropathy. In women with no proteinuria the incidence was 6%, those with microalbuminuria (24 hourly urinary albumin 30−300 mg) had a 42% incidence, and those with frank nephropathy (24 hourly urinary albumin >300 mg) a 64% incidence ($P < 0.001$) (Ekbom *et al.*, 2001).

Other risk factors for an increased risk of pre-eclampsia in women with type 1 diabetes include a longer duration of the diabetes, the co-existence of chronic hypertension, and poor glycemic control prior to 20 weeks gestation (Sibai, 2000). There is a direct relationship between the glycemic control in early pregnancy, based on HbA1c, and the risk of pre-eclampsia. Hiilesmaa and colleagues found an adjusted odds ratio of 1.6 (95% CI 1.3−2.0) for each 1% increment in the HbA1c measured in the first trimester. For each 1% fall in HbA1c achieved during the first half of pregnancy the odds ratio was 0.6 (95% CI 0.5−0.8) (Hiilesmaa *et al.*, 2000).

In gestational diabetes the risk of pre-eclampsia is doubled. A retrospective cohort study from Canada (Xiong *et al.*, 2001) of 2755 women with gestational diabetes found an increased risk of pre-eclampsia (RR = 2.58 95%, CI 2.04−3.28). In the South American study (Conde-Agudelo and Belizan, 2000a) the relative risk of pre-eclampsia was 1.93 in the women with gestational diabetes (95% CI 1.66−2.25). A similar direct relationship between degree of carbohydrate intolerance and the risk of pre-eclampsia is also seen in women without overt gestational diabetes but with impaired carbohydrate tolerance in pregnancy (Sermer et al., 1998).

Recently it has been argued that obesity is an important confounding variable and in one study gestational diabetes and obesity were not independent risk factors for hypertensive disorders in pregnancy (van Hoorn et al., 2002).

Management

In women with diabetes, it is important to document and quantify any prepregnancy (and/or early pregnancy) hypertension or proteinuria, since this allows not only a baseline on which to assess subsequent increases, but also accurate counseling regarding the risk of pre-eclampsia. The above data (Hiilesmaa et al., 2000; Sibai, 2000) provide a clear rationale for optimal control of diabetes before conception, in early pregnancy, and for the first half of pregnancy, since a reduction in HbA1c will reduce the risk of pre-eclampsia. There are many other reasons why good diabetic control before and throughout pregnancy is desirable, including the associated reduction in congenital abnormalities, macrosomia, perinatal morbidity and mortality.

Systemic lupus erythematosus and antiphospholipid syndrome

Pregnancy in systemic lupus erythematosus (SLE) is associated with an increased risk of pre-eclampsia (Khamashta and Hughes, 1997). However, this risk is largely attributable to the presence of certain risk factors, particularly the presence of antiphospholipid antibodies (APAs), renal involvement of the lupus with or without hypertension, and active disease at the time of conception (Nelson-Piercy and Khamashta, 2003). Thus for women with SLE without antiphospholipid antibodies, lupus nephritis, or hypertension whose disease is quiescent at the time of conception, the risk of pre-eclampsia is probably not increased compared to the background rate. One exception to this may be women who suffer a flare of their SLE in pregnancy or those requiring high doses of prednisolone (Huong et al., 2001a). Disease flare may be difficult to differentiate from pre-eclampsia and may also precipitate pre-eclampsia. High doses of prednisolone such as may be required to treat a severe flare of SLE in pregnancy have been associated with an increased risk of hypertension in pregnancy (Laskin et al., 1997).

Antiphospholipid syndrome (APS) is discussed below. Women with proteinuria (as above for diabetes) or renal impairment (see below) from any cause have an increased risk of super-imposed pre-eclampsia. Even quiescent renal lupus is associated with an increased risk of fetal loss, pre-eclampsia and IUGR, particularly if there is hypertension or proteinuria. In a study of 32 pregnancies in 22 women with biopsy proven lupus nephritis, 5 women (16%) developed pre-eclampsia even though all but one of the 22 women had a baseline serum creatinine of $<100\,mol\,l^{-1}$(1.13 mg dl^{-1}) and none had hypertension (Huong et al., 2001b).

Antiphospholipid syndrome (APS) is defined as the presence of lupus anticoagulant and/or anticardiolipin antibodies on two occasions 6 weeks apart in association with a clinical history of thrombosis (arterial, venous or thrombotic microangiopathy affecting the kidney) or adverse pregnancy outcome (one or more fetal death after 10 weeks, or three or more pre-embryonic/embryonic losses, delivery before 35 weeks because of pre-eclampsia or intrauterine growth restriction) (Wilson et al., 1999). Women with APS may or may not have associated SLE. Those without associated connective tissue disease are termed primary APS (PAPS). All women with APS, whether primary or associated with SLE, are at increased risk of pre-eclampsia, but this risk varies depending on the clinical characteristics of the APS (Ware-Branch and Khamashta, 2003). Those women diagnosed with APS because of recurrent miscarriage carry a lower risk of pre-eclampsia. Two studies of women with APS recruited from recurrent miscarriage clinics found incidences of pre-eclampsia of 3%

in 53 pregnancies (Granger and Farquharson, 1997) and 11% in 150 pregnancies (Backos et al., 1999). Women with APS with associated SLE, thromboses and previous late-pregnancy losses are at extremely high risk of pre-eclampsia, varying from 18% (Lima et al., 1996) to 51% (Ware-Branch et al., 1992). Furthermore, there is an association between APS and early onset severe pre-eclampsia (Huong et al., 2001a; Moodley et al., 1995; Ware-Branch et al., 1992). This is reflected in the updated clinical classification criteria for APS that now include premature birth before 35 weeks due to severe pre-eclampsia (Wilson et al., 1999).

The pathogenesis of fetal loss and pre-eclampsia in APS is not fully known, but is likely to be closely related to the pathogenesis of thrombosis in APS. There is typically massive infarction and thrombosis of the placental and decidual vessels, probably secondary to spiral artery vasculopathy. Platelet deposition and prostanoid imbalance may be implicated in a similar way to pre-eclampsia. It is hypothesized that adverse pregnancy outcome and pre-eclampsia relates to thrombosis within the placenta. aPLs cause thrombosis via a co-factor β_2-glycoprotein which is the target antigen for aCL. β_2-glycoprotein is an endogenous coagulation inhibitor and its binding by aCL may underlie APS-associated thrombosis (Ware-Branch, 1994). APLs may mediate interference with trophoblastic annexin V causing localized thrombosis in the placenta (Levine et al., 2002).

Management

The management of APS in pregnancy includes low-dose aspirin and unfractionated or low molecular weight heparin (LMWH) (Nelson-Piercy and Khamashta, 2003), although the additional benefit of LMWH over and above aspirin is controversial. The randomized studies examining the efficacy of such strategies have used fetal loss rates and live birth rates as outcome measures (Farquharson et al., 2002; Kutteh, 1996; Rai et al., 1997). Data relating to incidence of pre-eclampsia come predominantly from retrospective cohort studies.

Therefore it is difficult to be certain that treatment with aspirin and/or LMWH reduces the incidence of pre-eclampsia in women with APS. Indeed studies demonstrating a beneficial effect of aspirin and heparin find that this benefit relates mainly to a reduction in miscarriage, rather than a difference in birth weight or gestational age (and therefore a likely reduction in pre-eclampsia) within those women achieving a live birth. Furthermore, it may be the case that successful treatment to prevent fetal losses and miscarriage results in a paradoxically higher rate of pre-eclampsia as the pregnancy progresses into the third trimester. However, when women with APS and previous late losses, neonatal deaths and/or early-onset pre-eclampsia are treated with aspirin and LMWH in subsequent pregnancies, success is normally associated with at least a reduction in the severity of pre-eclampsia, if indeed it develops.

Treatment with intravenous immunoglobulin has been shown to confer no additional benefit over aspirin and LMWH (Triolo et al., 2003).

Renal disease

Renal disease, and particularly renal impairment from any cause, is associated with an increased risk of pre-eclampsia. This risk is directly related to the degree of renal impairment. Those with severe renal impairment (serum creatinine $> 250 \, \text{mol}\,\text{l}^{-1}$ [2.8 mg dl^{-1}]) and hypertension have a less than 50% chance of successful pregnancy, often developing severe, early onset pre-eclampsia with marked IUGR (Davison and Baylis, 2002; Epstein, 1996; Jones and Hayslett, 1996; Jungers and Chauveau, 1997).

This risk is also relevant for women who have received renal allografts that may not be functioning optimally or are experiencing chronic rejection (Armenti et al., 1995). Data from the UK National Transplant Registry of 377 pregnancies reveals an incidence of pre-eclampsia of 27% (Armenti et al., 1998).

Renal disease is often associated with hypertension and this further compounds the risk of superimposed pre-eclampsia. Meticulous control of any associated hypertension both prior to and during pregnancy is essential to protect the kidneys from further damage. Control prior to pregnancy may reduce the risk of pre-eclampsia.

Asthma

The association of asthma with an increased risk of pre-eclampsia is much more controversial. In a review of the incidence of pre-eclampsia in asthmatic women, Schatz and Dombrowski (2000) report significantly increased incidences (RR = 2.2–3.2) in three studies, but no increase in five studies. In a historical cohort analysis using hospital discharge data of 8672 cases of pregnant asthmatics in Canada, Wen and colleagues (2001) demonstrated an increased risk of pre-eclampsia (adjusted odds ratio 1.84, 95% CI 1.64, 2.05) in women with asthma compared to a control population.

There are several possible explanations for this association if indeed it is real. First the prevalence of pre-existing hypertension has been reported to be approximately 2–3.5-fold higher in pregnant asthmatic women (Schatz and Dombrowski, 2000). However, the study by Wen and coworkers controlled for pre-existing hypertension (Wen et al., 2001). Second there may be common pathogenic factors for asthma and pre-eclampsia, linking for example bronchial hyperactivity and vascular hyper-reactivity. Last the association may be a medication effect. This is supported by the fact that in some studies an increased incidence of pre-eclampsia is only demonstrated in subgroups of asthmatics treated with steroids. Using multivariate regression techniques, Schatz et al. (1997) reported an independent association (RR = 2.0, P = 0.027) between the use of oral corticosteroids and pre-eclampsia in asthmatic women. If oral corticosteroids do increase the risk of pre-eclampsia, as would be supported by the data for SLE (see above), this has implications for a possible increased risk of pre-eclampsia in women with other conditions that may require steroid therapy in pregnancy.

Management of women with medical conditions associated with an increased risk of pre-eclampsia

Management should begin with pre-pregnancy counseling. It is important that women understand the risk of pre-eclampsia. Since the above medical conditions are often associated with early onset and severe pre-eclampsia the associated risk of severe prematurity should be explained. The risk of pre-eclampsia may be modified by the pre-pregnancy control of diabetes and hypertension and by ensuring that SLE and renal disease are in remission or stable.

Antenatal management

Women with underlying medical conditions associated with an increased risk of pre-eclampsia require increased antenatal surveillance. One of the clinical problems arising in these women is the difficulty of reaching a diagnosis of pre-eclampsia when some of the features (e.g. hypertension, proteinuria, thrombocytopenia) may be present pre-pregnancy or may develop as a complication of the underlying medical disease as well as features of pre-eclampsia. Therefore it is extremely important that such women are managed in specialized units by clinicians with expertise in the differential diagnosis of pre-eclampsia and worsening medical diseases. Baseline and serial assessments of blood pressure, proteinuria and renal function, liver function, uric acid and platelet counts are recommended.

REFERENCES

Abalos, E., Duley, L., Steyn, D. W. and Henderson-Smart, D. J. (2003). Antihypertensive drug therapy for mild to moderate hypertension in pregnancy (Cochrane

Review). In *The Cochrane Library*, Issue 1, 2003. Oxford: Update Software.

ACOG Practice Bulletin #29, July 2001. Chronic Hypertension in Pregnancy.

Alfirevic, Z., Mousa, H. A., Martlew, V., Briscoe, L., Perez-Casal, M. and Toh, C. H. (2001). Postnatal screening for thrombophilia in women with severe pregnancy complications. *Obstet. Gynecol.*, **97**, 753–9.

Alfirevic, Z., Roberts, D. and Martlew, V. (2002). How strong is the association between maternal thrombophilia and adverse pregnancy outcome? A systematic review. *Eur. J. Obstet. Gynecol. Reprod. Biol.*, **101**, 6–14.

Armenti, V. T., Ahlswede, K. M., Ahlswede, B. A., *et al.* (1995). Variables affecting birth weight and graft survival in 197 pregnancies in cyclosporin treated female kidney transplant recipients. *Transplantation*, **59**, 476.

Armenti, V. T., Moritz, M. J. and Davison, J. M. (1998). Medical management of the pregnant transplant recipient. *Adv. Renal Reprod. Ther.*, **5**, 14–23.

Backos, M., Rai, R., Baxter, N., Chilcott, I. T., Cohen, H. and Regan, L. (1999). Pregnancy complications in women with recurrent miscarriage associated with antiphospholipid antibodies treated with low dose aspirin and heparin. *Br. J. Obstet. Gynaecol.*, **106**, 102–7.

Bianco, A. T., Stone, J., Lynch, L., Lapinski, R., Berkowitz, G. and Berkowitz, R. L. (1996). Pregnancy outcome at age 40 and older. *Obstet. Gynecol.*, **87**, 917–22.

Bianco, A. T., Smilen, S. W., Davis, Y., Lopez, S., Lapinski, R. and Lockwood, C. J. (1998). Pregnancy outcome and weight gain recommendations for the morbidly obese woman. *Obstet. Gynecol.*, **91**, 97–102.

Bobrowski, R. A. and Bottoms, S. F. (1995). Underappreciated risks of the elderly multipara. *Am. J. Obstet. Gynaecol.*, **172**, 1764.

Confidential Enquiries into Maternal and Child Health (2004). Why mothers die 2000–02. *6th Confidential Enquiry into Maternal Deaths in the United Kingdom*. London: RCOG Press.

Conde-Agudelo, A. and Belizan, J. M. (2000a). Risk factors for pre-eclampsia in a large cohort of Latin American and Caribbean women. *Br. J. Obstet. Gynaecol.*, **107**, 75–83.

Conde-Agudelo, A. and Belizan, J. M. (2000b). Maternal morbidity and mortality associated with interpregnancy interval: cross sectional study. *Br. Med. J.*, **321**, 1255–9.

Cooper, W. O., Hernandez-Dias, S., Arbogast, P. G., *et al.* (2006). Major congenital malformations after first-trimester exposure to ACE inhibitors. *N. Engl. J. Med.*, **354**, 2443–51.

Davison, J. and Baylis, C. (2002). Renal disease. In *Medical Disorders in Obstetric Practice*, 4th edn., ed. M. De Swiet. Oxford: Blackwell, pp. 198–266.

Department of Health, Welsh Office, Scottish Home and Health Department and Department of Health and Social Services, Northern Ireland. (2001). Confidential Enquiries into Maternal Deaths in the United Kingdom 1997–99. London: Royal College of Obstetricians and Gynaecologists.

Douglas, K. and Redman, C. W. (1994). British Eclampsia Survey. *Br. Med. J.*, **309**, 1395–400.

Drakeley, A. J., LeRoux, P. A., Anthony, J. and Penny, J. (2002). Acute renal failure complicating severe pre-eclampsia requiring admission to an obstetric intensive care unit. *Am. J. Obstet. Gynecol.*, **186**, 253–6.

Duckitt, K. and Harrington, D. (2005). Risk factors for pre-eclampsia at antenatal booking: a systematic review of controlled studies. *Br. Med. J.*, **330**, 565–7.

Ekbom, P., Damm, P., Feldt-Rasmussen, B., Feldt-Rasmussen, U., Molvig, J. and Mathiesen, E. R. (2001). Pregnancy outcome in type I diabetic women with microalbuminuria. *Diabetes Care*, **24**, 1739–44.

Epstein, F. H. (1996). Pregnancy and renal disease. *N. Engl. J. Med.*, **335**, 277–8.

Farquharson, R., Quenby, S. and Greaves, M. (2002). Antiphospholipid syndrome in pregnancy. A randomised, controlled trial of treatment. *Obstet. Gynaecol.*, **100**, 408–13.

Garner, P. R., D'Alton, M. E., Dudley, D. K., Huard, P. and Hardie, M. (1990). Pre-eclampsia in diabetic pregnancies. *Am. J. Obstet. Gynecol.*, **163**, 505–8.

Granger, K. A. and Farquharson, R. G. (1997). Obstetric outcome in antiphospholipid syndrome. *Lupus*, **6**, 509–13.

Hiilesmaa, V., Suhonen, L. and Teramo, K. (2000). Glycaemic control is associated with pre-eclampsia but not with pregnancy-induced hypertension in women with type I diabetes mellitus. *Diabetologia*, **43**, 1534–9.

Huong, D. L., Wechsler, B., Bletry, O., Vauthier-Brouzes, D., Lefebvre, G. and Piette, J. C. (2001a). A study of 75 pregnancies in patients with antiphospholipid syndrome. *J. Rheumatol.*, **28**, 2025–30.

Huong, D. L., Wechsler, B., Vauthier-Brouzes, D., Beaufils, H., Lefebvre, G. and Piette, J. C. (2001b). Pregnancy in past or present lupus nephritis: a study of 32 pregnancies from a single centre. *Ann. Rheum. Dis.*, **60**, 599–604.

Irgens, H. U., Reisaeter, L., Irgens, L. M. and Lie, R. T. (2001). Long-term mortality of mothers and fathers after pre-eclampsia: population based cohort study. *Br. Med. J.*, **323**, 1213–17.

Jones, D. C. and Hayslett, J. P. (1996). Outcome of pregnancy in women with moderate or severe renal insufficiency. *N. Engl. J. Med.*, **335**, 226–32.

Jungers, P. and Chauveau, D. (1997). Pregnancy in renal disease. *Kidney Int.*, **52**, 871–85.

Levine, J. S., Ware-Branch, D. and Rauch, J. (2002). The Antiphospholipid Syndrome. *N. Engl. J. Med.*, **346**, 752–63.

Khamashta, M. A. and Hughes, G. R. V. (1997). Pregnancy in systemic lupus erythematosus. *Curr. Opin. Rheumatol.*, **8**, 424–9.

Kutteh, W. H. (1996). Antiphospholipid antibody-associated recurrent pregnancy loss: treatment with heparin and low-dose aspirin is superior to low-dose aspirin alone. *Am. J. Obstet. Gynecol.*, **174**, 1574–89.

Laskin, C. A., Bombardier, C., Hannah, M. E., *et al.* (1997). Prednisone and aspirin in women with autoantibodies and unexplained recurrent fetal loss. *N. Engl. J. Med.*, **337**, 148–53.

Lee, C. J., Hsieh, T. T., Chiu, T. H., *et al.* (2000). Risk factors for pre-eclampsia in an Asian population. *Int. J. Gynecol. Obstet.*, **70**, 327–33.

Lehmann, D. K. and Chism, J. (1987). Pregnancy outcome in medically complicated and uncomplicated patients aged 40 years or older. *Am. J. Obstet. Gynecol.*, **157**, 738–42.

Lima, F., Khamashta, M. A., Buchanan, N. M., Kerslake, S., Hunt, B. J. and Hughes, G. R. (1996). A study of sixty pregnancies in patients with the antiphospholipid syndrome. *Clin. Exp. Rheumatol.*, **14**, 131–6.

Mabie, W. C., Pernoll, M. L. and Biswas, M. K. (1986). Chronic hypertension in pregnancy. *Obstet. Gynecol.*, **67**, 197–205.

Magee, L. A., Ornstein, M. P. and von Dadelszen, P. (1999). Management of hypertension in pregnancy. *Br. Med. J.*, **318**, 1332–6.

McCowan, L. M. E., Buist, R. G., North, R. A. and Gamble, G. (1996). Perinatal morbidity in chronic hypertension. *Br. J. Obstet. Gynaecol.*, **103**, 123–9.

Moodley, J., Bhoola, V., Duursma, J., Pudifin, D., Byrne, S. and Kenoyer, D. G. (1995). The association of APA with severe early-onset pre-eclampsia. *S. Afr. Med. J.*, **85**, 105–7.

Nelson-Piercy, C. (1999). Thrombophilia and adverse pregnancy outcome: has the time come for routine testing? *Br. J. Obstet. Gynaecol.*, **106**, 513–15.

Nelson-Piercy, C. (2006). Hypertension and pre-eclampsia. In *Handbook of Obstetric Medicine*, third edn., ed. C. Nelson-Piercy. London: Informa Healthcare.

Nelson-Piercy, C. and Khamastha, M. (2003). Autoimmune rheumatic disorders and vasculitis in pregnancy. In *Oxford Textbook of Medicine*, 4th edn., ed. D. Weatherall, J. Cunningham and J. Firth. Oxford: Oxford University Press.

O'Shaughnessy, K. M., Fu, B., Ferraro, F., Lewis, I., Downing, S. and Morris, N. H. (1999). Factor V Leiden and thermolabile methylenetetrahydrofolate reductase gene variations in an East Anglian preeclampsia cohort. *Hypertension*, **33**, 1338–41.

Powers, R. W., Minich, L. A., Lykins, D. L., Ness, R. B., Crombleholme, W. R. and Roberts, J. M. (1999). Methylenetetrahydrofolate reductase polymorphism, folate, and susceptibility to pre-eclampsia. *J. Soc. Gynecol. Invest.*, **6**, 74–9.

Rai, R., Cohen, H., Dave, M. and Regan, L. (1997). Randomized controlled trial of aspirin and aspirin plus heparin in pregnant women with recurrent miscarriage associated with phospholipid antibodies (or antiphospholipid antibodies). *Br. Med. J.*, **314**, 253–7.

Rey, E. and Couturier, A. (1994). The prognosis of pregnancy in women with chronic hypertension. *Am. J. Obstet. Gynecol.*, **171**, 410.

Rey, E., Kahn, S. R., David, M. and Shrier, I. (2003). Thrombophilic disorders and fetal loss: a meta-analysis. *Lancet*, **361**, 901–8.

Ros, H. S., Cnattingius, S. and Lipworth, L. (1998). Comparison of risk factors for pre-eclampsia and gestational hypertension in a population based cohort study. *Am. J. Epidemiol.*, **147**, 1062–70.

Salha, O., Sharma, V., Dada, T., *et al.* (1999). The influence of donated gametes on the incidence of hypertensive disorders of pregnancy. *Hum. Reprod.*, **14**, 2268–73.

Sattar, N., Clark, P., Lean, M., Holmes, A., Walker, I. and Greer, I. A. (2001). Antenatal waist circumference and hypertension risk. *Obstet. Gynaecol.*, **97**(2), 268–71.

Schatz, M., Zeiger, R. S., Harden, K., *et al.* (1997). The safety of asthma and allergy medications during pregnancy. *J. Allergy Clin. Immunol.*, **100**, 301–6.

Schatz, M. and Dombrowski, M. (2000). Outcomes of pregnancy in asthmatic women. *Immun. Allerg. Clin. N.A.*, **20**, 715–27.

Sermer, M., Naylor, C.D., Farine, D., *et al.* (1998). The Toronto Tri-Hospital Gestational Project. *Diabetes Care*, **21** (Suppl. 2), B33–42.

Sibai, B.M., Abdella, T.N. and Anderson, G.D. (1983). Pregnancy outcome in 211 patients with mild chronic hypertension. *Obstet. Gynecol.*, **61**, 571–6.

Sibai, B.M., Mabie, B.C., Harvey, R.N. and Gonzalez, A.R. (1987). Pulmonary edema in severe preeclampsia–eclampsia: analysis of thirty-seven consecutive cases. *Am. J. Obstet. Gynecol.*, **156**, 1174–9.

Sibai, B.M., Ramadan, M.K., Usta, I., Salama, M., Mercer, B.M. and Friedman, S.A. (1993). Maternal morbidity and mortality in 442 pregnancies with hemolysis, elevated liver enzymes, and low platelets (HELLP syndrome). *Am. J. Obstet. Gynecol.*, 1993, **169**, 1000–6.

Sibai, B.M., Ewell, M., Levine, R.J., *et al.* (1997). Risk factors associated with preeclampsia in healthy nulliparous women. The Calcium for Pre-eclampsia Prevention (CPEP) Study Group. *Am. J. Obstet. Gynecol.*, **177**, 1003–10.

Sibai, B.M. (2000). Risk factors, pregnancy complications, and prevalence of hypertensive disorders in women with pregravid diabetes mellitus. *J. Matern. Fetal. Med.*, **9**, 62–5.

Skjaerven, R., Wilcox, A.J. and Lie, R.T. (2002). The interval between pregnancies and the risk of pre-eclampsia. *N. Engl. J. Med.*, **346**, 33–8.

Smith, G.C.S., Pell, J.P. and Walsh, D. (2001). Pregnancy complications and maternal risk of ischaemic heart disease: a retrospective cohort study of 129,290 births. *Lancet*, **357**, 2002–6.

Triolo, G., Ferrante, A., Ciccia F., Accardo-Palumbo A., *et al.* (2003). Randomized study of subcutaneous low molecular weight heparin plus aspirin versus intravenous immunoglobulin in the treatment of recurrent fetal loss associated with antiphospholipid antibodies. *Arthritis Rheum.*, **48**, 728–31.

van Hoorn, J., Dekker, G. and Jeffries, B. (2002). Gestational diabetes versus obesity as risk factors for pregnancy-induced hypertensive disorders and fetal macrosomia. *Aust. N.Z. J. Obstet. Gynaecol.*, **42**, 29–34.

Wang, J.X., Knottnerus, A.M., Schuit, G., Norman, R.J., Chan, A. and Dekker, G.A. (2002). Surgically obtained sperm and the risk of gestational hypertension and pre-eclampsia. *Lancet*, **359**, 673–4.

Ware-Branch, D. (1994). Thoughts on the mechanism of pregnancy loss associated with the antiphospholipid syndrome. *Lupus*, **3**, 275–80.

Ware-Branch, D.W., Silver, R.M., Blackwell, J.L., Reading, J.C. and Scott, J.R. (1992). Outcome of treated pregnancies in women with antiphospholipid syndrome: an update of the Utah experience. *Obstet. Gynecol.*, **80**, 614–20.

Ware-Branch, D. and Khamashta, M.A. (2003). Antiphospholipid syndrome: obstetric diagnosis, management and controversies. *Obstet. Gynecol.*, **101**, 1333–44.

Wen, S.W., Demissie, K.W. and Liu, S. (2001). Adverse outcomes in pregnancies of asthmatic women: results from a Canadian population. *Ann. Epidemiol.*, **11**, 7–12.

Wilson, B.J., Watson, M.S., Prescott, G.J., *et al.* (2003). Hypertensive diseases of pregnancy and risk of hypertension and stroke in later life: results from cohort study. *Br. Med. J.*, **326**, 845–9.

Wilson, W.A., Gharavi, A.E., Koike, T., *et al.* (1999). International consensus statement on preliminary classification criteria for definite antiphospholipid syndrome: Report of an International workshop. *Arthritis Rheumat.*, **42**, 1309–11.

Xiong, X., Saunders, L.D., Wang, F.L. and Demianczuk, N.N. (2001). Gestational diabetes: prevalence, risk factors, maternal and fetal outcomes. *Int. J. Gynaecol. Obstet.*, **75**, 221–8.

23

The kidney and pre-eclampsia

M. C. Smith and J. M. Davison

The healthy kidney undergoes considerable vascular adaptation in pregnancy and it is therefore not surprising that pre-eclampsia, with widespread endothelial dysfunction, is associated with substantial renal consequences, an understanding of which provides insight into the overall vascular pathology. It is important to interpret impaired renal function secondary to pre-eclampsia in the context of the substantially enhanced renal performance of normal pregnancy, otherwise significant end organ damage in pre-eclamptic patients will go unrecognized.

The pathological renal characteristics of pre-eclampsia

It has been recognized for almost a century that pre-eclampsia is associated with morphological renal changes. Lohlein in 1918 noticed that glomeruli in autopsy specimens from pre-eclamptic patients were enlarged and had a thickened basement membrane. The precise nature of the pathological lesion was not determined until the introduction of the electron microscope. The classical pathology we now recognize to be associated with pre-eclampsia is that of endothelial vacuolization and hypertrophy of the cytoplasmic organelles classically described by Spargo *et al.* (1959) as "glomerular capillary endotheliosis." Many original studies used biopsy specimens but there is one particularly notable post-mortem series by Sheehan and Lynch (1973). This was remarkable in that the autopsies were generally performed

between 15 min and 2 h following death, thus minimizing histological artefact from tissue decomposition and biopsy techniques.

The ultrastructural renal consequences of pre-eclampsia are primarily seen in the glomerulus. The glomerulus is large and bloodless, an appearance compatible with gestational hypertension of any cause, but it is particularly marked in pre-eclamptic specimens. In pre-eclampsia the glomerular enlargement is seen in isolation, without any accompanying increases in the stroma or cells, distinguishing nephropathy of a pre-eclamptic origin from that associated with glomerulonephritis or diabetes.

The glomerular tuft can be seen to contain intracapillary and mesangial cells. In the early stages of the disease this intracapillary hypercellularity gives the appearance of capillary dilatation or "ballooning," then later in the disease the capillaries become longitudinally expanded in a characteristic "cigar-shaped" morphology. The increased capillary cellularity can eventually push several capillary loops into the proximal tubule – a phenomenon known as "pouting." Once again, this is seen in other hypertensive situations but is accentuated in pre-eclampsia. In severe cases the mesangial cells (particularly the lysosomes) can enlarge and may further infiltrate the endothelial cells and basement membrane contributing to the appearance of basement membrane thickening.

The glomeruli are effectively obstructed, giving rise to the bloodless appearance (Figures 23.1 and 23.2). It is therefore all the more remarkable that

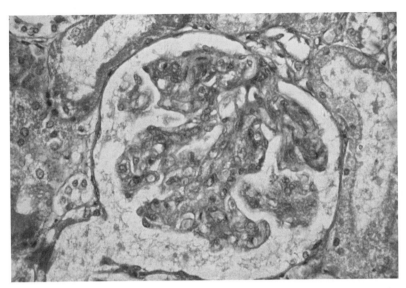

Figure 23.1 Glomerular appearance in pre-eclampsia (some artefactual debris from fixing techniques).

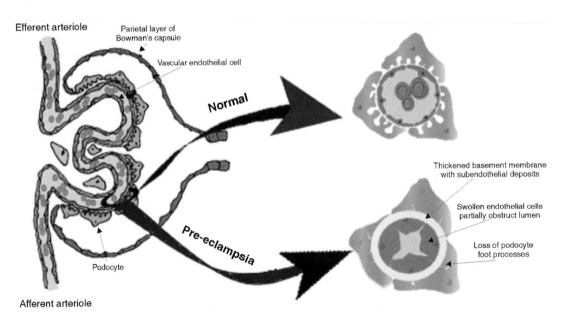

Figure 23.2 Schematic representation of glomerular changes in pre-eclampsia.

the glomerular filtration rate is preserved to the extent that it is, albeit much reduced compared to normal pregnancy. The pre-eclamptic renal lesion is restricted to the glomerulus although nonspecific tubular dilatation and flattening can be seen in cases with severe proteinuria. No typical histological features in renal epithelial cells or juxtaglomerular apparatus have been seen consistently in pre-eclampsia and their involvement in the renal lesion remains disputed.

The pre-eclamptic renal morphology begins to resolve in the early postpartum period and studies which have examined renal tissue remote from delivery support the view that resolution is complete (Bryans, 1966; Chesley, 1980) but the duration of the recovery period remains uncertain with estimates ranging from a few weeks to 6 months (Dennis *et al.*, 1968; Fadel *et al.*, 1969; Furukawa *et al.*, 1983; Oe *et al.*, 1980; Sheehan and Lynch, 1973).

Renal hemodynamics in normal pregnancy and pre-eclampsia

In 1951, Bucht's studies suggested that renal blood flow increased substantially in human pregnancy, and this was confirmed by subsequent investigators, but methodological variation resulted in considerable controversy regarding the timing and magnitude of the increment. The "best" studies were those where the same women were studied serially throughout pregnancy as well as prepregnancy and/or postnatally under standardized conditions with glomerular filtration rate (GFR) and effective renal plasma flow (ERPF) determined by para-aminohippurate (PAH) and inulin clearances, respectively (Assali *et al.*, 1959; Chapman *et al.*, 1997; de Alvarez, 1958; Dunlop, 1981; Milne *et al.*, 2002; Roberts *et al.*, 1996; Sims and Krantz, 1958).

From these studies it is acknowledged that ERPF and GFR increase markedly in the first part of pregnancy by 50–85% and 40–60%, respectively. The consensus is that this enhanced performance is maintained throughout pregnancy, possibly with a reduction in ERPF in late pregnancy (Ezimokhai *et al.*, 1981). From 24 h creatinine clearance as well as inulin measurements it is evident that GFR is increased in the luteal phase of the menstrual cycle and still further by 2 weeks (25%) and 6 weeks (41%) gestation (Chapman *et al.*, 1997; Davison and Noble, 1981).

Overall GFR is determined by the number of functioning nephrons and the rate of filtration in

each one. Each human kidney has approximately 1,000,000 glomeruli and it is believed that in the healthy kidney all the glomeruli are functioning all of the time. Variation in overall renal function is therefore a result of regulation of the filtration rate within individual glomeruli. Variables which influence the single nephron glomerular filtration rate (SNGFR) will necessarily modify renal function as a whole.

Four physical parameters have been identified which determine glomerular filtration rate (Figure 23.3):

- the trans-capillary hydrostatic pressure gradient;
- the characteristics of the membrane;
- the characteristics of the solutes; and
- glomerular hemodynamics.

Animal model studies allow direct measurement of renal parameters using micropuncture techniques and in pregnancy it seems likely that the gestational increases in GFR are a consequence of renal vasodilatation (Baylis, 1987; Conrad, 1984, 1987), with both afferent and efferent arterioles equally affected, thus increasing GFR without concomitant elevation in glomerular pressure (ΔP) (Baylis, 1980, 1994). Although such invasive studies are impossible in humans, mathematical estimations of the various parameters can be indirectly estimated (Deen *et al.*, 1979) and results using these methods accord with the animal work (Milne *et al.*, 2002; Moran *et al.*, 2003; Roberts *et al.*, 1996). The stimulus for gestational renal vasodilatation remains elusive but there is compelling evidence that it is mediated via nitric oxide pathways (Alexander *et al.*, 1999; Danielson and Conrad, 1995; Gandley *et al.*, 2001). Furthermore, work in rats has demonstrated that the ovarian hormone relaxin plays an important role (Baylis, 1999; Danielson *et al.*, 1999; Novak *et al.*, 2001) and its role in renal adaptation in human pregnancy is currently under investigation. As the failure to establish an appropriate hemodynamic response in early pregnancy can be associated with an increased tendency to develop fetal growth restriction and pre-eclampsia at a later gestation (Duvekot *et al.*, 1995; Easterling *et al.*, 1990), better understanding of the renal adaptation in normal pregnancy could provide further clues about the etiology of the pre-eclamptic process.

A recent review (Lindheimer, 1999) of studies investigating renal hemodynamic changes in pre-eclamptic and normal pregnancies showed that, on average, there is a 32% reduction in GFR and a 24% reduction in ERPF in pre-eclampsia compared to normal pregnancy values (Table 23.1). Although the perpetrator responsible for the reduced blood flow has not been identified, there is probably a selective increase in afferent arteriolar resistance (Baylis and Reckelhoff, 1991), explaining why filtration fraction (FF) is affected to a lesser extent than the other hemodynamic parameters.

Glomerular ultrafiltration, and its individual components, can be interrogated using models which apply theoretical principles of fluid properties to the glomerular vascular bed (Deen *et al.*, 1972, 1979, 1985). The ultrafiltration coefficient K_f represents the product of glomerular hydraulic permeability and filtration surface area and is thus an important determinant of GFR. Studies using both morphometric techniques (Lafayette *et al.*, 1998) and mathematical modeling of neutral dextran clearances (Moran *et al.*, 2003) predict a

40% reduction of K_f in pre-eclampsia compared to normal pregnancy. It is unlikely that the surface area is altered and therefore it has been suggested that the reduction in K_f is a consequence of reduced glomerular hydraulic permeability secondary to impaired structural integrity of the membrane or altered charge selectivity. The relative contribution of the two main determinants of renal function, namely blood flow and glomerular hydraulic permeability, to the reduced GFR seen in pre-eclampsia remains controversial.

Table 23.1. Comparison of renal hemodynamic function in nonpregnant women, normal pregnancy and pregnancy complicated by pre-eclampsia (mean values, summarized from Conrad and Lindheimer (1999) and Moran *et al.* (2003))

	Non-pregnant	Normal pregnancy	Pre-eclamptic pregnancy
GFR (ml min^{-1})	114	133	90
ERPF (ml min^{-1})	581	649	487
FF (%)	19.5	20.4	18.7
K_f (ml min^{-1}mmHg^{-1})	8.0	8.9	4.6

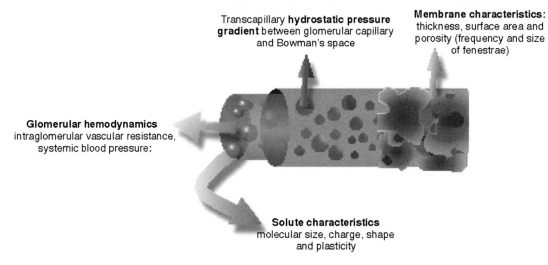

Transcapillary **hydrostatic pressure gradient** between glomerular capillary and Bowman's space

Membrane characteristics: thickness, surface area and porosity (frequency and size of fenestrae)

Glomerular hemodynamics intraglomerular vascular resistance, systemic blood pressure:

Solute characteristics molecular size, charge, shape and plasticity

Figure 23.3 Physical parameters determining glomerular filtration rate.

Volume and sodium homeostasis

Clinicians have been aware for a long time that plasma sodium levels and therefore plasma osmolality are significantly reduced by the fifth week of pregnancy, and reach a nadir by the tenth week, thence maintained for the duration of the pregnancy (Davison, 1984; Davison and Noble, 1981). The osmotic changes seen following the missed menstrual period have in fact been initiated prior to this and indeed are reflected to a lesser degree in the normal, luteal phase of the menstrual cycle (Chapman et al., 1997, 1998).

Outside of pregnancy plasma osmolality varies between 280 and 300 mosmol kg^{-1} and remains remarkably stable within any one individual. Under normal circumstances a drop comparable to that seen in pregnancy of 8–10 mosmol kg^{-1} would cause suppression of arginine vasopressin (AVP), stimulating polyuria and then polydipsia in an attempt to correct the shift. Pregnant women, however, continue to concentrate their urine and do not significantly increase their fluid intake. It was therefore postulated and demonstrated that the thresholds for AVP release and thirst were reset in pregnancy at approx. 9 mosmol kg^{-1} less than in the nonpregnant state, permitting the new gestational hypo-osmolar steady state to be maintained (Davison et al., 1984; Durr et al., 1987).

A transient form of Diabetes Insipidus (DI) is a rare presentation in the late stages of pregnancy (incidence 2–4 per 100,000 maternities), with the polyuria and polydipsia resistant to treatment with AVP, resolving following delivery. Most cases are seen in women who have pre-eclampsia, HELLP syndrome or acute fatty liver of pregnancy. This syndrome arises because AVP, eliminated in normal pregnancy by the placental enzyme vasopressinase (which is in turn eliminated by the liver), is even more depleted when liver function is impaired because vasopressinase levels rise even more. Interestingly, the syndrome is resistant to treatment with exogenous AVP (Durr et al., 1987) but responds well to desmopressin (dDAVP), a synthetic vasopressin analog which is resistant to vasopressinase (Durr and Lindheimer, 1996).

The characteristic hemodynamic adaptations to pregnancy, namely a reduction in systemic vascular resistance alongside increased cardiac output, necessitate increased plasma volume. This is effected by increasing renal tubule sodium retention 3–4 mmol day^{-1}, a remarkable accomplishment considering the massively increased GFR. In pre-eclampsia the ability to excrete sodium is impaired and it is unclear if this is a consequence of reduced renal tubular function or if it is an appropriate response to the comparatively reduced vascular volume. These subtle adjustments to sodium homeostasis are brought about by modifications to the renin–angiotensin–aldosterone system (RAAS) (see Chapter 5), with the maternal kidney being the principal source of active renin with increased levels in pregnancy along with other components of RAAS.

Renal tubular function

The physiological gestational increase in plasma volume will cause a small decrement in many plasma constituent concentrations. The increase in GFR is such that despite the lower plasma concentrations the filtered renal load of many solutes is increased, necessitating enhanced tubular reabsorption to maintain physiological levels. No specific renal tubular features have been identified in pre-eclampsia but secondary tubular damage may occur, possibly because of intratubular hemoglobin cast deposition or myoglobinuria after repeated eclamptic seizures. Hyperuricemia in pre-eclamptic patients is probably a result of increased tubular reabsorption and it has been suggested that this is linked to increased reabsorption of sodium in pre-eclampsia.

Renal handling of protein

In the healthy nonpregnant individual the glomerulus is relatively impermeable to large proteins and although smaller proteins (radius <30 Å) are freely filtered there is almost complete reabsorption in the proximal tubule such that daily renal excretion of protein is only 20–80 mg, 40% of which is albumin. In normal pregnancy, both the total protein excretion (TPE) and the urinary albumin excretion (UAE) are increased after 20 weeks gestation, attaining 200 mg 24 h^{-1} (upper limit 300 mg) and 12 mg 24 h^{-1} (upper limit 20 mg) (Higby et al., 1994; Taylor and Davison, 1997), respectively.

The normal renal handling of protein depends upon the integrity of both the glomerular barrier and protein reabsorption mechanisms in the proximal tubule. Proteinuria is a consequence of either reductions in the integrity of the glomerular barrier (restricting protein flux on the basis of molecular size), the electrical charge (glomerular anion) and the sterical conformation, or of impairment of tubular reabsorption. Models of the glomerulus, derived from hydrodynamic theories, explain its size-selective properties by considering the glomerular membrane to be perforated with a population of restrictive pores (Deen et al., 1985; Edwards et al., 1999). Some studies report that a log normal distribution of pore sizes would best explain the sieving characteristics of the membrane, whilst others have found that a bimodal model with a population of small pores of similar radius and a second population of larger, less restrictive "shunts" (isoporous + shunt model) best explain glomerular handling of macromolecules. To account for the changes seen in pregnancy, alterations in both the distribution of the size-selective pores as well as the charge selectivity of the membrane are such that high molecular weight proteins cross into the tubule more easily.

One of the classical signs of pre-eclampsia is proteinuria >500 mg 24 h^{-1} (Brown et al., 2001). Studies using clearance of neutral molecules (e.g. dextran) and mathematical modeling suggest that this degree of proteinuria seen in pre-eclampsia, particularly when the reduced GFR is taken into account, is much larger than can be explained by changes in size selectivity alone. Thus loss of charge selectivity must be the major cause of pre-eclamptic proteinuria; as the protein load delivered to the proximal tubule increases, it rapidly saturates the reabsorption transport mechanisms so that there is also cytoplasmic protein accumulation with the potential for interstitial inflammation and fibrosis (Lopez-Espinoza et al., 1986).

Renal considerations in the prediction and diagnosis

Early pregnancy assessment

It is difficult to predict in early pregnancy which women are at risk of developing pre-eclampsia or its renal complications. A history of renal complications in a previous pre-eclamptic pregnancy will obviously alert the obstetrician to an increased risk in the current pregnancy but, as pre-eclampsia is chiefly a disease of primiparity, this strategy alone will fail to anticipate the majority of subsequent problems. Other elements at the booking interview might highlight risk factors for pre-eclampsia but it is difficult to predict which of these women are at particular risk of renal complications.

Patients with pre-existing renal problems, during or independent of pregnancy, are more likely to develop pre-eclampsia and their antenatal surveillance should reflect this. In the past, patients with chronic renal disease were discouraged from pursuing pregnancy because of the high frequency of fetal and maternal complications including pre-eclampsia. Today the advice given depends largely upon the severity of existing renal disease and pregnancies in patients with mild disease (serum creatinine <1.4 mg dl^{-1} (125 μmol l^{-1})) with well-controlled hypertension generally have an optimistic prognosis. Katz et al. (1980) reported the outcome of 121 pregnancies in 89 women who had renal disease diagnosed on the basis of renal biopsy. All had normal or mildly impaired renal function prior to pregnancy. In 16% renal function deteriorated mildly during the course of the pregnancy but spontaneously resolved following delivery. Fifty percent of pregnancies were associated with proteinuria, which was frequently heavy, but this did not appear to exacerbate the underlying renal disease. Fetal outcome was good, with a live birth rate of 94%, although the incidence of preterm delivery and intrauterine growth restriction was increased compared to the normal population.

The prognosis is more guarded with severe renal impairment (certainly when serum creatinine $>180 \, \mu mol \, l^{-1}$ ($2 \, mg \, dl^{-1}$)) or when hypertension is poorly controlled. Such pregnancies are more often associated with considerable deterioration in renal function which may not be reversible following delivery. As well as the maternal considerations, there is an increased incidence of pregnancy loss, both in the first trimester and at later gestations, and poorer fetal outcome in live births. Control of hypertension before and during pregnancy in such cases is probably the best way to optimize pregnancy outcome. In patients with moderate and severe underlying renal pathology who experience deterioration of renal function during pregnancy, the extent of renal recovery following delivery is difficult to predict, and the implications, to both the woman and her family, of long-term renal replacement therapy are considerable. All women of reproductive age with renal impairment should be appropriately counseled and prepregnancy assessment strongly recommended. It is inevitable, however, that the obstetric team will have to manage patients who have not been adequately assessed prior to pregnancy, particularly because erratic menstrual cycles typical of severe renal disease frequently contribute to the late diagnosis of pregnancy.

Antenatal assessment

Routine antenatal assessments should include measurement of blood pressure and urinary protein analysis. Proteinuria associated with hypertension is strongly suggestive of pre-eclampsia although other causes, particularly urinary tract infection, must be excluded. Urinary protein excretion increases during normal pregnancy with an upper limit of $250 \, mg \, day^{-1}$ in the third trimester. Significant proteinuria ($>500 \, mg \, day^{-1}$) is seen with pre-eclampsia and levels may exceed $5 \, g \, 24 \, h^{-1}$ in severe cases.

Methods of assessing proteinuria

The "gold standard" method of assessing proteinuria is widely acknowledged to be 24 h urine collection. This method, however, is time-consuming, and can only be conducted where patients are highly motivated with easy access to hospital facilities. Furthermore, this method does not lend itself as a screening investigation to be applied to the antenatal population in general.

The most common method of screening for proteinuria is dipstick analysis. A positive result of +1 is interpreted as being equivalent to $300 \, mg \, 24 \, h^{-1}$ and if associated with hypertension is then followed up with a 24 h urine collection. This approach, although commonly employed, is far from ideal (Halligan et al., 1999). In the subgroup of patients who are hypertensive, proteinuria assessed using dipstick methods has high false positive (66%) and false negative (8–66%) rates (Meyer et al., 1994), which are unacceptable when used as to distinguish non-proteinuric hypertension from pre-eclampsia. The accuracy can be improved by formal training of clinic staff (Bell et al., 1999), using a mid stream sample and/or an automated reading system (Saudan et al., 1997). Whilst false positives will be identified if a subsequent 24 h collection is completed, this generates a significant number of unnecessary and costly investigations. More worryingly, the high false negative result with urine dipstick will result in a significant proportion of pre-eclamptic women being incorrectly diagnosed as non-proteinuric hypertensives.

In the nonpregnant population urinary protein to creatinine ratios are frequently used to quantify proteinuria. Reference ranges have been established for use in normal pregnancy (Waugh et al., 2003) and early reports of their use in pre-eclampsia are promising. Recently published guidelines for management of pre-eclampsia in the community (PRECOG) (Milne *et al.*, 2005) recommend using a threshold of ≥ 30 mg mmol^{-1} which has been shown to predict significant proteinuria in pregnancy with 93% sensitivity and 92% specificity (Saudan *et al.*, 1997). Random urinary PCR is a useful screening tool but does not replace 24 h urine collection for accurate quantification of proteinuria (Durnwald and Mercer, 2003).

Monitoring renal involvement in pre-eclampsia

Serum creatinine

Serum creatinine concentration, often used as a measure of renal function, has poor sensitivity because levels may remain within the normal range until renal function is compromised by more than 50%, particularly misleading in pregnancy if the lower average serum levels are not appreciated (Table 23.2). In addition, serum creatinine levels are influenced by diurnal variation and dietary factors. An isolated serum creatinine result above 75 μmol l^{-1} in pregnancy should prompt further renal investigation but such patients may have considerable renal compromise by this point.

Although para-aminohippurate (PAH) and inulin clearances remain the gold standard to assess renal function, impracticality excludes their routine performance in pregnancy. An alternative, the commonly used 24 h creatinine clearance, relies upon creatinine being freely filtered at the glomerulus and minimal tubular secretion. Consequently the increased renal perfusion in pregnancy causes the 24 h creatinine clearance to increase from nonpregnant mean values of 92 ml min^{-1} to maximal gestational levels of 125 ml min^{-1} in the mid trimester. Creatinine clearance is an approximation of function because it is assumed that the tubular secretion of creatinine is offset by the overestimation of plasma creatinine levels as a result of technical limitations of creatinine assays

Table 23.2. Mean serum levels of urea and creatinine in pregnancy

	Nonpregnant	First trimester	Second trimester	Third trimester
Serum creatinine (μmol l^{-1})	73	65	51	47
Serum urea (mmol l^{-1})	4.3	3.5	3.3	3.1

(chromagen is measured along with true creatinine). Under normal circumstances this assumption is valid but if GFR falls considerably creatinine clearance may overestimate GFR by as much as 25–50% (Smith, 1951).

Several groups have compared gestational GFR estimation using both inulin and creatinine clearances and the results are generally comparable with the possible exception of late pregnancy where 24 h creatinine clearance falls (Davison and Hytten, 1974; de Alvarez, 1958). This is not just due to posture-dependent pressure of the enlarged uterus on the renal vasculature but also there is some renal "de-adaptation" in the third trimester.

Clinicians caring for nonpregnant patients may be used to applying formulae to correct for patient age, height, sex and weight, which are not appropriate in pregnancy because body weight and size do not reflect an increase in functional renal mass (Conrad *et al.*, 1999; Hytten and Leitch, 1971).

Serum urea

Serum urea or blood urea nitrogen (BUN) indices are inaccurate surrogates for GFR. Although GFR will influence blood urea levels, other factors such as tubular reabsorption, dietary protein intake and liver protein metabolism are confounding variables. Urea results should be interpreted with the gestational reference ranges in mind (Table 23.2), but any isolated serum level greater than 4.5 mmol l^{-1} warrants further renal investigation. Serum urea levels are more useful clinically if GFR is reduced. If the decrement in GFR is attributable to dehydration or urinary tract obstruction the urea levels will be disproportionably raised compared to the creatinine levels because of low urine flow rates in the distal tubule.

Serum uric acid

The metabolism of purine produces uric acid which is freely filtered at the glomerulus, thence there is about 90% proximal reabsorption of the filtered load. Serum levels fall by 25% in early pregnancy because of reduced tubular resorbtion but increase toward nonpregnant concentrations by term. In pre-eclampsia hyperuricemia is one of the earliest signs and correlates well with disease severity. Isolated results, however, should be interpreted cautiously in view of diurnal fluxes in serum levels, higher levels in multifetal pregnancies and the considerable interindividual variation in normotensive pregnancy. Serum uric acid levels are therefore of limited use in the initial diagnosis of pre-eclampsia.

Once pre-eclampsia is definitely diagnosed, serial serum uric acid measurements are useful to monitor disease progression. Most investigators have found that there is a positive correlation between the degree of hyperuricemia and the severity of pre-eclampsia (Connon and Wadsworth, 1968; Dunlop et al., 1978; McFarlane, 1963; Pollak and Nettles, 1960; Widholm and Kuhlback, 1964). Of particular interest is the classic study by Pollock and Nettles in 1960 where they compared serum uric acid levels in normal pregnancy, pre-eclamptic pregnancy and pregnancies with hypertensive vascular disease. The diagnosis in the latter two groups was established using antepartum percutaneous renal biopsy (no longer widely practised). They found that serum uric acid was significantly raised ($P < 0.001$) in the pre-eclamptic group compared to the other two groups and moreover the degree of hyperuricemia correlated with the severity of the histological renal lesion.

A further importance of serum uric acid monitoring in pre-eclamptic pregnancies is its correlation with fetal outcome, first noted by Redman et al. in 1976 and subsequently confirmed in 1984 by Sagen et al., with both groups of investigators reporting that fetal growth restriction and mortality are increased in the presence of pre-eclampsia-induced hyperuricemia as well as there being an increased incidence of intrapartum fetal distress.

Serum Cystatin C

The limitations of creatinine and urea as serum markers of renal involvement in pre-eclampsia have prompted clinicians to consider other possibilities. In particular, serum Cystatin C has recently been introduced as an indicator of GFR which is independent of age, gender and muscle mass in the nonpregnant population (Coll et al., 2000; Dharnidharka et al., 2002; Dworkin, 2001). The low molecular weight protein is produced by all nucleated cells and is removed from the circulation exclusively by the kidney. Studies from Sweden have established reference ranges in pregnancy and suggest that it is a better diagnostic tool than creatinine or urea in pre-eclampsia, with increased sensitivity than existing methods to detect reduced GFR (Strevens et al., 2001, 2002). The same group have reported that the increased serum Cystatin C levels correlate well with the severity of glomerular endotheliosis (Strevens et al., 2003). Although such studies, using renal biopsies from healthy third-trimester pregnant women, are ethically questionable, they do underscore other evidence that serum Cystatin C is emerging as a promising marker for renal impairment in pregnancy, and pre-eclampsia in particular.

Proteinuria

Whilst the accurate assessment of proteinuria in the diagnosis of pre-eclampsia is important, the value of its serial monitoring of proteinuria following diagnosis is less clear. Proteinuria in pre-

Table 23.3. Renal considerations when prescribing drugs to treat hypertension in pregnancy

Drug	Dose	Renal cautions
Chronic treatment		
Methyldopa	500–3000 mg in 2–4 divided doses	Dose may need to be reduced if significant renal impairment
Labetolol	100–500 mg tds	
Nifedipine (SR)	10–40 mg bd	Care to avoid profound hypotension when used alongside magnesium sulfate
Acute treatment		
Hydralazine	5–10 mg IV or IM repeated if necessary	
Labetolol	20 mg IV repeated if necessary at 20 min intervals	
Nifedipine	10–20 mg repeated if necessary at 20 min intervals	Care to avoid profound hypotension when used alongside magnesium sulfate

eclampsia can be severe and reach nephrotic levels. Several studies (Chua and Redman, 1992; Newman et al., 2003; Odendaal et al., 1990; Schiff et al., 1996; Sibai et al., 1994) have tried to address the question of whether this degree of proteinuria which, outside of pregnancy, would be associated with significant renal damage has the same significance in pregnant women. It would seem that massive proteinuria alone does not increase maternal morbidity; rather, it is an indicator of early onset disease and subsequent progression to severe pre-eclampsia. After correction for gestational age there is no increased fetal morbidity associated with heavy proteinuria. It would seem reasonable, therefore, to monitor proteinuria in a pre-eclamptic pregnancy as a measure of disease progression, but there is no good evidence that delivery justified on heavy proteinuria alone will improve maternal or fetal outcome.

Renal considerations in the treatment of pre-eclampsia

The mainstay of antenatal pre-eclampsia maternal management is control of hypertension. It is important to remember that renal clearance of pharmacological substances may be reduced with impaired renal function and that the prescribed dose or dose interval may need to be adjusted. This situation is most likely to arise when treating a patient with chronic renal disease and superimposed pre-eclampsia, but it may also be relevant to a patient who has renal complications of pre-eclampsia.

Antihypertensive medication

See Table 23.3.

Hydralazine

Hydralazine is a commonly used antihypertensive useful in the acute management of hypertension. It acts as a direct vascular dilator and has a rapid onset of action. This vasodilation induces activation of the sympathetic nervous system and increased plasma renin and fluid retention. The drug is metabolized by the liver with renal excretion of inactive metabolites, so toxicity because of renal impairment is unlikely. Of more concern is the risk of precipitating renal ischemia because of rapid vasodilation superimposed on a contracted fluid volume, and it is for this reason that some authorities advise administration of a fluid bolus prior to hydralazine (Belfort et al., 1989).

Methyldopa

Methyldopa is probably the most commonly used agent for chronic control of gestational hypertension. It is a centrally acting α adrenergic agonist, which brings about reduced systemic vascular resistance via decreased sympathetic vascular tone. Its use in pregnancy is well established. Methyldopa is not associated with a reduction in glomerular filtration rate or renal blood flow, but caution should be exercised when it is prescribed to a patient with significant renal impairment because this will reduce renal clearance of the drug and dosages will need to be adjusted accordingly.

Beta-blockers

Beta-blockers can be used to treat hypertension in pregnancy in both the acute and chronic situation. The ongoing debate concerning the effectiveness of such treatment, particularly in the chronic situation, has centered upon the possible adverse fetal side effects of the drug. The commonest beta-blocker in obstetric practice is labetolol, a combined α and β adrenoreceptor blocker. As well as the β_2 receptor effect of peripheral vasodilation, β_1 receptors in cardiac tissue modulate the sympathetic response whilst renal receptors mediate changes in renin synthesis. This modest decrement in renin synthesis may contribute to the overall antihypertensive effect in some patients. Beta-blocker therapy has little effect upon renal function in the doses used to treat hypertension. Clearance of the drug is not impaired in patients with renal impairment because inactive metabolites are handled by the kidney.

ACE inhibitors

ACE inhibitors are commonly used outside of pregnancy to treat hypertension of renal origin and diabetic nephropathy. They work by inhibiting angiotensin-converting, enzyme (ACE) and therefore reduce production of angiotensin II (AII), reducing AII-mediated vasoconstriction. It is well-recognized that the RAS system is activated in pregnancy, albeit to a lesser extent in pre-eclampsia than in normal pregnancy, it might therefore seem that the ACE inhibitor might be an attractive antihypertensive. Unfortunately, there have been considerable problems related to fetal renal compromise associated with these drugs, with reports of a specific fetopathy including renal dysgenesis, oligohydramnios, and fatal anuric renal failure (Buttar, 1997; Pryde et al., 1993). ACE inhibitors are therefore avoided in pregnancy.

Diuretics

Diuretics are commonly used to manage hypertension in the general population and it was initially thought that they might be useful in the management of pre-eclampsia considering that the disease is usually associated with some degree of peripheral edema. As our understanding of the pathogenesis of preeclampsia has improved it has been realized that it is irrational to treat pre-eclampsia, a disorder associated with volume depletion, with an agent which reduces intravascular volume further by promoting naturesis. In addition, a diuretic-induced depleted vascular volume enhances proximal tubule function and will augment hyperuricemia, which can confuse the situation when monitoring pre-eclampsia. Diuretics are therefore not used to manage the hypertension of pre-eclampsia; however, they have an important role in the treatment of pre-eclamptic pulmonary edema.

Calcium channel antagonists

Calcium channel antagonists (e.g. nifedipine) are sometimes used in the chronic treatment of hypertension in pre-eclampsia although their use is restricted because of concerns about fetal side effects, precipitous drops in blood pressure and interactions with magnesium sulfate. These agents act by inhibiting Ca^{2+} influx into vascular myocytes and therefore inhibiting vasoconstriction.

The renal hemodynamic consequences of such drugs, particularly at the afferent arteriole and possibly the tubular circulation, cause natures and may contribute to a sustained antihypertensive effect. Nifedipine is primarily metabolized by the liver and inactive metabolites are excreted in the urine. Renal impairment would not therefore be expected to significantly affect the pharmacological actions of the drug.

Magnesium sulfate

Magnesium sulfate is widely recommended to treat and prevent eclamptic fits. It is largely metabolized by the kidneys and therefore the infusion rate should be titrated against plasma magnesium levels when treating patients with renal impairment to avoid magnesium toxicity.

Renal biopsy

The role of renal biopsy in the management of pre-eclampsia has been a controversial issue over the past 30 years. As it became apparent that the kidney has an important role in the pathogenesis of pre-eclampsia and that a typical histological appearance could be described, renal biopsy was used as a diagnostic tool. The procedure was associated with a perceived high complication rate, particularly in this group of women at risk of labile hypertension and coagulation derangement. As clinicians became aware that renal biopsy results were rarely useful in the acute management of pre-eclamptic patients, renal biopsy in pregnancy fell out of vogue until at one point pregnancy was a relative contraindication to renal biopsy. Although recent studies (Kuller et al., 2001; Packham and Fairley, 1987) would suggest that the complication rate is not as high as previously thought, the fact remains that histological analysis of renal tissue is of little use in the antenatal management of most patients. Most clinicians would consider renal biopsy in pregnancy to be useful in a few specific circumstances (Gaber and Lindheimer, 1999), such as unexplained sudden

deterioration of renal function or symptomatic nephritic syndrome presenting before 32 weeks gestation. Such women may respond to high-dose steroids, thus avoiding delivery at extreme prematurity. Problems presenting after 32 weeks gestation will rarely require renal biopsy as delivery after this gestation and subsequent postnatal renal biopsy is generally associated with a favorable maternal and fetal outcome. Proteinuria or hematuria alone are not considered to be indications for antenatal renal biopsy unless an ultrasound examination has suggested the possibility of a renal tumor.

Fluid management

The peripartum period is associated with considerable volume fluxes in the maternal circulation and meticulous fluid management in pre-eclamptic patients is crucial in management at this time. In pre-eclampsia, altered capillary permeability favors an increased interstitial volume and a 10–15% reduction in intravascular volume (Brown and Gallery, 1994; Davison, 1997). In addition, plasma oncotic pressure, already reduced in normal pregnancy, is lower secondary to proteinuria, thus contributing toward fluid shifts into the extravascular space. Plasma oncotic pressure may be further reduced peripartum following blood loss and/or administration of intravenous crystalloids. Increased peripheral vascular resistance impairs myocardial contractility and may encourage a cardiogenic component of pulmonary edema. As part of a normal postnatal hemodynamic response, extracellular fluid to move back into the intravascular space, causing an increase in pulmonary capillary wedge pressure prior to renal excretion. In pre-eclampsia, when the alveolar capillary epithelium is damaged this period of postpartum fluid shifts is a time when women are particularly susceptible to pulmonary edema.

Urine output, measured hourly using an indwelling catheter, should be maintained at $>100\,\mathrm{ml}\,4\,\mathrm{h}^{-1}$. Within our own unit we have found that a fluid regime of $85\,\mathrm{ml}\,\mathrm{h}^{-1}$ of crystalloid fluid will usually achieve this with minimal

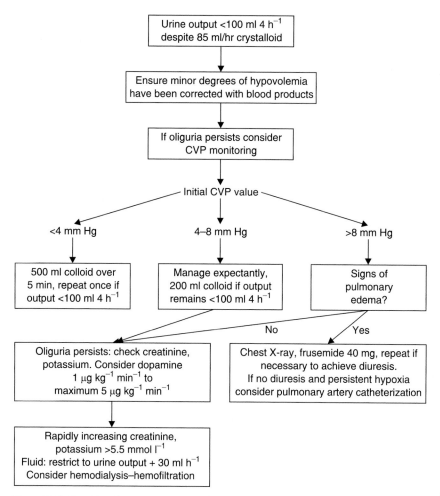

Figure 23.4 Algorithm for management of oliguria associated with pre-eclampsia. (Courtesy of Professor S. C. Robson, Royal Victoria Infirmary, Newcastle upon Tyne.)

associated risk of fluid overload. It is rare that diuretics are necessary to stimulate postpartum diuresis. Frusemide should only be considered if oliguria persists despite vasodilation and judicious volume expansion. Of patients with severe pre-eclampsia, 30% will have a relative oliguria during the first 24 h following delivery which will recover spontaneously. Careful assessment of oliguria is essential as these patients are often at risk of postoperative bleeding and poor renal function might be secondary to reduced circulating volume.

Repeated fluid challenges in pre-eclamptic patients cause pulmonary edema, a significant cause of maternal mortality in this group. An example of an algorithm used in our own department for fluid management in pre-eclamptic patients is given in Figure 23.4.

Control of blood pressure

Blood pressure should be carefully monitored during the peripartum period. If acute episodes of hypertension occur the aim of treatment should be to reduce blood pressure smoothly to avoid profound intermittent hypotensive episodes which may compromise peripheral perfusion, causing end-organ ischemic damage.

Acute renal failure (ARF)

ARF is a rare complication of pre-eclampsia in the developed world (Randeree *et al.*, 1995), with an estimated incidence of 1 in 10,000–15,000 pregnancies. Relative oliguria in the early postpartum period is common but this generally resolves spontaneously and can be treated conservatively, providing that the serum creatinine and urea levels are not rising alarmingly. ARF in the general obstetric population is most commonly secondary to massive hemorrhage and this must be excluded before an intrarenal cause of renal failure is diagnosed.

ARF in a pre-eclamptic patient who is otherwise well has a good prognosis, with full recovery being the norm. Patients who develop renal complications of pre-eclampsia superimposed upon pre-existing renal disease are at increased risk of bilateral renal cortical necrosis, which is associated with increased maternal mortality and persistent renal compromise. Renal failure due to pre-eclampsia in antenatal patients will almost always prompt delivery.

The initial treatment of ARF in the pre-eclamptic patient will depend upon the precipitating cause. Restoration of the intravascular volume with appropriate fluids should be carefully monitored to avoid precipitating pulmonary edema. The volume status in such patients can be very difficult to assess and this is a situation where central pressure monitoring can be useful. Diuretics are sometimes used to treat the oliguric phase of acute tubular necrosis, but there is no evidence that this will improve the speed of recovery or the eventual outcome (Brown *et al.*, 1981; Shilliday *et al.*, 1997). Meticulous attention to fluid balance should ensure that urine output is replaced along with

insensible losses (6–8 ml kg^{-1}24 h^{-1}), blood losses (from delivery) and other losses (diarrhea, vomiting). Fluid depletion secondary to pyrexia should be compensated for by 200 ml 24 h^{-1} normal saline for each 1°C temperature elevation. Potassium supplementation in fluid replacement is not advised because of the tendency toward hyperkalemia in patients with renal compromise. Serum electrolyte levels should be monitored at least once daily in order that the replacement fluids can be adjusted appropriately. Acidosis should be excluded, using arterial blood gases and serum bicarbonate levels, in critically ill patients. The diet should have a high protein content along with glucose to minimize protein catabolism and production of nitrogenous waste.

In the event of significant renal deterioration during pregnancy dialysis could be considered. Hemodialysis is generally preferred to peritoneal dialysis in an antenatal patient requiring dialysis for the first time. There is no evidence that dialysis speeds recovery in patients who would recover with conservative management, indeed dialysis may prolong recovery (Conger, 1990; Mindell and Chertow, 1997). As many as 80% of patients with underlying renal disease who develop renal failure associated with pre-eclampsia such that dialysis is required will proceed onto long-term renal replacement therapy. Although it is the exception for patients who had normal renal function prepregnancy to have long-term renal impairment even if dialysis had been required as a supportive measure, there is controversy as to whether or not the entire vascular tree fully recovers.

Postnatal management

A postnatal review at 6–12 weeks after delivery provides an opportunity to endorse the earlier diagnosis of pre-eclampsia (assuming the blood pressure has returned to normal) and to ensure that any systemic complications have resolved. Assessment of renal recovery involves establishing that serum electrolytes have returned to normal and performing dipstick analysis of a urine sample. Any unexplained persistent proteinuria should prompt referral for further renal investigation.

The importance of ensuring that renal impairment detected in hypertensive pregnancies is indeed attributable to pre-eclampsia has been highlighted by Ficher *et al.* (1981). Renal biopsies were taken in the postpartum period in 176 women who had been diagnosed in pregnancy as having renal complications of pre-eclampsia. An alternative diagnosis was established in a third of cases overall, and in the multiparous group alone almost two-thirds of patients had an alternative diagnosis established.

Severe pre-eclampsia has a recurrence rate of 30% in future pregnancies although generally the onset of problems is 2–3 weeks later and it is less severe than in the first pregnancy (Walker, 2000). Patients who are identified as having underlying renal or hypertensive problems will be at a higher risk of recurrence of superimposed pre-eclampsia and will be more likely to have further renal complications. Such patients should be advised to attend for prepregnancy counseling before embarking on further pregnancies to ensure that hypertension is controlled optimally and that the extent of any renal impairment can be assessed in order that they can be advised with regards to the risks of further pregnancy.

Summary

The renal system is important in both the pathogenesis and pathological sequelae of pre-eclampsia. All pre-eclamptic patients will have renal involvement to some degree and this should be monitored against the background of what would be the normal enhanced renal function in pregnancy. Even patients who have severe renal compromise during the peripartum period can generally be expected to make an excellent recovery with negligible residual renal impairment, providing there has been appropriate blood pressure control and meticulous fluid management.

Given the significant number of patients who will have pre-eclampsia superimposed on previously unsuspected renal disease it is important to assess patients in the postnatal period to exclude ongoing problems which may impact a future pregnancy.

REFERENCES

Alexander, B.T., Miller, M.T., Kassab, S., *et al.* (1999). Differential expression of renal nitric oxide synthase isoforms during pregnancy in rats. *Hypertension*, **33**, 435–9.

Assali, N., Dignam, W. and Dasgupta, K. (1959). Renal function in human pregnancy. *J. Lab. Clin. Med.*, **54**, 394–408.

Baylis, C. (1980). The mechanism of the increase in glomerular filtration rate in the twelve-day pregnant rat. *J. Physiol.*, **305**, 405–14.

Baylis, C. (1987). The determinants of renal hemodynamics in pregnancy. *Am. J. Kidney Dis.*, **9**, 260–4.

Baylis, C. (1994). Glomerular filtration and volume regulation in gravid animal models. *Baill. Clin. Obstet. Gynaecol.*, **8**, 235–64.

Baylis, C. (1999). Relaxin may be the "elusive" renal vasodilatory agent of normal pregnancy. *Am. J. Kidney Dis.*, **34**, 1142–4; discussion 1144–5.

Baylis, C. and Reckelhoff, J.F. (1991). Renal hemodynamics in normal and hypertensive pregnancy: lessons from micropuncture. *Am. J. Kidney Dis.*, **17**, 98–104.

Belfort, M., Uys, P., Dommisse, J. and Davey, D.A. (1989). Haemodynamic changes in gestational proteinuric hypertension: the effects of rapid volume expansion and vasodilator therapy. *Br. J. Obstet. Gynaecol.*, **96**, 634–41.

Bell, S.C., Halligan, A.W., Martin, A., *et al.* (1999). The role of observer error in antenatal dipstick proteinuria analysis. *Br. J. Obstet. Gynaecol.*, **106**, 1177–80.

Brown, C.B., Ogg, C.S. and Cameron, J.S. (1981). High dose frusemide in acute renal failure: a controlled trial. *Clin. Nephrol.*, **15**, 90–6.

Brown, M.A. and Gallery, E.D. (1994). Volume homeostasis in normal pregnancy and pre-eclampsia: physiology and clinical implications. *Baill. Clin. Obstet. Gynaecol.*, **8**, 287–310.

Brown, M.A., Lindheimer, M.D., de Swiet, M., Van Assche, A. and Moutquin, J.M. (2001). The classification and diagnosis of the hypertensive disorders of pregnancy: statement from the International Society for the Study of Hypertension in Pregnancy (ISSHP). *Hypertens. Pregn.*, **20**, IX–XIV.

Bryans, C. I., Jr. (1966). The remote prognosis in toxemia of pregnancy. *Clin. Obstet. Gynecol.*, **9**, 973–90.

Bucht, H. (1951). Studies on renal function in man with special reference to glomerular filtration and renal plasma flow in pregnancy. *Scand. J. Clin. Lab. Invest.*, **3** (Suppl.), 1–64.

Buttar, H. S. (1997). An overview of the influence of ACE inhibitors on fetal–placental circulation and perinatal development. *Mol. Cell. Biochem.*, **176**, 61–71.

Chapman, A. B., Zamudio, S., Woodmansee, W., *et al.* (1997). Systemic and renal hemodynamic changes in the luteal phase of the menstrual cycle mimic early pregnancy. *Am. J. Physiol.*, **273**, F777–82.

Chapman, A. B., Abraham, W. T., Zamudio, S., *et al.* (1998). Temporal relationships between hormonal and hemodynamic changes in early human pregnancy. *Kidney Int.*, **54**, 2056–63.

Chesley, L. C. (1980). Hypertension in pregnancy: definitions, familial factor, and remote prognosis. *Kidney Int.*, **18**, 234–40.

Coll, E., Botey, A., Alvarez, L., *et al.* (2000). Serum cystatin C as a new marker for noninvasive estimation of glomerular filtration rate and as a marker for early renal impairment. *Am. J. Kidney Dis.*, **36**, 29–34.

Conger, J. (1990). Does haemodialysis delay recovery from acute renal failure? *Semin. Dial.*, **3**, 146–7.

Connon, A. F. and Wadsworth, R. J. (1968). An evaluation of serum uric acid estimations in toxaemia of pregnancy. *Aust. N. Z. J. Obstet. Gynaecol.*, **8**, 197–201.

Conrad, K. P. (1984). Renal hemodynamics during pregnancy in chronically catheterized, conscious rats. *Kidney Int.*, **26**, 24–9.

Conrad, K. P. (1987). Possible mechanisms for changes in renal hemodynamics during pregnancy: studies from animal models. *Am. J. Kidney Dis.*, **9**, 253–9.

Conrad, K. P. and Lindheimer, M. D. (1999). Renal and cardiovascular alterations. In *Chesleys Hypertensive Disorders of Pregnancy*, ed. F. G. Cunningham. Stanford, CT: Appleton & Lange.

Chua, S. and Redman, C. W. (1992). Prognosis for pre-eclampsia complicated by 5 g or more of proteinuria in 24 hours. *Eur. J. Obstet. Gynecol. Reprod. Biol.*, **43**, 9–12.

Danielson, L. A. and Conrad, K. P. (1995). Acute blockade of nitric oxide synthase inhibits renal vasodilation and hyperfiltration during pregnancy in chronically instrumented conscious rats. *J. Clin. Invest.*, **96**, 482–90.

Danielson, L. A., Sherwood, O. D. and Conrad, K. P. (1999). Relaxin is a potent renal vasodilator in conscious rats. *J. Clin. Invest.*, **103**, 525–33.

Davison, J. M. (1984). Renal haemodynamics and volume homeostasis in pregnancy. *Scand. J. Clin. Lab. Invest. Suppl.*, **169**, 15–27.

Davison, J. M. (1997). Edema in pregnancy. *Kidney Int. Suppl.*, **59**, S90–6.

Davison, J. M. and Hytten, F. E. (1974). Glomerular filtration during and after pregnancy. *J. Obstet. Gynaecol. Br. Commonw.*, **81**, 588–95.

Davison, J. M. and Noble, M. C. (1981). Serial changes in 24 hour creatinine clearance during normal menstrual cycles and the first trimester of pregnancy. *Br. J. Obstet. Gynaecol.*, **88**, 10–17.

Davison, J. M., Gilmore, E. A., Durr, J., Robertson, G. L. and Lindheimer, M. D. (1984). Altered osmotic thresholds for vasopressin secretion and thirst in human pregnancy. *Am. J. Physiol.*, **246**, F105–9.

de Alvarez, R. (1958). Renal glomerulotubular mechanisms during normal pregnancy. *Am. J. Obstet. Gynecol.*, **75**, 931–44.

Deen, W. M., Robertson, C. R. and Brenner, B. M. (1972). A model of glomerular ultrafiltration in the rat. *Am. J. Physiol.*, **223**, 1178–83.

Deen, W. M., Bohrer, M. P. and Brenner, B. M. (1979). Macromolecule transport across glomerular capillaries: application of pore theory. *Kidney Int.*, **16**, 353–65.

Deen, W. M., Bridges, C. R., Brenner, B. M. and Myers, B. D. (1985). Heteroporous model of glomerular size selectivity: application to normal and nephrotic humans. *Am. J. Physiol.*, **249**, F374–89.

Dennis, E. J., McIver, F. A. and Smythe, C. M. (1968). Renal biopsy in pregnancy. *Clin. Obstet. Gynecol.*, **11**, 473–86.

Dharnidharka, V. R., Kwon, C. and Stevens, G. (2002). Serum cystatin C is superior to serum creatinine as a marker of kidney function: a meta-analysis. *Am. J. Kidney Dis.*, **40**, 221–6.

Dunlop, W. (1981). Serial changes in renal haemodynamics during normal human pregnancy. *Br. J. Obstet. Gynaecol.*, **88**, 1–9.

Dunlop, W., Hill, L. M., Landon, M. J., Oxley, A. and Jones, P. (1978). Clinical relevance of coagulation and renal changes in pre-eclampsia. *Lancet*, **2**, 346–9.

Durnwald, C. and Mercer, B. (2003). A prospective comparison of total protein/creatine ratio versus 24-hour urine protein in women with suspected pre-eclampsia. *Am. J. Obstet. Gynecol.*, **189**(3), 848–52.

Durr, J. A. and Lindheimer, M. D. (1996). Diagnosis and management of diabetes insipidus in pregnancy. *Endocrine Practice*, **2**, 353–61.

Durr, J. A., Stamoutsos, B. and Lindheimer, M. D. (1981). Osmoregulation during pregnancy in the rat. Evidence for resetting of the threshold for vasopressin secretion during gestation. *J. Clin. Invest.*, **68**, 337–46.

Durr, J. A., Hoggard, J. G., Hunt, J. M. and Schrier, R. W. (1987). Diabetes insipidus in pregnancy associated with abnormally high circulating vasopressinase activity. *N. Engl. J. Med.*, **316**, 1070–4.

Duvekot, J. J., Cheriex, E. C., Pieters, F. A. and Peeters, L. L. (1995). Severely impaired fetal growth is preceded by maternal hemodynamic maladaptation in very early pregnancy. *Acta Obstet. Gynecol. Scand.*, **74**, 693–7.

Dworkin, L. D. (2001). Serum cystatin C as a marker of glomerular filtration rate. *Curr. Opin. Nephrol. Hypertens.*, **10**, 551–3.

Easterling, T. R., Benedetti, T. J., Schmucker, B. C. and Millard, S. P. (1990). Maternal hemodynamics in normal and preeclamptic pregnancies: a longitudinal study. *Obstet. Gynecol.*, **76**, 1061–9.

Edwards, A., Daniels, B. S. and Deen, W. M. (1999). Ultrastructural model for size selectivity in glomerular filtration. *Am. J. Physiol.*, **276**, F892–902.

Ezimokhai, M., Davison, J. M., Philips, P. R. and Dunlop, W. (1981). Non-postural serial changes in renal function during the third trimester of normal human pregnancy. *Br. J. Obstet. Gynaecol.*, **88**, 465–71.

Fadel, H. E., Sabour, M. S., Mahran, M., Seif el-Din, D. and el-Mahallawi, M. N. (1969). Reversibility of the renal lesion and functional impairment in preeclampsia diagnosed by renal biopsy. *Obstet. Gynecol.*, **33**, 528–34.

Fisher, K. A., Luger, A., Spargo, B. H. and Lindheimer, M. D. (1981). Hypertension in pregnancy: clinical–pathological correlations and remote prognosis. *Medicine*, **60**, 267–76.

Furukawa, T., Shigematsu, H., Aizawa, T., Oguchi, H. and Furuta, S. (1983). Residual glomerular lesions in postpartal women with toxemia of pregnancy. *Acta Pathol. Jpn.*, **33**, 1159–69.

Gaber, L. W. and Lindheimer, M. D. (1999). Pathology of the kidney, liver and brain. In *Chesley's Hypertensive Disorders in Pregnancy*, ed. F. G. Cunningham. Stamford, CT: Appleton & Lange.

Gandley, R. E., Conrad, K. P. and McLaughlin, M. K. (2001). Endothelin and nitric oxide mediate reduced myogenic reactivity of small renal arteries from pregnant rats. *Am. J. Physiol. Regul. Integr. Comp. Physiol.*, **280**, R1–7.

Halligan, A. W., Bell, S. C. and Taylor, D. J. (1999). Dipstick proteinuria: caveat emptor. *Br. J. Obstet. Gynaecol.*, **106**, 1113–15.

Higby, K., Suiter, C. R., Phelps, J. Y., Siler-Khodr, T. and Langer, O. (1994). Normal values of urinary albumin and total protein excretion during pregnancy. *Am. J. Obstet. Gynecol.*, **171**, 984–9.

Hytten, F. E. and Leitch, I. (1971). *The Physiology of Human Pregnancy*. London: Blackwell Scientific.

Katz, A. I., Davison, J. M., Hayslett, J. P., Singson, E. and Lindheimer, M. D. (1980). Pregnancy in women with kidney disease. *Kidney Int.*, **18**, 192–206.

Kuller, J. A., D'Andrea, N. M. and McMahon, M. J. (2001). Renal biopsy and pregnancy. *Am. J. Obstet. Gynecol.*, **184**, 1093–6.

Lafayette, R. A., Druzin, M. and Sibley, R., *et al.* (1998). Nature of glomerular dysfunction in pre-eclampsia. *Kidney Int.*, **54**, 1240–9.

Lindheimer, M. D., Cunningham, F. G., Roberts, J. M. and Chesley, L. C. (1999). *Chesley's Hypertensive Disorders in Pregnancy*. Stamford, CT: Appleton & Lange.

Lohlein, M. (1918). Zur Pathogense der Neirenkrankheiten; Nephritis und Nephrose mit besonderer Berucksichtigung der Nephropathia gravidarum. *Deut. Med. Wochenschr.*, **44**, 1187–9.

Lopez-Espinoza, I., Dhar, H., Humphreys, S. and Redman, C. W. (1986). Urinary albumin excretion in pregnancy. *Br. J. Obstet. Gynaecol.*, **93**, 176–81.

McFarlane, C. N. (1963). An evaluation of the serum uric acid level in pregnancy. *J. Obstet. Gynaecol. Br. Emp.*, **70**, 63–8.

Meyer, N. L., Mercer, B. M., Friedman, S. A. and Sibai, B. M. (1994). Urinary dipstick protein: a poor predictor of absent or severe proteinuria. *Am. J. Obstet. Gynecol.*, **170**, 137–41.

Milne, F., Redman, C., Walker, J., *et al.* (2005). The pre-eclampsia community guideline (PRECOG): how to screen for and predict onset of pre-eclampsia in the community. *Br. Med. J.*, **330**(7491), 576–80.

Milne, J. E., Lindheimer, M. D. and Davison, J. M. (2002). Glomerular heteroporous membrane modeling in third trimester and postpartum before and during amino acid infusion. *Am. J. Physiol. Renal Physiol.*, **282**, F170–5.

Mindell, J. A. and Chertow, G. M. (1997). A practical approach to acute renal failure. *Med. Clin. North Am.*, **81**, 731–48.

Moran, P., Baylis, P. H., Lindheimer, M. D. and Davison, J. M. (2003). Glomerular ultrafiltration in normal and pre-eclamptic pregnancy. *J. Am. Soc. Nephrol.*, **14**, 648–52.

Newman, M. G., Robichaux, A. G., Stedman, C. M., *et al.* (2003). Perinatal outcomes in preeclampsia that is complicated by massive proteinuria. *Am. J. Obstet. Gynecol.*, **188**, 264–8.

Novak, J., Danielson, L. A., Kerchner, L. J., *et al.* (2001). Relaxin is essential for renal vasodilation during pregnancy in conscious rats. *J. Clin. Invest.*, **107**, 1469–75.

Odendaal, H. J., Pattinson, R. C., Bam, R., Grove, D. and Kotze, T. J. (1990). Aggressive or expectant management for patients with severe preeclampsia between 28–34 weeks' gestation: a randomized controlled trial. *Obstet. Gynecol.*, **76**, 1070–5.

Oe, P. L., Ooms, E. C., Uttendorfsky, O. T., Stolte, L. A., van Delden, L. and Graaff, P. (1980). Postpartum resolution of glomerular changes in edema–proteinuria–hypertension gestosis. *Ren. Physiol.*, **3**, 375–9.

Packham, D. and Fairley, K. F. (1987). Renal biopsy, indications and complications in pregnancy. *Br. J. Obstet. Gynaecol.*, **94**, 935–9.

Pollak, V. and Nettles, J. (1960). The kidney in toxaemia of pregnancy: a clinical and pathological study based on renal biopsy. *Medicine*, **39**, 469–525.

Pryde, P. G., Sedman, A. B., Nugent, C. E. and Barr, M., Jr. (1993). Angiotensin-converting enzyme inhibitor fetopathy. *J. Am. Soc. Nephrol.*, **3**, 1575–82.

Randeree, I. G., Czarnocki, A., Moodley, J., Seedat, Y. K. and Naiker, I. P. (1995). Acute renal failure in pregnancy in South Africa. *Ren. Fail.*, **17**, 147–53.

Roberts, M., Lindheimer, M. D. and Davison, J. M. (1996). Altered glomerular permselectivity to neutral dextrans and heteroporous membrane modeling in human pregnancy. *Am. J. Physiol.*, **270**, F338–43.

Rodriguez-Thompson, D. and Lieberman, E. S. (2001). Use of a random urinary protein-to-creatinine ratio for the diagnosis of significant proteinuria during pregnancy. *Am. J. Obstet. Gynecol.*, **185**, 808–11.

Redman, C. W., Beilin, L. J., Bonnar, J. and Wilkinson, R. H. (1976). Plasma-urate measurements in predicting fetal death in hypertensive pregnancy. *Lancet*, **1**, 1370–3.

Sagen, N., Haram, K. and Nilsen, S. T. (1984). Serum urate as a predictor of fetal outcome in severe pre-eclampsia. *Acta Obstet. Gynecol. Scand.*, **63**, 71–5.

Saudan, P. J., Brown, M. A., Farrell, T. and Shaw, L. (1997). Improved methods of assessing proteinuria in hypertensive pregnancy. *Br. J. Obstet. Gynaecol.*, **104**, 1159–64.

Schiff, E., Friedman, S. A., Kao, L. and Sibai, B. M. (1996). The importance of urinary protein excretion during conservative management of severe preeclampsia. *Am. J. Obstet. Gynecol.*, **175**, 1313–16.

Shilliday, I. R., Quinn, K. J. and Allison, M. E. (1997). Loop diuretics in the management of acute renal failure: a prospective, double-blind, placebo-controlled, randomized study. *Nephrol. Dial. Transplant.*, **12**, 2592–6.

Sibai, B. M., Mercer, B. M., Schiff, E. and Friedman, S. A. (1994). Aggressive versus expectant management of severe preeclampsia at 28 to 32 weeks' gestation: a randomized controlled trial. *Am. J. Obstet. Gynecol.*, **171**, 818–22.

Sims, E. A. H. and Krantz, K. (1958). Serial studies of renal function during pregnancy and the pverperium in normal women. *J. Clin. Invest.*, **37**, 1764–74.

Smith, H. (1951). *The Kidney.* New York: Oxford University Press.

Sheehan, H. and Lynch, J. (1973). *Pathology of Toxaemia of Pregnancy.* Baltimore: Williams & Wilkins Co.

Spargo, B., Potter, E. and McCartney, C. (1973). Renal biopsies from patients with toxaemia of pregnancy. *Arch. Pathol.*, **13**, 593–9.

Strevens, H., Wide-Swensson, D. and Grubb, A. (2001). Serum cystatin C is a better marker for preeclampsia than serum creatinine or serum urate. *Scand. J. Clin. Lab. Invest.*, **61**, 575–80.

Strevens, H., Wide-Swensson, D., Torffvit, O. and Grubb, A. (2002). Serum cystatin C for assessment of glomerular filtration rate in pregnant and non-pregnant women. Indications of altered filtration process in pregnancy. *Scand. J. Clin. Lab. Invest.*, **62**, 141–7.

Strevens, H., Wide-Swensson, D., Ingemarsson, I., Grubb, A., Wilner, J. and Horn, T. (2003). Serum Cystatin C reflects glomerular endotheliosis in normal, hypertensive and preeclamptic pregnancies. *Society of Maternal–Fetal Medicine.* San Francisco, California.

Taylor, A. A. and Davison, J. M. (1997). Albumin excretion in normal pregnancy. *Am. J. Obstet. Gynecol.*, **177**, 1559–60.

Walker, J. J. (2000). Severe pre-eclampsia and eclampsia. *Baill. Best Pract. Res. Clin. Obstet. Gynaecol.*, **14**, 57–71.

Waugh, J., Bell, S. C., Kilby, M. D., *et al.* (2003). Urinary microalbumin/creatinine ratios: reference range in uncomplicated pregnancy. *Clin. Sci. (Lond.)*, **104**, 103–7.

Widholm, O. and Kuhlback, B. (1964). The prognosis of the fetus in relation to the serum uric acid in toxaemia of pregnancy. *Acta Obstet. Gynecol. Scand.*, **43**, 137–9.

24

Management of mild pre-eclampsia

Tracey Glanville and James J. Walker

Introduction

The hypertensive disorders of pregnancy affect more than 10% of the antenatal population. Each year they complicate 80,000 pregnancies in the United Kingdom and account for between 12 and 24% of antenatal admissions (Twaddle and Harper, 1992). Frequent outpatient measurement of blood pressure and urinalysis for proteinuria are the basis of routine antenatal care. The purpose of these tests is to screen for the development of pre-eclampsia, which remains one of the largest causes of maternal and perinatal mortality and morbidity (Walker, 2000). In order to make sure that potential at-risk cases are not missed, the thresholds for diagnosis are kept low and there is a high false positive rate. This means that a further assessment system needs to be in place as a further filter. Many women, especially late in the third trimester, develop transient hypertension that is not sustained, and, therefore, does not contribute to adverse perinatal or maternal outcome. This method of stepwise care helps to diagnose those at-risk of severe pre-eclampsia early, allowing management and intervention which has done much to reduce the maternal mortality rate in the last 30 years (Walker, 2000).

Walker (1987) and Walker et al. (1989) in separate studies examined the progression of hypertension in women attending an outpatient Antenatal Day Unit (ADU) setting from 28 weeks of gestation. These women attended because of a diastolic blood pressure (DBP) greater than 90 mmHg recorded at the antenatal clinic. At the ADU, they were classified at the first visit based on blood pressure measurement, urinalysis hematology and biochemistry. The majority remained at the same level of severity of disease as classified at the first visit. However, half of the women finally classified as severe (DBP > 110 mmHg, proteinuria > 0.5 mg l^{-1}) were initially less severe and 7% of those initially classified as normal and 30% of those with mild disease progressed to a more advanced disease. The percentage of those that progressed to a more severe disease increased the earlier the presenting gestation, suggesting duration of disease as an important contributing factor.

Prediction of disease

The success of outpatient management of hypertension in pregnancy is based on the accuracy and predictive value of the screening tests. The ideal test should allow detection of those who will develop significant disease weeks or months before the onset of clinical symptoms. Currently, the main screening tests are based on the clinical manifestations of pre-eclampsia such as hypertension (Waugh et al., 2001), proteinuria (Murray et al., 2002) and weight gain (Ellison and Holliday, 1997) through the weeks of pregnancy. However, the value of these and their accuracy are not well established. Generally, once certain threshold levels have been reached, further studies are required to assess seriousness as there is a high false positive rate. This is best done in an ADU.

Since the pathogenesis of pre-eclampsia is thought to be related to abnormal placentation, various studies have focused on the use of Doppler studies of the uterine and arcuate arteries. Screening has been assessed in selected and unselected populations, using increased impedance (resistance index of more than 0.58) and/or the presence of a diastolic notch. Increased impedance in uterine artery flow in an unselected population can detect those at increased risk of developing intrauterine growth restriction and pre-eclampsia (Harrington et al., 1991). However, the value of these tests have been largely disappointing in the low-risk population but may be of value in the high-risk pregnancy where the information can be additive (Venkat-Raman et al., 2001).

Platelet consumption is one of the main pathological changes seen in developing pre-eclampsia (Redman et al., 1978). Changes in platelet size is seen prior to the clinical manifestations of the disease (Missfelder-Lobos et al., 2002; Walker et al., 1989). Similarly, uric acid rises in many cases of severe disease but it does not appear to be predictive before the disease is manifest (Ries et al., 2000) but is useful once clinical hypertension is present (Voto et al., 1988).

Other serum markers have also been investigated, with varied results. Most appear to be able to predict around 50% of those who will develop pre-eclampsia (Krauss et al., 2002; Wald and Morris, 2001), but at present these do not appear to be better than traditional antenatal care and are not useful in clinical practice.

Therefore, currently there is no investigation or combination of investigations that fulfills the attributes of an ideal screening test for pre-eclampsia. With greater understanding of the pathogenesis of the disease, hopefully this situation will change. In the meantime, screening is achieved by providing regular antenatal assessment of blood pressure and urinalysis for protein for the early signs of the disease.

Risk factors

There are clinical risk factors that can increase the possibility of disease development and associated morbidity. These include a high BMI (Thadhani et al., 1999), older age (Barton et al., 1997), lower social group (Ceron-Mireles et al., 2001), a family history or past history of pre-eclampsia (Gonzalez et al., 2000). These women may be referred for closer monitoring purely because of these factors alone or in addition to clinical findings.

It is important, however, that the definitions of the thresholds are clear for all carers to follow.

Definitions

Pregnancy hypertension

Pregnancy-related hypertension is usually defined as an absolute systolic blood pressure (SBP) of at least 140 mmHg and a DBP of at least 90 mmHg, on two occasions more than 4 h apart or a DBP of >110 mmHg on a single occasion, after 20 weeks of pregnancy (Davey and MacGillivray, 1988). Since it is the rise in blood pressure that may be important, rather than the absolute value, some definitions include a SBP of 30 mmHg above the earliest recorded pregnancy reading or a diastolic increase of 15–25 mmHg. In women with chronic hypertension, whose blood pressure may already exceed the above thresholds, these increases over blood pressure at booking may be used to aid the diagnosis of superimposed pre-eclampsia but an elevation of blood pressure above a threshold level of 140/90 mmHg may be enough for referral. Pre-eclampsia requires the presence of newly developed proteinuria of at least 0.3 g in 24 h. Once diagnosed, there is no consensus on the subclassification of pre-eclampsia according to severity, but most would consider blood pressures of >160/110 mmHg to indicate severe disease requiring immediate admission and intervention. A further complication for the "pure" diagnosis of pre-eclampsia is the need for the disappearance of these signs after delivery, but this has no place in the clinical management of the condition which is concerned with the acute presentation.

There remains some controversy regarding whether DBP should be recorded as the fourth (muffling, K4) or fifth (disappearance, K5) Korotkoff sound. A recent study has shown that a change from the use of K4 to K5 would mean one fewer case of severe diastolic hypertension recorded for every six hypertensive pregnancies (Brown *et al.*, 1998). The frequency of severe systolic hypertension, or simultaneous severe systolic and diastolic hypertension, did not differ between the two groups. There were no differences in laboratory parameters, need for antihypertensive therapy, fetal birth weight, or incidence of fetal growth restriction, or perinatal morbidity. The K4/5 difference is smaller in hypertensive than in normotensive pregnant women, and K5 is closer to the actual intra-arterial pressure, is more reliably detected and is reproducible (Halligan *et al.*, 1996). Therefore, the adoption of K5 to record DBP should be introduced universally. This would help to standardize the classifications worldwide.

The most important factor about BP measurement is that the method used should be consistent and documented (Natarajan *et al.*, 1999). The blood pressure cuff should be of the appropriate size and placed at the level of the heart. Because of the normal blood pressure variation, an average of several readings should be used to confirm the diagnosis and not single absolute levels (Walker, 2000).

Gestational hypertension

Gestational hypertension is usually characterized by the onset of hypertension, after 20 weeks gestation, in the absence of signs or symptoms suggesting pre-eclampsia or chronic hypertension. It may be the pre-protein phase of pre-eclampsia, the return to the high blood pressure levels of essential hypertension after the normal physiological nadir of the second trimester, or the heralding of a latent hypertensive problem that will develop in later life. No matter what the underlying pathology, any woman who develops a blood pressure above 140/90 mmHg should be seen to be at risk of progression to pre-eclampsia and assessed accordingly (Walker, 2000, 2003).

Pre-eclampsia

Pre-eclampsia is defined as the occurrence of hypertension and proteinuria after 20 weeks of pregnancy. It is the presence of proteinuria that distinguishes pre-eclampsia from hypertension alone. This finding is generally associated with the classic pathological finding of glomeruloendotheliosis (McCartney, 1968), which is not permanent but recovers after delivery. Proteinuria is defined as urinary protein $>0.3\,\text{g}\,24\,\text{h}^{-1}$ (Davey and MacGillivray, 1988). This is most accurately confirmed with a quantitative urinary collection over a 24 h period. Semi-quantitative dipstick urinalysis is commonly used to identify abnormal proteinuria in the clinic setting. Measurements greater than 1+ are considered positive. Studies have shown a poor correlation between dipstick urinalysis and 24 h quantitative measurements (Brown, 1995; Meyer *et al.*, 1994). The protein/creatinine ratio is a better measurement and can be used as an alternative but it is highly variable and, where possible, a 24 h quantitative measurement should still be obtained (Lindow and Davey, 1992).

The presence of proteinuria confirms the diagnosis of pre-eclampsia and the associated rise in risk for both the woman and the fetus. The risk is related to the presence of proteinuria; it is not affected by the absolute value or any increase in the urinary protein excretion (Ferrazzani *et al.*, 1990).

In some cases, there is an absence of either hypertension or proteinuria but other signs such as thrombocytopenia, abnormal liver function or seizures. These can often present with the classic symptoms of abdominal pain and headache (HELLP syndrome) (Weinstein, 1982). This emphasizes the importance of detailed history taking and the consideration of pre-eclampsia as the diagnosis in all cases where there are unusual presenting signs and symptoms.

Stepwise management

Traditionally, when the threshold for hypertension was detected, the women were admitted to hospital for further observation and assessment. This management was based on the fear of progression to severe disease and eclampsia and was not evidence-based. However, because the majority of these women will not progress to severe disease, and because this progression is unpredictable in terms of timescale and severity, the concept of outpatient management was suggested (Mathews *et al.*, 1971; Walker, 1993). It was found that as long as the monitoring could be provided as an outpatient, this could be safely carried out without the need for hospital admission in the majority of cases (Walker, 1987).

One of the reasons for hospital admission was the belief that it was beneficial due to the therapeutic value of bed rest. Crowther *et al.* (1992) performed a randomized study of 218 women with hypertension without proteinuria between 28 and 38 weeks gestation to hospital bed rest or routine outpatient care. Those in hospital were allowed ambulation if desired but were encouraged to rest in bed. Those allocated to outpatient management were encouraged to continue normal daily activities. They were asked to check urine for protein on a daily basis. Weekly outpatient assessment for hypertension was arranged. Admission to hospital was arranged if blood pressure was greater than 160/110 mmHg, >1+ or greater of protein on dipstick, change in fetal movements, or symptoms of pre-eclampsia. Those allocated to hospital care had a lower incidence of progression to severe hypertension but there were no other significant findings for maternal outcome. The mean gestational age at delivery was similar for the two groups (38.3 weeks for hospital, 38.2 for home). There was a significant difference in the preterm delivery rate, which was lower in the hospital group. Otherwise there was no difference in the neonatal morbidity. The conclusion was that outpatient management of nonproteinuric hypertension was a safe alternative to hospitalization as long as close monitoring could be maintained.

Antenatal daycare units

In 1981, the first ADU was opened in Glasgow, Scotland (Walker, 1993). The purpose of this unit was to provide inpatient monitoring on an outpatient basis. It allowed a "third way" of caring for women with hypertension in pregnancy between full outpatient management and inpatient care. It is now accepted practice in the UK, with most hospitals providing this service. It has led to the dramatic reduction in inpatient stay in the management of hypertension and mild pre-eclampsia (Table 24.1). An ADU offers advantages over outpatient visits since it allows repeated blood pressure measurements over a period of time as well as single site access for full assessment of the mother and fetus.

Tuffnell *et al.* (1992) randomized 54 women who presented at 26 weeks of pregnancy or later with nonproteinuric hypertension (SBP 150–170 mmHg and/or DBP 90–105 mmHg on two occasions at least 15 min apart) to either ADU or routine care (clinicians without access to daycare who manage according to established practice). Women randomized to routine care spent on average 4.6 times longer as inpatients (difference in mean stay 4.0 days, 95% confidence interval 2.1–5.9 days) than the group allocated to daycare and were 8.8 times (95% CI 3.0–25.8) more likely to be admitted to hospital. Induction of labor was 4.9 times (95% CI 1.6–13.8) more likely in the routine group compared to the daycare group. The authors concluded that these women could be safely managed in an ADU, with less intervention and with no difference in the deterioration of the underlying disease process.

Since daycare has become more widespread in the management of hypertension in pregnancy, there has been a need to assess the implications of the economic and social value on its use in the health service and also on the women involved (Rosenberg and Twaddle, 1990). The introduction of these services has reduced inpatient workload and the associated costs. Twaddle and Harper (1992) evaluated the efficiency of daycare in the management of hypertension compared to inpatient management with prior domiciliary visits. The comparison was between two maternity teaching hospitals, one with an established daycare and one without. The findings showed that the daycare

Table 24.1. Changes in number of admissions to the antenatal ward because of Hypertension in Pregnancy, Antenatal Day Unit referrals and total average bed occupancy in The Royal Maternity Hospital in Glasgow, a 4500 delivery unit, between the years 1980 and 1989. The ADU was opened in August 1981

Year	80	81	82	83	84	85	86	87	88	89
Daycare referrals	0	25	75	245	423	456	485	492	482	473
Admissions	352	343	256	184	146	134	121	135	120	115
Antenatal bed occupancy		57	55	46	34	27	24	27	22	20

management of hypertension is more efficient than inpatient care with prior domiciliary visits for most women, but less efficient for women with transient or previous hypertension. One important question in the analyses is whether any potential cost savings that can be identified can be translated into actual savings to the health service. For the full cost savings of a daycare system to be realized requires certain conditions to be in place. Beds freed must be closed and not redeployed for other uses. The study showed that there is a lower cost per pregnancy for certain groups of women under a daycare system, although the differences were not significant. A system that could screen out transient hypertension before proceeding to the more expensive daycare system may offer an even more cost-effective solution. Overall, daycare was found to be a very acceptable, safe method of assessment to the women involved.

Home monitoring programs

An alternative to daycare is monitoring in the home environment. This involves variations of home self-monitoring and home visits by midwives or nurse (Leung et al., 1998). This can utilize the increasingly available home blood pressure monitors and self-testing of urine using stix (Barton et al., 1994; Waugh et al., 2001). Although concerns have been expressed about the difficulty of antepartum self-testing and compliance to medical recommendations, particularly in certain at-risk groups (Barton et al., 1997, 2002), the overall benefits of reduced hospitalization with no change in outcome appears uniform (Barton et al., 1994; Crowther et al., 1992;

Leung et al., 1998; Mathews et al., 1971; Waugh et al., 2001).

Blood pressure recordings can be carried out by the women themselves. A study by Waugh et al. (2001) recruited 72 women from the antenatal hypertension clinic in a university teaching hospital. All were high-risk for pre-eclampsia and were asked to measure and record their blood pressure three times per day at home using a validated blood pressure device with an internal memory. 979 measurements were taken, and of these only 2.9% appeared to be inaccurate. These were restricted to three women who admitted family members using the device. The true nonconcordance was therefore 1.4%. The authors concluded that blood pressure recording taken and documented by high-risk women at home were accurate. This allows a method of taking more frequent measurements without the inconvenience of additional visits to hospital and may therefore lead to the earlier detection of progression of pre-eclampsia (Waugh et al., 2001).

There have also been studies into the use of 24 h ambulatory blood pressure monitoring pregnancy, which, if successful will get round the problem of "white coat" hypertension. Brown et al. (1998) demonstrated that normal ambulatory blood pressure in pregnancy showing the expected rise as pregnancy progresses and diurnal variations. Awake measurements are higher than "clinic" measurements recorded under relaxed conditions. It was felt that outpatient ambulatory blood pressure determination may improve the predictive value of blood pressure measurements (Biswas et al., 1997; Penny et al., 1998). However, further studies suggest that the differences seen are small and give no benefit over traditional screening methods (Higgins et al., 1997). A recent Cochrane review concluded that there is no randomized controlled evidence to support the use of ambulatory blood pressure monitoring during pregnancy. Further studies with adequate design and sample sizes are required to establish the usefulness of ambulatory blood pressure monitoring for those at risk of the disease and also in those with established hypertension. They also commented that these trials should not only evaluate clinical outcomes, but also the use of healthcare resources and the women's views (Bergel et al., 2002).

Clinical assessment

The ultimate management of pre-eclampsia is the delivery of the fetus. However, delivery too soon may be detrimental to the fetus because of complications of prematurity. Management of pre-eclampsia is therefore based on detection of those at risk, monitoring of mother and fetus, stabilization of the maternal condition and timing of delivery that is optimum for both mother and her baby. Many studies have demonstrated that prolongation of pregnancy can safely be aimed for with the appropriate selection of women and targeted treatment (Barton et al., 1994; Magee et al., 1999; Visser and Wallenburg, 1995; Walker, 1987). The starting point of this care is the appropriate assessment of the maternal and fetal risk. This requires the women to be flagged and referred to a monitoring system, e.g. an ADU.

Assessment of mother

The purpose of the ADU is to triage those women who have transient hypertension, or mild pregnancy-induced hypertension from those with true pre-eclampsia. This is done by a mixture of clinical assessment, biophysical monitoring and blood analysis (Table 24.2). Fetal assessment is carried out using standard techniques of CTG (NST) and ultrasound (Table 24.2). When the ADU was first started all the tests were carried out in all

Table 24.2. Antenatal Day Unit investigations in St James University Hospital, Leeds

Patient	Investigation
Mother	Full history, including specific questions on symptoms
	Blood pressure level (average of at least three readings)
	Proteinuria (confirms pre-eclampsia; increased fetal risk)
	Platelet count
	Uric acid
	Liver function tests (alanine aminotransferase)
	Creatinine
Fetus	Cardiotocograph (Nonstress test)
	Ultrasound:
	Umbilical artery Doppler
	Liquor volume
	Growth studies

women. It became clear that this was not necessary and a stepwise approach was developed. Initially, a history is taken to assess maternal wellbeing and maternal appreciation of fetal movements. Any symptoms, such as headache, abdominal pain, nausea, flu-like symptoms and visual disturbances should be taken seriously and the management is guided by this. If they are significant, admission to hospital is mandatory. If all is well, four blood pressure readings are taken, 30 min apart, and averaged to assess the average blood pressure level. The reason for this is that blood pressure is an inherently variable parameter and the average gives a better idea of what the true blood pressure is (Pickering, 1993). Urine is tested for the presence of protein. A CTG (NST) is normally carried out at the same time while the woman is waiting to have her blood pressure checked. It was found that 60% of women attending an ADU will have no clinical symptoms, normal blood pressure averages, no proteinuria and a reactive CTG (Walker, 1993). These women do not have any increased risk at this time and can be referred back to the antenatal care system. If the average diastolic blood pressure

Table 24.3. Threshold levels of normality in the assessment of pre-eclampsia

Patient	Investigation
Mother	Diastolic blood pressure $>90\,mmHg$
	Proteinuria $>0.3\,g\,day^{-1}$
	Uric acid $>2\,SD$
	Platelet count $<150 \times 109\ l^{-1}$
	Alanine aminotransferase $\geq 32\,u\,l^{-1}$
Symptoms	
	Headache
	Abdominal pain
Fetus	Intrauterine growth restriction
	AC <10th centile
	UA PI > 2 SD
	MVP ≤ 2 cm
	Or
	AFI < 5

is above 90, there is evidence of proteinuria, or signs of fetal compromise, further testing is carried out (Table 24.2). This consists of tests looking for changes associated with progressive pre-eclampsia, platelet count (Redman *et al.*, 1978), uric acid (Redman *et al.*, 1977) and abnormalities of liver function (Weinstein, 1982). None of these parameters should be taken in isolation and should be considered together. If there is any cause for concern (Table 24.3) admission should be arranged for continued monitoring and management decisions. Around 20% of those that attend ADU will be admitted but not necessarily on the first visit. The other 20%, plus any that return from the antenatal care service, are seen through the ADU for signs of progression. The frequency of visits will in general be determined on an individual basis but for women with stable disease the number of visits is likely to be once to twice per week. The development of proteinuria, increasing edema, signs of systemic involvement which can be assessed by decreasing platelet count, rise in uric acid concentration, abnormal liver function, or the presence of clinical symptoms such as headache, visual disturbance, or epigastric pain should prompt careful assessment with probable admission.

Women should be warned of the symptoms associated with worsening disease in order that they can self refer if they occur between visits.

Therefore, the majority of women attend the ADU once for triage and are either admitted or discharged back into the community. Only 20–25% of women have repeated visits, either to verify the assessment or monitor for signs of progression (Table 24.1).

Use of antihypertensive therapy

In women who have an elevated blood pressure but do not have true pre-eclampsia and do not require admission to hospital, antihypertensive therapy can be introduced. In the United Kingdom during the past 20 years, the use of antihypertensive drugs has increased (Walker, 2000). This has been associated with a reduction in the incidence of cerebral vascular accident as a cause of maternal mortality, although other factors may be involved.

If blood pressure is above 160/100 mmHg, treatment is started in an effort to reduce the risk of hypertensive crisis, the need for further antihypertensive therapy and the need for a hospital admission. Methyldopa and labetalol are the most common antihypertensive therapies used in pregnancy (Magee *et al.*, 1999). Methyldopa has proven safety in terms of long-term follow up of delivered babies (Ounsted *et al.*, 1980). Labetalol would appear to be at least equally safe (Magee and Duley, 2000) but atenalol is associated with an increase in fetal growth restriction. Because of fears concerning fetal affects, angiotensin-converting enzyme (ACE) inhibitors are contraindicated beyond the first trimester (Magee, 2001) although there are case reports of successful outcome where there is no alternative (Muller and James, 2002; Tomlinson *et al.*, 2000).

Although some have suggested starting treatment at lower levels, delaying the treatment of hypertension in pregnancy until DBP is 100 mmHg is not associated with additional maternal or fetal risk and reduces the number requiring treatment by 50% (Walker, 1991).

Since methyldopa has significant maternal side effects, it has been the authors' practice to use labetalol starting at 200 mg bd increasing in increments to a maximum of 1200 mg a day (Walker, 1991). In a prospective double-blind randomized placebo-controlled study of 144 women who developed mild pre-eclampsia after 20 weeks gestation, labetalol significantly lowered blood pressure and reduced the incidence of progression to pre-eclampsia. However, there did not appear to be a benefit in late-onset disease, and therefore the appropriateness of pharmacologic therapy for late onset mild pre-eclampsia may be questioned (Pickles *et al.*, 1992). Labetalol does appear to be well-tolerated with no significant maternal toxicity (Cruickshank *et al.*, 1992). Various studies have demonstrated that in labetalol-treated patients there is less progression to severe disease and a reduction in hospital inpatient antenatal stay without any detrimental effect on fetal outcome. There is a trend toward prolongation of pregnancy, reduction in emergency Cesarean sections and an increase in vaginal deliveries.

Therefore, as long as there is no immediate reason to admit to hospital, antihypertensive therapy can be started safely as an outpatient in the ADU where continued monitoring of the mother and baby can be made on a weekly basis. This appears to be associated with a reduction in hospital admission, prolongation of pregnancy and a reduction of progression to more severe disease (Magee *et al.*, 1999).

Assessment of the fetus

In pregnancy there are two patients, the mother and the fetus. Just because the mother is well, the baby is not necessarily well and vice versa. The main problem for the baby is the associated placental insufficiency (Walker, 2000). Because of this, specific monitoring of the baby is required (Table 24.2). In general, if the mother has no hypertension or proteinuria at ADU attendance no fetal monitoring is required unless there are specific problems like lack of fetal movements. In most ADUs a CTG (NST) is carried out while the

woman is waiting for her blood pressure measurement. Although there is little evidence of clinical benefit (Pattison and McCowan, 2000) it can be beneficial as part of a combined assessment (Begum and Buckshee, 1998) and it is also reassuring to the mother and her carers.

The mainstay of fetal assessment for the at-risk fetus is ultrasound, either in the form of amniotic fluid volume assessment or Doppler ultrasound. Amniotic fluid volume can be measured in various ways, all assessing the amount of fluid present in relation to the fetal and uterine size. This is either done by measurement of the largest single pool or the amniotic fluid index, which is addition of the largest pool sizes in each quadrant. This methodology is useful in the assessment of women with pregnancy hypertension. Depending on the definition used, the incidence of oligohydramnios ranges from 10 to 30% in hypertensive patients. An AFI 5.0 cm or less predicts growth restriction and changes occur with serial assessment (O'Brien *et al.*, 1993). Oligohydramnios is associated with fetal compromise and poor maternal outcome (Banks and Miller, 1999) but a normal AFI does not exclude fetal compromise and other parameters must be taken into account (Magann *et al.*, 1999).

Umbilical artery Doppler waveforms are a better early sign of fetal impairment and are useful in the assessment of fetus wellbeing. A review of 12 randomized, controlled trials of Doppler waveform analysis of the umbilical artery in high-risk pregnancies reported that in the Doppler group, there was a significant reduction in the number of antenatal admissions, induction of labor, and Cesarean section for fetal distress. The clinical action guided by Doppler studies reduced the odds of perinatal death by 38% (95% confidence interval 15–55%). Post hoc analyses also showed a reduction in elective delivery, intrapartum fetal distress, and hypoxic encephalopathy. The study concluded that there was compelling evidence that umbilical artery Doppler should be an integral part of the assessment in high-risk pregnancies affected by pre-eclampsia and suspected growth restriction (Neilson and Alfirevic, 2000). This form of monitoring is used in those pregnancies that are followed up through the ADU (Table 24.2).

Growth-restricted fetuses are at risk of hypoxia and acidemia. In fetal hypoxia there is an increase in the blood supply to the brain, myocardium and adrenal glands, with a reduction in perfusion to kidneys, gastrointestinal tract, and extremities. This compensation is likely to be mediated by chemoreceptors sensitive to changes in the partial pressures of oxygen and carbon dioxide. Cerebral vasodilatation can be monitored through the pulsatility index (PI) of the cerebral vessels, and the middle cerebral artery is commonly used for the assessment of compensatory redistribution of the fetal circulation. However, changes can occur up to 2 weeks before the fetus is jeopardized (Chandran et al., 1993; Severi et al., 2002). Fetal wellbeing can be further assessed using fetal venous Doppler (Hofstaetter et al., 2002) and biophysical profile (Manning et al., 1982). However, if this level of surveillance is required, admission to hospital is usually required. The purpose of outpatient monitoring of the mother and her baby is to assess the progression of risk and consider the need for admission, and ultimately, delivery.

Planning of delivery

Delivery is the ultimate cure for pre-eclampsia. The decision when to deliver is made when the benefits of delivery outweigh those associated with prolonging pregnancy. Timing of the intervention will depend on a number of different parameters relating to either maternal or fetal condition. If there is any evidence of deterioration of the clinical condition after 37 weeks, admission to hospital for delivery may be decided rather than admission to the antenatal ward for further monitoring. From 37 weeks gestation there is little benefit from prolonging pregnancy if there is any degree of concern but stabilization of the maternal condition prior to delivery is still important (Walker, 2000). Also, delaying delivery to allow use of prostaglandins to aid in the induction process, and increase the chances of vaginal delivery, is preferable.

Women with pre-eclampsia have a poorer outcome to the induction process compared to nonpre-eclamptic women (Xenakis et al., 1997). This is partly due to an increased risk of fetal distress, but even when several variables were controlled for by logistic regression, pre-eclamptic women had fourfold higher risk of failed induction and a twofold higher risk of Cesarean section. Therefore, where maternal disease is stable, with no evidence of fetal growth restriction, there is justification to await spontaneous labor, with close continuous monitoring through the ADU. Intervention is then as for other post-date pregnancies.

If antihypertensive therapy is being used, this should be continued throughout labor and into the postnatal period as long as it is required. An epidural, by allowing adequate pain relief, can reduce the rise in blood pressure commonly associated with labor. It also allows a planned delivery and easy transition to surgical intervention if required.

One of the remaining areas of controversy in the management of hypertension in pregnancy is the use of magnesium sulfate. The Collaborative Eclampsia Trial provides compelling evidence that magnesium sulfate is the anticonvulsant of choice in the presence of eclampsia (Duley et al., 1995). More recently, the MAGPIE study suggested the benefit of using magnesium sulfate in pre-eclampsia (The Magpie Trial Collaboration, 2002). This was supported by the recent Cochrane review, which included the findings from the MAGPIE study, and showed that the use of magnesium sulfate was associated with more than halving of the risk of eclampsia (relative risk 0.41, 95% CI 0.29–0.58; number needed to treat 100, 95% CI 50–100) (Duley et al., 2003). There was a non-significant reduction in the risk of maternal death which was not related to convulsion. Side effects, in particular flushing, were more common with magnesium sulfate. There was no overall difference in the risk of stillbirth or neonatal death. However, when data from women in developed countries were analysed, the benefits are less clear. Therefore, there is little evidence that magnesium sulfate is of use in women with mild pre-eclampsia in developed countries (Livingston et al., 2003). The guidelines used in the authors' unit only uses magnesium sulfate prophylaxis in women with diastolic blood pressures above 100 mg Hg and proteinuria. Therefore, those women admitted from the ADU for delivery rarely require this therapy. However, where there is a concern regarding the development of eclampsia, there should be a low threshold for its use.

Postpartum management

Most postnatal pathology, including convulsions, occur in the first 24 h after delivery. Therefore, after delivery the women with mild gestational hypertension and pre-eclampsia should be observed closely for 24–48 h. If being used, the dose of antihypertensive drugs should be lowered after delivery depending on the blood pressure levels. Sometimes the blood pressure does not settle for some weeks after delivery and antihypertensive drugs need to be continued after discharge. The postnatal follow-up should again be carried out through the ADU. If the blood pressure has not returned to normal by 6 weeks postnatally, consideration should be made to investigate the cause further as it may not be pre-eclampsia and the possibility of chronic hypertension, renal disease and other causes should be evaluated.

Conclusion

An Antenatal Day Unit allows the ambulatory management of mild to moderate hypertension through a low-intervention care system but maintains the appropriate monitoring of the mother and baby. It allows continuity of care by experienced trained professionals who are used to the decision-making required and can provide total care including postnatal assessment.

REFERENCES

Banks, E. H. and Miller, D. A. (1999). Perinatal risks associated with borderline amniotic fluid index. *Am. J. Obstet. Gynecol.*, **180**(6 Pt. 1), 1461–3.

Barton, J. R., Stanziano, G. J., et al. (1994). Monitored outpatient management of mild gestational hypertension remote from term. *Am. J. Obstet. Gynecol.*, **170**(3), 765–9.

Barton, J. R., Bergauer, N. K., et al. (1997). Does advanced maternal age affect pregnancy outcome in women with mild hypertension remote from term? *Am. J. Obstet. Gynecol.*, **176**(6), 1236–40; discussion 1240–3.

Barton, C. B., Barton, J. R., et al. (2002). Mild gestational hypertension: differences in ethnicity are associated with altered outcomes in women who undergo outpatient treatment. *Am. J. Obstet. Gynecol.*, **186**(5), 896–8.

Begum, F. and Buckshee, K. (1998). Foetal compromise by spontaneous foetal heart rate deceleration in reactive non-stress test and decreased amniotic fluid index. *Bangl. Med. Res. Council Bull.*, **24**(3), 60–6.

Bergel, E., Carroli, G., et al. (2002). Ambulatory versus conventional methods for monitoring blood pressure during pregnancy. *Cochrane Database of Systematic Reviews* (2); CD001231.

Biswas, A., Choolani, M. A., et al. (1997). Ambulatory blood pressure monitoring in pregnancy induced hypertension. *Acta Obstet. Gynecol. Scand.*, **76**(9), 829–33.

Brown, M. A. (1995). The physiology of pre-eclampsia. *Clin. Exp. Pharmacol. Physiol.*, **22**(11), 781–91.

Brown, M. A., Robinson, A., et al. (1998). Ambulatory blood pressure monitoring in pregnancy: what is normal? *Am. J. Obstet. Gynecol.*, **178**(4), 836–42.

Ceron-Mireles, P., Harlow, S. D., et al. (2001). Risk factors for pre-eclampsia/eclampsia among working women in Mexico City. *Paed. Perinat. Epidemiol.*, **15**(1), 40–6.

Chandran, R., Serra-Serra, V., et al. (1993). Fetal cerebral Doppler in the recognition of fetal compromise. *Br. J. Obstet. Gynaecol.*, **100**(2), 139–44.

Crowther, C. A., Bouwmeester, A. M., et al. (1992). Does admission to hospital for bed rest prevent disease progression or improve fetal outcome in pregnancy complicated by non-proteinuric hypertension? *Br. J. Obstet. Gynaecol.*, **99**(1), 13–17.

Cruickshank, D. J., Robertson, A. A., et al. (1992). Does labetalol influence the development of proteinuria in pregnancy hypertension? A randomised controlled study. *Eur. J. Obstet. Gynecol. Reprod. Biol.*, **45**(1), 47–51.

Davey, D. A. and MacGillivray, I. (1988). The classification and definition of the hypertensive disorders of pregnancy. *Am. J. Obstet. Gynecol.*, **158**(4), 892–8.

Duley, L., Carroli, G., et al. (1995). Which anticonvulsant for women with eclampsia – evidence from the collaborative eclampsia trial. *Lancet*, **345**, 1455–63.

Duley, L., Gulmezoglu, A. M., *et al.* (2003). Magnesium sulphate and other anticonvulsants for women with pre-eclampsia. *Cochrane Database Syst Rev* (2): CD000025.

Ellison, G. T. and Holliday, M. (1997). The use of maternal weight measurements during antenatal care. A national survey of midwifery practice throughout the United Kingdom. *J. Eval. Clin. Pract.*, **3**(4), 303–17.

Ferrazzani, S., Caruso, A., *et al.* (1990). Proteinuria and outcome of 444 pregnancies complicated by hypertension. *Am. J. Obstet. Gynecol.*, **162**(2), 366–71.

Gonzalez, A. L., Ulloa Galvan, G., *et al.* (2000). Risk factors for preeclampsia. Multivariate analysis. *Ginecol. Obstet. Mex.*, **68**, 357–62.

Halligan, A., Shennan, A., *et al.* (1996). Diurnal blood pressure difference in the assessment of preeclampsia. *Obstet. Gynecol.*, **87**(2), 205–8.

Harrington, K. F., Campbell, S., *et al.* (1991). Doppler velocimetry studies of the uterine artery in the early prediction of pre-eclampsia and intra-uterine growth retardation. *Eur. J. Obstet. Gynecol. Reprod. Biol.*, **42**(Suppl.), S14–20.

Higgins, J. R., Walshe, J. J., *et al.* (1997). Can 24-hour ambulatory blood pressure measurement predict the development of hypertension in primigravidae? *Br. J. Obstet. Gynaecol.*, **104**(3), 356–62.

Hofstaetter, C., Gudmundsson, S., *et al.* (2002). Venous Doppler velocimetry in the surveillance of severely compromised fetuses. *Ultrasound Obstet. Gynecol.*, **20**(3), 233–9.

Krauss, T., Emons, G., *et al.* (2002). Predictive value of routine circulating soluble endothelial cell adhesion molecule measurements during pregnancy. *Clin. Chem.*, **48**(9), 1418–25.

Leung, K. Y., Sum, T. K., *et al.* (1998). Is in-patient management of diastolic blood pressure between 90 and 100 mmHg during pregnancy necessary? *Hong Kong Med. J.*, **4**(2), 211–17.

Lindow, S. W. and Davey, D. A. (1992). The variability of urinary protein and creatinine excretion in patients with gestational proteinuric hypertension. *Br. J. Obstet. Gynaecol.*, **99**(11), 869–72.

Livingston, J. C., Livingston, L. W., *et al.* (2003). Magnesium sulfate in women with mild preeclampsia: a randomized controlled trial. *Obstet. Gynecol.*, **101**(2), 217–20.

Magann, E. F., Kinsella, M. J., *et al.* (1999). Does an amniotic fluid index of ≤5 cm necessitate delivery in high-risk pregnancies? A case-control study. *Am. J. Obstet. Gynecol.*, **180**(6 Pt. 1), 1354–9.

Magee, L. A. (2001). Treating hypertension in women of child-bearing age and during pregnancy. *Drug Safety*, **24**(6), 457–74.

Magee, L. A. and Duley, L. (2000). Oral beta-blockers for mild to moderate hypertension during pregnancy. *Cochrane Database Syst. Rev.* (4): CD002863.

Magee, L. A., Ornstein, M. P., *et al.* (1999). Fortnightly review: management of hypertension in pregnancy. *Br. Med. J.*, **318**(7194), 1332–6.

Manning, F. A., Morrison, I., *et al.* (1982). Antepartum determination of fetal health: composite biophysical profile scoring. *Clin. Perinatol.*, **9**(2), 285–96.

Mathews, D. D., Patel, I. E., *et al.* (1971). Outpatient management of toxaemia. *J. Obstet. Gynaecol. Br. Com.*, **78**, 610–14.

McCartney, C. P. (1968). Renal morphology and function among patients with preeclampsia and gravidas with essential hypertension. *Clin. Obstet. Gynecol.*, **11**, 506–21.

Meyer, W. J., Gauthier, D., *et al.* (1994). Ultrasonographic detection of abnormal fetal growth with the gestational age-independent, transverse cerebellar diameter/abdominal circumference ratio. *Am. J. Obstet. Gynecol.*, **171**(4), 1057–63.

Missfelder-Lobos, H., Teran, E., *et al.* (2002). Platelet changes and subsequent development of pre-eclampsia and fetal growth restriction in women with abnormal uterine artery Doppler screening. *Ultrasound Obstet. Gynecol.*, **19**(5), 443–8.

Muller, P. R. and James, A. (2002). Pregnancy with prolonged fetal exposure to an angiotensin-converting enzyme inhibitor. *J. Perinatol.*, **22**(7), 582–4.

Murray, N., Homer, C. S., *et al.* (2002). The clinical utility of routine urinalysis in pregnancy: a prospective study. *Med. J. Aust.*, **177**(9), 477–80.

Natarajan, P., Shennan, A. H., *et al.* (1999). Comparison of auscultatory and oscillometric automated blood pressure monitors in the setting of preeclampsia. *Am. J. Obstet. Gynecol.*, **181**(5 Pt. 1), 1203–10.

Neilson, J. P. and Alfirevic, Z. (2000). Doppler ultrasound for fetal assessment in high risk pregnancies. *Cochrane Database Syst. Rev.* (2): CD000073.

O'Brien, J. M., Mercer, B. M., *et al.* (1993). Amniotic fluid index in hospitalized hypertensive patients managed expectantly. *Obstet. Gynecol.*, **82**(2), 247–50.

Ounsted, M., Moar, V., *et al.* (1980). Infant growth and development following treatment of maternal hypertension. *Lancet*, **1**, 705.

Pattison, N. and McCowan, L. (2000). Cardiotocography for antepartum fetal assessment. *Cochrane Database of Syst. Rev.* (2): CD001068.

Penny, J. A., Halligan, A. W., *et al.* (1998). Automated, ambulatory, or conventional blood pressure measurement in pregnancy: which is the better predictor of severe hypertension? *Am. J. Obstet. Gynecol.*, **178**(3), 521–6.

Pickering, T. G. (1993). Blood pressure variability and ambulatory monitoring. *Curr. Opin. Nephrol. Hypertens.*, **2**(3), 380–5.

Pickles, C. J., Broughton Pipkin, F., *et al.* (1992). A randomised placebo controlled trial of labetalol in the treatment of mild to moderate pregnancy induced hypertension. *Br. J. Obstet. Gynaecol.*, **99**(12), 964–8.

Redman, C. W. G., Williams, G. F., *et al.* (1977). Plasma urate and serum deoxycytidylate deaminase measurements for the early diagnosis of pre-eclampsia. *Br. J. Obstet. Gynaecol.*, **84**, 904–8.

Redman, C., Bonnar, J., *et al.* (1978). Early platelet consumption in pre-eclampsia. *Br. Med. J.*, **1**, 467–9.

Ries, A., Kopelman, J. N., *et al.* (2000). Laboratory testing for preeclampsia: result trends and screening recommendations. *Mil. Med.*, **165**(7), 546–8.

Rosenberg, K. and Twaddle, S. (1990). Screening and surveillance of pregnancy hypertension – an economic approach to the use of daycare. *Baill. Clin. Obstet. Gynaecol.*, **4**(1), 89–107.

Severi, F. M., Bocchi, C., *et al.* (2002). Uterine and fetal cerebral Doppler predict the outcome of third-trimester small-for-gestational age fetuses with normal umbilical artery Doppler. *Ultrasound in Obstet. Gynecol.*, **19**(3), 225–8.

Thadhani, R., Stampfer, M. J., *et al.* (1999). High body mass index and hypercholesterolemia: risk of hypertensive disorders of pregnancy. *Obstet. Gynecol.*, **94**(4), 543–50.

The Magpie Trial Collaboration (2002). Do women with pre-eclampsia, and their babies, benefit from magnesium sulphate? The Magpie Trial: a randomised placebo-controlled trial. *Lancet*, **359**(9321), 1877–90.

Tomlinson, A. J., Campbell, J., *et al.* (2000). Malignant primary hypertension in pregnancy treated with lisinopril. *Ann. Pharmacotherapy*, **34**(2), 180–2.

Tuffnell, D. J., Lilford, R. J., *et al.* (1992). Randomised controlled trial of day care for hypertension in pregnancy. *Lancet*, **339**(8787), 224–7.

Twaddle, S. and Harper, V. (1992). An economic evaluation of daycare in the management of hypertension in pregnancy. *Br. J. Obstet. Gynaecol.*, **99**, 459–63.

Venkat-Raman, N., Backos, M., *et al.* (2001). Uterine artery Doppler in predicting pregnancy outcome in women with antiphospholipid syndrome. *Obstet. Gynecol.*, **98**(2), 235–42.

Visser, W. and Wallenburg, H. C. (1995). Maternal and perinatal outcome of temporizing management in 254 consecutive patients with severe pre-eclampsia remote from term. *Eur. J. Obstet. Gynecol. Reprod. Biol.*, **63**(2), 147–54.

Voto, L. S., Illia, R., *et al.* (1988). Uric acid levels: a useful index of the severity of preeclampsia and perinatal prognosis. *J. Perinat. Med.*, **16**(2), 123–6.

Wald, N. J. and Morris, J. K. (2001). Multiple marker second trimester serum screening for pre-eclampsia. *J. Med. Screen.*, **8**(2), 65–8.

Walker, J. J. (1987). The case for early recognition and intervention in pregnancy induced hypertension. *Hypertension in Pregnancy. Proceedings Sixteenth Study Group of the Royal College of Obstetricians and Gynaecologists*, ed. F. Sharp and E. M. Symonds. New York: Perinatology Press, pp. 289–99.

Walker, J. J. (1991). Hypertensive drugs in pregnancy. Antihypertension therapy in pregnancy, preeclampsia, and eclampsia. *Clin. Perinatol.*, **18**(4), 845–73.

Walker, J. J. (1993). Day care obstetrics. *Br. J. Hosp. Med.*, **50**(5), 225–6.

Walker, J. J. (2000). Pre-eclampsia. *Lancet*, **356**(9237), 1260–5.

Walker, J. J. (2003). Stepwise management. In *Pre-eclampsia*, ed. H. Critchley, A. MacLean, L. Poston and J. Walker. London, RCOG, pp. 370–386.

Walker, J. J., Cameron, A. D., *et al.* (1989). Can platelet volume predict progressive hypertensive disease in pregnancy? *Am. J. Obstet. Gynecol.*, **161**(3), 676–9.

Waugh, J., Bosio, P., *et al.* (2001). Home monitoring of blood pressure in pregnancy at high risk of pre-eclampsia. *Eur. J. Obstet. Gynecol. Reprod. Biol.*, **99**(1), 109–11.

Weinstein, L. (1982). Syndrome of hemolysis, elevated liver enzymes, and low platelet count: a severe consequence of hypertension in pregnancy. *Am. J. Obstet. Gynecol.*, **142**(2), 159–67.

Xenakis, E. M., Piper, J. M., *et al.* (1997). Preeclampsia: is induction of labor more successful? *Obstet. Gynecol.*, **89**(4), 600–3.

25

Management of severe pre-eclampsia

Kristin H. Coppage and Baha M. Sibai

Introduction

Hypertensive disorders are the most common medical complication of pregnancy, affecting 6–8% of all pregnancies (National High Blood Pressure Working Group, 2000). Approximately 30% of hypertensive disorders in pregnancy are due to chronic hypertension and 70% are due to gestational hypertension–pre-eclampsia. The spectrum of disease ranges from mildly elevated blood pressures with minimal clinical significance to severe hypertension and multi-organ dysfunction.

Severe pre-eclampsia is a clinical syndrome that can progress rapidly to an obstetric emergency. It embraces a spectrum of signs and symptoms, primarily systolic or diastolic blood pressure (BP) exceeding 160 or 110 mmHg, respectively, significant proteinuria (>5 g in a 24 h specimen), and evidence of end-organ damage. In healthy nulliparous women, the rate of severe pre-eclampsia is 2–3% (Sibai et al., 1993). It accounts for a significant proportion of indicated preterm deliveries and contributes to maternal and neonatal morbidity and mortality (Kurkinen-Raty et al., 2000; Mackay et al., 2001; Waterstone et al., 2001). Until recently, women with severe pre-eclampsia were delivered without delay regardless of gestational age. When pre-eclampsia occurred remote from term, this practice usually resulted in a nonviable fetus or an extremely low-birthweight infant. Not until the early 1980s was expectant management considered a legitimate option for severe pre-eclampsia. Since most neonatal complications in patients with severe, early-onset pre-eclampsia are caused by prematurity (Derham et al., 1989; Friedman et al., 1995), prolonging a pregnancy for 1 to 2 weeks – or even 1 to 2 days for the administration of corticosteroids – may improve neonatal outcome without increasing maternal morbidity or mortality. This chapter will review the diagnosis and management of severe pre-eclampsia.

Defining severe pre-eclampsia

Pre-eclampsia is severe when it manifests itself with a systolic or diastolic BP exceeding 160 or 110 mmHg, respectively. Pre-eclampsia may also be severe when it involves a systolic or diastolic BP above 140 or 90 mmHg, respectively, accompanied by abnormal hemostasis or end-organ dysfunction, such as headache, visual disturbances, and right upper quadrant pain with nausea or vomiting. The criteria used to diagnose severe pre-eclampsia are listed in Table 25.1 (ACOG Practice Bulletin, 2001). Intrauterine growth restriction (IUGR) was excluded from the criteria in 2000 by the National High Blood Pressure in Pregnancy Working Group because of inconsistencies in its definition.

Severe pre-eclampsia was once thought to have a beneficial effect on the preterm fetus as a result of intrauterine stress. That stress was said to accelerate neonatal lung maturity and neurologic development. However, Schiff and colleagues (1993) reported no significant difference in fetal lung maturity tests between women with

Table 25.1. Classification of pre-eclampsia

Mild pre-eclampsia	Severe pre-eclampsia
Blood pressure ≥140/90 – two occasions 6 h apart (not more than 1 week apart)	Blood pressure ≥160/110 – two occasions at least 6 h apart
Proteinuria ≥300 mg 24 h^{-1} sample	Proteinuria ≥ 5 g 24 h^{-1} sample
Or	Or
≥1+ on two urine samples 6 h apart (not more than 1 week apart)	≥3+ on two urine samples 6 h apart (not more than 1 week apart)
	Oliguria < 500 cc 24 h^{-1}
	Thrombocytopenia < 100,000 mm^{-3}
	Epigastric or right upper quadrant pain
	Pulmonary edema
	Persistent cerebral or visual disturbances

pre-eclampsia and controls. While the rate of respiratory distress syndrome (RDS) was greater in the pre-eclampsia group than the control group, this difference was not significant. Neurologic and physical development, as defined by the Ballard score, were not found to be accelerated at the time of delivery in infants born to women with pre-eclampsia (Chari *et al.*, 1996). In a matched cohort study, Friedman and colleagues (1995) found no significant differences in regard to neonatal death, RDS, severe intraventricular hemorrhage, necrotizing enterocolitis, and sepsis between premature neonates born to women with pre-eclampsia at 24–35 weeks' gestation, and those born to normotensive women with preterm labor. In that study, results were similar for severe pre-eclampsia. These data underscore the fact that neonatal complications in preterm infants are related to prematurity rather than pre-eclampsia.

Severe pre-eclampsia – immediate delivery vs. expectant management

The clinical course of severe pre-eclampsia may be characterized in some patients by progressive deterioration in both maternal and fetal condition. Pregnancies complicated by severe pre-eclampsia are associated with increased rates of perinatal mortality, and increased risks of maternal morbidity and mortality. As a result, there is universal

agreement that all such patients should be delivered if the disease develops after 34 weeks' gestation, or prior to that time if there is evidence of maternal or fetal distress. There is also agreement on delivery of such patients prior to 35 weeks' gestation in the presence of any of the following: premature rupture of membranes, labor, or fetal growth restriction (less than tenth percentile for age). In this situation, appropriate management consists of parenteral medication to prevent convulsions, control of maternal blood pressure within a safe range, and then induction of labor to achieve delivery. If delivery of a preterm infant (less than 36 weeks' gestation) is anticipated at a level I or level II hospital, the mother should be transferred to a tertiary care center with adequate neonatal intensive care facilities.

On the other hand, there is considerable disagreement about management of patients with severe disease prior to 34 weeks' gestation. Some authors consider delivery as the definitive therapy for all cases, regardless of gestational age, whereas others recommend prolonging pregnancy in all severe pre-eclamptic gestations remote from term until either development of fetal lung maturity, fetal or maternal distress, or gestational age of 36 weeks is achieved.

One of the earliest studies dealing with conservative management was that by Nochimson and Petrie (1979). They delayed delivery of patients with severe hypertension at 27–33 weeks for 48 h to permit steroid acceleration of fetal lung maturity. Rick *et al.* (1980) also delayed delivery for 48–72 h when lecithin/sphyngomyelin (L/S) ratio revealed immature fetal lungs.

Martin and Tupper (1975) described the results of conservative management in 55 women with severe pre-eclampsia before 36 weeks gestation. The patients were treated with bed rest, oral phentobarbital, diuretics, and antihypertensive agents. Parenteral $MgSO_4$ was used if there was maternal hyperreflexia or if maternal blood pressure exceeded 170 over 110 mmHg. These authors reported that they could prolong such pregnancies for an average of 19.2 days. Their study was, however, complicated by three stillbirths and two neonatal deaths, resulting in a perinatal mortality of 8.9%. In addition, 56.6% of the neonates were severely growth restricted and 9% were asphyxiated.

Pattinson *et al.* (1988) studied 34 patients with severe pre-eclampsia before 28 weeks managed conservatively with bed rest, antihypertensive drugs, and frequent fetal and maternal evaluation. All 11 pregnancies less than 24 weeks resulted in perinatal deaths. The 34 patients with a gestational age between 24 and 27 weeks had a 38% survival rate.

Odendaal *et al.* (1990) performed the first recent randomized control study, and reported their results of individualized management in 58 women with severe pre-eclampsia at 28–34 weeks' gestation. These patients were treated initially with magnesium sulfate, hydrazine, and corticosteroids for fetal lung immaturity. All received intensive maternal and fetal evaluation in a high-risk obstetric ward. Non-stress tests were done at least three times daily and laboratory tests were evaluated at least twice weekly. Twenty of the 58 women were delivered because of maternal and/or fetal reasons within 48 h after hospitalization. The remaining 38 were then randomized to either aggressive or expectant management ($n=20$). Patients assigned to the aggressive management group received steroids and were delivered within 72 h. Patients assigned to the expectant management group were treated with hydrazine to maintain blood pressure between 140 over 90 and 150 over 100 mmHg. In addition, they received frequent evaluation of maternal and fetal wellbeing. These patients were delivered at 34 weeks' gestation or before in the presence of maternal or fetal distress. The authors found lower neonatal complications and lower number of days spent in the neonatal intensive care unit in the expectant management group.

Fenakel *et al.* (1991) conducted a randomized clinical trial in which patients with severe pre-eclampsia between 26 weeks' and 36 weeks' gestation were assigned to be treated with either nifedipine ($n=24$) or hydrazine ($n=25$). Patients assigned to the nifedipine group received 10 mg to 30 mg sublingually initially, then 40 mg to 120 mg per day orally. Those assigned to the hydrazine group received 6.25 mg to 12.5 mg intravenously initially. Maternal evaluation included frequent measurements of blood pressure, heart rate, platelet indices, urine output, and laboratory tests. Fetal evaluation included daily fetal heart rate monitoring, biophysical profile three times a week, and weekly ultrasonographic assessment of fetal growth. The authors found better control of blood pressure and a lower incidence of fetal distress in the group managed with nifedipine. In addition, the group receiving nifedipine had a better perinatal outcome than those receiving hydrazine. They concluded that nifedipine is a safe and effective drug in the management of patients with severe pre-eclampsia remote from term.

Sibai and co-workers (1994) studied 95 women with severe pre-eclampsia at 28–32 weeks' gestation who were randomly assigned to either aggressive management (AM) ($n=46$) or expectant management (EM) ($n=49$). The two groups were similar at the time of randomization with respect to several clinical and laboratory findings. The average pregnancy prolongation in the EM group was 15.4 ± 6.6 days (range 4–36 days), which was significantly higher than the average in the AM group of 2.6 days ($P < 0.0001$, range 2–3 days). Indications for delivery in the EM group were maternal reasons ($n=16$), fetal compromise ($n=13$), attainment

Table 25.2. Pregnancy outcome in the management of severe pre-eclampsia (Sibai *et al.*, 1994)

	Aggressive management (N=46)	Expectant management (N=49)	Significance
Gestational age at delivery (weeks)	30.8 ± 1.7	32.9 ± 1.5	P < 0.0001
Placental weight (g)	355 ± 88	435 ± 117	P < 0.01
Birth weight (g)	1233 ± 287	1622 ± 360	P = 0.0004
Cesarean section N (%)	39 (85)	36 (73)	NS
Abruptio placentae N (%)	2 (4.3)	2 (4.1)	NS
HELLP, N (%)	1 (2.1)	2 (4.1)	NS
Postpartum stay (days)	5.3 ± 2.1	5.1 ± 1.9	NS

HELLP = hemolysis, elevated liver enzymes, and low platelets.

of 34 weeks' gestation ($n=10$), preterm labor or rupture of membranes ($n=7$), or vaginal bleeding ($n=3$). The maternal indications for delivery were thrombocytopenia ($n=5$), uncontrolled severe hypertension ($n=3$), headache/blurred vision ($n=3$), epigastric pain ($n=2$), severe ascites ($n=1$), and maternal demand ($n=2$). Table 25.2 compares the pregnancy outcomes in the two groups. Gestational age at delivery, placental weight, and birth weight were significantly higher in the EM group. The two cases of abruptio placentae in the AM group were found at time of Cesarean section, whereas the two cases in the EM group were suspected because of abnormal fetal heart rate testing and vaginal bleeding. There were no cases of eclampsia, pulmonary edema, renal failure, or disseminated coagulopathy in either group. No fetal or neonatal deaths occurred in either group. The number of infants admitted to neonatal care unit (37% vs. 46%), average duration of stay in that unit (20% vs. 37%), the frequency of respiratory distress syndrome (22% vs. 50%), and necrotizing enterocolitis (0% vs. 11%) were all significantly lower in the EM group.

The majority of the studies mentioned above have only shown that expectant management is possible and beneficial in a select group of patients with severe pre-eclampsia, and have excluded patients with severe IUGR and HELLP syndrome. The presence of intrauterine growth restriction (IUGR) appears to be detrimental rather than protective for neonatal survival in severe pre-eclampsia and limits expectant management (Chammas *et al.*, 2000; Witlin *et al.*, 2000). In a retrospective study, Witlin and others (2000) reported that the rate of IUGR increased with an increase in gestational age and latency period during expectant management in a series of 195 neonates born of women with severe pre-eclampsia. In multivariate ($P=0.038$; OR, 13.2; 95% CI 1.16–151.8) and univariate analysis ($P=0.001$; OR, 5.88; 95% CI 1.81–192), IUGR decreased survival. Because prolongation of an adverse intrauterine environment may worsen rather than improve fetal outcome, patients with severe IUGR, oligohydramnios and nonreassuring antenatal testing should be excluded from expectant management.

Chammas and colleagues (2000) recommend delivery of an IUGR neonate 48 h after the first dose of betamethasone. In this retrospective study, patients with severe pre-eclampsia <34 weeks' gestation were managed expectantly at the authors' institution. On admission, 19% and 11% of the fetuses were below the 5th percentile and between the 5th and 10th percentiles for estimated fetal weights by ultrasound, respectively. The mean gestational age on admission was 31.1 ± 1.9 for women suspected of having IUGR and 29.3 ± 2.8 ($P=0.034$) for those without growth restriction. The mean latency interval was 3.1 ± 2.1 days for IUGR neonates, which was significantly shorter than the latency for neonates with no IUGR, 6.6 ± 6.1 days. The rates for maternal and fetal indications were similar in both groups. There were no differences in Apgar scores, cord pH and length of stay in the neonatal intensive care unit between the groups. There were two neonatal deaths due to prematurity but none occurred in the IUGR group. Because the mean latency period for IUGR neonates was only 3.1 + 2.1 days, Chammas concluded that IUGR neonates did not benefit by delaying delivery for 1 to 2 days after steroids took effect.

Initial evaluation/management

At the University of Cincinnati, patients with severe pre-eclampsia are admitted initially to the labor and delivery area for continuous evaluation of maternal and fetal condition (Figure 25.1). During observation, they receive a continuous infusion of magnesium sulfate to prevent convulsions, and bolus IV doses of hydrazine (5–10 mg) or oral

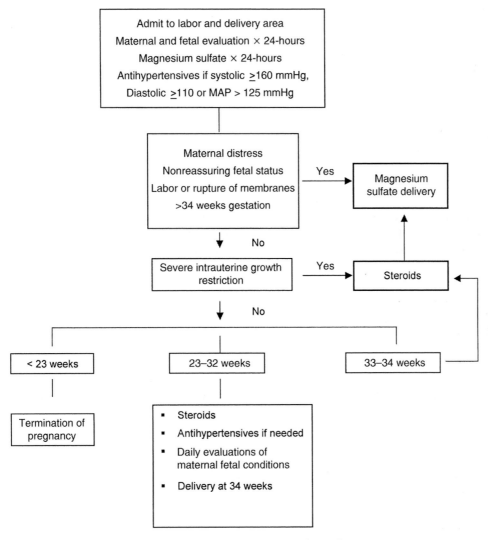

Figure 25.1 Recommended management of severe pre-eclampsia (from Sibai, 2003).

Table 25.3. Maternal/fetal guidelines for severe pre-eclampsia management

	Maternal	Fetal
Expeditious delivery (within 72 h)	One or more of the following:	One or more of the following:
	Uncontrolled severe hypertension[+]	Repetitive late or severe variable decels
	Eclampsia	Biophysical profile <4 on two occasions 4 h apart
	Platelet count <100,000 mm^{-3}	Amniotic Fluid Index <2 cm
	AST or ALT >2x upper limit of normal with RUQ or epigastric pain	Ultrasound EFW <5th percentile
	Pulmonary edema	Reverse umbilical artery diastolic flow
	Compromised real function	
	Abruptio placentae	
	Persistent severe headache or visual changes	
Consider expectant management	One or more of the following:	One or more of the following:
	Controlled hypertension	Biophysical profile >6
	Urinary protein of any amount	Amniotic Fluid Index >2
	Oliguria (<0.5 ml kg^{-1}h^{-1}) which resolves with po intake or IVF	Ultrasound EFW >5th percentile
	AST/ALT >2x upper limit of normal without RUQ or epigastric pain	

[+]Blood pressure persistently >160/110 despite maximum recommended doses of two anti-hypertensive medications.

nifedipine (10 mg) as needed to keep their diastolic blood pressure below 110 mmHg. Maternal evaluation includes continuous monitoring of blood pressure, heart rate, urine output, cerebral status, and the presence of epigastric pain. Laboratory evaluation includes a platelet count and liver enzymes. Fetal evaluation includes continuous fetal heart monitoring, a biophysical profile, and ultrasonographic assessment of fetal anatomy and an estimated fetal weight. Patients with resistant severe hypertension or other signs of maternal or fetal deterioration are delivered within 48 h, irrespective of gestational age or fetal lung maturity (Table 25.3). In addition, patients in labor, or those with fetuses with a gestational age older than 34 weeks, and those with evidence of fetal lung maturity (by amniocentesis) at 33–34 weeks also are delivered within 24 h. Patients at 33–34 weeks' gestation with immature lung studies receive steroids to accelerate fetal lung maturity and are delivered 24 h after the last dose of steroids in the absence of any change in maternal or fetal

condition. Patients at 28–32 weeks' gestation receive individualized management based on their clinical response during the observation period. All of these patients receive steroids to accelerate fetal lung maturity. Some demonstrate marked diuresis and improvement in blood pressure during the observation period. If the blood pressure remains below 100 mmHg diastolic (without antihypertensive therapy) after the observation period, magnesium sulfate is discontinued, and the patients are followed closely on the high-risk ward until fetal maturity is achieved. During hospitalization, they receive antihypertensive drugs (usually oral nifedipine 40–120 mg day^{-1}) to keep their diastolic blood pressure between 90 and 100 mmHg with daily evaluation of maternal and fetal wellbeing. Steroids are usually used as indicated. In general, most of these patients will require delivery within 2 weeks. However, some patients may continue their pregnancies for several weeks. It is important to note that such pregnancies should be managed at tertiary care centers because the course of pregnancy in these women is very unpredictable.

Intrapartum management of severe pre-eclampsia

The goals of management of women with pre-eclampsia are early detection of fetal heart rate abnormalities and prevention of maternal complications. Pregnancies complicated by pre-eclampsia, particularly those with severe disease and/or fetal growth restriction, are at risk for reduced fetal reserve and abruptio placentae. Therefore, all women with pre-eclampsia should receive continuous monitoring of fetal heart rate and uterine activity with special attention to hyperstimulation and development of vaginal bleeding during labor. The presence of uterine irritability and/or recurrent variable or late decelerations may be the first sign of abruptio placentae in these women.

All women with severe pre-eclampsia should have blood pressure recordings at least every hour during labor. Maternal pain relief during labor and delivery can be provided by either systemic opioids or segmental epidural anesthesia. Although there is no unanimity of opinion regarding the use of epidural anesthesia in women with severe pre-eclampsia, a significant body of evidence indicates that epidural anesthesia is safe in these women (National High Blood Pressure Working Group, 2000; Schiff et al., 1994). A randomized trial of 116 women with severe pre-eclampsia receiving either epidural analgesia or patient controlled analgesia reported no differences in Cesarean delivery rates, and the group receiving epidural had significantly better pain relief during labor (Hogg et al., 1999). The use of either epidural, spinal, or combined techniques or regional anesthesia is considered by most obstetric anesthesiologists to be the method of choice during Cesarean delivery. In women with severe pre-eclampsia, general anesthesia increases the risk of aspiration, failed intubation due to airway edema, and is associated with marked increases in systemic and cerebral pressures during intubation and extubation (National High Blood Pressure Working Group, 2000). Women with airway or laryngeal edema may require awake intubation under fiber optic observation with the availability of immediate tracheostomy. Changes in systemic and cerebral pressures may be attenuated by pretreatment with labetalol or nitroglycerine injections. It is important to emphasize that regional anesthesia is contraindicated in the presence of coagulopathy or severe thrombocytopenia (platelet count <50,000 mm^{-3}).

Mode of delivery

There are no randomized trials comparing the optimal method of delivery in women with pre-eclampsia. A plan for vaginal delivery should be considered in all women with severe disease particularly those beyond 30 weeks' gestation (National High Blood Pressure Working Group, 2000). The decision to perform Cesarean delivery should be based on fetal gestational age, fetal condition, presence of labor and cervical Bishop score. In general, the presence of severe pre-eclampsia is not an indication for Cesarean delivery. Our policy is to recommend elective Cesarean delivery for all women with severe pre-eclampsia below 30 weeks gestation who are not in labor and in whom the Bishop score is below five. In addition, we recommend elective Cesarean delivery to those with severe pre-eclampsia plus fetal growth restriction if the gestational age is below 32 weeks in the presence of an unfavorable cervical Bishop score.

Prevention of convulsions

Magnesium sulfate is the drug of choice to prevent convulsions in women with pre-eclampsia. The results of two recent randomized trials revealed that magnesium sulfate is superior to placebo for prevention of convulsions in women with severe pre-eclampsia (Coetzee *et al.*, 1998; Magpie Trial Collaborative Group, 2002). One of the largest randomized trials to date enrolled 10,141 women with pre-eclampsia in 33 nations, largely in the third world (Magpie Trial Collaborative Group, 2002). Almost all of the enrolled patients had severe disease by United States standards: 50% received antihypertensive drugs before randomization, 75% received antihypertensive agents after randomization, and the remainder had severe pre-eclampsia or imminent eclampsia. Among all of the enrolled women, the rate of eclampsia was significantly lower in those assigned to magnesium sulfate (0.8% vs. 1.9%, RR; 0.42; 95% Confidence Interval, 0.29–0.60). However, among the 1560 women enrolled in the Western world, the rates of eclampsia were 0.5% in the magnesium group versus 0.8% in the placebo, a difference that was not significant (RR 0.67; 95% CI 1.19–2.37).

There are two randomized placebo-controlled trials evaluating the efficacy and safety of magnesium sulfate in women with mild pre-eclampsia (Livingston *et al.*, 2003; Witlin *et al.*, 1997). One trial included only135 women and the other only 222 women. Both studies were underpowered to detect a significant difference in seizure rate. There were no instances of eclampsia in either group in these trials. In addition, the findings of both studies suggest that magnesium sulfate does not affect the duration of labor and that it does not affect the rate of Cesarean delivery. The benefit of magnesium sulfate in women with mild pre-eclampsia remains unclear, and a randomized trial to answer this question is urgently needed.

The policy at the University of Cincinnati is to give IV magnesium sulfate during labor and postpartum for all women with diagnosed severe pre-eclampsia. We do not use this therapy in women with mild gestational hypertension or pre-eclampsia in the absence of symptoms. In women having elective Cesarean delivery, magnesium sulfate is given at least 2 h prior to the procedure and continued during surgery and for at least 12 h postpartum.

Control of severe hypertension

The objective of treating acute severe hypertension is to prevent potential cerebrovascular and cardio-vascular complications such as encephalopathy, hemorrhage, and congestive heart failure (National High Blood Pressure Working Group, 2000). For obvious ethical reasons, there are no randomized trials to determine the level of hypertension to treat in order to prevent these complications. The point at which to begin antihypertensive drug therapy is not clear. Antihypertensive therapy is recommended by some for sustained systolic blood pressure values of $\geq$180 mmHg, and for sustained diastolic values of $\geq$110 mmHg. Some experts recommend treating systolic levels of $\geq$160 mmHg, others recommend treating diastolic levels of $\geq$105 mmHg, whereas others use a mean arterial blood pressure of $\geq$126–130 mmHg (ACOG Practice Bulletin, 2001; National High Blood Pressure Working Group, 2000). The definition of sustained hypertension is not clear and ranges from 30 min to 2 h.

The most commonly used and advocated agent for the treatment of severe hypertension in pregnancy is intravenous hydralazine given as bolus injections of 5–10 mg every 15–20 min for a maximum dose of 30 mg. Recently, several drugs have been compared to hydralazine in small, randomized trials. The results of these trials were the subject of a recent systematic review that suggested that intravenous labetalol or oral nifedipine are as effective as each other, and that these two drugs have fewer side effects than intravenous hydralazine (Duley *et al.*, 2000). The recommended dose of labetalol is 20–40 mg IV every 10–15 min for a maximum of 220 mg, and the dose of nifedipine is 10–20 mg orally every 30 min for a maximum dose of 50 mg (National High Blood Pressure Working Group, 2000). We generally use sustained blood pressure values of $\geq$170 mmHg systolic or $\geq$110 mmHg diastolic to initiate therapy intrapartum. For women with thrombocytopenia and those in the postpartum period we use systolic values of $\geq$160 mmHg or diastolic of $\geq$105 mmHg.

Table 25.4. Acute treatment of hypertension

Medication	Onset of action	Dose
Hydralazine	10–20 min	5–10 mg IV every 20 min up to max. dose of 30 mg
Labetalol	10–15 min	10–20 mg IV, then 40–80 mg every 10 min up to max dose of 300 mg
		Or
		Continuous infusion 1–2 mg min^{-1}
Nifedipine	5–10 min	10 mg po, repeated in 30 min prn, then 10–20 mg q 4–6 h
		Max. dose 240 mg 24 h^{-1}
Sodium nitroprusside	0.5–5 min	0.25–5 mcg kg^{-1} min^{-1} IV infusion
		Risk of fetal cyanide poisoning with prolonged treatment

Table 25.5. Chronic treatment with antihypertensive medications

Medication	Dose	Maximum	Half life
Methyldopa	250–500 mg po q 6–12 h	4 g 24 h^{-1}	2 h
Labetalol	100 mg po bid	2400 mg 24 h^{-1}	5–8 h
Thiazide diuretic	12.5 mg po bid	50 mg 24 h^{-1}	3 h
Nifedipine	10–20 mg po q 4–6 h	240 mg 24 h^{-1}	2 h

Our first line agent is IV labetalol, and if maximum doses are ineffective, oral nifedipine is added. Tables 25.4 and 25.5 list the most commonly used antihypertensive medications.

Maternal and perinatal outcome

Maternal and perinatal outcomes in pre-eclampsia are usually dependent on one or more of the following: gestational age at onset of pre-eclampsia, as well as at time of delivery, the severity of the disease process, the presence of a multifetal gestation, and the presence of pre-existing medical conditions such as pregestational diabetes, renal disease or thrombophilia. Perinatal mortality and morbidities, as well as the rates of abruptio placentae, are substantially increased in women with severe pre-eclampsia (Sibai, 2003). The rate of neonatal complications is markedly increased in those who develop severe pre-eclampsia in the second trimester, whereas it is minimally increased

in those with severe pre-eclampsia beyond 35 weeks' gestation.

Severe pre-eclampsia is also associated with an increased risk of maternal mortality (0.2%), and increased rates of maternal morbidity (5%) with conditions such as convulsions, intracranial hemorrhage/infarction, pulmonary edema, acute renal or liver failure, liver hemorrhage, pancreatitis, and disseminated intravascular coagulopathy (DIC). These complications are usually seen in women who develop pre-eclampsia before 32 weeks' gestation and in those with pre-existing medical conditions (Sibai, 2003).

Summary

Patients with pre-eclampsia are at great risk for maternal and neonatal morbidity and mortality. Every effort should be made to maximize the care for both. The risk to the fetus relates largely to the gestational age at delivery. The risk to the mother can be significant and includes the possible development of disseminated intravascular coagulation, intracranial hemorrhage, renal failure, retinal detachment, pulmonary edema, liver rupture, abruptio placentae, and death. Therefore, the risks and benefits of immediate delivery versus expectant management must be weighed carefully. Chapters such as this can, and should, only be regarded as a guideline. The providers involved in each individual patient's care should rely on their clinical judgment to determine which strategy is best for any particular patient. The ultimate goal should always be safety of the mother first, and delivery of a mature infant who will not require intensive and prolonged neonatal care.

REFERENCES

ACOG Practice Bulletin No. 33. (2001). Diagnosis and management of preeclampsia and eclampsia. American College of Obstetricians and Gynecologists. *Obstet. Gynecol.*, **98**, 159–67.

Chammas, M. F., Nguyen, T. M., Li, M. A., Nuwayhid, B. S. and Castro, L. C. (2000). Expectant management of severe preterm preeclampsia: is intrauterine growth restriction an indication for immediate delivery. *Am. J. Obstet. Gynecol.*, **183**, 853–8.

Chari, R. S., Friedman, S. A., Schiff, E., Frangieh, A. T. and Sibai, B. M. (1996). Is fetal neurologic and physical development accelerated in preeclampsia? *Am. J. Obstet. Gynecol.*, **174**, 829–32.

Coetzee, E. J., Dommisse, J. and Anthony, J. (1998). A randomized controlled trial of intravenous magnesium sulfate versus placebo in the management of women with severe preeclampsia. *Br. J. Obstet. Gynaecol.*, **105**, 300–3.

Derham, R. J., Hawkins, D. F., de Vries, L. S., Aber, V. R. and Elder, M. G. (1989). Outcome of pregnancies complicated by severe hypertension and delivered before 34 weeks; stepwise logistic regression analysis of prognostic factors. *Br. J. Obstet. Gynaecol.*, **96**, 1173–81.

Duley, L. and Henderson-Smart, D. J. (2000). Drugs for rapid treatment of very high blood pressure during pregnancy (Cochrane Review). *Cochrane Library*, **2**.

Fenakel, K., Fenakel, E., Appleman, Z., *et al.* (1991). Nifedipine in the treatment of severe preeclampsia. *Obstet. Gynecol.*, **77**, 331.

Friedman, S. A., Schiff, E., Koa, L. and Sibai, B. M. (1995). Neonatal outcome after preterm delivery for preeclampsia. *Am. J. Obstet. Gynecol.*, **172**, 1785–92.

Hogg, B., Hauth, J. C., Caritis, S. N., Sibai, B. M., Lindheimer, M., *et al.* (1999). Safety of labor epidural anesthesia for women with severe hypertensive disease. National Institute of Child Health and Human Development Maternal–Fetal Medicine Units Network. *Am. J. Obstet. Gynecol.*, **181**, 1096–101.

Kurkinen-Raty, M., Koivisto, M. and Jouppila, P. (2000). Preterm delivery for maternal or fetal indications: maternal morbidity, neonatal outcome and late sequelae in infants. *Br. J. Obstet. Gynaecol.*, **137**, 616–22.

Livingston, J. C., Livingston, L. W., Ramsey, R., Mabie, B. C. and Sibai, B. M. (2003). Magnesium sulfate in women with mild preeclampsia: a randomized, double blinded, placebo-controlled trial. *Obstet. Gynecol.*, **101**(2), 217–20.

Mackay, A. P., Berg, C. J. and Atrash, H. K. (2001). Pregnancy-related mortality from preeclampsia and eclampsia. *Obstet. Gynecol.*, **97**, 533–83.

The Magpie Trial Collaborative Group. (2002). Do women with pre-eclampsia, and their babies, benefit from magnesium sulfate? The Magpie trial: a randomized placebo-controlled trial. *Lancet*, **359**, 1877–90.

Martin, T. N. and Tupper, W. R. C. (1975). The management of severe toxemia in patients less than 36 weeks gestation. *Obstet. Gynecol.*, **54**, 602–5.

Report of the National High Blood Pressure Education Program. (2000). Working Group Report on High Blood Pressure in Pregnancy. *Am. J. Obstet. Gynecol.*, **183**, S1–22.

Nochimson, D. J. and Petrie, R. H. (1979). Glucocorticoid therapy for induction of pulmonary maturity in severely hypertensive gravid women. *Am. J. Obstet. Gynecol.*, **133**, 449.

Odendaal, H. J., Pattinson, R. C., Bam, R., *et al.* (1990). Aggressive or expectant management of patients with severe preeclampsia between 28–34 weeks' gestation: a randomized controlled trial. *Obstet. Gynecol.*, **76**, 1070.

Pattinson, R. C., Odendaal, H. J. and Du Toit, R. (1988). Conservative management of severe proteinuria hypertension before 28 weeks' gestation. *S. Afr. Med. J.*, **73**, 516–18.

Rick, P. S., Elliot, J. P. and Freeman, R. K. (1980). Use of corticosteroids in pregnancy-induced hypertension. *Obstet. Gynecol.*, **55**, 206.

Schiff, E., Friedman, S. A., Mercer, B. M. and Sibai, B. M. (1993). Fetal lung maturity is not accelerated in preeclamptic pregnancies. *Am. J. Obstet. Gynecol.*, **169**, 1096–101.

Schiff, E., Friedman, S. A. and Sibai, B. M. (1994). Conservative management of severe preeclampsia remote from term. *Obstet. Gynecol.*, **84**, 620–30.

Sibai, B. M., Caritis, S. N., Thom, E., *et al.* (1993). Prevention of preeclampsia with low-dose aspirin in healthy, nulliparous pregnant women. *N. Engl. J. Med.*, **329**, 1213–18.

Sibai, B. M., Mercer, M. M., Schiff, E. and Friedman, S. A. (1994). Aggressive versus expectant management of severe preeclampsia at 28–32 weeks' gestation: a randomized controlled trial. *Am. J. Obstet. Gynecol.*, **171**, 818.

Sibai, B. M. (2003). Diagnosis and management of gestational hypertension–preeclampsia. *Obstet. Gynecol.*, **102**, 181–92.

Waterstone, M., Bewley, S. and Wolfe, C. (2001). Incidence and predictors of severe obstetric morbidity: case-control study. *Br. Med. J.*, **322**, 1089–94.

Witlin, A. G., Friedman, S. A. and Sibai, B. M. (1997). The effect of magnesium sulfate therapy on the duration of labor in women with mild preeclampsia at term: a randomized, double-blind, placebo-controlled trial. *Am. J. Obstet. Gynecol.*, **176**, 623–7.

Witlin, A. G., Saade, G. R., Mattar, F. and Sibai, B. M. (2000). Predictors of neonatal outcome in women with severe preeclampsia or eclampsia between 24 and 33 weeks' gestation. *Am. J. Obstet. Gynecol.*, **182**, 607–11.

26

The differential diagnosis of pre-eclampsia and eclampsia

Michael Varner

Of the four dominant worldwide causes of maternal mortality (hemorrhage, infection, pre-eclampsia/eclampsia, obstructed labor), pre-eclampsia/eclampsia is the only one whose etiology remains poorly understood. Although the syndrome is now well defined (ACOG, 1996), it is clear that it represents a final common pathway for multiple etiologies. It is also a systemic disorder with potential effects on every organ system in the pregnant woman's body. As a result, pre-eclampsia could be expected to have many and varied presenting signs and symptoms, a reality known well to experienced clinicians. Indeed, the observation that "the most common multi-system disease in late pregnancy is pre-eclampsia" is truly germane to this discussion. On the other hand, women at any time in pregnancy may develop signs and symptoms of virtually any medical condition that might be otherwise unrelated to pregnancy.

A recent review has characterized the differential diagnosis of this syndrome based on the ACOG criteria for severe pre-eclampsia (Varner, 2002). It is thus the purpose of this chapter to examine the differential diagnoses that can mimic this pregnancy complication, with emphasis on those conditions more likely to be associated with clinically significant end-organ involvement. Because real-life clinical practice routinely distinguishes between symptoms and signs and incorporates these findings with laboratory and imaging results, this chapter will review each major organ system by symptoms, signs, laboratory findings and imaging findings, recognizing that some organ systems may

not have any relevant findings. In each case, the assumption will be made that a woman HAS pre-eclampsia/eclampsia and the discussions will address the differential diagnoses of each symptom and sign.

I. Cardiovascular

Cardiovascular symptoms

Chest pain

Chest pain is a symptom that is universally recognized as abnormal by patients as well as by their friends and families. Chest pain invokes concerns about myocardial ischemia. While myocardial ischemia can occur in association with pre-eclampsia, it is rare and usually occurs in women with underlying predisposing risks (age, hypertension or other vascular diseases, etc.). The pain associated with myocardial ischemia is typically described as "pressure" or "squeezing," often radiates to the neck, jaw or ulnar aspects of the arms, and is not characteristically pleuritic. Chest pain in women with pre-eclampsia is more commonly associated with pulmonary edema and/or congestive heart failure.

Chest pain in pregnancy can also represent other rare complications of pre-eclampsia such as pulmonary hypertension, pericarditis or dissecting aortic aneurysm. Individuals with pulmonary hypertension may have pain similar to that seen with myocardial ischemia or infarction. Patients with pericarditis often report pain that is worse when lying down, particularly when lying on their left side. Dissecting aortic aneurysms usually produce severe, relentless anterior chest pain that, depending on the location and extent of the aneurysm, radiates to the back and/or abdomen.

Other causes of chest pain that can be seen in pregnant women include pleuritic pain (sharp in character, related to breathing, and localized) or chest wall pain (pleuritic, but constant and associated with tenderness to palpation).

Shortness of breath

Shortness of breath, or dyspnea, is difficult to define precisely and impossible to quantify. It is often described in terms such as "suffocating" or "inability to take a deep breath" or "chest tightness." The shortness of breath associated with pre-eclampsia is virtually always a result of pulmonary edema. Most frequently this symptom develops over a few hours, although it can develop acutely.

The sudden development of dyspnea should raise concerns about pulmonary embolism, spontaneous pneumothorax, or anxiety. Dyspnea that awakens individuals from a sound sleep is called paroxysmal nocturnal dyspnea and should suggest some degree of left ventricular failure and/or chronic pulmonary disease. Orthopnea, or the onset or worsening of dyspnea upon assuming a supine position, should also suggest some degree of left ventricular failure and/or chronic pulmonary disease. In both cases the dyspnea associated with chronic pulmonary disease can be produced by pooling of secretions and/or gravity-induced decreases in lung volumes.

Cardiovascular signs

Hypertension

It is now clear that persistent systolic blood pressures above 160 mmHg and/or diastolic blood pressures above 110 mmHg represent thresholds above which the risks progressively increase for both mother and baby (NHBPEP, 2000).

Clinical experience dictates that the new onset of hypertension in the latter half of pregnancy always be considered the onset of pre-eclampsia, at least until proven otherwise, particularly in young (<age 25) previously healthy primigravidas. On the other hand, the renal biopsy findings from the University of Chicago studies demonstrate clearly that a sizable proportion of such women will also have other underlying causes for hypertension such as chronic renal disease, chronic hypertension or autoimmune disease (Fisher et al., 1981). The possibility of underlying microvascular disease either mimicking or complicating pre-eclampsia should be particularly considered in pregnant women whose hypertension is present in the first half of pregnancy, who develop pre-eclampsia in other than their first viable pregnancy or whose pre-eclampsia is early and severe in onset.

Women with chronic hypertension commonly have elevated blood pressures prior to pregnancy. Many individuals with chronic hypertension will have a positive family history of hypertension and its complications, including congestive heart failure, coronary artery disease, stroke and renal dysfunction. However, chronic hypertension may also be first suspected when hypertension is identified prior to 20 weeks gestation.

There has been substantial interest in the past decade in the influence of the intrauterine environment on long-term cardiovascular function (Barker and Osmond, 1986). There is also evidence that several gene polymorphisms, such as nitric oxide synthase (Hingorani, 2003) and angiotensinogen (Lalouel et al., 2001; Procopciuc et al., 2002), are more common both in pregnancies complicated by pre-eclampsia and in individuals with hypertension and/or atherosclerotic vascular disease, also suggesting that this association might represent different phenotypes of the same genotype.

Underlying renal disease should be suspected when the serum creatinine equals or exceeds $1.0 \, mg \, dl^{-1}$, the creatinine clearance is $<100 \, ml \, min^{-1}$ or an active urinary sediment is seen. Likewise, a sudden acceleration of hypertension, with blunted response to antihypertensives, should suggest the possibility of renovascular hypertension.

Significant blood pressure differences between upper and lower extremities, significant lag between radial and femoral pulses and/or significant blood pressure differences between upper extremities are all suggestive of coarctation of the aorta. Mild-to-moderate coarctations may not become symptomatic until subjected to the major physiologic challenges of pregnancy.

A history of intermittent and/or paroxysmal hypertension, headaches, palpitations, hyperhidrosis, or tremor associated with anxiety should suggest pheochromocytoma. These women may also report visual disturbances, chest or abdominal pain or unusual reactions to medications mediating catecholamines. With extreme hypertension they may also experience convulsions or intracranial hemorrhage. Unexplained myocardial infarction in a pregnant woman should prompt a search for pheochromocytoma. Although most authorities suggest that pregnancy does not affect the disease, the increased cardiac output and blood volume, as well as the mechanical effects of the third-trimester uterus, may exacerbate the signs and symptoms of pheochromocytoma. The additional vascular stimulation and stress associated with labor and delivery may also induce a hypertensive crisis. Pheochromocytoma diagnosed in pregnancy may be treated either surgically or medically. Ninety percent of these tumors are located in the adrenal medulla, but 10% are extra-adrenal and may be difficult to locate. Ten percent are malignant. Surgery is best reserved for the first half of pregnancy, both for considerations of visualization and maternal vascular volume and for consideration of fetal well-being. Ten percent of pheochromocytomas will recur after surgical removal and the patient should be made aware of this fact. The tumor can also be treated by alpha-adrenergic blockade using oral phenyxybenzamine (starting at 10 mg per day and increasing every 2 days to a maximum of $1 \, mg \, kg^{-1} day^{-1}$) for maintenance

therapy and IV phentolamine or nitroprusside for emergency blood pressure control.

Primary hyperaldosteronism is a rare cause of hypertension in pregnancy (Solomon et al., 1996). Occasionally this hypertension can be severe, and can be confused with pre-eclampsia. In addition, the degree of hypertension can be variable and can significantly worsen in first 6 weeks of the postpartum period.

Patients with classic aldosteronism present with hypertension, hypokalemia, and elevated urine potassium levels (Baron et al., 1995; Hammond et al., 1982; Laurel and Kabadi, 1997). Before biochemical diagnosis, hypokalemia should be corrected because a low potassium level suppresses aldosterone. When making the diagnosis potassium replacement should be initiated, all diuretics should be discontinued for at least 2 weeks, and high doses of beta-blockers should be reduced because they reduce renin production. Calcium channel blockers should not be used for at least 2–3 h before testing (Laurel and Kabadi, 1997).

Ultrasonography and MRI are the preferred imaging methods in pregnant women for localizing the tumor, but if necessary any appropriate imaging modality should be used to confirm the presence of a tumor.

If an adrenal adenoma is detected, the preferred treatment is unilateral adrenalectomy (Baron et al., 1995). Cases of successful adrenalectomy in the second trimester have been reported. Early delivery may need to be considered in the third trimester since spironolactone and angiotensin-converting enzyme inhibitors are generally avoided in pregnancy. The goals of therapy are to reduce blood pressure and replace potassium and while alpha-methyldopa, beta-blockers, and calcium channel blockers can be used they have variable success rates.

Pulmonary edema

Pulmonary edema is among the least frequently diagnosed criteria for severe pre-eclampsia.

While this may be because most pre-eclamptic women are delivered before they develop this complication, it may also reflect the infrequency with which obstetric care providers search for and recognize this problem. Pulmonary edema is particularly prone to develop postpartum, when the patient begins her diuresis phase and serum osmolality is further decreased by intrapartum blood loss.

Pulmonary edema usually presents with a nonproductive cough, wheezing, tachypnea and dyspnea. As fluid further accumulates in the capillaries, rales and rhonchi can be heard, initially in the lower lobes, then extending upward as severity of the disease increases. By this point, women are usually acutely dyspneic, pale, sweating, agitated and producing pink or blood-tinged sputum.

The differential diagnosis of pulmonary edema associated with pre-eclampsia includes congestive heart failure, hypertensive cardiomyopathy, or pulmonary embolism. Congestive heart failure and cardiomyopathy can be distinguished by echocardiography. Pulmonary embolism is usually associated with an abrupt onset of new cardiopulmonary symptoms.

Pre-eclamptic women must always have careful attention paid to fluid intake and output. They are perfect candidates for single-page bedside flow sheets on which all of the patient's providers can record and follow her fluid status. This will minimize the risk of iatrogenic fluid overload.

Peripheral edema

The decreasing serum osmolality during pregnancy results in a physiologic expansion of extracellular fluid volume. As a result, almost all pregnant women have some clinically perceptible edema. This is characteristically restricted to the distal extremities and tends to increase through the course of the day.

However, edema in late pregnancy may be the result of many other underlying conditions. In fact, the National High Blood Pressure Education Program Working Group on High Blood Pressure in Pregnancy states that edema in late pregnancy is sufficiently non-specific that it should not be considered a diagnostic criterion for pre-eclampsia (NHBPEP, 2000).

Facial edema, particularly involving the eyelids, is not a prominent finding in normal pregnancy. Women with severe pre-eclampsia may complain of visual disturbances, or even blindness, as a result of prominent eyelid edema. Eyelid edema, particularly when out of proportion to other potential symptoms/signs of pre-eclampsia should suggest the possibility of venous thrombosis, migraine, cellulitis, infiltrative disease or allergic reactions.

Cardiovascular laboratory findings

Troponins

Troponin T and I are sensitive markers of cardiac muscle damage. These assays are widely used in the evaluation of chest pain and have high sensitivity and specificity, having different amino acid sequences from skeletal muscle troponins (Zimmerman et al., 1999).

Normal pregnancy is not associated with any change in serum troponin levels. However, troponin I levels have been shown to be modestly elevated in pregnancies complicated by pre-eclampsia (Fleming et al., 2000), indicating some degree of cardiac myofibrillary damage. Despite these findings, it should never be assumed that any elevation in serum troponin levels in a pre-eclamptic woman is merely a manifestation of her obstetric complication. A thorough cardiac evaluation to exclude intrinsic myocardial disease should be considered in such situations.

Catecholamines

The laboratory criteria for the diagnosis of pheochromocytoma are not affected by the physiologic changes of pregnancy. The hallmark laboratory findings are elevated vanillylmandelic acid, catecholamines and metanephrines in a 24 h urine collection. Importantly, these values may be affected by concurrent alpha-methyldopa, clonidine, labetalol, sotalol, tricyclic antidepressant or levodopa administration and a full disclosure of all medications (and potential alcohol or illicit drug exposures) should be provided to the laboratory with the urine specimen. Other laboratory findings may include erythrocytosis, hyperglycemia and hypercalcemia. As with Cushing's syndrome, pheochromocytoma is not characterized by progressive proteinuria. Because of the risk of associated conditions such as medullary thyroid carcinoma and hyperparathyroidism, an endocrinology workup is important.

Aldosterone, renin levels and renin activity

The measurement of plasma aldosterone levels may not be useful in the diagnosis of hyperaldosteronism in pregnant women because of the physiological increase in aldosterone levels in pregnancy. The levels measured during normal pregnancy are often within the primary hyperaldosteronism range. Pregnant women may have less urinary potassium wasting than other patients with primary hyperaldosteronism because of the antagonizing effects of progesterone. Another factor that may complicate the diagnosis in pregnancy is that plasma renin levels in normal pregnancy are increased. In primary hyperaldosteronism plasma renin levels are usually decreased, and in pregnancy the decrease may be attenuated. Outside of pregnancy salt-loading studies are desirable to confirm the autonomous secretion of aldosterone, but during pregnancy there are concerns about volume overload, worsening of hypokalemia, and the lack of specific reference ranges for pregnancy. One test that can be used in pregnancy involves prolonged positioning of the patient in an upright posture. This usually causes a modest increase in plasma renin activity. However, if there is primary hyperaldosteronism, the renin activity remains suppressed.

Cardiovascular imaging findings

Echocardiography

The increased cardiac output in pregnancy is known to be associated with cardiac remodeling, with load-independent comparisons of left ventricular function (end-systolic stress, rate-corrected velocity of circumferential fiber shortening) demonstrating that left ventricular hypertrophy seen in normotensive and pre-eclamptic pregnancy matches the changes in cardiac work, with preservation of left ventricular contractility (Simmons et al., 2002).

Ultrasonographic assessments of cardiac output have also been developed and in many centers have replaced the traditional thermodilution calculations. Caution must be used when interpreting ultrasonographic assessments of cardiac output in women with severe pre-eclampsia, as this technique has been shown to predictably and significantly underestimate actual thermodilution-measured cardiac output (Basdogan et al., 2000).

A low cardiac output in late pregnancy cannot be attributed to pre-eclampsia and must be explained by another etiology. Conditions commonly associated with low cardiac output include intrinsic myocardial disease, significant valvular or supravalvular stenosis, hypertension, coronary arteriosclerosis or pericardial disease.

Likewise, clinical heart failure can be seen in the presence of a normal, or even high, cardiac output. Diagnostic considerations in this category include hyperthyroidism, anemia and various forms of arteriovenous fistulae.

Pre-eclamptic patients with suspected pulmonary edema require intensive monitoring and represent one of the few generally agreed indications for pulmonary artery catheterization. Initial examination with an echocardiogram will quickly reveal those patients with a poor ejection fraction and systolic dysfunction (i.e. hypertensive cardiomyopathy) or those with diastolic dysfunction and high filling pressures. Undiagnosed valvular disease can also be elucidated with echocardiography. In those women with cardiogenic pulmonary edema, ARDS or sepsis, or who are hemodynamically unstable, a pulmonary artery catheter may be important.

Electrocardiography

The electrocardiogram in the later stages of normal pregnancy demonstrates a characteristic 10–15 degree left axis deviation as a result of diaphragmatic elevation. No left ventricular hypertrophy should be seen. Any other changes on an electrocardiogram require an explanation other than pregnancy and/or pre-eclampsia.

II. Pulmonary

Pulmonary symptoms

Cough

Coughing is an important defense mechanism that protects the airways from the adverse effects of inhaled irritants and/or retained secretions. Most people recognize coughing as abnormal and will seek medical advice more commonly for this symptom than for many others.

Coughing is a common presenting symptom for pulmonary edema, a finding that is particularly prone to present in the immediate puerperium in pre-eclamptic women (Sibai *et al.*, 1987). Pulmonary edema can occur as part of the evolving disease process in which decreasing serum osmolality and increasing capillary permeability result in increased extracellular fluid volumes. However, pulmonary edema in pre-eclampsia is frequently iatrogenic and may result from inattention to fluid balance and/or further decrease in serum osmolality associated with peripartum blood loss. Pre-eclampsia-associated pulmonary edema may present both antepartum and postpartum, so careful attention to the fluid status of puerperal pre-eclamptic women should be maintained until the disease process has clearly abated.

Pregnant women may also develop coughing for reasons unrelated to pre-eclampsia, sometimes even concurrent with evolving pre-eclampsia. A careful history will frequently identify such concurrent problems. In particular, a cough that is worse at night may be the result of congestive heart failure. A cough that is worse after meals should suggest gastroesophageal disease, usually reflux. A cough associated with wheezing should suggest some degree of airway obstruction, most commonly asthma.

Other associated symptoms are appreciably less likely in pregnant women but might include a worsening upon awaking (suggesting overnight pooling of secretions as with severe bronchitis or bronchiectasis).

Hemoptysis

Hemoptysis is not a symptom that is characteristically associated with pre-eclampsia. However, the pink, usually frothy, sputum production associated with pulmonary edema may be mistaken for hemoptysis. In any case, a patient complaint of hemoptysis, or possible hemoptysis, requires prompt evaluation. Hemoptysis in pregnancy should also raise the suspicion of pulmonary embolism, mitral stenosis or pulmonary arteriovenous malformation (Esplin and Varner, 1997).

Chest pain

(See Chest Pain discussion under *Cardiovascular Symptoms.*)

Pulmonary signs

Tachypnea

Increasing fetal respiratory requirements result in an increased respiratory rate during normal pregnancy. Despite the progressive elevation of the diaphragm during pregnancy, diaphragmatic excursion is not characteristically affected and there is a characteristic increase in minute respiratory volume in pregnancy (Contreras *et al.*, 1991). However, resting respiratory rates above 20–25 breaths per minute require further evaluation. Pulmonary edema is characteristically associated with rapid breathing as well as coughing.

Pulmonary laboratory findings

Pulmonary function testing

Given the increased oxygen requirements imposed by the fetus, predictable changes can be seen in pulmonary function testing through the course of pregnancy. Tidal volume, minute ventilatory volume and minute oxygen uptake all increase through the course of pregnancy. However, forced or timed vital capacities are not altered and the functional residual capacity and residual volume of air are decreased as a result of diaphragmatic elevation.

Pre-eclamptic women have been shown to have inspiratory flow limitations (Connolly *et al.*, 2001) as a result of upper airway narrowing in both upright and supine postures (Izci *et al.*, 2003). These changes could contribute to the upper airway resistance episodes during sleep in patients with pre-eclampsia, which may further increase their blood pressure and also contribute to the known increased incidence of snoring in women with pre-eclampsia (Connolly *et al.*, 2001; Izci *et al.*, 2003).

Perhaps a larger concern is the potential effects of magnesium sulfate on pulmonary function. Herpolsheimer and colleagues (1991) demonstrated a significant decrease in pulmonary function tests in term pre-eclamptic patients receiving magnesium sulfate for seizure prophylaxis. These changes included a decrease in maximal inspiratory pressure (an indicator of generalized respiratory muscle weakness), maximal expiratory pressure (an indicator of expiratory muscle strength), functional vital capacity and forced expiratory volume.

Pulmonary imaging findings

Chest X-ray

The aforementioned physiologic changes in the respiratory system during pregnancy produce predictable changes on the chest X-ray in late pregnancy. These include an elevation of the diaphragm, increased cardiac silhouette (in part due to diaphragmatic elevation and in part due to increased blood volume) and increased pulmonary vascular markings. These changes are normal in pregnancy and do not necessarily represent congestive heart failure or fluid overload.

Other X-ray findings of fluid overload and/or congestive heart failure can never be attributed to pregnancy per se and include Kerley's B lines, alveolar edema and pleural effusions. These findings should suggest fluid overload, a condition that is most commonly of iatrogenic origin.

III. Gastrointestinal

Gastrointestinal symptoms

As with other chronic diseases, most women with gastrointestinal diseases will have had symptoms that antedate the pregnancy. However, it is certainly possible both to develop the new onset of a gastrointestinal disease during pregnancy and/or to develop gastrointestinal symptoms associated with pre-eclampsia during a pregnancy. As a result, a careful and accurate history is essential for the correct interpretation of gastrointestinal symptoms during pregnancy. This includes specific inquiries about previous episodes of the current symptoms as well as any previous diagnoses (including the method(s) by which the diagnoses were established) and any history of abdominal surgery. In addition, specific descriptions of the duration, nature and location of the symptoms and connections, if any, between the waxing and waning of symptoms and external factors such as eating, fatigue, activity or stress can be vitally important to establishment of the correct diagnoses.

Nausea

Certain clinical entities associated with the new onset of nausea in late pregnancy require specific evaluation for their exclusion. These include intra-abdominal (most common), intracranial and metabolic diseases. It must be emphasized that the onset of nausea beyond the first trimester should NEVER be ascribed to hyperemesis.

Nausea due to intra-abdominal conditions is usually associated with other gastrointestinal symptoms, characteristically vomiting and/or abdominal pain. Nausea that is exacerbated by food intake should suggest the possibility of cholelithiasis and/or cholecystitis, as this condition is a relatively common cause for non-obstetric surgical intervention during pregnancy. The nausea, vomiting and abdominal pain associated with acute cholecystitis is characteristically exacerbated by food intake and may radiate to the back, particularly if there is common duct obstruction (and associated pancreatitis).

Intracranial hypertension is commonly associated with nausea. While classically associated with early morning projectile vomiting, the nausea can occur at any time and these women should have a fundoscopic examination to exclude papilledema.

A careful history will often identify the concurrent ingestion of other medications, herbal preparations or toxins (recognized or unrecognized) that may be responsible for nausea.

Vomiting

In pregnant women with vomiting a careful history can often be very helpful in identifying or excluding concurrent gastrointestinal disease. Concurrent medications or ingestion of toxins, recognized or unrecognized, may be associated with vomiting, as can concurrent psychogenic disorders.

When a patient vomits during or immediately after a meal it is frequently psychogenic in origin, although the possibility of pyloric obstruction, usually due to an associated ulcer, must be

considered. The possibility of structural distortion of the pancreas by a pseudocyst or tumor could also be considered. These women would be expected to have concurrent pain that, in contradistinction to women with ulcer disease, would not be relieved by vomiting.

Vomiting that occurs an hour or more after eating is characteristic of pancreatitis, gastric outlet obstruction or motility disorders such as gastroparesis diabetacorum. These individuals may have enlarged stomachs that can be palpated or percussed on physical examination.

Idiopathic intracranial hypertension, previously called pseudotumor cerebrii, is also associated with vomiting, as can be other causes of increased intracranial pressure such as mass lesions. While classically associated with early morning projectile vomiting, vomiting can occur at any time. These patients can be easily identified by examination of the optic fundus, where papilledema should be readily apparent.

The contents of the vomitus should also be evaluated. Undigested food would suggest a gastric outlet obstruction, whereas the presence of bile should suggest a postpyloric condition. Likewise, the presence of blood should suggest an inflammatory, or rarely malignant, origin although prolonged vomiting in pregnancy may also lead to hematemesis secondary to gastroesophageal junction lacerations (Mallory-Weiss syndrome).

Finally, consideration must be given to the possibility of iatrogenic causes of vomiting, primarily as side effects of concurrently administered medication. Magnesium sulfate is notorious for causing nausea and vomiting in pregnant women, whether administered for seizure prophylaxis or for treatment of premature labor. The list of additional medications is lengthy and can arguably include many of the medications commonly used in the treatment of pre-eclampsia and/or eclampsia.

Abdominal pain

The abdominal pain classically associated with pre-eclampsia is epigastric and/or right-upper quadrant in location and is not characteristically affected by food intake. The pain associated with visceral and/or hepatic ischemia is characteristically epigastric in location and does not radiate. The pain associated with hepatic hemorrhage may be more localized if the hemorrhage is contained within the liver parenchyma or may be diffuse if it has progressed to hemoperitoneum.

Patients, as well as their friends and families, all recognize that abdominal pain is abnormal and tend to report more promptly for evaluation of this symptom than for many others. Pain resulting from hollow viscera is characteristically dull, poorly localizable but described as midline and associated with nausea and/or vomiting. Esophageal pain may be confused with chest pain (see Chest Pain under *Pulmonary Signs*). As mentioned above, the pain associated with biliary tract disease is characteristically right-upper quadrant and postprandial in nature and is not associated with hypertension or proteinuria. The pain associated with cholecystitis is more constant, may radiate to the back (should suggest secondary pancreatitis) and is often accompanied by fever. Viral hepatitis may be associated with right-upper quadrant abdominal pain but is almost always associated with clinically apparent jaundice and is not characterized by proteinuria or hypertension. Pain from small bowel involvement (ischemia, obstruction, etc.) is characteristically periumbilical in location whereas pain from colonic sources is characteristically lowered abdominal in location. Pregnancy does not increase the risk of appendicitis over that expected in non-pregnant women of reproductive age. However, appendicitis in pregnant women is more likely to be associated with complications.

While recent cautions about vaginal delivery following previous Cesarean delivery have resulted in fewer attempts at subsequent vaginal birth, uterine rupture following previous Cesarean is still a recognized complication of subsequent pregnancies. In contrast to the gradual onset of pre-eclampsia, uterine rupture is an acute, often catastrophic, event generally occurring in labor and with maternal shock, fetal distress and vaginal bleeding. The sudden onset during labor and associated vaginal bleeding generally make this distinction obvious.

Pre-eclampsia clearly predisposes pregnant women to placental abruption. Abruption may also present as abdominal pain. However, physical examination generally identifies the uterus, rather than the upper abdomen, as the source of pain. Likewise, vaginal bleeding, although not invariably present, generally directs diagnostic consideration away from maternal visceral ischemia.

It must be emphasized that pain caused by conditions restricted to the viscera, i.e. without peritoneal involvement, is NOT affected by coexistent pregnancy and will be perceived in the same manner and locations as in the non-pregnant state.

As visceral inflammation and/or ischemia progresses, however, abdominal pain will characteristically shift from poorly localized visceral descriptions to the site of the involved peritoneal irritation. Appendicitis in pregnancy represents an instructive example. While the condition is no more or less common in pregnancy than during any other interval for women of reproductive age, it is likely to be more serious if it occurs during pregnancy, in part because of reluctance to perform the appropriate diagnostic and therapeutic interventions in a timely fashion because of concerns for the pregnancy, in part because the peritoneal irritation associated with the condition is characteristically right-upper quadrant in location, at least in late pregnancy, and is frequently confused with cholelithiasis/cholecystitis, and in part because the peritonitis associated with appendiceal rupture is less likely to be contained by the omentum because of the enlarged uterus.

Specific attention must also be directed to the patient's behavior during the pain. Pain caused by the stretching of smooth muscle (not only the intestinal tract but also the biliary tract and the ureter) is colicky in nature, not affected by movement, and affected patients tend to be restless. In contradistinction, patients whose pain is associated with peritoneal irritation tend to avoid movement, since this makes their pain worse.

Gastrointestinal signs

The presence or absence of associated findings is equally important in the consideration of gastrointestinal system findings in pregnant women who have pre-eclampsia and/or gastrointestinal disease. For example, the development of fever, arthritis, uveitis and/or conjunctivitis in a pregnant woman with hypertension and proteinuria would suggest at least a concurrent underlying autoimmune condition such as systemic lupus erythematosus.

Although palmar erythema and spider telangiectasias should suggest underlying liver disease outside of pregnancy, this association does not hold in pregnancy. Over half of all pregnant women will have these findings as a reflection of their high circulating estrogen levels.

Jaundice

Serum bilirubin levels may be moderately elevated in pre-eclampsia, usually in association with hemolysis and associated increases in lactate dehydrogenase and characteristic peripheral smear findings. The hyperbilirubinemia associated with pre-eclampsia seldom exceeds 5.0 mg% and is usually below 2–2.5 mg%. These latter values are the general range above which jaundice can be clinically detected. As a result, jaundice is seldom clinically evident. Clinically apparent jaundice should raise suspicions of other underlying conditions (Table 26.1).

The hyperbilirubinemia associated with the hypertensive disorders of pregnancy is characteristically unconjugated and is therefore not seen in the urine. Clinical detection of bilirubinuria, characteristic of conjugated hyperbilirubinemia, should suggest extrahepatic obstruction or severe intrahepatic cholestasis. If also associated with pruritis, particularly pruritis that involves the palms of the hands and the soles of the feet and is worse at night, the possibility of intrahepatic cholestasis of pregnancy should be strongly considered.

Ascites

The capillary endothelial disruption associated with pre-eclampsia results in the characteristic edema that has long been associated with the disease. However, edema has been recognized as being a sufficiently variable finding that it is not included in current diagnostic criteria (NHBPEP, 2000). This variability of extracellular fluid accumulation is also seen in the peritoneal cavity. Previous clinical evaluations of women with severe pre-eclampsia as manifested by the HELLP syndrome have shown that the presence of ascites was associated with a sixfold increase in the incidence of congestive heart failure and a ninefold increase in the incidence of adult respiratory distress syndrome, both of which usually became clinically apparent within 24 h postpartum. Those HELLP syndrome patients without ascites at surgery developed congestive heart failure or adult respiratory distress syndrome infrequently (Woods et al., 1992).

In the presence of fetal hydrops, either immune or non-immune, secondary maternal ascites can develop as part of the "mirror syndrome." In this condition, maternal pre-eclampsia with significant hydrops develops presumably as a result of placental edema secondary to fetal hydrops. If the fetal hydrops is reversible, as with a fetal cardiac arrhythmia or acute fetal anemia, it is possible for the mirror syndrome to resolve following treatment (Duthie and Walkinshaw, 1995). This possibility again underscores the importance of a thorough fetal evaluation in any woman with suspected pre-eclampsia.

Non-obstetric causes of ascites must always be considered when clinically significant ascites are encountered in the setting of pre-eclampsia. Conditions to be considered should include cirrhosis of the liver, intra-abdominal malignancy, nephritic syndrome and/or tuberculosis

Table 26.1. The differential diagnosis of hepatocellular dysfunction in late pregnancy

Condition	Symptoms/signs	Laboratory findings	Clinical considerations
Pre-eclampsia	Usually none Hypertension If symptomatic, then by definition is severe pre-eclampsia	Proteinuria (>300 mg 24 h^{-1}) sample, ≥2+ on dipstick, or a urinary protein:creatinine ratio of more that 0.35	The most common multisystem disease in late pregnancy
HELLP syndrome	Upper abdominal pain Nausea and vomiting	Hemolysis Bilirubin LDH Elevated Liver Function Tests SGOT LDH Low platelets <100,000	Often seen in multiparous women who initially have only modest hypertension
Acute fatty metamorphosis of pregnancy	Abdominal pain Malaise Hypertension Proteinuria	Clinically apparent jaundice May be hypoglycemic Clinically apparent coagulopathy is common	Euglycemia suggests residual hepatic function Hypoglycemic women are at increased mortality risk Suspect this condition whenever a significant coagulopathy is seen in a pre-eclamptic woman in the absence of an abruption
Pre-eclampsia-associated hepatic rupture	Sudden right upper quadrant abdominal pain Nausea and vomiting Right shoulder pain from diaphragmatic irritation	Obtundation and shock Progressive coagulopathy Ultrasound may reveal intrahepatic hematoma or hemoperitoneum	90% involve the right lobe Often initially misdiagnosed as an abruption, ruptured uterus or perforated viscus
Long-chain 3-hydroxyacyl-Coenzyme A Dehydrogenase deficiency (LCHAD deficiency)	Abdominal pain Malaise Hypertension Proteinuria	Clinically apparent jaundice May be hypoglycemic Clinically apparent coagulopathy is common	Frequently associated with early significant fetal growth restriction (usually means the fetus is homozygous-positive) (Thyi *et al.*, 1998)
Viral hepatitis	Fatigue, anorexia, nausea and vomiting Pruritis, jaundice, and steatorrhea	Serologic testing may be positive for hepatitis viruses (A through E), the herpesvirus viruses (cytomegalovirus, Epstein–Barr virus, herpes and varicella) or human immunodeficiency virus Clinically apparent hyperbilirubinuria	Hypertension and proteinuria are not present in otherwise uncomplicated hepatitis

Table 26.1. *(cont.)*

Condition	Symptoms/signs	Laboratory findings	Clinical considerations
Cholecystitis	Right upper quadrant pain that sometimes radiates to the back Postprandial nausea and vomiting	Laboratory evidence of obstructive jaundice but not usually clinically jaundiced	The most common incorrect diagnosis in HELLP syndrome
Sepsis	Usually associated with localized pain	Gram stain of infected tissue is helpful for the prompt diagnosis of clostridial or Group A streptococcal sepsis	Should be considered with persistent tachycardia
Cocaine abuse	Often associated with hypertension, convulsions, abruption or preterm labor	Positive maternal or newborn toxicology screen	
Budd–Chiari syndrome	Most common in the first few weeks postpartum	Best diagnosed with Doppler ultrasound imaging of the hepatic veins	
	Painless ascites and rapid abdominal distension	Such patients require evaluation for pregnancy-associated thrombophilias	

(Semshyshyn, 1977). In any such patient the upper abdomen and pelvis should be carefully explored at the time of surgery.

Gastrointestinal laboratory findings

Elevated liver function tests (LFTs)

The liver is frequently involved in women with severe pre-eclampsia and eclampsia. Although transaminases may be elevated to $2000–3000\,U\,l^{-1}$, they are usually $<500\,U\,l^{-1}$. Bilirubin levels may be modestly elevated (2–3 mg%, occasionally to 5 mg%); women with pre-eclampsia are not obviously jaundiced. Intrahepatic and subcapsular hemorrhage may occur and can lead to hepatic rupture.

The description and popularization of the subset of women with severe pre-eclampsia presenting with Hemolysis, Elevated Liver function tests and Low Platelets, or HELLP syndrome (Weinstein,

1982) (Table 26.1) has helped to draw attention to the differential diagnostic considerations of elevated liver function tests in late pregnancy. These women are usually symptomatic (nausea, vomiting, upper abdominal pain) and may not always have dramatic hypertension or proteinuria, at least on initial presentation. They are often initially misdiagnosed as having cholecystitis. However, women with cholecystitis are not thrombocytopenic. This frequent diagnostic error again emphasizes the dictum that "the most common multisystem disease in the later half of pregnancy is pre-eclampsia."

The corollary to the aforementioned dictum is, of course, that other pregnancy-specific conditions can masquerade in late pregnancy as, or be confused with, pre-eclampsia. As outlined in Table 26.1, these include acute fatty metamorphosis of pregnancy (AFMP) and long-chain 3-hydroxyacyl-coenzyme A dehydrogenase deficiency (LCHAD deficiency).

AFMP is a multisystem syndrome characterized by abdominal pain, malaise, confusion or encephalopathy, hypertension and proteinuria that characteristically has its onset in the third trimester. In contrast to pre-eclampsia, these women are clinically jaundiced and have severe hepatocellular dysfunction. This hepatocellular dysfunction frequently manifests itself not only by elevated transaminases but also by obvious coagulopathy and hypoglycemia. This latter finding is ominous and associated with an increased mortality risk. Up to 50% of these women will also develop renal failure and pancreatitis. As with pre-eclampsia, the only known cure for AFMP is delivery. LCHAD deficiency can produce a clinical syndrome resembling AFMP or HELLP syndrome, particularly if the fetus is affected. It can sometimes also resemble persistent hyperemesis gravidarum (Wilcken et al., 1993).

In addition, there are a number of other medical conditions, any of which might co-exist with late pregnancy that should also be considered in the differential diagnosis of pre-eclampsia. In each case, there are other clinical and/or laboratory findings that can help diagnose or exclude these conditions (Table 26.1).

Gastrointestinal imaging findings

Ultrasound

Ultrasound remains particularly well suited to obstetrics because of the direct proximity of the fluid and solid filled uterus to the abdominal wall. In contrast, ultrasound is not at all helpful in the evaluation of gas-filled structures (i.e. bowel, lungs) and has the potential to cause harm. In these structures, the acoustic energy of ultrasound can be converted into mechanical energy, resulting in microbubble motion. This subsequent mechanical energy can result in localized very high temperatures, shockwave generation and free radical production (Miller et al., 1998).

Ultrasound may be helpful for identification of cholelithiasis or a dilated biliary tree. However, the presence of cholelithiasis does not exclude the co-existence of pre-eclampsia.

Ultrasound can also be helpful for identification of subcapsular (usually under the diaphragmatic surface of the right lobe) or intrahepatic hematomas or for hemoperitoneum.

Abdominal CT

Computed tomography remains a valuable modality for imaging the solid organs of the gastrointestinal tract and is most valuable for evaluating the liver for suspected subcapsular or intrahepatic hematoma. It can be of value in assessing patients with an acute abdomen, particularly in the immediate puerperium.

Radiation exposure is between 3 and 5 cGy per examination and should not preclude use of the technique during pregnancy if otherwise indicated in an equivalent setting outside of pregnancy. Complications related to CT are uncommon and are associated with the use of IV contrast agents, primarily as nephrotoxicity (defined as an increase in serum creatinine by more than 1 mg% in the ensuing 48 h) or anaphylactoid reactions ($\sim$1/2500).

IV. Renal

Renal symptoms

Pre-eclampsia and chronic renal disease share the characteristic of often remaining asymptomatic until their respective conditions are advanced.

Renal signs

Most women with underlying renal disease also have few signs until their conditions are far advanced. However, women with renovascular disease may have hypertension of sudden onset. Outside of pregnancy individuals with renovascular hypertension will frequently be found to have upper abdominal high-pitched continuous bruits.

The physical changes of pregnancy make such a physical finding much less likely.

Hypertension

(See Hypertension section in *Cardiovascular Signs* above.)

Renal laboratory findings

Proteinuria

Although normal pregnancy is associated with increased urine protein excretion (up to $300\,mg\,24\,h^{-1}$ as compared to $<100\,mg\,24\,h^{-1}$ non-pregnant), clinically significant proteinuria, particularly in the first half of pregnancy, should strongly suggest underlying renal disease. An obstetric ultrasound should be performed to exclude either gestational trophoblastic disease or multiple pregnancy, both of which have been reported to cause pre-eclampsia prior to 20 weeks gestation. On the other hand, the presence of proteinuria and hypertension late in pregnancy in a woman who has not to that point received prenatal care presents a difficult differential diagnosis, particularly if she has evidence of other multisystem organ dysfunction (thrombocytopenia, acute liver failure, etc.). While the diagnosis of pre-eclampsia should be considered seriously, this diagnosis can only be confirmed via either renal biopsy or puerperal resolution of signs and symptoms.

Otherwise healthy young adults may have postural proteinuria, present when upright but absent when recumbent, but this seldom exceeds $750–1000\,mg\,24\,h^{-1}$. Likewise extreme exertion, fever, seizures (eclamptic or non-eclamptic), antibiotic injury or congestive heart failure may produce proteinuria. However, proteinuria in excess of $1000\,mg\,24\,h^{-1}$ in pregnancy should always be considered an indicator of parenchymal renal disease.

While pre-eclampsia is associated with parenchymal renal disease, it is not associated with active urinary sediment. Hematuria is frequently associated with concurrent systemic disorders such as coagulopathies, sepsis or hemoglobinopathies. It can also be the result of urinary tract trauma, tumors or urolithiasis. Hematuria is often seen in acute-onset renal diseases, both interstitial and glomerular, and in renal infarction. Red cell casts are often seen with glomerular diseases.

Likewise, proteinuria associated with pyuria should suggest an inflammatory process, usually infectious in origin, in the urinary tract. If leukocyte casts also accompany the pyuria, renal parenchymal inflammation is usually present.

Although reported only rarely, the onset of acute glomerulonephritis in late pregnancy may closely mimic pre-eclampsia, since both are characterized by hypertension, proteinuria and edema. A positive streptococcal culture/rapid test, elevated anti-streptolysin O titer and low C3 or C4 complement levels may aid in the diagnosis. Hematuria is common with distorted red cells from glomerular bleeding (as opposed to red cells with normal morphology when the bleeding is from the lower urinary tract). Pregnancy may also occur in women known to have glomerulonephritis prior to conception. These pregnancies are generally well tolerated if maternal blood pressure is normal and the creatinine clearance is at least $70\,ml\,min^{-1}$ (Jungers *et al.*, 1995).

Hyperuricemia

The increase in renal blood flow normally seen in pregnancy results in a decrease in serum uric acid levels, generally to the range of $3–4\,mg\,dl^{-1}$. Presumably in response to the decreased renal perfusion seen in pre-eclampsia a characteristic progressive increase in serum uric acid is seen in women developing the syndrome. However, there is substantial variability between patients and absolute values are not particularly useful.

Elevated uric acid levels in late pregnancy may also be due to many other causes. These are primarily associated with increased nucleic acid turnover such as chronic hemolysis or polycythemia or decreased renal clearance from other causes including intrinsic renal disease, inhibition of urate secretion and/or enhanced reabsorption by drugs, toxins or endogenous metabolic products.

Elevated creatinine/decreased creatinine clearance

Because of the increased renal blood flow and glomerular filtration rate that occurs during pregnancy, creatinine and blood urea nitrogen (BUN) levels are lower during pregnancy, with normal serum creatinine and BUN levels decreasing to approximately $0.5\,\mathrm{mg\,dl^{-1}}$ and 6–$8\,\mathrm{mg\,dl^{-1}}$, respectively. Pre-eclampsia does not increase serum creatinine or BUN until the condition is far advanced. Thus a creatinine of $\geq 1.0\,\mathrm{mg\,dl^{-1}}$ or a $\mathrm{BUN} \geq 12\,\mathrm{mg\,dl^{-1}}$, although within the normal range on most laboratory reports (since the normal values during pregnancy are almost never stated), must be interpreted as elevated during pregnancy. In women whose serum creatinine is $\geq 1.5\,\mathrm{mg\,dl^{-1}}$ in the first trimester, the possibilities of fetal loss and accelerated deterioration of maternal function increase progressively (Cunningham et al., 1990).

Increased renal blood flow and glomerular filtration also result in a characteristic increase in creatinine clearance, almost always greater than $100\,\mathrm{ml\,min^{-1}}$ in the latter half of pregnancy. The specific values will vary substantially based on the muscle mass of the woman. Caution should be exercised in the situation where a serum creatinine is normal but the creatinine clearance is decreased. This is most commonly the result of an inadequate 24 h sample collection and can be evaluated by the amount of creatinine in the 24 h sample. Normal should be between 1.0 and $1.4\,\mathrm{g\,24\,h^{-1}}$ (again depending on maternal muscle mass), with lower values usually representing incomplete sample collection.

Just as proteinuria may also signify underlying renal disease, elevated serum chemistries, especially if present in the first half of pregnancy, may also be a harbinger of underlying maternal renal disease. Indeed, the clinical triad of pre-eclampsia (hypertension, proteinuria, edema) is also seen in many non-pregnant women with intrinsic renal disease. If these findings are present before 20 weeks gestation the likelihood of intrinsic renal disease is very high. The two potential obstetric confounders that can present at this early gestational age are multiple gestation and gestational trophoblastic disease.

The definitive initial diagnosis of renal disease usually requires renal biopsy. However, the aforementioned physiologic changes during pregnancy make this procedure unacceptably dangerous and clinicians are therefore generally obliged to operate on a presumed clinical diagnosis. Previous renal biopsy studies (Fisher et al., 1981) have demonstrated that the majority of primigravidas with apparent pre-eclampsia have the characteristic biopsy findings. On the other hand, multigravidas with the pre-eclampsia syndrome may have only that (38%) but may also have underlying renal disease (26%) or chronic hypertension (24%).

Intrinsic renal disease is not characteristically associated with abnormal liver function tests or thrombocytopenia. The association of these abnormalities with impaired renal function in the latter half of pregnancy further supports the suspicion of pre-eclampsia, although acute fatty metamorphosis of pregnancy (AFMP), hemolytic uremic syndrome (HUS) or thrombotic thrombocytopenic purpura (TTP) should be considered.

Although women with acute fatty metamorphosis of pregnancy (AFMP) may have significant renal impairment, they are also clinically jaundiced, a very uncommon sign in pre-eclampsia.

Although HUS is primarily seen in children, the condition can occur in women of reproductive age. Women of reproductive age with HUS usually have prominent renal failure, impressive gastrointestinal features, and fewer neurologic signs and symptoms. Women with TTP usually have mucous membrane bleeding and petechiae, fluctuating neurologic symptoms and jaundice. Laboratory evidence of microangiopathic hemolysis is present. Hematuria is often a prominent component, a complication not characteristically present in pre-eclampsia.

Microscopic urinalysis

Both pregnancy and pre-eclampsia are associated with quiet urinary sediment. The finding of active urinary sediment, such as casts or significant white cells or red cells, should suggest underlying renal disease. Red cell casts are generally indicative of glomerular injury, while white cell casts are suggestive of parenchymal inflammation.

Hematuria is not a characteristic finding in pre-eclampsia. The finding of hematuria should suggest systemic disorders (hemoglobinopathies, coagulation disorders, sepsis), inflammatory and/ or necrotizing glomerular diseases, structural abnormalities (neoplasia, trauma, urolithiasis) or inflammatory disorders (infection).

Renal imaging findings

Ultrasound

Ultrasound examination of the maternal kidneys is not helpful for the diagnosis of pre-eclampsia per se. However, abnormalities encountered on renal ultrasound may well suggest underlying renal disease. These findings can include renal parenchymal disease (dysplasia, polycystic kidney disease, hydronephrosis, etc.), nephrolithiasis and/or adrenal disease (adenomas, hyperplasia, pheochromocytoma, etc.).

Angiography

Renovascular hypertension is confirmed by the finding of significant renal artery stenosis on angiography. Fibromuscular dysplasia is by far the most common cause in women of reproductive age, although atherosclerosis can occasionally be seen. Definitive diagnosis of functionally significant renal artery stenosis requires selective renal angiography and differential renal vein renin measurements. The venous effluent from the involved kidney should have at least 1.5 times the renin activity of the uninvolved kidney. Outside of pregnancy this difference can be enhanced with the administration of angiotensin-converting enzyme (ACE) inhibitors. Because of their documented adverse fetal effects (Hanssens *et al.*, 1991), ACE inhibitors should be avoided during pregnancy.

V. Hematologic

Hematologic symptoms

The majority of women with pre-existing hematologic disease will be sufficiently familiar with their condition that they can describe their symptoms quite precisely (sickle crisis, paroxysmal nocturnal hemoglobinuria, thalassemias, etc.). Their perception of their symptoms will be unchanged by pregnancy.

Symptoms of hematologic disease whose onset occurs during pregnancy (hemolysis, aplastic anemia, thrombocytopenia, etc.) are characteristically non-localizing (fatigue, weakness, etc.). They are not characteristically associated with pre-eclampsia. Prominent complaints of this type, when accompanied by findings of pre-eclampsia (and prior to magnesium sulfate therapy), should raise the possibility of other underlying conditions. A complete blood count (CBC) is almost universally obtained in the evaluation of presumed pre-eclampsia and would identify any obvious hematologic abnormalities (anemia, leukocytosis, thrombocytopenia, etc.). If these complaints are accompanied by a normal CBC, consideration should also be given to other metabolic or endocrine conditions (see *Endocrine Symptoms* section below).

Hematologic signs

Petechiae

Petechiae are pinpoint lesions resulting from breakage or increased permeability of arterioles, capillaries or venules. They appear at pressure points and mucosal surfaces and are characteristically observed in patients with thrombocytopenia. Purpura is the term applied to confluent petechiae and is also associated with thrombocytopenia. Neither of these are associated with normal pregnancy and require further evaluation.

Hematologic laboratory findings

Thrombocytopenia

Thrombocytopenia (defined as a platelet count of less than the normal range of 150,000 – 400,000 ul^{-1}) is common in late pregnancy, with one large series reporting an incidence of 7.6% (Burrows and Kelton, 1990). The most common cause of isolated thrombocytopenia in pregnancy is gestational thrombocytopenia. Gestational thrombocytopenia characteristically has its onset earlier in gestation than does pre-eclampsia and is commonly detected as part of routine prenatal screening. The thrombocytopenia is generally mild and only rarely falls below 70,000 ul^{-1}.

Thrombocytopenia in pre-eclamptic women is most commonly the result of thrombus formation and/or membrane damage from contact with abnormal surfaces resulting in premature removal from the circulation. The thrombocytopenia in severe pre-eclampsia does not commonly fall below 50,000 ul^{-1} (Pritchard et al., 1976) and when the platelet count is below this level, other diagnoses should be considered.

The single most common differential consideration for thrombocytopenia in pre-eclampsia is disseminated intravascular coagulation (DIC). Because DIC is always a secondary phenomenon, the management should be directed to the identification, and resolution, of the instigating condition. Relatively common concurrent obstetric complications predisposing to DIC include hemorrhage and infection. These conditions must be appropriately and aggressively treated. Besides bacterial sepsis, concurrent viral infections, including HIV, should also be considered.

Conditions associated with microangiopathic hemolytic anemia such as thrombotic thrombocytopenic purpura (TTP) or hemolytic uremic syndrome (HUS) must also be considered in the thrombocytopenic pre-eclamptic pregnant woman. TTP is characterized by hemolytic anemia, thrombocytopenia, neurologic symptoms, renal abnormalities and fever. Women with this condition usually have mucous membrane bleeding and petechiae, fluctuating neurologic symptoms and jaundice. There is prominent laboratory evidence of microangiopathic hemolysis. Some degree of renal failure is usually present, with elevated serum BUN and creatinine as well as proteinuria developing early in the disease. Hematuria is often a prominent component, a complication not characteristically present in pre-eclampsia. Neurologic findings are variable but can include paresis, aphasia, headache, obtundation and seizures. Although patients early in the disease often do not have evidence of disseminated intravascular coagulation (DIC), progression of the disease to hepatic and renal failure is frequently associated with DIC.

The pathognomonic lesions of TTP are arteriolar and capillary hyaline thrombi. These thrombi are not associated with inflammatory reaction or vasculitis. The lesions are thought to consist of dense platelet aggregates surrounded by fibrin and can usually be found in biopsies of petechial sites. TTP has recently been shown to be related to increased circulating von Willebrand multimers. von Willebrand multimers are normally present in small amounts and their circulating levels are regulated by an enzyme that breaks them down, von Willebrand factor (vWf) metalloproteinase. If vWf levels increase, systemic platelet aggregation occurs with microcirculation obstruction and non-inflammatory necrosis in organs such as the brain, heart, kidney, pancreas and adrenal gland.

Optimal treatment of TTP consists of plasma administration in the rare cases of relapsing chronic familial TTP, and plasmapheresis in the more commonly encountered acute idiopathic TTP. High-dose steroid therapy is also important, as is the avoidance of platelet transfusions, or the use of heparin or DDAVP (vaospressin). Consultation with a hematologist experienced in the management of this disease is important.

Although similar in many respects to TTP, HUS is characterized by more prominent hypertension and renal failure with fewer neurologic signs and symptoms. HUS occurs primarily in children and is often preceded by gastroenteritis or viral upper respiratory tract infection within the preceding 7–10 days. The elevated liver function tests are primarily the result of microangiopathic hemolysis. Elevated fibrin split products are seen more commonly in HUS than in TTP.

Although most children with HUS recover completely in the course of a few weeks with supportive treatment alone, adults with HUS have a relatively worse prognosis because of their characteristically more severe renal involvement, often progressing to bilateral cortical necrosis.

It is not clear that any therapies are effective for HUS, although plasma exchange, steroids, anti-platelet agents and aspirin may all be of benefit.

Another relatively common (0.2% of pregnancies) differential consideration of thrombocytopenia in young women is immune thrombocytopenic purpura (also called autoimmune thrombocytopenic purpura) (Rouse et al., 1998). This condition is the result of immune-mediated platelet destruction and is often, but not always, associated with maternal IgG antiplatelet antibodies. It is clinically characterized by persistent thrombocytopenia, normal or increased numbers of megakaryocytes on bone marrow examination, exclusion of other systemic disorders or drugs known to be associated with thrombocytopenia and absence of splenomegaly (ACOG, 1999). The majority of these women will have had this diagnosis established prior to pregnancy, usually as a result of easy bruising, petechiae, epistaxis, gingival bleeding or meno- or metrorrhagia. This condition is not usually exacerbated by pregnancy and is not associated with hypertension or proteinuria.

Systemic lupus erythematosus can masquerade as pre-eclampsia and may be associated with thrombocytopenia. In fact, thrombocytopenia may be the initial presenting feature and may antedate other manifestations by months or years. The antiphospholipid- and anticardiolipin-antibody syndromes must also be considered, particularly in women with early onset severe pre-eclampsia.

Certain medications can also cause thrombocytopenia. These include, but are not limited to, heparin, quinine, quinidine, zidovudine and sulfonamides.

VI. Neurologic

Neurologic symptoms

Headache

Headache has long been recognized as a harbinger of eclampsia. The precise mechanism of these headaches is not certain although hypertensive encephalopathy, cerebral vasospasm and abnormal cerebral perfusion pressure are intimately involved (Belfort et al. 1999). However, pre-eclampsia can develop in women with pre-existing headache disorders. All pre-eclamptic women should be questioned about underlying or pre-existing medical problems, including headaches. A previous history of headaches similar in kind to the present headache should suggest a primary headache syndrome. Vascular or tension headaches often begin in childhood and migraine headaches most commonly have their onset around puberty.

The temporal course of the pre-existing headache syndrome may also be helpful for establishing or confirming a diagnosis. Migraine headaches usually begin while awake, often have a prodrome or aura and characteristically build over minutes to hours. Vascular, or tension, headaches typically occur daily, progress through the day and are often associated with depression and/or pharmacologic rebound. The combination of a positive headache history and the absence of other signs or symptoms of severe pre-eclampsia could justify continued careful observation, particularly if remote from term.

The new onset of headache during pregnancy should increase the suspicion of underlying pathology. The primary symptom associated with intracranial hemorrhage is the sudden onset of either "the worst headache of my life" or of loss of consciousness. Intracranial hemorrhage in women of reproductive age is usually due either to arteriovenous malformations (AVMs) or arterial aneurysms, with AVMs being relatively more common in younger pregnant women and aneurysms being more common in the mature spectrum of the reproductive years.

AVMs are relatively more likely to have produced antecedent central nervous system symptoms than other considerations in the eclampsia differential diagnosis. They often present as recurrent unilateral migraine headaches or progressive neurologic disorders. The increase in blood volume and cardiac output, as well as the progressive arteriolar collagen reorganization, is widely thought to make AVMs more likely to become symptomatic in pregnancy.

Cerebral venous thrombosis is often associated with fluctuating symptoms and levels of consciousness. Although occurring more commonly in the puerperium, cerebral venous thrombosis does occur during pregnancy. Intracranial tumors may first become symptomatic during pregnancy, although this most commonly occurs in the first trimester. Intracranial tumors are also often associated with fluctuating symptoms that are affected by changes in position.

Altered consciousness

Neurologists define consciousness as a state expressed in two dimensions: wakefulness and the self-aware cognition of past events and future anticipations which accompanies the normal wakeful state. Altered consciousness can take many forms, including coma, stupor, obtundation, delirium, dementia and persistent vegetative state. The subtleties of these diagnoses are clearly beyond the scope of this chapter but do emphasize the fact that none of them should be persistent in women whose pregnancy is complicated by pre-eclampsia–eclampsia.

There are situations in pre-eclampsia–eclampsia where transient or reversible altered consciousness may be seen. These are: (1) the post-ictal recovery following an eclamptic convulsion and (2) the administration of substantial amounts (often excessive) of magnesium sulfate for seizure prophylaxis. In the former condition, gradual recovery should be expected within a few hours. Gradual recovery should be expected within a few hours in the latter condition as well unless the dosage of magnesium was extremely high or unless the woman has concurrent renal dysfunction, in which case it may take somewhat longer for the magnesium levels to return toward normal.

In pre-eclamptic women with persistent altered consciousness, the major diagnostic considerations are outlined in Table 26.2. Intracranial hemorrhage is the single most common cause for persistent altered consciousness in women with severe pre-eclampsia or eclampsia. If persistent altered consciousness is suspected a head CT scan should be performed promptly for evaluation of intracranial blood. CT scans are widely available, can be performed rapidly and are still the best imaging technique for identifying or excluding recent intracranial hemorrhage. If altered consciousness persists and there is no evidence of bleeding, the other causes listed in Table 26.2 should be pursued.

Blurred vision

Blurred vision is a term applied by patients to a variety of ophthalmologic symptoms. It is important to distinguish between these symptoms because the etiologies and clinical implications vary substantially (Table 26.3).

It is also important to distinguish between pre-magnesium sulfate symptoms and those that have developed after initiation of magnesium

Table 26.2. The differential diagnosis of persistent altered consciousness

---

I. Supratentorial lesions
   Cerebral hemorrhage (intraparenchymal,
     subdural, epidural)
   Cerebral infarction
   Brain tumor

II. Infratentorial lesions
   Pontine or cerebellar hemorrhage
   Brain stem infarction
   Tumor
   Abscess

III. Metabolic and/or diffuse lesions
   Anoxia
   Hypoglycemia
   Endogenous toxin (organ failure or deficiency)
   Exogenous poin or toxin
   Infection (meningitis, encephalitis)
   Electrolyte disturbances
   Concussion

IV. Psychogenic

---

sulfate therapy. Magnesium sulfate commonly produces not only blurred vision and diplopia but ptosis, accommodative and convergence insufficiencies and abnormal papillary responsiveness (Digre *et al.*, 1990).

Neurologic signs

Seizure

The grand mal seizures that distinguish eclampsia from pre-eclampsia are appropriately considered an indication to proceed with delivery. Otherwise uncomplicated clamptic convulsions are not associated with an aura and, in the absence of associated hemorrhage, do not result in localizing neurologic deficits. Likewise, eclamptic convulsions do not characteristically result in prolonged obtundation or coma or status epilepticus.

When these, or other, signs or symptoms are present other causes of grand mal seizures must be considered in the late-pregnant woman. Likewise, grand mal seizures in the recently delivered woman, particularly those more than 24 h postpartum, have an extended differential diagnosis. The following conditions must be considered, particularly if the woman has any localizing neurologic deficit(s) or suffers prolonged obtundation or coma (see also Table 26.2).

While it is possible to have the initial onset of epilepsy in pregnancy, women with pre-existing grand mal seizure disorders, or epilepsy, will usually be known or identified at the time of their seizure. In such women, the association of the seizure with known stimulatory factors such as flashing lights, music, video games, or sleep deprivation may also be of diagnostic value. Importantly, epileptic convulsions are not associated with hypertension, proteinuria or other microvascular dysfunction.

Cerebral venous thrombosis is a notorious imitator of eclampsia. Pregnancy, and particularly the immediate puerperium, is a hypercoagulable state. Pregnant women with underlying microvascular diseases, trauma or infection are at particularly increased risk. Depending on the extent and location of the lesion(s), cerebral venous thrombosis can produce increased intracranial pressure, multifocal regions of brain ischemia or cerebral infarction. Superior sagittal sinus thrombosis often presents with generalized seizures or focal seizures that alternatively involve one and then the other side of the body. Motor deficits are common. These women often also have fever, headache, papilledema and various ophthalmoplegias, visual field deficits or expressive/receptive neurologic deficits.

Vasculitis can also mimic eclampsia, being potentially associated with hypertension, proteinuria and convulsions. Systemic lupus is the most common such vasculitis in women of reproductive age. Convulsions with lupus are usually associated with extreme hypertension (Lupus cerebritis flare).

The initial onset of seizures in a pregnant woman with no evidence of hypertension or proteinuria should raise the questions of head trauma, central

Table 26.3. The differential diagnosis of visual symptoms in pre-eclampsia

Term	Definition	Localization	Clinical implication(s)
Amblyopia	Dimness or partial loss of vision usually from birth	Unknown	Usually none
Amaurosis fugax, or transient monocular blindness	Blindness in one eye that can occur as the result of a vascular embolism, or vasospasm, transient loss of blood flow to the optic disk	Retina and optic nerve blood flow	Can lead to permanent loss depending on the cause
Scotoma	Areas of relative or complete vision loss isolated within a comparatively better total field of vision for the particular eye	Usually retina	Can be demonstrated on Amsler Grid
Diplopia	Two separate images that are extinguished by covering one eye	From muscle weakness to nerve dysfunction (sixth nerve)	Can be due to drugs (e.g. magnesium); also due to increased intracranial pressure
Field defect	Loss of vision in a portion of one or both eyes	Monocular visual loss is due to lesions of the eye and/or optic nerve. Binocular visual loss can be anywhere between the retina and the occipital cortex	Can be associated with cortical blindness

nervous system (CNS) infection, poisoning or metabolic disturbances, or vascular disease. CNS trauma sufficient to cause seizures should be obvious to examination. Brain abscess should be considered in the presence of other chronic infections, especially those near the brain (chronic middle ear disease, sinusitis) and those associated with a high risk of bacteremia such as endocarditis. Acute meningitis and/or encephalitis are characteristically accompanied by high fever, malaise or myalgia and other systematic complaints that frequently focus on the respiratory or gastrointestinal tracts.

Recreational drug abuse, particularly cocaine and metamphetamine, may result in seizures and obtundation. Pregnant women who are using these substances will frequently continue usage through the course of pregnancy and may first present late in pregnancy with these symptoms. Particularly in the absence of hypertension or proteinuria or the absence of prenatal care, consideration should

be given to testing for substances of abuse. The requirements for informed consent vary between jurisdiction and practitioners should be aware of their local regulations before ordering these tests.

Known histories of alcohol or other recreational substance abuse should raise the possibility of withdrawal symptoms.

Somatization disorders can occasionally be confused for grand mal seizures. While these conditions may be accompanied by other appropriate complaints such as headache or epigastric pain, they are not associated with other physical findings. Hypertension, proteinuria, edema or other laboratory abnormalities are not characteristically present. These patients often also have childhood histories of neglect and/or abuse and domestic violence is common. Personal and family histories of alcoholism and/or substance abuse, multiple divorces, multiple surgeries are also common in such patients.

The differential diagnosis of eclamptic convulsions is summarized in Table 26.4.

Hypertension

Unless accompanied by pre-existing pre-eclampsia, the blood pressure in pregnant women with AVMs and berry aneurysms is often normal until the bleed and then rises suddenly and persistently thereafter. Likewise, these individuals will have localizing symptoms related to the location and volume of their intracranial bleeding. Please also see the discussion of Hypertension in *Cardiovascular Signs*.

Nuchal rigidity

Nuchal rigidity is not a characteristic finding of pre-eclampsia. If present, it should increase the suspicion of intracranial hemorrhage or infection.

Visual field defects

The evaluation of visual field defects should first be distinguished from diplopia. Diplopia, or double vision, is extinguished by covering one eye and is seen with magnesium sulfate therapy and/or with increased intracranial pressure.

Visual field defects should prompt a careful evaluation for localization of the lesion(s). Monocular visual disturbances suggest a more anterior localization (eye or optic nerve) whereas binocular visual disturbances are more characteristically posterior in location. This should suggest the possibility of cortical defects (i.e. ischemia).

Facial edema, particularly involving the eyelids, is not a prominent finding in normal pregnancy. Women with severe pre-eclampsia may complain of visual disturbances, or even blindness, as a result of prominent eyelid edema. Eyelid edema, particularly when out of proportion to other potential symptoms/signs of pre-eclampsia, should suggest the possibility of venous thrombosis, migraine, cellulitis, infiltrate disease or allergic reactions.

Neurologic laboratory findings

Cerebrospinal fluid

There is very little information available on cerebrospinal fluid contents in otherwise uncomplicated pre-eclampsia. Intuition suggests that there should not be any significant findings.

Cerebrospinal fluid analysis can still be of value for confirmation of the diagnosis of meningitis (culture, Gram stain, glucose), subarachnoid hemorrhage (red cells, xanthochromia – particularly in a clinically suspicious setting but without obvious neuroimaging findings) or multiple sclerosis (oligoclonal bands). These diagnostic considerations should not be affected by coexistent or superimposed pre-eclampsia.

Neurologic imaging findings

Computed tomography

Cerebral CT scan is often the first imaging procedure performed in consideration of possible intracranial hemorrhage. A head CT scan should be performed promptly when intracranial hemorrhage is considered. Cerebral CT demonstrates hemorrhage, linear hyperdensities consistent with thrombosed veins on precontrast scans and filling defects with contrast enhancement. It remains the diagnostic procedure of choice both because of accuracy and widespread availability. Cerebral CT is safe during pregnancy and should be used in any indicated situation irrespective of pregnancy.

Magnetic resonance imaging

There are no known maternal or fetal risks associated with magnetic resonance imaging. Vascular and space-occupying lesions are best identified with this technique. Cerebral venous thrombosis is best diagnosed via magnetic resonance venography. The newer diffusion-weighted and FLAIR (Fluid-Attenuated Inversion Recovery) techniques are particularly helpful for

Table 26.4. The differential diagnosis of eclamptic convulsions

Condition	Symptoms	Exam findings	Laboratory	Comments
Eclampsia	No auras with convulsions	No localizing findings	Elevated liver function tests Thrombocytopenia Proteinuria	Consider CNS imaging if localizing physical findings are present or if obtundation is prolonged
	Occurs in second half of pregnancy or soon after delivery	Post-ictal obtundation usually only for minutes to a few hours		
Intracranial hemorrhage	Sudden onset of the "worst headache of my life" or loss of consciousness	Normal blood pressures until onset of bleeding	Blood in cerebrospinal fluid	CT scan is best for identification of recent CNS bleeding
	Aneurysms often associated with antecedent nausea or dizziness	Nuchal rigidity and/or photophobia		AVMs often have history of antecedent CNS symptoms Aneurysms seen more commonly in women with known atherosclerosis or polycystic kidney disease
Cerebral vascular disease	Variable symptoms that are dependent on the location of the thrombus (i). Often with headache, behavioral changes, and/or visual changes	Fluctuating deficits	Often associated with concurrent infection, major surgery, hemorrhage, trauma and/or microvascular disease	90% occur postpartum
Vasculitis	Usually known before pregnancy	May have hypertension and proteinuria that antedates the pregnancy		May be seen with prolonged recreational drug use
Epilepsy	Usually known before pregnancy Often have an antecedent aura Exacerbated by known stimuli	Not associated with hypertension or coexistent microvascular disease	Not associated with elevated liver function tests, thrombocytopenia or proteinuria	
Behavioral disturbances		Not associated with hypertension coexistent microvascular disease	Not associated with elevated liver function tests, thrombocytopenia or proteinuria	Often have a history of abuse, neglect, and/or domestic violence Higher frequency of multiple surgeries, multiple divorces or substance abuse

identifying areas of ischemia or infarction (Perkins *et al.*, 2001).

Angiography

Cerebral angiography is more invasive and is now uncommonly employed. When performed, specific attention should be directed to delayed filling of the venous sinuses and veins.

VII. Endocrine

Endocrine symptoms

Weakness

Weakness is not a characteristic symptom of pre-eclampsia per se but is extremely common in women with pre-eclampsia who are hospitalized and receiving magnesium sulfate seizure prophylaxis. Weakness, prior to magnesium prophylaxis, could suggest the possibility of an underlying endocrine problem such as primary aldosteronism or Cushing's syndrome.

Primary aldosteronism is frequently also accompanied by muscle cramping. Treatment is usually surgical for unilateral aldosterone producing cortical adenoma and medical for bilateral adrenal hyperplasia. The preferred medical treatments for bilateral adrenal hyperplasia (spironolactone and ACE inhibitors) are contraindicated in pregnancy. Alternative drugs that may be used include calcium antagonists and low-dose thiazide diuretics.

Cushing's syndrome is classically accompanied by truncal obesity, prominent striae and hypertension. Pregnancies complicated by Cushing's syndrome are known to be at increased risk for spontaneous premature labor and delivery. Cushing's syndrome is not associated with proteinuria or abnormalities of serum chemistries. This distinction can be of clinical value in assessing the possibility of superimposed pre-eclampsia.

Endocrine signs

Tachycardia

Sinus tachycardia is defined when the resting heart rate exceeds 100 beats per minute (bpm) and rarely exceeds 200 bpm. In addition to the potential endocrine causes (primarily thyrotoxicosis), sinus tachycardia represents a physiologic response to a variety of stresses including fever, volume depletion, anxiety, hypoxemia and/or hypotension. Sinus tachycardia associated with thyrotoxicosis is also characterized by a widened pulse pressure.

Sudden, or paroxysmal, increases in heart rate should suggest an underlying arrhythmia.

Endocrine laboratory findings

Hypokalemia

The partially compensated respiratory alkalosis of pregnancy often results in a low-normal serum potassium level. Potassium levels below the normal range, particularly if associated with muscle cramps, weakness, palpitations, glucose intolerance, polydipsia and/or polyuria should raise the possibility of hyperaldosteronism. The definitive test for primary aldosteronism is the measurement of aldosterone excretion after 3 days of salt loading. Patients with primary aldosteronism will have aldosterone excretion rates of at least $14\,\mu g\,24\,h^{-1}$. Hyperaldosteronism is almost always the result of either an adrenal cortical adenoma (usually unilateral) or adrenal cortical hyperplasia (usually bilateral).

Hyperglycemia

Insulin resistance is increased in pregnancy as a result of the progressively increasing levels of multiple steroid hormones. While pre-eclampsia is more common in women with underlying microvascular diseases (including diabetes), hyperglycemia is not more common in pre-eclampsia per se. The finding of hyperglycemia in a pre-eclamptic woman requires an alternative explanation, the most common of which is previously unrecognized or inadequately treated diabetes. Cushing's syndrome should also be considered, particularly if associated with prominent skin striae, truncal obesity and a buffalo hump.

Alkalosis

The progesterone-mediated hyperventilation of pregnancy produces a characteristic partially compensated respiratory alkalosis. Importantly, pregnancy does not produce a metabolic alkalosis. A metabolic alkalosis should raise suspicions of hyperaldosteronism, particularly when associated with refractory hypertension.

Endocrine imaging findings

Adrenal glands

Most patients with primary aldosteronism will have an adrenal cortical adenoma and the majority of the remainder will have bilateral adrenal hyperplasia. The adenoma group characteristically has more severe hypertension, more extreme aldosterone elevation and more marked electrolyte imbalances. Adrenal cortical adenomas can usually be visualized via adrenal CT scanning but sometimes selective adrenal venous sampling for aldosterone levels is required.

REFERENCES

American College of Obstetricians and Gynecologists. (1996). *Hypertension in Pregnancy.* ACOG Technical Bulletin 219. Washington, DC: ACOG.

American College of Obstetricians and Gynecologists. (1999). *Thrombocytopenia in Pregnancy.* ACOG Practice Bulletin #6. Washington, DC: ACOG.

Barker, D. J. and Osmond, C. (1986). Infant mortality, childhood nutrition, and ischaemic heart disease in England and Wales. *Lancet,* **1**, 1077–81.

Baron, F., Sprauve, M. E., Huddleston, J. F. and Fishe, A. J. (1995). Diagnosis and surgical treatment of primary hyperaldosteronism in pregnancy. *Obstet. Gynecol.,* **86**, 644.

Basdogan, F., Visser, W., Struijk, P. C., *et al.* (2000). Automated cardiac output measurements by ultrasound are inaccurate at high cardiac outputs. *Ultrasound Obstet. Gynecol.,* **15**, 508–12.

Belfort, M. A., Saade, G. R., Grunewald, C., *et al.* (1999). Association of cerebral perfusion pressure with headache in women with pre-eclampsia. *Br. J. Obstet. Gynaecol.,* **106**, 814–21.

Burrows, R. F. and Kelton, J. G. (1990). Thrombocytopenia at delivery: a prospective survey of 6715 deliveries. *Am. J. Obstet. Gynecol.,* **162**, 731–4.

Connolly, G., Razak, A. R., Hayanga, A., Russell, A., McKenna, P., McNicholas, W. T. (2001). Inspiratory flow limitation during sleep in pre-eclampsia: comparison with normal pregnant and nonpregnant women. *Eur. Respir. J.,* **18**, 672–6.

Contreras, G., Gutierrez, M., Beroiza, T., *et al.* (1991). Ventilatory drive and respiratory muscle function in pregnancy. *Am. Rev. Respir. Dis.,* **144**, 837–41.

Cunningham, F. G., Cox, S. M., Harstad, T. W., Mason, R. A. and Pritchard, J. A. (1990). Chronic renal disease and pregnancy outcome. *Am. J. Obstet. Gynecol.,* **163**, 453–9.

Digre, K. B., Varner, M. W. and Schiffman, J. S. (1990). Neuro-ophthalmologic effects of intravenous magnesium sulfate. *Am. J. Obstet. Gynecol.,* **163**, 1848–52.

Duthie, S. J. and Walkinshaw, S. A. (1995). Parvovirus associated fetal hydrops: reversal of pregnancy induced proteinuric hypertension by in utero fetal transfusion. *Br. J. Obstet. Gynaecol.,* **102**, 1011–13.

Esplin, M. S. and Varner, M. W. (1997). Progression of pulmonary arteriovenous malformation during pregnancy: case report and review of the literature. *Obstet. Gynecol. Survey,* **52**, 248–53.

Fisher, K., Luger, A., Spargo, B. H. and Lindheimer, M. D. (1981). Hypertension in pregnancy: clinical–pathological correlations and remote prognosis. *Medicine,* **60**, 267–76.

Fleming, S. M., O'Gorman, T., Finn, J., Grimes, H., Daly, K. and Morrison, J. J. (2000). Cardiac troponin I in pre-eclampsia and gestational hypertension. *Br. J. Obstet. Gynaecol.,* **107**, 1417–20.

Hammond, T. G., Buchanan, J. G., Scoggins, B. A., *et al.* (1982). Primary hyperaldosteronism in pregnancy. *Aus. N. Z. J. Med.,* **12**, 537.

Hanssens, M., Keirse, M.J.N.C., Vankelecom, F. and Van Assche, F.A. (1991). Fetal and neonatal effects of treatment with angiotensin-converting enzyme inhibitors in pregnancy. *Obstet. Gynecol.*, **78**, 128–35.

Herpolsheimer, A., Brady, K., Yancey, M.K., Pandian, M. and Duff, P. (1991). Pulmonary function of preeclamptic women receiving intravenous magnesium sulfate seizure prophylaxis. *Obstet. Gynecol.*, **78**, 241–4.

Hingorani, A.D. (2003). Endothelial nitric oxide synthase polymorphisms and hypertension. *Curr. Hypertens. Rep.*, **5**, 19–25.

Izci, B., Riha, R.L., Martin, S.E., *et al.* (2003). The upper airway in pregnancy and pre-eclampsia. *Am. J. Respir. Crit. Care Med.*, **15**, 137–40.

Jungers, P., Houillier, P., Forget, D., *et al.* (1995). Influence of pregnancy on the course of primary chronic glomerulonephritis. *Lancet*, **346**, 1122–4.

Lalouel, J.M., Rohrwasser, A., Terreros, D., Morgan, T. and Ward, K. (2001). Angiotensinogen in essential hypertension: from genetics to nephrology. *J. Am. Soc. Nephrol.*, **12**, 606–15.

Laurel, M.T. and Kabadi, U.M. (1997). Primary hyperaldosteronism. *Endocrine. Pract.*, **3**, 47.

Miller, M.W., Brayman, A.A. and Abramowicz, J.S. (1998). Obstetric ultrasonography: a biophysical consideration of patient safety – the rules have changed. *Am. J. Obstet. Gynecol.*, **179**, 241–54.

National High Blood Pressure Education Program Working Group on High Blood Pressure in Pregnancy. (2000). Report of the National High Blood Pressure Education Program Working Group on High Blood Pressure in Pregnancy. *Am. J. Obstet. Gynecol.*, **183**, S1–22.

Perkins, C.J., Kahya, E., Roque, D.T., Roche, P.E. and Newman, G.C. (2001). Fluid-attenuated inversion recovery and diffusion- and perfusion-weighted MRI abnormalities in 117 consecutive patients with strope symptoms. *Stroke*, **32**, 2774–81.

Pritchard, J.A., Cunningham, F.G. and Mason, R.A. (1976). Coagulation changes in eclampsia: their frequency and pathogenesis. *Am. J. Obstet. Gynecol.*, **124**, 855–64.

Procopciuc, L., Jebeleanu, G., Surcel, I. and Puscas, M. (2002). Angiotensinogen gene M235T variant and pre-eclampsia in Romanian pregnant women. *J. Cell. Mol. Med.*, **6**, 383–8.

Rouse, D.J., Owen, J. and Goldenberg, R.L. (1998). Routine maternal platelet count: an assessment of technologically driven practice. *Am. J. Obstet. Gynecol.*, **179**, 573–6.

Semshyshyn, S. (1977). Ascites in toxemia. *Am. J. Obstet. Gynecol.*, **129**, 925–6.

Sibai, B.M., Mabie, B.C., Harvey, C.J. and Gonzalez, A.R. (1987). Pulmonary edema in severe preeclampsia–eclampsia: analysis of thirty-seven consecutive cases. *Am. J. Obstet. Gynecol.*, **156**, 1174–9.

Simmons, L.A., Gillin, A.G. and Jeremy, R.W. (2002). Structural and functional changes in left ventricle during normotensive and preeclamptic pregnancy. *Am. J. Physiol. Heart Circ. Physiol.*, **283**, H1627–33.

Solomon, G.C., Thiet, M., Moore, F. and Seely, E.W. (1996). Primary hyperaldosteronism in pregnancy. *Obstet. Gynecol.*, **41**, 255.

Tyni, T., Ekholm, E. and Pihko, H. (1998). Pregnancy complications are frequent in long-chain 3-hydroxyacyl-coenzyme A dehydrogenase deficiency. *Am. J. Obstet. Gynecol.*, **178**, 603–8.

Varner, M.W. (2002). The differential diagnosis of preeclampsia and eclampsia. In *Hypertension in Pregnancy*, ed. M.A. Belfort, M. Thornton and G.R. Saade. New York: Marcel Dekker, pp. 57–83.

Weinstein, L. (1982). Syndrome of hemolysis, elevated liver enzymes and low platelet count; a consequence of hypertension in pregnancy. *Am. J. Obstet. Gynecol.*, **142**, 159–67.

Wilcken, B., Leung, K.C., Hammond, J., Kamath, R. and Leonard, J.V. (1993). Pregnancy and fetal long-chain 3-hydroxyacyl-CoA dehydrogenase deficiency. *Lancet*, **341**, 407–8.

Woods, J.B., Blake, P.G., Perry, K.G. Jr., Magann, E.F., Martin, R.W. and Martin, J.N. Jr. (1992). Ascites: a portent of cardiopulmonary complications in the preeclamptic patient with the syndrome of hemolysis, elevated liver enzymes, and low platelets. *Obstet. Gynecol.*, **80**, 87–91.

Zimmerman, J., Fromm, R., Meyer, D., *et al.* (1999). Diagnostic marker cooperative study for the diagnosis of myocardial infarction. *Circulation*, **99**, 1671–7.

27

Complications of pre-eclampsia

Gary A. Dildy III and Michael A. Belfort

Introduction

Pre-eclampsia complicates 5–8% of pregnancies and significantly contributes to maternal mortality in the United States (Berg *et al.*, 2003; Chang *et al.*, 2003), the United Kingdom (de Swiet, 2000; Scott and Owen, 1996), Europe (Hogberg *et al.*, 1994; Schuitemaker *et al.*, 1998) and, most notably, in developing nations (Bouvier-Colle *et al.*, 2001). Pre-eclampsia is a disease unique to human pregnancy, with pathophysiologic effects which may compromise cardiovascular, renal, hematologic, neurologic, hepatic, and other organ systems. Early-onset pre-eclampsia is associated with greater morbidity (Murphy and Stirrat, 2000). The classification of hypertensive diseases and the pathophysiology of pre-eclampsia are comprehensively addressed in other sections of this book. The purpose of this chapter is to provide a practical guide to clinicians caring for patients with complications of pre-eclampsia.

Eclampsia

The incidence of eclampsia in the United Kingdom and the United States is approximately 5 per 10,000 births (Atrash *et al.*, 1990; Douglas and Redman, 1994). However, at teaching hospitals in Africa, the eclampsia rate is reported around 50 per 10,000 deliveries (Adze *et al.*, 2001; Majoko and Mujaji, 2001), likely an effect of home births and late medical care. Contemporary maternal mortality rates of eclampsia are under 2% in developed countries but are significantly higher in developing nations (Table 27.8). In the Dallas series of 245 eclamptics, one maternal death occurred, which was attributed to magnesium overdose (Cunningham *et al.*, 1984). In the Memphis series of 254 eclamptics, there was one maternal death in a woman who arrived to hospital in a moribund state (Sibai, 1990). In the United Kingdom during 1992, a 1.8% maternal case mortality rate was reported for eclamptics (Douglas and Redman, 1994).

Until relatively recently there remained considerable controversy regarding the best agent for eclampsia prophylaxis and treatment. During the late 1990s several important randomized clinical trials of magnesium sulfate for prevention or control of eclamptic seizures were published and are summarized in Table 27.1. The Cochrane Review of randomized clinical trials has found magnesium superior to lytic cocktail (Duley and Gulmezoglu, 2001), diazepam (Duley and Henderson-Smart, 2000), and phenytoin (Duley and Henderson-Smart, 2000) for prevention and/or treatment of eclampsia. Based upon these recent data, magnesium sulfate is currently the agent of choice for prophylaxis of severe pre-eclamptics and treatment of eclamptics (ACOG Practice Bulletin, 2002; Arnott *et al.*, 1996; Burgess *et al.*, 1997; Cunningham *et al.*, 2001). The role of magnesium sulfate seizure prophylaxis for mild pre-eclampsia remains undefined (Livingston *et al.*, 2003; Scott, 2003; Sibai, 2003).

Eclampsia typically produces fetal bradycardia, which usually normalizes upon resolution of the

Table 27.1. Randomized trials comparing magnesium sulfate ($MgSO_4$) with other agents for prophylaxis (preventing eclampsia in pre-eclamptics) and treatment (preventing recurrent seizures) of eclampsia. Modified from Dildy (2004)

Authors	Study population	N	$MgSO_4$ (%)	Placebo (%)	Phenytoin (%)	Diazepam (%)	Lytic cocktail (%)	Nimodipine (%)
Bhalla *et al.*, 1994	Eclamptics	91	2.2	–	–	–	24.4	–
Lucas, 1995	Mixed pre-eclamptics	2138	0	–	0.9	–	–	–
ETCG, 1995	Eclamptics	905	13.2	–	–	27.9	–	–
	Eclamptics	775	5.7	–	17.1	–	–	–
Coetzee, 1998	Severe pre-eclamptics	685	0.3	3.2	–	–	–	–
Belfort, 2003	Severe pre-eclamptics	1650	0.8	–	–	–	–	2.6

seizure. Appropriate steps should be taken to enhance maternal–fetal well-being, including maintenance of maternal airway, oxygen administration, and maternal lateral positioning. A magnesium sulfate loading dose consisting of 4–6 g is administered intravenously (IV) over 20 min, followed by an IV maintenance infusion at 2–3 g h^{-1}. If control of seizures is not successful after the initial IV bolus, a second 2 g bolus of magnesium sulfate may be cautiously administered. No more than a total of 8 g of magnesium sulfate is recommended at the outset of treatment.

Seizures may recur despite apparently appropriate maintenance magnesium therapy. The incidence of recurrent seizures ranges from 8 to 13% and half of such patients are found to have a subtherapeutic magnesium level (Anderson *et al.*, 1986). Seizures refractory to magnesium sulfate may be treated with a slow IV administration of thiopental sodium 100 mg, diazepam 1–10 mg, or sodium amobarbital up to 250 mg. Lucas and colleagues described a simplified regimen of phenytoin; an IV infusion rate of 16.7 mg min^{-1} over 1 h provides an initial dose of 1000 mg and an additional 500 mg is administered orally 10 h after treatment to maintain therapeutic levels for an additional 14 h (Cunningham, *et al.*, 1984).

Dunn and associates recommended that eclamptic patients with repetitive seizures despite therapeutic magnesium levels have head CT

evaluation, because five of seven such patients had abnormalities including cerebral edema and cerebral venous thrombosis (Cotton *et al.*, 1986c). However, Sibai reported 20 cases of eclampsia with neurologic signs or repetitive seizures who all had normal CT findings (Anderson *et al.*, 1985). We generally reserve CT imaging for patients with late-onset postpartum pre-eclampsia, repetitive seizures despite adequate magnesium levels, or those patients with focal neurologic deficits.

Eclamptic patients require delivery regardless of gestational age (Cunningham and Grant, 1994). Cesarean delivery should be reserved for obstetric indications or deteriorating maternal condition. As demonstrated in Table 27.8 vaginal delivery may be achieved in at least half of eclamptic patients. Pritchard and colleagues reported successful vaginal delivery in 82% of oxytocin-induced patients (Cunningham *et al.*, 1984).

Magnesium toxicity

Plasma magnesium levels maintained at 4–7 mEq l^{-1} are believed to be therapeutic in preventing eclamptic seizures. Patellar reflexes usually are lost at 8–10 mEq l^{-1}, and respiratory arrest may occur at 13 mEq l^{-1} (Pritchard, 1955). Urine output, patellar reflexes, and respiratory rates should be routinely monitored during magnesium administration. Serial serum magnesium levels are advised for patients with renal dysfunction. Calcium gluconate should be available in the event of magnesium toxicity; a 1 g dose (10 ml of a 10% solution) is given IV over a period of 2 min. Oxygen saturation monitoring, supplemental oxygen administration, and endotracheal intubation are provided as indicated.

Bohman and Cotton reported a case of supra-lethal magnesemia (38.7 mg dl^{-1}) with patient survival and no adverse sequelae (Bohman and Cotton, 1990). Prevention and resuscitation of toxic magnesemia are summarized in Table 27.4.

Amaurosis (temporary blindness)

Temporary blindness may complicate 1–3% of cases of pre-eclampsia and has been reported in 15% of women with eclampsia at Parkland Hospital; cases of permanent visual impairment have been reported (Cunningham *et al.*, 1995a; Do *et al.*, 2002; Ekbladh *et al.*, 1980; Moseman and Shelton, 2002). Pregnancy-related blindness has been associated with eclampsia, cavernous sinus thrombosis, hypertensive encephalopathy, and occipital lobe edema (Beal and Chapman, 1980; Beck *et al.*, 1980; Beeson and Duda, 1982; Devoe *et al.*, 1985). The injury is usually the result of severe damage to the retinal vasculature or occipital lobe ischemia (Beal and Chapman, 1980).

Transient blindness usually resolves spontaneously after delivery of the fetus. Nevertheless, focal neurologic deficits such as this require ophthalmologic and neurologic consultation and CT or MRI of the brain. Generally, management is supportive and does not differ from pre-eclamptics without this complication (Cunningham *et al.*, 1995a). Associated conditions, such as cerebral edema, should be treated as indicated.

Malignant hypertension

In the previously normotensive patient, cerebral autoregulation is lost and the risk of intracranial bleeding increases when the mean arterial pressure (MAP) exceeds 140–150 mmHg (Zimmerman, 1995). Intracranial hemorrhage may result from the combination of severe hypertension and hemostatic compromise (Hobbins *et al.*, 1988). Belfort and colleagues hypothesize that uncontrolled cerebral perfusion pressure may cause barotrauma and vessel damage, leading to hypertensive encephalopathy and overperfusion injury (Belfort *et al.*, 2002). The maternal mortality associated with intracranial hemorrhage is substantial (Bullock *et al.*, 1987, 1988). Among 704 eclamptic women managed during a 15-year period in Mexico, the most common single cause of death among 86 fatal cases of eclampsia was cerebrovascular damage (Lopez-Llera, 1982).

The *Working Group Report on High Blood Pressure in Pregnancy* recommends medical intervention when severe hypertension (systolic BP ≥ 160 mmHg and/or diastolic BP ≥105 mmHg) is sustained (Report of the National High Blood Pressure Education Program Working Group on High Blood Pressure in Pregnancy, 2000). Although a variety of antihypertensive agents is available, we will confine our discussion to those most commonly used for acute hypertensive crisis in pregnancy (Table 27.2). In many centers throughout the United States, hydralazine remains the most popular initial agent for treatment of severe hypertension during pregnancy. Hydralazine will be effective in restoring BP to a desired range (160–130/110–80 mmHg) in the majority of cases. The administration of hydralazine may result in maternal hypotension and a nonreassuring fetal heart rate pattern (Anderson *et al.*, 1986). For this reason, we administer an initial IV dose of 5 mg, followed by observation of hemodynamic effects. If appropriate change in BP is not achieved, 5–10 mg doses may be administered IV at 20 min intervals to a total acute dose of 20 mg. When maximum doses of hydralazine (20 mg IV or 30 mg IM) (Report of the National High Blood Pressure Education Program Working Group on High Blood Pressure in Pregnancy, 2000) have not corrected severe hypertension, we then proceed to labetalol. In the

Table 27.2. Pharmacologic agents for antihypertensive therapy in pre-eclampsia–eclampsia. Modified from Dildy (2004)

Generic name	Trade name	Mechanism of action	Dosage	Comment
Hydralazine	Apresoline	Arterial vasodilator	5 mg IV, then 5–10 mg IV/20 min up to total dose of 40 mg; titrated IV infusion 5–10 mg h^{-1}	Must wait 20 min for response between IV doses; possible maternal hypotension
Labetalol	Normodyne Trandate	Selective alpha- and nonselective beta-antagonist	20 mg IV, then 40–80 mg IV/10 min to 300 mg total dose; titrated IV infusion 1–2 mg min^{-1}	Less reflex tachycardia and hypotension than with hydralazine
Nifedipine	Procardia Adalat	Calcium channel blocker	10 mg PO, may repeat after 30 min	Oral route only; possible exaggerated effect if used with MgSO$_4$
Nitroglycerin	Nitrostat IV Tridil Nitro-Bid IV	Relaxation of venous (and arterial) Vascular smooth muscle	5 µg min^{-1} infusion; double every 5 min	Requires arterial line for continuous BP monitoring; potential methemoglobinemia
Sodium nitroprusside	Nipride Nitropress	Vasodilator	0.25 µg kg^{-1}min^{-1} infusion; increase 0.25 µg kg^{-1}min^{-1} 5 min^{-1}	Requires arterial line for continuous blood pressure monitoring; potential cyanide toxicity
Diazoxide	Hyperstat	Peripheral arteriolar vasodilator	30–60 mg IV/5 min; titrated IV infusion 10 mg min^{-1}	Possible rapid hypotension, hyperglycemia, decreased uterine contractility

rare cases when these agents are ineffective, we use nitroglycerin or nitroprusside.

Calcium channel blockers such as nifedipine (Procardia, Adalat) lower BP primarily by relaxing arterial smooth muscle. An initial oral dose of 10 mg is administered, which may be repeated after 30 min, if necessary, for the acute management of severe hypertension; 10–20 mg may then be administered orally every 3–6 h as needed (Naden and Redman, 1985). Principal side effects in severe pre-eclamptics include headache and cutaneous flushing. A beneficial effect may be seen on urine output in women with severe pre-eclampsia who are treated with nifedipine (Aali and Nejad, 2002; Chauhan et al., 1999).

Labetalol (Normodyne, Trandate) is a combined alpha- and beta-adrenoceptor antagonist that may be used to decrease BP via decreased SVR (Lund-Johansen, 1984). Reports on the efficacy and safety of labetalol in the treatment of hypertension during pregnancy have been favorable (Amon et al., 1987; Fredholm et al., 1982). Mabie and co-workers compared bolus IV labetalol with IV hydralazine in the acute treatment of severe hypertension. They found that labetalol had a quicker onset of action and did not result in reflex tachycardia (Amon et al., 1987). An initial dose of 20 mg is given and is followed by progressively increasing doses (40, 80 mg) every 10 min, to a total dose of 300 mg. Lunell and co-workers studied the effects of labetalol on uteroplacental perfusion in hypertensive pregnant women and noted increased uteroplacental perfusion and decreased uterine vascular resistance (Lewander et al., 1984).

Nitroglycerin (Nitrostat IV, Nitro-Bid IV, Tridil) is a rapidly acting potent antihypertensive agent with a very short hemodynamic half-life. Nitroglycerin relaxes predominantly venous vascular smooth muscle, decreasing preload at low doses and afterload at high doses (Herling, 1984). Using invasive hemodynamic monitoring, Cotton and associates (Cotton et al., 1986a, b, c) noted that the ability to control BP was dependent on volume status; although larger doses were required following volume expansion, the ability to effect a smoother and more controlled drop in BP required prevasodilator hydration. Nitroglycerin is administered via an infusion pump at an initial rate of $5\,\mu g\,min^{-1}$ and may be doubled every 5 min. Methemoglobinemia may result from high dose $(7\,\mu g\,kg^{-1}min^{-1})$ IV infusion (Hoppelshauser and Pasch, 1983). Patients with normal arterial oxygen saturation who appear cyanotic should be evaluated for toxicity, defined as a methemoglobin level greater than 3% (Herling, 1984).

Sodium nitroprusside (Nipride, Nitropress) is another potent antihypertensive agent that may be used to control severe PIH. A dilute solution may be administered by infusion pump at $0.25\,\mu g\,kg^{-1}min^{-1}$ and titrated by increasing the dose $0.25\,\mu g\,kg^{-1}min^{-1}$ every 5 min. Arterial blood gases should be monitored to watch for developing metabolic acidosis, which may be an early sign of cyanide toxicity. In nonpregnant subjects, infusion rates of less than $2\,\mu g\,kg^{-1}min^{-1}$ for several hours are nontoxic (Hoppelshauser et al., 1983). Correction of hypovolemia prior to initiation of nitroprusside infusion is necessary to avoid profound hypotension.

Hypertensive cardiomyopathy

During pregnancy, pregnant women show an increase in left ventricular muscle mass index and

a decrease in fractional shortening. When studied with echocardiography, many normal pregnant women show a degree of "physiologic" diastolic dysfunction. Schannwell et al. (2001) demonstrated affected LV relaxation with a reduction in peak early diastolic flow and an increase of isovolumetric relaxation time at 33 weeks gestation in normal pregnant women. In pregnant patients with mild chronic hypertension they showed definite signs of diastolic dysfunction with delayed relaxation noted as early as the beginning of the gestation. Some patients with pregnancy-associated hypertension developed diastolic dysfunction at midgestation, while others only showed this abnormality at term. They concluded that in healthy pregnant women, the increased preload associated with normal pregnancy results in a reversible physiologic left ventricular hypertrophy, a significant alteration in diastolic left ventricular function (disturbed relaxation pattern) and a temporary decrease in the efficacy of systolic function. In women with chronic hypertension, however, there is delayed LV relaxation demonstrable at the beginning of pregnancy and in as many as 50% of cases signs of restrictive cardiomyopathy may develop.

Desai et al. (1996) used echocardiography to show that 25% (4/16) of patients they studied with pulmonary edema and hypertensive crisis in pregnancy had impaired left ventricular systolic function. The remaining 75% (12/16) had abnormal left ventricular diastolic filling.

Diastolic dysfunction in patients with severe hypertension from pre-eclampsia needs to be recognized as a potential cause for fulminant pulmonary edema, cardiac failure and sudden death. It is important that the obstetrician understand that diastolic dysfunction can occur despite normal left ventricular systolic function, and in the face of an elevated blood pressure. Pulmonary edema from diastolic dysfunction occurs frequently with severe hypertension, and "cardiac failure" is not always associated with hypotension or a diminished ejection fraction. In fact, up to 40% of hypertensive patients presenting with clinical signs of congestive heart failure have normal systolic left ventricular function. The concept that a pre-eclamptic patient with elevated blood pressure cannot be in cardiac failure needs to be discarded. Likewise, the idea that a pre-eclamptic patient who develops severe pulmonary edema always has peripartum cardiomyopathy should be questioned. Peripartum cardiomyopathy is a distinct entity that carries significant implications for long-term therapy and future pregnancies. Pre-eclamptic women who develop pulmonary edema due to diastolic dysfunction and hypertensive cardiomyopathy should not be labeled as having had peripartum cardiomyopathy. The pathophysiology is different, and in most cases of hypertensive cardiomyopathy associated with pre-eclampsia the ejection fraction rapidly returns to normal after treatment of the pre-eclampsia. It is highly unlikely that a pre-eclamptic patient with severely elevated blood pressure who develops pulmonary edema is then delivered and recovers rapidly within 24–48 h has peripartum cardiomyopathy. The most likely diagnosis in this scenario is that of hypertensive cardiomyopathy and diastolic dysfunction. Witlin *et al.* (1997b) have shown that patients with severe myocardial dysfunction due to peripartum cardiomyopathy are unlikely to regain normal cardiac function on follow-up. In addition, the same group showed that pre-eclampsia and chronic hypertension are likely to unmask underlying cardiac abnormalities (Witlin *et al.*, 1997a). In situations where it is unclear why the patient is in pulmonary edema echocardiography can be very useful. Not only does it allow an assessment of the systolic and diastolic function, as well as cardiac output, but the state of filling of the vasculature can also be evaluated. This is especially important in a severely pre-eclamptic patient who may have intravascular dehydration but pulmonary congestion and increased capillary permeability. Mabie *et al.* (1988) showed that obese women with chronic hypertension are at particular risk of underlying cardiac abnormality and diastolic dysfunction.

Malignant ventricular arrhythmias

Ventricular arrhythmias are not a commonly noted feature of severe pre-eclampsia. This is perhaps more due to the fact that we do not monitor for these arrhythmias than that they do not occur. Naidoo *et al.* (1991) studied 24 patients with hypertensive crises during pregnancy with continuous electrocardiographic monitoring over a period of 24 h to detect the presence of serious ventricular arrhythmias. They excluded three patients from the analysis because of low serum potassium levels. Of the remaining 21 patients, 13 (62%) had ventricular tachycardia on subsequent analysis of the electrocardiogram. These arrhythmias subsided after induction of anesthesia when blood pressure control was optimal. The authors of this paper felt that their finding may explain, in part, the pathogenesis of pulmonary edema and sudden death in some patients with malignant hypertension in pre-eclampsia. The high rate of ventricular arrhythmia in this study may be explained by the fact that many of these patients had little or no prenatal care and were admitted with severe, prolonged hypertensive crises. Hopefully, in an environment where prenatal care is more prevalent, we are less likely to see such ventricular dysfunction. Another explanation as to why this complication is less frequently seen in the USA is that beta-blocker use is common and we use hydralazine (not dihydralazine) for blood pressure control. Regardless of the potential pathophysiology, this paper underlines the importance of expeditious control of the blood pressure in severely hypertensive pregnant women.

The same group (Bhorat *et al.*, 1993) studied the effects of beta-adrenergic blockade during the peripartum period on their previously observed high incidence of ventricular arrhythmias in 40 eclamptic postpartum patients. Cardiac rhythm was assessed by blinded analysis of a 24-h Holter record using the Lown classification of arrhythmias. They showed a significantly higher incidence of serious ventricular arrhythmias in patients receiving dihydralazine (81%) than in those receiving labetalol (17%, $P < 0.0001$). Patients receiving labetalol showed a significant decrease in mean heart rate ($P < 0.0001$), whereas patients receiving dihydralazine showed a significant increase ($P < 0.0001$). They concluded that introduction of beta-adrenergic blockade into peripartum hypertensive management of eclampsia significantly reduced the incidence of dangerous ventricular arrhythmias. This may be on the basis of improved myocardial oxygen supply/demand ratio with beta-blockade. This paper makes a cogent argument for control of severely elevated blood pressure with labetalol instead of hydralazine or similar agents.

Pulmonary edema

Sibai and colleagues reported a 3% incidence of pulmonary edema in severe pre-eclampsia–eclampsia, the majority of cases developing postpartum (Gonzalez et al., 1987). Chronic hypertension was identified as an underlying factor in 90% of the cases that developed prior to delivery. A higher incidence of pulmonary edema was noted in older patients, multigravidas, and patients with underlying chronic hypertension. The development of pulmonary edema was also associated with the administration of excess colloid or crystalloid infusion.

The etiology of pulmonary edema in pre-eclamptic patients appears to be multifactorial; abnormal COP-PCWP gradient, increased pulmonary capillary permeability, and left ventricular failure were identified causes (Benedetti et al., 1985). The majority of patients develop pulmonary edema in the postpartum period. Pregnancy is known to lower COP and COP is lower in pre-eclamptic patients than in normal pregnant patients. Colloid osmotic pressure decreases further postpartum, secondary to supine positioning, bleeding at the time of delivery, and intrapartum infusion of crystalloid solutions (Henning et al., 1996).

The diagnosis of pulmonary edema is made on clinical grounds. Symptoms of dyspnea and chest discomfort are usually elicited. Tachypnea, tachycardia, and pulmonary rales are noted on examination. Chest radiograph and arterial blood gases confirm the diagnosis. Other serious conditions such as thromboembolism should be considered and ruled out as quickly as possible.

Initial management of pulmonary edema includes oxygen administration and fluid restriction. A pulse oximeter should be placed so that oxygen saturation may be monitored. Furosemide (Lasix) as a 10–40 mg dose IV is administered over 1–2 min for suspected fluid overload. An 80 mg dose may be administered if adequate diuresis does not commence within 1 h. In severe cases a diuresis of 2–3 l needs to be achieved before oxygenation begins to improve. Again, the degree of diuresis appropriate for these hemodynamically complex patients may be clarified by complete hemodynamic evaluation, using parameters derived by a pulmonary artery catheter. When hypoxemia persists mechanical ventilation may be required, pending correction of the underlying problem. Close monitoring of arterial blood gases should be performed. Fluid balance is maintained by careful monitoring of intake and output. An indwelling catheter with urometer should be placed to follow hourly urine output. Serum electrolytes should be monitored, especially in patients receiving diuretics.

The pulmonary artery (PA) catheter, introduced over 30 years ago, has been useful in the management of critically ill patients (Chonette et al., 1970). In cases of severe pre-eclampsia, most clinicians have obtained excellent results without invasive monitoring. The PA catheter may be considered for pre-eclamptic patients who do not respond to initial therapy, in order to distinguish between fluid overload, left ventricular dysfunction, and nonhydrostatic pulmonary edema, each of which may require different therapeutic approaches (Clark and Cotton, 1988).

Table 27.3. Hemodynamic profiles of nonpregnant women, normal women during the late third trimester, and severe pre-eclamptics. Modified from Dildy (2004)

	Normal non-pregnant ($n=10$) [126] (mean ± SD)	Normal late third trimester ($n=10$) [126] (mean ± SD)	Severe pre-eclampsia ($n=45$) [127] (mean ± SEM)	Severe pre-eclampsia ($n=49$) [128] (mean ± SEM)
Heart rate (beats min^{-1})	71 ± 10	83 ± 10	95 ± 2	94 ± 2
Systolic BP (mmHg)	N/A	N/A	193 ± 3	175 ± 3
Diastolic BP (mmHg)	N/A	N/A	110 ± 2	106 ± 2
Mean arterial BP (mmHg)	86.4 ± 7.5	90.3 ± 5.8	138 ± 3	130 ± 2
Pulse pressure (mmHg)	N/A	N/A	84 ± 2	70 ± 2
Central venous pressure (mmHg)	3.7 ± 2.6	3.6 ± 2.5	4 ± 1	4.8 ± 0.4
Pulmonary capillary wedge pressure (mmHg)	6.3 ± 2.1	7.5 ± 1.8	10 ± 1	8.3 ± 0.3
Pulmonary artery pressure (mmHg)	11.9 ± 2.0^{d}	12.5 ± 2.0*	17 ± 1	15 ± 0.5
Cardiac output (l min^{-1})	4.3 ± 0.9	6.2 ± 1.0	7.5 ± 0.2	8.4 ± 0.2
Stroke volume (ml)	N/A	N/A	79 ± 2	90 ± 2
Systemic vascular resistance (dynes sec cm^{-5})	1530 ± 520	1210 ± 266	1496 ± 64	1226 ± 37
Pulmonary vascular resistance (dynes sec cm^{-5})	119 ± 47	78 ± 22	70 ± 5	65 ± 3
Serum colloid osmotic pressure (mmHg)	20.8 ± 1.0	18.0 ± 1.5	19.0 ± 0.5	N/A
Body surface area (m^{2})	N/A	N/A	N/A	N/A
Systemic vascular resistance index (dynes sec cm^{-5} m^{2})	N/A	N/A	2726 ± 120	2293 ± 65
Pulmonary vascular resistance index (dynes sec cm^{-5} m^{2})	N/A	N/A	127 ± 9	121 ± 7
Right ventricular stroke work index (gm m m^{-2})	N/A	N/A	8 ± 1	10 ± 0.5
Left ventricular stroke work index (gm m m^{-2})	41 ± 8	48 ± 6	81 ± 2	84 ± 2
Cardiac index (l min^{-1} m^{2})	N/A	N/A	4.1 ± 0.1	4.4 ± 0.1
Stroke volume index (ml beat m^{2})	N/A	N/A	44 ± 1	48 ± 1
COP-PCWP (mmHg)	14.5 ± 2.5	10.5 ± 2.7	N/A	N/A

Table 27.3 summarizes hemodynamic findings in nonpregnant women, normal third-trimester pregnancy, and severe pre-eclamptics. Routine use of the pulmonary artery catheter in uncomplicated severe pre-eclampsia is not recommended, for the potential morbidity does not appear to be justified.

Laryngeal and glottic edema

Catastrophic laryngeal and/or glottic edema with acute respiratory failure can occur rarely. This is a life-threatening situation that demands immediate securing of an airway. Patients who have been intubated for a prolonged period of time (such as

Table 27.4. Prevention and treatment of magnesium toxicity

Prevention
    Monitor urine output, maternal respiration, patellar reflexes
    Serum magnesium levels (in certain cases)
    Infusion of intravenous magnesium in a buretrol-type system

Treatment
    Respiratory support as determined by clinical indicators (respiratory rate, SpO$_2$)
    Continuous cardiac monitoring
    Infusion of calcium salts
    Loop or osmotic diuretics
    Careful attention to fluid and electrolyte balance
    Recognition that toxic magnesium is neither anesthetic nor amnestic to the patient

may occur after status eclampticus) are at particular risk for this complication. Visualization of the larynx prior to extubation is important and if there is evidence of edema or swelling removal of the endotracheal tube should be delayed. Obviously, in such patients, it is essential that the eclampsia be controlled prior to extubation to reduce the need for re-intubation which may be very difficult with laryngeal or glottic edema.

HELLP syndrome

HELLP syndrome is characterized by hemolysis, elevated liver enzymes, and low platelets. The acronym was coined by Weinstein (1982), but the hematologic and hepatic abnormalities of three cases were described by Pritchard *et al.* (1954), who credited the association of thrombocytopenia to Stahnke in 1922 and the hepatic changes to Sheehan in 1950. HELLP syndrome is a variant of severe pre-eclampsia, affecting up to 12% of patients with pre-eclampsia–eclampsia. In one series of 442 cases of severe pre-eclampsia, the incidence of HELLP syndrome was 20% (Friedman *et al.*, 1993). HELLP syndrome may be the imitator of nonobstetric medical entities and serious medical–surgical pathology may be misdiagnosed as HELLP syndrome (Dillard *et al.*, 1975; Goodlin, 1991).

Patients may present with malaise, nausea, vomiting, and epigastric pain and tenderness. Some patients with HELLP do not present with significant hypertension. In one series of 112 women with severe pre-eclampsia–eclampsia complicated by HELLP syndrome, diastolic BP was less than 110 mmHg in 31% of cases and less than 90 mmHg in 15% at admission (el-Nazer *et al.*, 1986).

Laboratory studies are essential to making a correct diagnosis. The peripheral blood smear demonstrates burr cells and schistocytes, consistent with microangiopathic hemolytic anemia. Scanning electron microscopy demonstrates evidence of microangiopathic hemolysis in patients with HELLP syndrome due to passage of the red cells through thrombosed, damaged vessels (Cunningham *et al.*, 1985). Thrombocytopenia during pregnancy may be defined as a platelet count less than 100,000–150,000 μl^{-1}. Thrombocytopenia in pre-eclampsia occurs secondary to peripheral platelet destruction (Gibson *et al.*, 1989). In a retrospective review of 353 patients with pre-eclampsia, Romero and colleagues reported a 12% incidence of thrombocytopenia, defined as a platelet count less than 100,000 μl^{-1} (Lockwood *et al.*, 1989). Liver dysfunction, as defined by an elevated SGOT, was retrospectively identified in 21% of 355 patients with pre-eclampsia (Emamian *et al.*, 1988). Clotting parameters, such as the prothrombin time (PT), partial thromboplastin time (PTT), fibrinogen, and bleeding time (BT), in the patient with HELLP syndrome are generally normal in the absence of abruptio placenta or fetal demise. Elevation of alkaline phosphatase is seen in normal pregnancy; elevation of SGOT or SGPT indicates hepatic pathology.

Laboratory abnormalities usually return to normal within a short time after delivery; it is not unusual, however, to see transient worsening of both thrombocytopenia and hepatic function in the first 24–48 h postpartum (Contag et al., 1991). An upward trend in platelet count and a downward trend in lactate dehydrogenase concentration should occur in patients without complications by the fourth postpartum day. Martin and colleagues evaluated postpartum recovery in 158 women with HELLP syndrome at the University of Mississippi Medical Center (Blake et al., 1991). A return to a normal platelet count of $100,000\,\mu l^{-1}$ occurred in all women whose platelet nadir was below $50,000\,\mu l^{-1}$ by the eleventh postpartum day, and in all women whose platelet nadir was $50,000–100,000\,\mu l^{-1}$ by the sixth postpartum day. Consideration should be given to thrombotic thrombocytopenic purpura (TTP) in patients with suspected HELLP syndrome who do not show significant recovery within 72 h.

Complications associated with HELLP syndrome include placental abruption, acute renal failure, hepatic hematoma, and ascites. Placental abruption in HELLP syndrome patients occurs at a rate 20 times that seen in the general obstetric population; the reported incidence ranges from 7% to 20% (el-Nazer et al., 1986; Messer, 1987; Pritchard et al., 1954). Abruption in the presence of HELLP syndrome is frequently associated with fetal death and consumptive coagulopathy.

Pancreatitis

Pancreatitis has been observed in association with pre-eclampsia and HELLP syndrome, thought to be secondary to ischemia or possibly diuretics administered for oliguria (Badja et al., 1997; Girolami et al., 1999; Goodlin, 1987; Marcovici and Marzano, 2002). The association between diuretic use and postpartum pancreatitis is interesting. It is possible that pancreatic ischemia due to generalized vasoconstriction from pre-eclampsia is worsened by the use of loop diuretics in the setting of oliguria with renal failure. The authors suggest that in postpartum women with pregnancy-induced hypertension and acute renal failure, diuretics should be used cautiously because they may increase the risk of pancreatitis. In cases where unrelenting upper abdominal or chest pain is documented, especially where there is radiation to the back, it would be wise to consider pancreatitis and aortic dissection as differential diagnoses. Serum amylase and lipase levels should be checked and appropriate pancreatitis management regimens instituted in those cases where pre-eclampsia and pancreatitis coexist.

Liver rupture

Hepatic ischemia may lead to intrahepatic hemorrhage and subcapsular hematoma, which may rupture and result in shock and death. Subcapsular hematomas usually develop on the anterior and superior aspects of the liver (Brenner and Herbert, 1982). The diagnosis of a liver hematoma may be aided by use of ultrasonography, radionuclide scanning, computed tomography (CT), magnetic resonance imaging (MRI) and selective angiography (Brummelkamp et al., 1982). Contemporary maternal mortality is reported at 39% (Beinder et al., 2001).

When the diagnosis of liver hematoma is suspected prior to delivery, immediate exploratory laparotomy and Cesarean delivery should be performed in order to prevent potential rupture of the hematoma. When the diagnosis of liver hematoma is made in the postpartum period, conservative management with serial ultrasonography may be reasonable, particularly if the patient

Table 27.5. Differential diagnoses of HELLP syndrome, modified from Dildy (2004)

Autoimmune thrombocytopenic purpura
Chronic renal disease
Pyelonephritis
Cholecystitis
Gastroenteritis
Hepatitis
Pancreatitis
Thrombotic thrombocytopenic purpura
Hemolytic–uremic syndrome
Acute fatty liver of pregnancy

Table 27.6. Maternal outcomes in HELLP syndrome, modified from Dildy (2004)

Series	Location	Years	Cases (n)	Incidence (%)	Maternal mortality (%)	Cesarean rate (%)
MacKenna, 1983	Greenville, NC	1978–1982	27	12%[a]	0	N/A
Weinstein, 1985	Tucson, AZ	1980–1984	57	0.67%[b]	3.5	58
Sibai, 1986	Memphis, TN	1977–1985	112	9.7%[c]	1.8	63
Romero, 1988	New Haven, CT	1981–1984	58	21%[a]	N/A	57
Sibai and Ramadan, 1993	Memphis, TN	1977–1992	442	20%[d]	0.9	42

[a]Among all pre-eclamptic–eclamptic patients.
[b]Among all live births.
[c]Among severe pre-eclamptic–eclamptic pregnancies.
[d]Among severe pre-eclamptic women.
N/A, not available.

is hemodynamically stable and the hematoma is not expanding (Anderson *et al.*, 1985; Brummelkamp *et al.*, 1983). If ruptured or expanding hematoma is suspected after delivery, intervention is indicated. Hemostasis has been achieved by compression, simple suture, topical coagulant agents, arterial embolization, omental pedicles, ligation of the hepatic artery, or lobectomy, depending on the extent of the hepatic damage (Ledgerwood and Lucas, 1976). We believe that control of bleeding may be best achieved by packing and draining the rupture site.

Smith and colleagues reviewed the literature for the years 1976–1990 and reported their experience at Baylor College of Medicine for the years 1978–1990 (Carpenter *et al.*, 1991). The incidence of liver rupture during pregnancy was one per 45,145 live births in the Baylor series. A significant difference in maternal survival was seen among patients who were managed by packing and drainage, compared with those managed by hepatic lobectomy (82% versus 25%). A conservative surgical approach is supported by a report of 1000 consecutive cases of traumatic liver injury at the same institution (Bitondo *et al.*, 1986a, b; Feliciano *et al.*, 1981). Extensive resection of the liver or lobectomy with selective vascular ligation resulted in a 34% mortality rate, whereas conservative surgery (packing and drainage and/or use of topical hemostatic agents) resulted in a 7% mortality.

A few cases of pregnancy following hepatic rupture have been reported. There have been

Table 27.7. Perinatal outcomes in HELLP syndrome, modified from Dildy (2004)

Series	Location	Years	Cases (n)	Perinatal mortality (%)	Small for gestational age (%)	Respiratory distress syndrome (%)
MacKenna, 1983	Greenville, NC	1978–1982	27	11	N/A	8
Weinstein, 1985	Tucson, AZ	1980–1984	57	8	N/A	16
Sibai, 1986	Memphis, TN	1977–1985	112	33	32	N/A
Romero, 1988	New Haven, CT	1981–1984	58	7	41	31

Table 27.8. Eclampsia: maternal–fetal complications. Modified from Dildy (2004)

Series	Location	Years	N	Antepartum eclampsia (%)	Cesarean rate (%)	Maternal mortality (%)	Perinatal mortality (%)
Bryant and Fleming, 1940	Cincinnati, OH	1930–1940	120	62	0	1.7	29[a]
Zuspan, 1966	Augusta, GA	1956–1965	69	88	1.4[b]	2.9	32[a]
Harbert, 1968	Charlottesville, VA	1939–1963	168	78	6[b]	4.8	22[a]
Pritchard, 1975	Dallas, TX	1955–1975	154	82	23	0	15[b]
Lopez-Llera, 1982	Mexico City, Mexico	1963–1979	704	83	57[b]	14	27
Pritchard et al., 1984	Dallas, TX	1975–1983	91	91	33[b]	1.1	16[b]
Adetoro et al., 1989	Ilorin, Nigeria	1972–1987	651	N/A	N/A	14	N/A
Sibai, 1990	Memphis, TN	1977–1989	254	71	49[b]	0.4	12[a]
Douglas and Redman, 1994	United Kingdom	1992	383	56	54[b]	1.8	7[a]
Majoko and Mujaji, 2001	Harare, Zimbabwe	1997–1998	151	68	63[a]	27	15[b]
Onwuhafua et al., 2001	Kaduna State, Nigeria	1990–1997	45	60	53[a]	42	44[a]

[a]All cases.
[b]Antepartum and intrapartum cases only.
N/A, not available.

several reported cases of nonrecurrence in subsequent pregnancies and one case of recurrence with survival in a subsequent pregnancy (Boyer et al., 1994). Orthotopic liver transplantation can be life-saving (Behnda et al., 1995). Spontaneous splenic rupture associated with pre-eclampsia has also been reported (Adair et al., 1999).

Acute renal failure

Acute renal failure and pre-eclampsia are uncommon (Krane, 1988). In a series of 245 cases of eclampsia, none required dialysis for renal failure (Cunningham et al., 1984). However, 7% of 435 women with HELLP syndrome developed acute renal failure; long-term prognosis was generally favorable in the absence of pre-existing chronic hypertension (Sibai and Ramadan, 1993). Acute renal failure secondary to pre-eclampsia is usually the result of acute tubular necrosis but may be secondary to bilateral cortical necrosis. Precipitating factors include abruption, coagulopathy, hemorrhage, and severe hypotension (Grunfeld and Pertuiset, 1987). Severe renal dysfunction in pre-eclampsia is most commonly initially manifested as oliguria, defined as urinary output less than $25-30\,\mathrm{ml\,h^{-1}}$ over 2 consecutive hours. This often parallels a rise in serum creatinine and BUN. The urine sediment may show granular casts and renal tubular cells (Gallery, 1993; Krane, 1988).

Close monitoring of fluid intake and output is of paramount importance in all patients diagnosed with pre-eclampsia. If urine output falls below $25-30\,\mathrm{ml\,h^{-1}}$ over 2 consecutive hours, a management plan should be instituted. Given the fact that plasma volume is diminished in pre-eclamptics, the cause of oliguria may be considered prerenal in most instances (Aldahl *et al.*, 1986; Chesley, 1972; Gallery *et al.*, 1979). A fluid challenge of $500-1000\,\mathrm{ml}$ of normal saline or lactated Ringer's solution may be administered over 30 min. If urine output does not respond to an initial fluid challenge, additional challenges may be given under echocardiographic monitoring of cardiac function and IVC diameter (Belfort *et al.*, 1994).

Abruptio placentae

Hypertensive patients are at higher risk for abruption. The pathophysiology of placental abruption in pre-eclamptic patients has been proposed to result from thrombotic lesions in the placental vasculature, leading to decidual necrosis, separation, and hemorrhage. A vicious cycle then continues as the decidual hemorrhage results in further separation. This cycle may be aggravated by coexisting hemostatic compromise. Abdella and colleagues evaluated 265 cases of abruption and estimated an incidence of approximately 1% in the total obstetric population, of which a quarter of cases were complicated by a hypertensive disorder. Pre-eclamptics, chronic hypertensives, and eclamptics were found to have a 2%, 10% and 24% incidence of abruption, respectively (Abdella *et al.*, 1984; Hertzberg *et al.*, 1983).

Primary management goals for abruption include delivery, restoration of red blood cell volume, and correction of hemostatic defects.

Conclusion

In conclusion, pre-eclampsia–eclampsia has the potential to produce significant maternal complications of most organ systems. Prompt recognition of pathophysiologic changes and evolving complications will allow minimization of perinatal morbidity and mortality.

REFERENCES

Aali, B. S. and Nejad, S. S. (2002). Nifedipine or hydralazine as a first-line agent to control hypertension in severe preeclampsia. *Acta Obstet. Gynecol. Scand.*, **81**, 25–30.

Abdella, T. N., Anderson, G. D., Hays, J. M. Jr. and Sibai, B. M. (1984). Relationship of hypertensive disease to abruptio placentae. *Obstet. Gynecol.*, **63**, 365–70.

ACOG Practice Bulletin. (2002). Diagnosis and management of preeclampsia and eclampsia. ACOG Committee on Practice Bulletins. *Obstet. Gynecol.*, **99** (Suppl.), 159–67.

Adair, D., Barrilleaux, P. S., Johnson, G. and Lewis, D. F. (1999). Splenic rupture associated with severe preeclampsia. A case report. *J. Reprod. Med.*, **44**, 899–901.

Adetoro, O. O. (1989). A sixteen year survey of maternal mortality associated with eclampsia in Ilorin, Nigeria. *Int. J. Gynaecol. Obstet.*, **30**, 117–21.

Adze, J., Mairami, Z., Onwuhfua, A. and Onwuhafua, P. I. (2001). Eclampsia in Kaduna State of Nigeria – a proposal for a better outcome. *Niger. J. Med.*, **10**, 81–4.

Aldahl, D., Clark, S. L., Greenspoon, J. S. and Phelan, J. P. (1986). Severe preeclampsia with persistent oliguria: management of hemodynamic subsets. *Am. J. Obstet. Gynecol.*, **154**, 490–4.

Allen, J. C. Jr., Anthony, J., Belfort, M. A. and Saade, G. R. (2003). A comparison of magnesium sulfate and nimodipine for the prevention of eclampsia. *N. Engl. J. Med.*, **348**, 304–11.

Amon, E., Gonzalez, A. R., Mabie, W. C. and Sibai, B. M. (1987). A comparative trial of labetalol and hydralazine in the acute management of severe hypertension complicating pregnancy. *Obstet. Gynecol.*, **70**, 328–33.

Anderson, G. D., Lewis, J. A., Sibai, B. M., Spinnato, J. A. and Watson, D. L. (1985). Eclampsia. IV. Neurological findings and future outcome. *Am. J. Obstet. Gynecol.*, **152**, 184–92.

Anderson, G.D., Sibai, B.M., Abdella, T.N. and Spinnato, J.A. (1986). Eclampsia. V. The incidence of nonpreventable eclampsia. *Am. J. Obstet. Gynecol.*, **154**, 581–6.

Anderson, G.D., Sibai, B.M. and Spinnato, J.A. (1986). Fetal distress after hydralazine therapy for severe pregnancy-induced hypertension. *South. Med. J.*, **79**, 559–62.

Anderson, J.C., Goodlin, R.C. and Hodgson, P.E. (1985). Conservative treatment of liver hematoma in the postpartum period. A report of two cases. *J. Reprod. Med.*, **30**, 368–70.

Anthony, J., Coetzee, E.J. and Dommisse, J. (1998). A randomised controlled trial of intravenous magnesium sulphate versus placebo in the management of women with severe pre-eclampsia. *Br. J. Obstet. Gynaecol.*, **105**, 300–3.

Anthony, J., Field, N.T., Gilbert, W.M. and Towner, D.R. (2000). The safety and utility of pulmonary artery catheterization in severe preeclampsia and eclampsia. *Am. J. Obstet. Gynecol.*, **182**, 1397–403.

Appelman, Z., Fenakel, G., Fenakel, K., Katz, Z., Lurie, S. and Shoham, Z. (1991). Nifedipine in the treatment of severe preeclampsia. *Obstet. Gynecol.*, **77**, 331–7.

Appignani, B., Chaves, C., Hinchey, J., *et al.* (1996). A reversible posterior leukoencephalopathy syndrome. *N. Engl. J. Med.*, **334**, 494–500.

Arnott, N., Chien, P.F. and Khan, K.S. (1996). Magnesium sulphate in the treatment of eclampsia and pre-eclampsia: an overview of the evidence from randomised trials. *Br. J. Obstet. Gynaecol.*, **103**, 1085–91.

Assali, N.S., Kaplan, S., Oighenstein, S. and Suyemoto, R. (1953). Hemodynamic effects of 1-hydrazinophthalazine (Apresoline) in human pregnancy: results of intravenous administration. *J. Clin. Invest.*, **32**, 922–30.

Atrash, H.K., Franks, A.L., Olson, D.R., Pokras, R. and Saftlas, A.F. (1990). Epidemiology of preeclampsia and eclampsia in the United States, 1979–1986. *Am. J. Obstet. Gynecol.*, **163**, 460–5.

Badja, N., Benhamou, D., Troche, G. and Zazzo, J.F. (1997). Acute pancreatitis and preeclampsia–eclampsia: a case report. *Am. J. Obstet. Gynecol.*, **176**, 707–9.

Beal, M.F. and Chapman, P.H. (1980). Cortical blindness and homonymous hemianopia in the postpartum period. *J. Am. Med. Ass.*, **244**, 2085–7.

Beck, R.W., Berman, G., Gamel, J.W. and Willcourt, R.J. (1980). Acute ischemic optic neuropathy in severe preeclampsia. *Am. J. Ophthalmol.*, **90**, 342–6.

Beeson, J.H. and Duda, E.E. (1982). Computed axial tomography scan demonstration of cerebral edema in eclampsia preceded by blindness. *Obstet. Gynecol.*, **60**, 529–32.

Beinder, E., Bussenius-Kammerer, M., Hohenberger, W., Muller, V., Ott, R. and Reck, T. (2001). Surgical treatment of HELLP syndrome-associated liver rupture – an update. *Eur. J. Obstet. Gynecol. Reprod. Biol.*, **99**, 57–65.

Belfort, M.A., Rokey, R., Saade, G.R. and Moise, K.J. Jr. (1994). Rapid echocardiographic assessment of left and right heart hemodynamics in critically ill obstetric patients. *Am. J. Obstet. Gynecol.*, **171**(4), 884–92.

Belfort, M.A., Dizon-Townson, D.S., Grunewald, C., Nisell, H. and Varner, M.W. (2002). Cerebral perfusion pressure, and not cerebral blood flow, may be the critical determinant of intracranial injury in preeclampsia: a new hypothesis. *Am. J. Obstet. Gynecol.*, **187**, 626–34.

Behnda, J.A., Hunter, S.K., Martin, M. and Zlatnik, F.J. (1995). Liver transplant after massive spontaneous hepatic rupture in pregnancy complicated by pre-eclampsia. *Obstet. Gynecol.*, **85**, 819–22.

Benedetti, T.J., Kates, R. and Williams, V. (1985). Hemodynamic observations in severe preeclampsia complicated by pulmonary edema. *Am. J. Obstet. Gynecol.*, **152**, 330–4.

Berg, C.J., Callaghan, W.M., Chang, J. and Whitehead, S.J. (2003). Pregnancy-related mortality in the United States, 1991–1997. *Obstet. Gynecol.*, **101**, 289–96.

Bhalla, A.K., Dhall, G.I. and Dhall, K. (1994). A safer and more effective treatment regimen for eclampsia. *Aust. N.Z. J. Obstet. Gynaecol.*, **34**, 144–8.

Bhorat, I.E., Naidoo, D.P., Rout, C.C. and Moodley, J. (1993). Malignant ventricular arrhythmias in eclampsia: a comparison of labetalol with dihydralazine. *Am. J. Obstet. Gynecol.*, **168**(4), 1292–6.

Bhorat, I., Desai, D.K., Moodley, J. and Naidoo, D.P. (1996). Cardiac abnormalities in pulmonary oedema associated with hypertensive crises in pregnancy. *Br. J. Obstet. Gynaecol.*, **103**, 523–8.

Bitondo, C.G., Burch, J.M., Feliciano, D.V., Jordan, G.L. Jr. and Mattox, K.L. (1986a). Packing for control of hepatic hemorrhage. *J. Trauma*, **26**, 738–43.

Bitondo, C.G., Burch, J.M., Cruse, P.A., Feliciano, D.V., Jordan, G.L. Jr. and Mattox, K.L. (1986b). Management of 1000 consecutive cases of hepatic trauma (1979–1984). *Ann. Surg.*, **204**, 438–45.

Blake, P.G., Hess, L.W., Martin, J.N., Jr., Martin, R.W., McCaul, J.F. and Perry, K.G. Jr. (1991). The natural history of HELLP syndrome: patterns of disease progression and regression. *Am. J. Obstet. Gynecol.*, **164**, 1500–9; discussion 1509–13.

Bohman, V. R. and Cotton, D. B. (1990). Supralethal magnesemia with patient survival. *Obstet. Gynecol.*, **76**, 984–6.

Bouvier-Colle, M. H., Decam, C., Dumont, A., Salanave, B., Ouedraogo, C. and Vangeenderhuysen, C. (2001). Maternal mortality in West Africa. Rates, causes and substandard care from a prospective survey. *Acta Obstet. Gynecol. Scand.*, **80**, 113–19.

Boyer, T. D., Greenstein, D. and Henderson, J. M. (1994). Liver hemorrhage: recurrent episodes during pregnancy complicated by preeclampsia. *Gastroenterology*, **106**, 1668–71.

Brame, R. G., Dover, N. L. and MacKenna, J. (1983). Preeclampsia associated with hemolysis, elevated liver enzymes, and low platelets – an obstetric emergency? *Obstet. Gynecol.*, **62**, 751–4.

Brenner, W. E. and Herbert, W. N. (1982). Improving survival with liver rupture complicating pregnancy. *Am. J. Obstet. Gynecol.*, **142**, 530–4.

Broering, D. C., Bloechle, C., Strate, T., *et al.* (2000). Orthotopic liver transplantation for complicated HELLP syndrome. Case report and review of the literature. *Arch. Gynecol. Obstet.*, **264**, 108–11.

Brummelkamp, W. H., Buller, H. R., Henny, C. P., Lim, T. E. and ten Cate, J. W. (1982). Spontaneous rupture of Glisson's capsule during pregnancy. An acute surgical emergency. *Neth. J. Surg.*, **34**, 72–5.

Brummelkamp, W. H., Buller, H. R., Henny, C. P., Lim, A. E. and ten Cate, J. W. (1983). A review of the importance of acute multidisciplinary treatment following spontaneous rupture of the liver capsule during pregnancy. *Surg. Gynecol. Obstet.*, **156**, 593–8.

Bryant, R. D. and Fleming, J. G. (1940). Veratrum viride in the treatment of eclampsia: II. *J. Am. Med. Ass.*, **115**, 1333–9.

Bullock, M. R., Downing, J. W., Moodley, J. and Richards, A. M. (1987). Maternal deaths from neurological complications of hypertensive crises in pregnancy. *S. Afr. Med. J.*, **71**, 487–90.

Bullock, R., Graham, D. and Richards, A. (1988). Clinicopathological study of neurological complications due to hypertensive disorders of pregnancy. *J. Neurol. Neurosurg. Psychiat.*, **51**, 416–21.

Burgess, E., Lange, I. R., Leduc, L., LeLorier, J. and Rey, E. (1997). Report of the Canadian Hypertension Society Consensus Conference: 3. Pharmacologic treatment of hypertensive disorders in pregnancy. *Canadian Medical Association Journal*, **157**, 1245–54.

Camera, M. I., Martinotti, A., Mayorga, L. M., Vignolo, C. A. and Waisman, G. D. (1988). Magnesium plus nifedipine: potentiation of hypotensive effect in preeclampsia? *Am. J. Obstet. Gynecol.*, **159**, 308–9.

Carpenter, R. J. Jr., Dildy, G. A., III, Moise, K. J. Jr. and Smith, L. G. Jr. (1991). Spontaneous rupture of liver during pregnancy: current therapy. *Obstet. Gynecol.*, **77**, 171–5.

Chang, J., Elam-Evans, L. D., Berg, C. J., *et al.* (2003). Pregnancy-related mortality surveillance – United States, 1991–1999. *MMWR Surveill. Summ.*, **52**, 1–8.

Chauhan, S. P., Newman, R. B., Scardo, J. A. and Vermillion, S. T. (1999). A randomized, double-blind trial of oral nifedipine and intravenous labetalol in hypertensive emergencies of pregnancy. *Am. J. Obstet. Gynecol.*, **181**, 858–61.

Chesley, L. C. (1972). Plasma and red cell volumes during pregnancy. *Am. J. Obstet. Gynecol.*, **112**, 440–50.

Chonette, D., Diamond, G., Forrester, J., Ganz, W., Marcus, H. and Swan, H. J. (1970). Catheterization of the heart in man with use of a flow-directed balloon-tipped catheter. *N. Engl. J. Med.*, **283**, 447–51.

Claiborne, H. A., Harbert, G. M., McGaughey, H. S., Thornton, W. N. and Wilson, L. A. (1968). Convulsive toxemia. *Am. J. Obstet. Gynecol.*, **100**, 336–42.

Clark, S. L., Horenstein, J. M., Montag, T. W., Paul, R. H. and Phelan, J. P. (1985). Experience with the pulmonary artery catheter in obstetrics and gynecology. *Am. J. Obstet. Gynecol.*, **152**, 374–8.

Clark, S. L. and Cotton, D. B. (1988). Clinical indications for pulmonary artery catheterization in the patient with severe preeclampsia. *Am. J. Obstet. Gynecol.*, **158**, 453–8.

Clark, S. L., Cotton, D. B., Lee, W., *et al.* (1989). Central hemodynamic assessment of normal term pregnancy. *Am. J. Obstet. Gynecol.*, **161**, 1439–42.

Contag, S. A., Coustan, D. R. and Neiger, R. (1991). The resolution of preeclampsia-related thrombocytopenia. *Obstet. Gynecol.*, **77**, 692–5.

Cotton, D. B., Dorman, K. F. and Gonik, B. (1985). Cardiovascular alterations in severe pregnancy-induced hypertension seen with an intravenously given hydralazine bolus. *Surg. Gynecol. Obstet.*, **161**, 240–4.

Cotton, D. B., Dorman, K. F., Jones, M. M., Joyce, T. H., Longmire, S. and Tessem, J. III (1986a). Role of intravenous nitroglycerin in the treatment of severe pregnancy-induced hypertension complicated by pulmonary edema. *Am. J. Obstet. Gynecol.*, **154**, 91–3.

Cotton, D. B., Dorman, K. F., Jones, M. M., Joyce, T. H., Longnire, S. and Tessem, J. III (1986b). Cardiovascular alterations in severe pregnancy-induced hypertension: effects of intravenous nitroglycerin coupled with blood volume expansion. *Am. J. Obstet. Gynecol.*, **154**, 1053–9.

Cotton, D. B., Dunn, R. and Lee, W. (1986c). Evaluation by computerized axial tomography of eclamptic women with seizures refractory to magnesium sulfate therapy. *Am. J. Obstet. Gynecol.*, **155**, 267–8.

Cotton, D. B., Lee, W. and Gonik, B. (1987). Urinary diagnostic indices in preeclampsia-associated oliguria: correlation with invasive hemodynamic monitoring. *Am. J. Obstet. Gynecol.*, **156**, 100–3.

Cotton, D. B., Kirshon, B., Lee, W. and Mauer, M. B. (1988b). Effects of low-dose dopamine therapy in the oliguric patient with preeclampsia. *Am. J. Obstet. Gynecol.*, **159**, 604–7.

Cotton, D. B., Dorman, K. F., Huhta, J. C. and Lee, W. (1988a). Hemodynamic profile of severe pregnancy-induced hypertension. *Am. J. Obstet. Gynecol.*, **158**, 523–9.

Cunningham, F. G., Pritchard, J. A. and Pritchard, S. A. (1984). The Parkland Memorial Hospital protocol for treatment of eclampsia: evaluation of 245 cases. *Am. J. Obstet. Gynecol.*, **148**, 951–63.

Cunningham, F. G., Guss, S., Lowe, T. and Mason, R. (1985). Erythrocyte morphology in women with severe preeclampsia and eclampsia. Preliminary observations with scanning electron microscopy. *Am. J. Obstet. Gynecol.*, **153**, 358–63.

Cunningham, F. G., DePalma, R. T., Leveno, L. K., *et al.* (1994). A simplified phenytoin regimen for preeclampsia. *Am. J. Perinatol.*, **11**, 153–6.

Cunningham, F. G. and Gant, N. F. (1994). Management of eclampsia. *Semin. Perinatol.*, **18**, 103–13.

Cunningham, F. G., Fernandez, C. O. and Hernandez, C. (1995a). Blindness associated with preeclampsia and eclampsia. *Am. J. Obstet. Gynecol.*, **172**, 1291–8.

Cunningham, F. G., Leveno, K. J. and Lucas, M. J. (1995b). A comparison of magnesium sulfate with phenytoin for the prevention of eclampsia. *N. Engl. J. Med.*, **333**, 201–5.

Cunningham, F. G., Gant, N. F., Gilstrap, L. C., Hauth, J. C., Leveno, K. J. and Wenstrom, K. D. eds. (2001). Hypertensive disorders in pregnancy. In: *Williams Obstetrics*. New York: McGraw-Hill.

de Swiet, M. (2000). Maternal mortality: confidential enquiries into maternal deaths in the United Kingdom. *Am. J. Obstet. Gynecol.*, **182**, 760–6.

Desai, D. K., Moodley, J., Naidoo, D. P. and Bhorat, I. (1996). Cardiac abnormalities in pulmonary oedema associated with hypertensive crises in pregnancy *Br. J. Obstet. Gynaecol.*, **103**(6), 523–8.

Devoe, L. D., Elgammal, T. A. and Hill, J. A. (1985). Central hemodynamic findings associated with cortical blindness in severe preeclampsia. A case report. *J. Reprod. Med.*, **30**, 435–8.

Dierker, L. R., Lazebnik, N., Pazmino, R., Takaoka, Y. and Warf, B. C. (1989). Maternal intracranial hemorrhage complicating severe superimposed preeclampsia. A case report. *J. Reprod. Med.*, **34**, 857–60.

Dildy, G. A. (2004). Complications of preeclampsia. In *Critical Care Obstetrics*, ed. G. A. Dildy, M. A. Belfort, G. R. Saade, J. P. Phelan, G. D. V. Hankins and S. L. Clark. Boston: Blackwell Scientific Publications.

Dillard, S. H., Killam, A. P., Patton, R. C. and Pederson, P. R. (1975). Pregnancy-induced hypertension complicated by acute liver disease and disseminated intravascular coagulation. Five case reports. *Am. J. Obstet. Gynecol.*, **123**, 823–8.

Do, D. V., Nguyen, Q. D. and Rismondo, V. (2002). Reversible cortical blindness in preeclampsia. *Am. J. Ophthalmol.*, **134**, 916–18.

Douglas, K. A. and Redman, C. W. (1994). Eclampsia in the United Kingdom. *Br. Med. J.*, **309**, 1395–400.

Duley, L. and Henderson-Smart, D. (2000a). *Magnesium sulphate versus diazepam for eclampsia.* Cochrane Database Syst Rev:CD000127.

Duley, L. and Henderson-Smart, D. (2000b). *Magnesium sulphate versus phenytoin for eclampsia.* Cochrane Database Syst Rev:CD000128.

Duley, L. and Gulmezoglu, A. M. (2001). *Magnesium sulphate versus lytic cocktail for eclampsia.* Cochrane Database Syst Rev:CD002960.

Ekbladh, L. E., Grimes, D. A. and McCartney, W. H. (1980). Cortical blindness in preeclampsia. *Int. J. Gynaecol. Obstet.*, **17**, 601–3.

el-Nazer, A., Amon, E., Mabie, B. C., Ryan, G. M., Sibai, B. M. and Taslimi, M. M. (1986). Maternal–perinatal outcome associated with the syndrome of hemolysis, elevated liver enzymes, and low platelets in severe preeclampsia–eclampsia. *Am. J. Obstet. Gynecol.*, **155**, 501–9.

Emamian, M., Romero, R., Vizoso, J., *et al.* (1988). Clinical significance of liver dysfunction in pregnancy-induced hypertension. *Am. J. Perinatol.*, **5**, 146–51.

Feliciano, D. V., Jordan, G. L. Jr. and Mattox, K. L. (1981). Intra-abdominal packing for control of hepatic hemorrhage: a reappraisal. *J. Trauma*, **21**, 285–90.

Fredholm, B., Hjemdahl, P., Lunell, N. O., *et al.* (1982). Labetalol, a combined alpha- and beta-blocker, in hypertension of pregnancy. *Acta Med. Scand. Suppl.*, **665**, 143–7.

Friedman, S. A., Mercer, B. M., Ramadan, M. K., Salama, M., Sibai, B. M. and Usta, I. (1993). Maternal morbidity and mortality in 442 pregnancies with hemolysis, elevated liver enzymes, and low platelets (HELLP syndrome). *Am. J. Obstet. Gynecol.*, **169**, 1000–6.

Gallery, E. D., Gyory, A. Z. and Hunyor, S. N. (1979). Plasma volume contraction: a significant factor in both pregnancy-associated hypertension (pre-eclampsia) and chronic hypertension in pregnancy. *Q. J. Med.*, **48**, 593–602.

Gallery, E. D., Gyory, A. Z. and Ross, M. (1993). Urinary red blood cell and cast excretion in normal and hypertensive human pregnancy. *Am. J. Obstet. Gynecol.*, **168**, 67–70.

Gibson, B., Hunter, D., Kelton, J. G. and Neame, P. B. (1989). Thrombocytopenia in preeclampsia and eclampsia. *Semin. Thromb. Hemost.*, **8**, 234–47.

Girolami, A., Paternoster, D. M., Rodi, J., Santarossa, C., Simioni, P. and Vanin, M. (1999). Acute pancreatitis and deep vein thrombosis associated with HELLP syndrome. *Minerva Ginecol.*, **51**, 31–3.

Gonzalez, A. R., Harvey, C. J., Mabie, B. C. and Sibai, B. M. (1987). Pulmonary edema in severe preeclampsia–eclampsia: analysis of thirty-seven consecutive cases. *Am. J. Obstet. Gynecol.*, **156**, 1174–9.

Goodlin, R. C. (1987). The effect of severe pre-eclampsia on the pancreas: changes in the serum cationic trypsinogen and pancreatic amylase. *Br. J. Obstet. Gynaecol.*, **94**, 1228.

Goodlin, R. C. (1991). Preeclampsia as the great impostor. *Am. J. Obstet. Gynecol.*, **164**, 1577–80; discussion 1580–1.

Grunfeld, J. P. and Pertuiset, N. (1987). Acute renal failure in pregnancy. *Am. J. Kidney Dis.*, **9**, 359–62.

Harbert, G. M. Jr., Claiborne, H. A. Jr., McGaughey, H. S. Jr., Wilson, L. A. Jr. and Thornton, W. N. Jr. (1968). Convulsive toxemia. A report of 168 cases managed conservatively. *Am. J. Obstet. Gynecol.*, **100**(3), 336–42.

Henderson, D. W., Milne, K. J., Nichol, P. M. and Vilos, G. A. (1984). The role of Swan-Ganz catheterization in severe pregnancy-induced hypertension. *Am. J. Obstet. Gynecol.*, **148**, 570–4.

Henning, R. J., Puri, V. K. and Weil, M. H. (1996). Colloid oncotic pressure: clinical significance. *Crit. Care. Med.*, **7**, 113–16.

Herling, I. M. (1984). Intravenous nitroglycerin: clinical pharmacology and therapeutic considerations. *Am. Heart J.*, **108**, 141–9.

Hertzberg, V., Hurd, W. W., Lavin, J. P. and Miodovnik, M. (1983). Selective management of abruptio placentae: a prospective study. *Obstet. Gynecol.*, **61**, 467–73.

Hobbins, J. C., Lockwood, C., Oyarzun, E. and Romero, R. (1988). Toxemia: new concepts in an old disease. *Semin. Perinatol.*, **12**, 302–23.

Hogberg, U., Innala, E. and Sandstrom, A. (1994). Maternal mortality in Sweden, 1980–1988. *Obstet. Gynecol.*, **84**, 240–4.

Hoppelshauser, G. and Pasch, T. (1983). Methaemoglobin levels during nitroglycerin infusion for the intraoperative induction of controlled hypotension. *Arzneimittelforschung*, **33**, 879–82.

Hoppelshauser, G., Pasch, T. and Schulz, V. (1983). Nitroprusside-induced formation of cyanide and its detoxication with thiosulfate during deliberate hypotension. *J. Cardiovasc. Pharmacol.*, **5**, 77–85.

Koch-Weser, J. (1976). Medical intelligence drug therapy. *N. Engl. J. Med.*, **295**, 320–3.

Krane, N. K. (1988). Acute renal failure in pregnancy. *Arch. Intern. Med.*, **148**, 2347–57.

Ledgerwood, A. M. and Lucas, C. E. (1976). Prospective evaluation of hemostatic techniques for liver injuries. *J. Trauma.*, **16**, 442–51.

Lewander, R., Lunell, N. O., Mamoun, I., Nylund, L., Sarby, S. and Thornstrom, S. (1984). Uteroplacental blood flow in pregnancy induced hypertension. *Scand. J. Clin. Lab. Invest. Suppl.*, **169**, 28–35.

Livingston, J. C., Livingston, L. W., Mabie, B. C., Ramsey, R. and Sibai, B. M. (2003). Magnesium sulfate in women with mild preeclampsia: a randomized controlled trial. *Obstet. Gynecol.*, **101**, 217–20.

Lockwood, C. J., Mazor, M., Romero, R., *et al.* (1989). Clinical significance, prevalence, and natural history of thrombocytopenia in pregnancy-induced hypertension. *Am. J. Perinatol.*, **6**, 32–8.

Lopez-Llera, M. (1982). Complicated eclampsia: fifteen years' experience in a referral medical center. *Am. J. Obstet. Gynecol.*, **142**, 28–35.

Lund-Johansen, P. (1984). Pharmacology of combined alpha-beta-blockade. II. Haemodynamic effects of labetalol. *Drugs*, **28**(Suppl. 2), 35–50.

Mabie, W. C., Ratts, T. E., Ramanathan, K. B. and Sibai, B. M. (1988). Circulatory congestion in obese hypertensive women: a subset of pulmonary edema in pregnancy. *Obstet. Gynecol.*, **72**(4), 553–8.

Mabie, W. C., Ratts, T. E. and Sibai, B. M. (1989). The central hemodynamics of severe preeclampsia. *Am. J. Obstet. Gynecol.*, **161**, 1443–8.

Majoko, F. and Mujaji, C. (2001). Maternal outcome in eclampsia at Harare Maternity Hospital. *Cent. Afr. J. Med.*, **1**, 123–8.

Marcovici, I. and Marzano, D. (2002). Pregnancy-induced hypertension complicated by postpartum renal failure and pancreatitis: a case report. *Am. J. Perinatol.*, **19**, 177–9.

Messer, R. H. (1987). Observations on bleeding in pregnancy. *Am. J. Obstet. Gynecol.*, **156**, 1419–20.

Moore, W. D. and Sakala, E. P. (1986). Successful term delivery after previous pregnancy with ruptured liver. *Obstet. Gynecol.*, **68**, 124–6.

Moseman, C. P. and Shelton, S. (2002). Permanent blindness as a complication of pregnancy induced hypertension. *Obstet. Gynecol.*, **100**, 943–5.

Murphy, D. J. and Stirrat, G. M. (2000). Mortality and morbidity associated with early-onset preeclampsia. *Hypertens. Pregnan.*, **19**, 221–31.

Naden, R. P. and Redman, C. W. (1985). Antihypertensive drugs in pregnancy. *Clin. Perinatol.*, **12**, 521–38.

Naidoo, D. P., Bhorat, I., Moodley, J., Naidoo, J. K. and Mitha, A. S. (1991). Continuous electrocardiographic monitoring in hypertensive crises in pregnancy. *Am. J. Obstet. Gynecol.*, **164**(2), 530–3.

Onwuhafua, P. I., Onwuhafua, A., Adze, J. and Mairami, Z. (2001). Eclampsia in Kaduna State of Nigeria – a proposal for a better outcome. *Niger. J. Med.*, **10**(2), 81–4.

Pritchard, J. A., Ratnoff, O. D., Vosburgh, G. J. and Weisman, R. (1954). Intravascular hemolysis, thrombocytopenia, and other hematologic abnormalities associated with severe toxemia of pregnancy. *N. Engl. J. Med.*, **150**, 89–98.

Pritchard, J. A. (1955). The use of the magnesium ion in the management of eclamptogenic toxemias. *Surg. Gynecol. Obstet.*, **100**, 131–40.

Pritchard, J. A. and Pritchard, S. A. (1975). Standardized treatment of 154 consecutive cases of eclampsia. *Am. J. Obstet. Gynecol.*, **123**, 543–52.

Pritchard, J. A., Cunningham, F. G. and Pritchard, S. A. (1984). The Parkland Memorial Hospital protocol for treatment of eclampsia: evaluation of 245 cases. *Am. J. Obstet. Gynecol.*, **148**(7), 951–63.

Report of the National High Blood Pressure Education Program Working Group on High Blood Pressure in Pregnancy. (2000). *Am. J. Obstet. Gynecol.*, **183**, S1–22.

Schannwell, C. M., Schmitz, L., Schoelsel, F. C., Zimmermann, T., Marx, R., Plehn, G., Leschke, M. and Strauer, B. E. (2001). Alterations of left ventricular function in hypertensive pregnant women. *Z. Cardiol.*, **90**(6), 427–36.

Schuitemater, N. O., van Roosmalen, J., Dekker, G., van Dongen, P., van Geijn, H. and Bennebroek Gravenhorst, J. (1998). Confidential enquiry into maternal deaths in The Netherlands 1983–92. *Eur. J. Obstet. Gynecol. Reprod. Biol.*, **79**, 57–62.

Scott, A. and Owen, P. (1996). Recent advances in the aetiology and management of pre-eclampsia. *Br. J. Hosp. Med.*, **55**, 476–8.

Scott, J. R. (2003). Magnesium sulfate for mild preeclampsia. *Obstet. Gynecol.*, **101**, 213.

Sibai, B. M. (1990). Eclampsia. VI. Maternal–perinatal outcome in 254 consecutive cases. *Am. J. Obstet. Gynecol.*, **163**, 1049–54; discussion 1054–5.

Sibai, B. M. and Ramadan, M. K. (1993). Acute renal failure in pregnancies complicated by hemolysis, elevated liver enzymes, and low platelets. *Am. J. Obstet. Gynecol.*, **168**, 1682–7; discussion 1687–90.

Sibai, B. M. (2003). Diagnosis and management of gestational hypertension and preeclampsia. *Obstet. Gynecol.*, **102**, 181–92.

Witlin, A. G., Mabie, W. C. and Sibai, B. M. (1997a). Peripartum cardiomyopathy: an ominous diagnosis. *Am. J. Obstet. Gynecol.*, **176**(1, Pt. 1), 182–8.

Witlin, A. G., Mabie, W. C. and Sibai, B. M. (1997b). Peripartum cardiomyopathy: a longitudinal echocardiographic study. *Am. J. Obstet. Gynecol.*, **177**(5), 1129–32.

Weinstein, L. (1982). Syndrome of hemolysis, elevated liver enzymes, and low platelet count: a severe consequence of hypertension in pregnancy. *Am. J. Obstet. Gynecol.*, **142**, 159–67.

Weinstein, L. (1985). Preeclampsia/eclampsia with hemolysis, elevated liver enzymes, and thrombocytopenia. *Obstet. Gynecol.*, **66**, 657–60.

Which anticonvulsant for women with eclampsia? Evidence from the Collaborative Eclampsia Trial. (1995). *Lancet*, **345**, 1455–63.

Zimmerman, J. L. (1995). Hypertensive crisis: emergencies and urgencies. In *Textbook of Critical Care*, ed. S. M. Ayers. Philadelphia: WB Saunders.

Zuspan, F. P. (1966). Treatment of severe preeclampsia and eclampsia. *Clin. Obstet. Gynecol.*, **9**, 954–72.

28

Central nervous system findings in pre-eclampsia and eclampsia

Diane Twickler and F. Gary Cunningham

Introduction

Eclampsia is one of the most severe forms of central nervous system (CNS) involvement in the pre-eclampsia syndrome. Although pre-eclampsia has been known to be a multisystem disorder for over 100 years, much of the pathophysiology, including its molecular manifestations, has only come to light in the past 20 years. This is exemplified by the fact that the prominent causative role of endothelial activation has only been recently appreciated (Redman *et al.*, 1999; Roberts and Redman, 1993; Roberts *et al.*, 1989; Taylor and Roberts, 1999). Currently, the CNS findings in eclampsia can be grouped in two ways: (1) Cerebral blood flow changes associated with gestational hypertension resulting in either hyperperfusion or hypoperfusion, either of which can cause edema and ischemia. (2) Characteristic anatomical lesions documented with either computed-tomographic (CT) scanning or magnetic resonance imaging (MRI) with diffusion-weighted techniques (Brown *et al.*, 1988; Cunningham and Twickler, 2000; Dahmus *et al.*, 1992; Digre *et al.*, 1993; Hauser *et al.*, 1988; Morriss *et al.*, 1997; Port *et al.*, 1998; Schwartz *et al.*, 1992, 2000; Zeeman *et al.*, 2004). These groupings are obviously artificial and there is a large amount of overlap. Specifically, endothelial injury and subsequent leakage of plasma from the intravascular compartment may be associated with manifestations of both functional flow abnormalities and discreet anatomical lesions. In our current understanding of the vascular involvement of the brain in eclampsia, we assume that the cerebral blood vessels are directly involved – in a similar fashion to the peripheral circulation in pre-eclampsia (Hankins *et al.*, 1984). Despite the fact that in most cases of pre-eclampsia cerebral autoregulation appears to remain intact, it has been shown that occasionally the middle cerebral artery fails to protect its distal circulation, and that this failure in autoregulation can be confined to only one side of brain, or to smaller areas within one hemisphere (Taylor, 1988). This may explain the regional nature of the imaging findings in eclampsia, where localized areas of cerebral edema, apparently at the gray–white matter interface, are frequently seen.

In this review of the CNS findings in eclampsia, we focus on three areas: (1) cerebrovascular hemodynamics, (2) hemodynamic changes during pregnancy, and (3) hemodynamic pathophysiology associated with eclampsia to include cerebrovascular alterations and imaging studies.

Central nervous system hemodynamics

The internal carotid and vertebral arteries are the main source of blood flow to the brain. These large vessels supply the Circle of Willis, which is the anastomotic ring at the base of the brain distributing blood flow to the cerebral cortex (Taylor, 1988) via the anterior, middle and posterior cerebral arteries. These paired arteries are responsible for the regional blood flow to the cerebral cortex, relative to their anatomic locations (Figure 28.1). They branch soon after exiting the Circle of Willis, forming a vast network of main

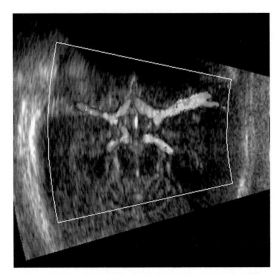

Figure 28.1 Doppler image of the anatomy of the Circle of Willis.

branches, terminal branches, arterioles, and end capillaries.

The hemodynamics of this network are complex, and blood flow to the brain is dependent on both the physical properties of the pulsatile flow of a complex fluid in a branching system, and the effects of autoregulation (Burns, 1988). It has been stated that the blood flow to the CNS is kept relatively constant by the vasoactive capabilities of the arterioles, which maintain cerebral perfusion at a relatively steady state, and protect the brain from acute hemodynamic perturbations (Port and Beauchamp et al., 1998). Significant decreases or increases in blood pressure or flow, however, may overwhelm the autoregulatory system, resulting in hemorrhagic or ischemic infarction (Hauser et al., 1988; Port and Beauchamp et al., 1998; Schwartz et al., 2000).

At the capillary level, changes in blood flow may cause disruption of the end-capillary pressures with subsequent increase in hydrostatic pressure and resultant vasogenic edema (Hauser et al., 1988; Port and Beauchamp et al., 1998; Schwartz et al., 2000). Vasogenic edema is a common endpoint to nonspecific insults to the brain, and if severe

enough can result in cellular ischemia, and irreversible cell death (cytotoxic edema) (Hackett et al., 1998).

Cerebral blood flow in pregnancy

Pregnancy results in increased maternal cardiac output to allow for the increased demands of the placental–fetal unit. With the increased maternal cardiac output and blood flow to the gravid uterus, it is expected that other maternal organs such as brain, adrenals, kidneys and heart maintain metabolic equilibrium. These vascular beds are thought to have relatively low vascular resistance to ensure adequate perfusion throughout most of the cardiac cycle, in order to maintain the high oxygen demands in these organs (Hackett et al., 1988; Hauser et al., 1988). It is difficult to study precise end-organ blood flow and perfusion in normal pregnant women, and much of our knowledge regarding blood flow and perfusion is based on indirect information. Of late, with the development of Doppler ultrasound technology, this modality has been extensively applied to the evaluation of the maternal uterus, brain and kidneys in normal and abnormal pregnancies (Boemi et al., 1996; Fleischer et al., 1986; Harrington et al., 1977, 1996; Kublickas et al., 1996; Levine et al., 1992; Liberati et al., 1994).

Doppler studies of the CNS are centered around the velocity of red blood cells flowing in the middle cerebral arteries. These pulsatile velocities are felt to indirectly represent flow in the middle cerebral arteries and also reflect changes in resistance in the vasoactive downstream arterioles (Burns, 1988). This is based on a somewhat oversimplified equation (flow = mean velocity multiplied by cross-sectional area of the vessel). There are, however, many confounding factors that influence this assumption. These include (but are not limited to) changes in the velocity as a result of decreased/ increased cardiac output and stroke volume; decreased viscosity of blood (anemia); changes in the luminal areas of large arteries and distal arterioles during the cardiac cycle due to vessel wall elasticity and perfusion pressure. Elevations in the middle cerebral artery Doppler velocity have been shown to reflect vasospasm in patients with subarachnoid hemorrhage (Giller et al., 1998; Hatab et al., 1997). Middle cerebral artery velocity elevation has also been reported in severe pre-eclampsia, and this observation caused many to favor the vasospasm model for the etiology of eclampsia (Aaslid et al., 1986; Belfort et al., 1999a, 1999b, 2001; Ikeda and Nori, 1990; Serra-Serra et al., 1995; Williams and Galerneau, 2003; Williams and McLean, 1993).

Belfort et al. and other investigators (Aaslid et al., 1986; Belfort et al., 1999a, 1999b, 2001; Ikeda and Nori, 1990; Serra-Serra et al., 1995; Williams and Galerneau, 2003; Williams and McLean, 1993), using transcranial Doppler ultrasound, have shown that in normal pregnancy there are decreases in the maximum and mean middle cerebral artery velocities, as well as in the Resistance Index (systolic–diastolic velocity/systolic velocity) as the pregnancy progresses. This finding has been noted in other central nervous system arteries (ophthalmic artery), confirming a general reduction in resistance in the CNS vasculature during pregnancy. Most studies based on Doppler technology assume a constant vessel diameter in the larger vessels such as the middle cerebral artery. This assumption has recently been supported by Zeeman et al. (2003), who demonstrated no significant change in middle cerebral artery cross-sectional area before and after pregnancy.

With the advent of Doppler ultrasound measurements of blood velocity in the middle cerebral artery, and the capability of simultaneously measuring maternal systemic blood pressure, it has become possible to derive a calculated cerebral perfusion pressure. Belfort et al. developed a Doppler equation using a method based on that validated in humans by Aaslid et al. (1986). They measured velocity in the middle cerebral artery (Doppler ultrasound), and intraventricular pressure and radial arterial blood pressure (direct strain gauge transducers) in 10 patients undergoing a supratentorial shunt procedure. They estimated cerebral perfusion pressure (CPP) using a ratio of the (mean flow velocity)/(pulsatile amplitude of flow velocity) multiplied by the arterial blood pressure. To increase the accuracy, only the amplitude of the first harmonic of the pulsatility in both flow–velocity and arterial blood pressure recordings were used in the analysis. They expressed their calculations as:

$$CPP = \frac{V_0}{V_1} \times ABP_1$$

where V_0 is the mean and V_1 is the amplitude of the first harmonic of the velocity waveform, and ABP_1 is the first harmonic of the arterial pressure wave. Their experimental results confirmed the validity of the method. The standard deviation between estimated CPP (CPP_e) and measured CPP (CPP_m) was 8.2 mmHg at a CPP of 40 mmHg, and the mean deviation was only 1 mmHg.

Belfort et al. (2000) adapted the Aaslid method by using the area under the pulsatile amplitude of the flow velocity and arterial blood pressure waveforms rather than the first harmonic of the velocity and pressure recordings. They validated their formula in 19 normal pregnant women. Their equation using areas under pulsatile amplitudes, which shows an $R = 0.92$, $R^2 = 0.85$ and $P = 0.001$, is as follows:

$$CPP = \frac{Velocity_{mean}}{Velocity_{mean} - Velocity_{diastolic}} \times (BP_{mean} - BP_{diastolic})$$

Using this formula and technique, Belfort et al. and other investigators have demonstrated a marked increase in middle artery perfusion pressure in normal pregnant women during gestation (Aaslid et al., 1986; Belfort et al., 1999a). Assuming the cerebral perfusion pressure is actually an indirect measure of blood flow and perfusion to the brain, Belfort suggested an increase in blood flow by as much as 50% during normal pregnancy (Belfort et al., 1999a).

Recently, studies with MR velocity encoded phase contrast imaging have revealed the finding of decreased maternal calculated blood flow in middle and posterior cerebral arteries as normal pregnancies progressed (Figure 28.2A) (Zeeman et al., 2003). One of the advantages of MR is the ability to measure the cross-sectional area of the vessels arising from the Circle of Willis, including the posterior cerebral artery. In addition, MR allows instantaneous determination of the blood velocity (Enzmann et al., 1993; Marks et al., 1992) and calculation of blood flow from velocity-encoded phase contrast and cross-sectional area has been validated in both

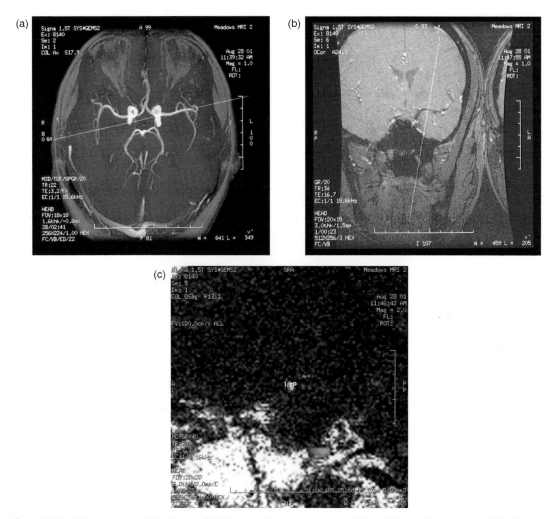

Figure 28.2A MR angiogram of the Circle of Willis (a), with coronal image of the middle cerebral artery (MCA) (b), and velocity encoded phase contrast MR showing the area of the MCA in the sagittal plane (c) in cross-section with region of interest and area of $5.84m^2$.

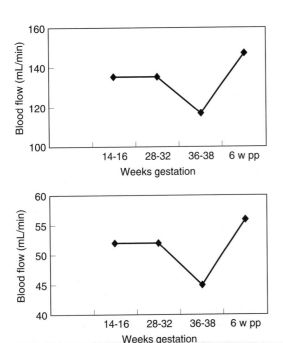

Figure 28.2B Graphs of the middle and posterior cerebral artery MR calculated blood flow as a function of gestational age. (From Zeeman, 2003, *Am. J. Obstet. Gynecol.*, **189**(4), 968–72.)

large and small lumen arteries in humans (Hundley *et al.*, 1995, 1996). Zeeman and coauthors explained that diminished calculated blood flow in the large vessels of the Circle of Willis may be secondary to the improved oxygen extraction and vasoactive properties of distal arterioles of the central nervous system in pregnancy (Zeeman *et al.*, 2003).

On the surface it appears that cerebral blood flow estimations from Doppler-measured CPP and from MR during normal pregnancy in large cerebral vessels blood flow show opposite findings. The two techniques are, however, very different and both are extrapolations from instantaneous measurements. Despite agreement with regard to velocity changes during pregnancy, flow measurements will require further comparative studies between Doppler and MR before the answer to this question will be known.

Central nervous system findings in severe pre-eclampsia and eclampsia

There is some difficulty in relating the histopathologic data from eclamptic individuals with the hemodynamic information being collected today. By necessity, the CNS histopathology of eclampsia is based on autopsy specimens from women who died from the condition, while the hemodynamic data are taken from surviving patients with pre-eclampsia and eclampsia. The autopsy specimens show cortical and subcortical edema, petechial hemorrhages, and infarctions (Chester *et al.*, 1978; Govan, 1961; Sheehan and Lynch, 1973). The hemodynamic data are derived from Doppler ultrasound (Aaslid *et al.*, 1986; Belfort *et al.*, 1999a, 1999b, 2001; Ikeda and Nori, 1990; Serra-Serra *et al.*, 1995; Williams and Galerneau, 2003; Williams and McLean, 1993), other imaging studies, including CT and MRI (Brown *et al.*, 1988; Cunningham and Twickler, 2000; Dahmus *et al.*, 1992; Digre *et al.*, 1993; Hauser *et al.*, 1988; Morriss *et al.*, 1997; Port and Beauchamp, 1998; Schwartz *et al.*, 1992, 2000; Zeeman and Twickler, 2004), and arteriography (Ito *et al.*, 1995; Kanayama *et al.*, 1993; Tajima *et al.*, 1999). The severity of the imaging findings appears to be proportionately related to the clinical severity of the pregnancy-induced hypertension (Cunningham and Twickler, 2000; Morriss *et al.*, 1997).

Doppler studies in pregnancy-induced hypertension have shown decreases in middle cerebral artery velocities compared to normal pregnant cohorts (Belfort *et al.*, 1999; Williams and Galerneau, 2003; Williams and Mclean, 1993). In addition, both increases and decreases in perfusion and flow velocity (as measured with MCA Doppler and systemic brachial artery pressures) have been demonstrated, with increases most frequently reported in severe pre-eclampsia (Belfort *et al.*, 1999, 2001; Williams and Galerneau, 2003; Williams and McLean, 1993, 1994; Zunker *et al.*, 2001). Very recent data with MRI reveals calculated flow in the middle cerebral and posterior cerebral arteries to be significantly increased in women with severe pre-eclampsia compared to the normal woman in the third trimester (Zeeman *et al.*, 2004b). In this regard, Doppler and MRI show similar findings.

CT and MRI findings are less frequently abnormal in women with severe pre-eclampsia in comparison to those with eclampsia. Morriss *et al.* found subtle changes in the peritrigonal gray matter on T-2 weighted images in only 2 of 10 severely pre-eclamptic women, based on increased signal intensity, compared to markedly abnormal findings of increased signal intensity in a number of locations in all women with eclampsia (Morris *et al.*, 1997) (Figure 28.3).

Measurements of middle and posterior cerebral artery calculated flow and vessel area were not significantly different in 8 eclamptic and 10 severely pre-eclamptic women studied on two occasions – the first within 24 h of delivery and the second 6 weeks postpartum. In addition to

no flow or area differences, there was no evidence of vasospasm in the large vessels of the Circle of Willis in these 18 women (Morris *et al.*, 1997). The authors concluded that pre-eclampsia does not appear to cause significant cerebral blood flow changes, and specifically that vasospasm is unlikely to be the etiology of eclampsia. The interpretation of these findings must be somewhat tempered by the fact that many of these patients had been treated with magnesium sulfate and antihypertensive agents prior to imaging. Such vasoactive drugs may render the findings difficult to extrapolate to untreated patients, and thus elude etiology. This may explain the differing findings of Kobayashi *et al.* who found middle cerebral artery vasospasm in 12 of 15 pre-eclamptic and eclamptic women; the therapy and timing of imaging in relation to the therapy was not discussed (Kobayashi *et al.*, 2001). Williams and McLean (1994) reported significantly higher antepartum Doppler blood flow velocities

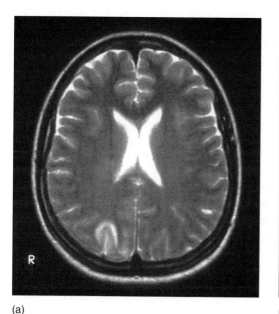

(a)

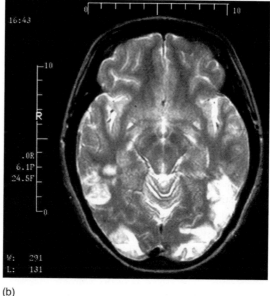

(b)

Figure 28.3 Examples of variation of severity of MR findings of T-2 weighted edema. (a) Mild, single focus edema of the right occipital region in eclampsia. (b) Larger and multiple areas of edema in eclampsia (Morris, 1997).

in women with pre-eclampsia compared to normo-tensive antepartum women, and a significant increase in postpartum velocity measurements in pre-eclamptic patients.

Cunningham and Twickler (2000) found clini-cally symptomatic global and multifocal cerebral edema in 6% of eclamptic women studied with CT and MR. Schwartz et al. evaluated 28 women with pre-eclampsia–eclampsia with MR and associated cerebral edema with abnormalities in specific endothelial markers, most specifically with abnor-mal red blood cell morphology (Schwartz et al., 2000). This same group showed, using PET scans, that patients with hypertensive encephalopathy demonstrated increased cerebral perfusion (Schwartz et al., 1992). Since some of their patients had pregnancy-induced hypertension, this study supported the hypothesis that eclampsia may be the result of hypertensive encephalopathy and cerebral overperfusion. Most recently, Zeeman et al. (2004a) demonstrated increased large vessel cerebral blood flow in severe pre-eclampsia using velocity encoded phase-contrast MRI. They demonstrated that the velocity flow was signifi-cantly higher in pre-eclamptic women, versus normotensive controls, in both the middle cere-bral and posterior cerebral arteries. This work supports the notion of hypertensive encephalo-pathy as an important contributor to the etiology of eclampsia.

One of the problems with CT scanning and conventional MRI has been that it is not possible to distinguish vasogenic and cytotoxic edema. Both have similar appearance in the acute phase and only long term studies will show permanent infarction. Zeeman et al., (2004a), using a series of MR acquisitions including diffusion-weighted imaging (DWI), apparent diffusion coefficient mapping (ADC), and fluid attenuated inversion recovery (FLAIR), were able to further characterize the lesions seen in eclamptic women. These specialized MR findings suggested a continuum of pathology that was proportionately associated with the severity of the clinical findings. They were able to identify 23 women who had cerebral

edema. Using the DWI, ADC and FLAIR techniques they were able to distinguish reversible vasogenic edema in all 23, and in 6 cases they were also able to show evidence of cytotoxic edema and cerebral infarction (Figure 28.4). These data are important since they lend support to the notion that pre-eclampsia/eclampsia may result in permanent cerebral lesions.

Belfort et al. (2002) have proposed that CPP in the middle cerebral artery may be an indicator of impending barotrauma injury even when cerebral blood flow is normal. This hypothesis is different to the traditional thinking which has relied on absolute cerebral blood flow (CBF) (either high or low) as the primary cause of pathology. Their hypothesis allows for significant pathology in the region and distribution of the middle (or posterior) cerebral artery (on the basis of arterial barotrauma and damage) within the constraint of maintained normal brain blood flow. They demonstrated that the majority of pre-eclamptic women have normal cerebral blood flow (which is in keeping with the findings of both Morriss et al. and Zeeman et al.) but that women with severe pre-eclampsia, if they do have abnormal CBF, are much more likely to have increased CBF than decreased CBF. They also showed that many women with severe pre-eclampsia have an abnormally high CPP. This elevated CPP is either required to maintain the normal blood flow in the face of abnormal vasospasm, or alternatively the abnormally high CPP (a result of the elevated MAP and diastolic velocity) is resisted by functioning autoregulation in the downstream resistance bed. They further demonstrate that despite a normal blood pressure, patients with severe pre-eclampsia can still have elevated CPP, presumably mediated by abnormal autoregulation and increased diastolic velocity. This is an important finding, since it suggests that in such patients, where CPP is almost unregulated and fluctuates in concert with mean arterial pressure, protection of the cerebral circulation is still required despite what appears to be a normal blood pressure. This may explain those situations where eclampsia occurs despite low blood

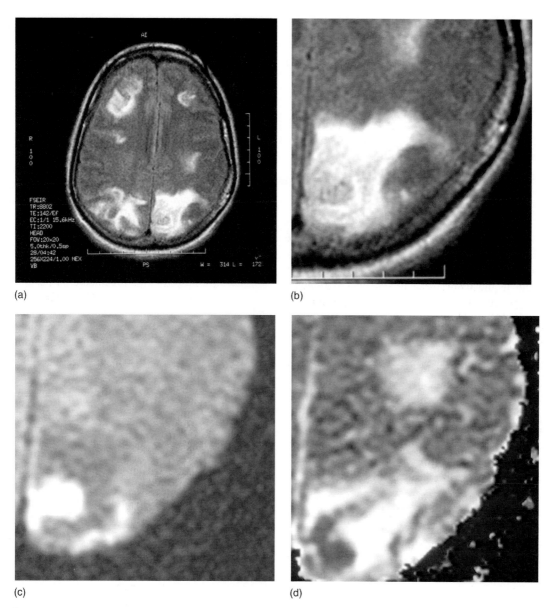

(a)

(b)

(c)

(d)

Figure 28.4 MR images of a woman with eclampsia with T-2 (a, b), diffusion weighted images (DWI) (c), and apparent diffusion coefficient (ADC) (d) images. Areas of edema on T2 weighted images may represent both vasogenic and cytotoxic edema(a, b). Areas that are hyperintense on DWI (c) and lower intensity with ADC(d) are areas of restricted diffusion and suggestive of cytotoxic edema and infarction. (Zeeman *et al.*, 2004a, *Am. J. Obstet. Gynecol.*)

pressure, and highlights the need for treating these women with drugs that are more likely to lower CPP than increase it. Regardless of whether the CPP is elevated as a result of high systemic mean arterial pressure or a failed autoregulatory mechanism that allows a pathological increase in the diastolic flow, persistently elevated intramural pressure can ultimately damage the endothelium and muscle of a conducting artery/arteriole and lead to extravasation of blood/serum into the surrounding brain (vasogenic edema and hypertensive encephalopathy).

In pre-eclamptic women with significant elevation of CPP one explanation of the progression of events is that initial protective vasoconstriction in the resistance vessels will limit overperfusion of the brain in the tissue distal to the middle cerebral artery. This concept is consistent with the findings of the Morriss et al. study, where cerebral blood flow was unchanged. Their studies may have been done at a time when the autoregulation was still intact. As the CPP increases or remains persistently elevated, the MCA (and its smaller branches) is damaged by the barotrauma. As each smaller MCA branch becomes involved the increased pressure is propagated further and further into the peripheral brain tissue and into smaller diameter vessels less capable of protecting themselves from the increased pressure. Ultimately, autoregulation is overwhelmed and distal overperfusion leads to hypertensive encephalopathy. This is consistent with the increased cerebral blood flow reported by Zeeman et al., which implies that the MR was performed at a time that the autoregulation had been overwhelmed. Once this happens vasogenic edema supervenes. At this time there may be persistent hypertensive encephalopathy, rupture of small vessels and intracranial hemorrhage, or severe conducting vessel trauma that causes pathologic vasospasm and regional or global cerebral ischemia. In this model initial overperfusion may result in either hypertensive encephalopathy or ischemia. The "cerebral barotrauma" model of Belfort et al. also explains the higher cerebral perfusion pressure seen in women with severe pre-eclampsia and a low cerebral blood flow.

Therapeutic agents and central nervous system effects

Doppler and MR studies have been performed to evaluate the effects of magnesium sulfate on the large arteries (MCA, and in some cases PCA) of the central nervous system. Belfort and Moise found intravenous administration of 6 g magnesium sulfate reduced the Doppler pulsatility index in the MCA in women with pregnancy induced hypertension. Based on these data they suggested that magnesium acted by vasodilating arterioles distal to the insonated MCA artery (Belfort and Moise, 1992). This study did not address the effect of magnesium sulfate on flow. Other data have emerged suggesting that magnesium sulfate decreases perfusion pressure in the MCA. If the concept of the MCA as a resistance vessel holds true, then the idea of intact autoregulation maintaining constant flow beyond the MCA in the smaller and more fragile distal vasculature is an attractive one. In such a model, magnesium sulfate would not be expected to necessarily reduce distal flow, but rather by its effect on perfusion pressure it should maintain flow while at the same time protecting the brain from overperfusion. A recent study by Zeeman et al. supports this by showing no difference in the calculated MR blood flow in women with severe pre-eclampsia before and after the administration of intravenous magnesium sulfate (Zeeman et al., 2002).

A recent clinical trial comparing the seizure prophylactic efficacy of magnesium sulfate and nimodipine found magnesium sulfate to be superior to nimodipine in the prevention of eclamptic seizures in severely pre-eclamptic women (Belfort et al., 2003). Since nimodipine is well known to vasodilate the cerebral circulation and increase cerebral perfusion pressure, as opposed to magnesium sulfate which reduces CPP, this clinical study has important etiologic implications. The lower seizure rate in the magnesium sulfate-treated patients supports the contention that at least one of the functions of magnesium sulfate is to reduce perfusion pressure and abrogate hypertensive encephalopathy and cerebral overperfusion. While this vascular effect is clearly important it is unlikely to be the only action of this drug. Some have hypothesized that magnesium sulfate acts at the endothelial level as a cell membrane stabilizer (Belfort *et al.*, 2003; Redman *et al.*, 1999; Roberts and Redman, 1993; Roberts *et al.*, 1989; Taylor and Roberts, 1999) while others have shown that magnesium's effect on NMDA receptors may play an important role (Hallack *et al.*, 1996). Still other investigators have implicated sympathetic nervous overactivity (Schobel *et al.*, 1996) and glucose metabolism (Zunker *et al.*, 2003) in the etiology of eclampsia. Magnesium sulfate is known to affect these pathways as well. It is an amazing fact that after more than four decades of use, the mechanism of action of magnesium sulfate in women with eclampsia and pre-eclampsia is yet to be determined. Regardless of this, the drug is clearly the most effective agent currently in our armamentarium (Duley, 1995, 2002; Goldman and Finkbeiner, 1988; Lucas *et al.*, 1995; Sadeh, 1989). This does not mean that further research into the etiology of eclampsia should be forestalled. The revelation that hypertensive encephalopathy may be an important etiologic factor in eclampsia suggests that the use of drugs that reduce cerebral perfusion pressure in pre-eclamptic women (such as labetalol) (Belfort *et al.*) may be of benefit. This field of research is something that deserves further attention.

In summary, middle and posterior cerebral artery blood flow (as determined by MRI), and MCA velocity and CPP are all increased in women with severe pre-eclampsia when compared with normotensive pregnant women. These women are different from normotensive women, who have decreases in the MR-calculated blood flow in large arteries (MCA and PCA) and Doppler calculated velocities with increasing gestational age. MR findings of focal and generalized vasogenic edema are more apparent in eclampsia than in severe pre-eclampsia, and permanent infarction with the development of cytotoxic edema was demonstrated in about 20% of women with eclampsia in whom MR of the brain was performed. Current data suggest that hypertensive encephalopathy and overperfusion of the brain occurs in women with pre-eclampsia; this overperfusion is coupled with capillary leak and vasogenic edema in most cases of eclampsia, and may in some cases of severe eclampsia result in local areas of infarction (cytotoxic edema). The role of vasospasm as the primary mechanism of eclampsia in women with severe pre-eclampsia is challenged by the more recent data which suggest hypertensive encephalopathy as the initiating injury. Secondary vasospasm may well then follow the primary pathophysiology, and the reported vasospasm in cases of eclampsia may be a reflection of the severity of the case, the long interval between the seizure and the imaging, and the development of cytotoxic edema and cerebral infarction. Empiric therapy trials for seizure prophylaxis have also supported the hypertensive encephalopathy and endothelial damage model of pathogenesis. Magnesium remains the seizure prophylaxis of choice, not for its role as a vasodilator, but rather as a drug that reduces CPP and acts as a membrane stabilizer in the brain. Further research is warranted to better understand the pathologic mechanisms, imaging findings, and therapeutic interventions in women with pregnancy induced hypertensive diseases.

REFERENCES

Aaslid, R., Lundar, T., Lindegaard, K. F. and Nornes, H. (1986). Estimation of cerebral perfusion pressure from arterial blood pressure and transcranial Doppler recordings. In *Intracranial Pressure VI*, ed. J. D. Miller, G. M. Teasdale, J. O. Rowan, S. I. Galbraith and A. D. Mendelow. Berlin: Springer-Verlag, pp. 226–9.

Belfort, M. A. and Moise, K. J., Jr. (1992). Effect of magnesium sulfate on maternal brain blood flow in preeclampsia: a randomized placebo-controlled study. *Am. J. Obstet. Gynecol.*, **167**, 661–6.

Belfort, M. A., Grunewald, C., Saade, G. R., Varner, M. and Nisell, H. (1999a). Preeclampsia may cause both overperfusion and underperfusion of the brain. *Acta Obstet. Gynecol. Scand.*, **78**, 586–91.

Belfort, M. A., Giannina, G. and Herd, J. A. (1999b). Transcranial and orbital Doppler ultrasound in normal pregnancy and preeclampsia. *Clin. Obstet. Gynecol.*, **42**, 479–506.

Belfort, M. A., Tooke-Miller, C., Varner, M., *et al.* (2000). Evaluation of a non-invasive transcranial Doppler and blood pressure method for the assessment of cerebral perfusion pressure in pregnant women. *Hypertens. Pregn.*, **19**(3), 331–40.

Belfort, M. A., Tooke-Miller, C., Allen, Jr., J. C., *et al.* (2001). Pregnant women with chronic hypertension and superimposed pre-eclampsia have high cerebral perfusion pressure. *Br. J. Obstet. Gynaecol.*, **108**, 1141–7.

Belfort, M. A., Varner, M. W., Dizon-Townson, D. S., Grunewald, C. and Nisell, H. (2002). Cerebral perfusion pressure, and not cerebral blood flow, may be the critical determinant of intracranial injury in preeclampsia: a new hypothesis. *Am. J. Obstet. Gynecol.*, **187**, 626–34.

Belfort, M. A., Anthony, J., Saade, G. R. and Allen, J. C. (2003). A comparison of magnesium sulfate and nimodipine for the prevention of eclampsia. *N. Engl. J. Med.*, **348**, 304–11.

Boemi, G., Bruno, M. T., La Ferrera, G., *et al.* (1996). Maternal renal and interlobar arteries waveforms evaluation with color Doppler ultrasound in pregnancy-induced hypertension. *Fetal Diagn. Ther.*, **11**, 132–6.

Brown, C. E., Purdy, P. and Cunningham, F. G. (1988). Head computed tomographic scans in women with eclampsia. *Am. J. Obstet. Gynecol.*, **159**, 915–20.

Burns, P. N. (1988). *Hemodynamics; Clinical Applications of Doppler Ultrasound.* New York, Raven Press, pp. 46–75.

Chester, E. M., Agamanolis, D. P., Banker, B. Q. and Victor, M. (1978). Hypertensive encephalopathy: a clinicopathologic study of 20 cases. *Neurology*, **28**, 928–39.

Cunningham, F. G. and Twickler, D. (2000). Cerebral edema complicating eclampsia. *Am. J. Obstet. Gynecol.*, **182**, 94–100.

Dahmus, M. A., Barton, J. R. and Sibai, B. M. (1992). Cerebral imaging in eclampsia; magnetic resonance imaging versus computed tomography. *Am. J. Obstet. Gynecol.*, **167**, 935–41.

Digre, K. B., Varner, M. W., Osborn, A. G. and Crawford, S. (1993). Cranial magnetic resonance imaging in severe preeclampsia vs eclampsia. *Arch. Neurol.*, **50**, 3999–406.

Duley, L. (1995). Which anticonvulsant for women with eclampsia? Evidence from the collaborative eclampsia trial. *Lancet*, **345**, 1455–63.

Duley, L. (2002). Do women with pre-eclampsia, and their babies, benefit from magnesium sulphate? The magpie trial: a randomized placebo-controlled trial. *Lancet*, **359**, 1877–90.

Enzmann, D. R., Marks, M. P. and Pelc, N. J. (1993). Comparison of cerebral artery blood flow measurements with gated cine and ungated phase-contrast techniques. *J. Magn. Res. Imag.*, **3**, 705–12.

Fleischer, A., Schulman, H., Farmakides, G., *et al.* (1986). Uterine artery Doppler velocimetry in pregnant women with hypertension. *Am. J. Obstet. Gynecol.*, **154**, 806–13.

Giller, C. A., Hatab, M. R. and Giller, A. M. (1998). Estimation of vessel flow and diameter during cerebral vasospasm using transcranial Doppler indices. *Neurosurgery*, **42**, 1076–82.

Goldman, R. S. and Finkbeiner, S. M. (1988). Therapeutic use of magnesium sulfate in selected cases of cerebral ischemia and seizure. *N. Engl. J. Med.*, **319**, 1224–5.

Govan, A. (1961). The pathogenesis of eclamptic lesions. *J. Pathol. Microbiol.*, **24**, 561–75.

Hackett, P. H., Yarnell, P. R., Hill, R., Reynard, K., Heit, J. and McCormick, J. (1998). High-altitude cerebral edema evaluated with magnetic resonance imaging. *J. Am. Med. Ass.*, **280**, 1920–5.

Hallak, M., Irtenkauf, S. M. and Cotton, D. B. (1996). Effect of magnesium sulfate on excitatory amino acid receptors in the rat brain. I. *N*-methyl-D-aspartate receptor channel complex. *Am. J. Obstet. Gynecol.*, **175**(3, Pt. 1), 575–81.

Hankins, G. D., Wendel, G. D. Jr., Cunningham, F. G. and Leveno, K. J. (1984). Longitudinal evaluation of hemodynamic changes in eclampsia. *Am. J. Obstet. Gynecol.*, **150**(5, Pt. 1), 506–12.

Harrington, K., Carpenter, R. G., Goldfrad, C. and Campbell, S. (1977). Transvaginal Doppler ultrasound of the uteroplacental circulation in the early prediction of pre-eclampsia and intrauterine growth retardation. *Br. J. Obstet. Gynaecol.*, **104**, 674–81.

Harrington, K., Cooper, D., Lees, C., Hecher, K. and Campbell, S. (1996). Doppler ultrasound of the uterine arteries: the importance of bilateral notching in the prediction of pre-eclampsia, placental abruption or delivery of a small-for-gestational-age baby. *Ultrasound Obstet. Gynecol.*, **7**, 182–8.

Hatab, M. R., Giller, C. A. and Clarke, G. D. (1997). Evaluation of cerebral arterial flow with transcranial Doppler ultrasound: theoretical development and phantom studies. *Ultrasound Med. Biol.*, **23**, 1025–31.

Hauser, R. A., Lacey, D. M. and Knight, M. R. (1988). Hypertensive encephalopathy: magnetic resonance imaging demonstration of reversible cortical and white matter lesions. *Arch. Neurol.*, **45**, 1078–83.

Hundley, W. G., Hong, F. L., Hillis, L. D., *et al.* (1995). Quantitation of cardiac output with velocity-encoded, phase-difference magnetic resonance imaging. *Am. J. Cardiol.*, **75**, 1250–5.

Hundley, W. G., Lange, R. A., Clarke, G. D., *et al.* (1996). Assessment of coronary arterial flow and flow reserve in humans with magnetic resonance imaging. *Circulation*, **93**, 1502–8.

Ikeda, T. and Nori, N. (1990). Assessment of cerebral hemodynamics in pregnant women by internal carotid artery pulsed Doppler velocimetry. *Am. J. Obstet. Gynecol.*, **163**, 494–8.

Ito, I., Sasaki, T., Inagawa, S., Utsu, M. and Bun, T. (1995). MR angiography of cerebral vasospasm in preeclampsia. *Am. J. Neuroradiol.*, **16**, 1344–6.

Kanayama, N., Nakajima, A., Maehara, K., *et al.* (1993). Magnetic resonance imaging angiography in a case of eclampsia. *Gynecol. Obstet. Invest.*, **36**, 56–8.

Kobayashi, T., Tokunaga, N., Isoda, H., Kanayama, N. and Terao, T. (2001). Vasospasms are characteristic in cases with eclampsia/preeclampsia and HELLP syndrome: proposal of an angiospastic syndrome of pregnancy. *Semin. Thromb. Hemost.*, **27**, 131–5.

Kublickas, M., Lunell, N. O., Nisell, H. and Westgren, M. (1996). Maternal renal artery blood flow velocimetry in normal and hypertensive pregnancies. *Acta Obstet. Gynecol. Scand.*, **76**, 715–19.

Levine, A. B., Lockwood, C. J., Chitkara, U. and Berkowitz, R. L. (1992). Maternal renal artery Doppler velocimetry in normotensive pregnancies and pregnancies complicated by hypertensive disorders. *Obstet. Gynecol.*, **79**, 264–7.

Liberati, M., Rotmensch, S., Zannoli, P. and Bellati, U. (1994). Doppler velocimetry of maternal renal interlobar arteries in pregnancy-induced hypertension. *Int. J. Gynecol. Obstet.*, **44**, 129–33.

Lucas, M. J., Leveno, K. J. and Cunningham, F. G. (1995). A comparison of magnesium sulfate with phenytoin for the prevention of eclampsia. *N. Engl. J. Med.*, **333**, 201–5.

Marks, M. P., Norbert, J. P., Ross, M. R. and Enzmann, D. R. (1992). Determination of cerebral blood flow with a phase-contrast cine MR imaging technique: evaluation of normal subjects and patients with arteriovenous malformations. *Radiology*, **182**, 477–81.

Morriss, M. C., Twickler, D. M., Hatab, M. R., Clarke, G. D., Peshock, M. R. and Cunningham, F. G. (1997). Cerebral blood flow and cranial magnetic resonance imaging in eclampsia and severe preeclampsia. *Obstet. Gynecol.*, **89**, 561–8.

Port, J. D. and Beauchamp, Jr., N. J. (1998). Reversible intracerebral pathologic entities mediated by vascular autoregulatory dysfunction. *RadioGraphics*, **18**, 353–67.

Redman, C. W., Sacks, G. P. and Sargent, I. L. (1999). Preeclampsia: an excessive maternal inflammatory response to pregnancy. *Am. J. Obstet. Gynecol.*, **180**, 499–506.

Roberts, J. M. and Redman, C. W. (1993). Preeclampsia: more than pregnancy-induced hypertension. *Lancet*, **341**, 1447–51.

Roberts, J. M., Taylor, R. N., Musci, T. J., Rogers, G. M., Hubel, C. A. and McLaughlin, M. K. (1989). Preeclampsia: an endothelial cell disorder. *Am. J. Obstet. Gynecol.*, **161**, 1200–4.

Sadeh, M. (1989). Action of magnesium sulfate in the treatment of preeclampsia–eclampsia. *Stroke*, **20**, 1273–5.

Schobel, H. P., Fischer, T., Heuszer, K., Geiger, H. and Schmieder, R. E. (1996). Preeclampsia – a state of sympathetic overactivity. *N. Engl. J. Med.*, **335**(20), 1480–5.

Schwartz, R. B., Jones, K. M., Kolina, P., *et al.* (1992). Hypertensive encephalopathy; findings on CT, MR imaging and SPECT imaging in 14 cases. *Am. J. Radiogr.*, **159**, 379–83.

Schwartz, R. B., Feske, S. K., Polak, J. F., *et al.* (2000). Preeclampsia–eclampsia; clinical and neuroradiographic correlates and insights into the pathogenesis of hypertensive encephalopathy. *Radiology*, **217**, 371–6.

Serra-Serra, V., Chandran, R., Kyle, P. M. and Redman, C. W. G. (1995). Cerebral hemodynamic changes during severe orthostatic hypotension in pregnancy. *Acta Obstet. Gynecol. Scand.*, **74**, 656–9.

Sheehan, J. L. and Lynch, J. B. (1973). *Pathology of Toxemia of Pregnancy.* New York, NY: Churchill Livingstone.

Tajima, Y., Isonishi, K., Kashiwaba, T. and Tashiro, K. (1999). Two similar cases of encephalopathy, possibly a reversible posterior leukoencephalopathy syndrome: serial findings of magnetic resonance imaging, SPECT and angiography. *Intern. Med.*, **38**, 54–8.

Taylor, K. J. W. (1988). *Clinical Applications of Carotid Doppler Ultrasound. Clinical Applications of Doppler Ultrasound.* New York, Raven Press, pp. 120–61.

Taylor, R. N. and Roberts, J. M. (1999). Endothelial cell dysfunction (Chap. 12). In *Chesley's Hypertensive Disorders in Pregnancy*, 2nd edn, ed. M. D. Lindheimer, J. M. Roberts and F. G. Cunningham. Stamford, CT: Appleton & Lange, pp. 395–429.

Williams, K. and Galerneau, F. (2003). Maternal transcranial Doppler in pre-eclampsia and eclampsia. *Ultrasound Obstet. Gynecol.*, **21**, 507–13.

Williams, K. and McLean, C. (1994). Transcranial assessment of maternal cerebral blood flow velocity in normal vs hypertensive states variations with maternal posture. *J. Reprod. Med.*, **39**, 685–8.

Williams, K. P. and McLean, C. (1993). Peripartum changes in maternal cerebral blood flow velocity in normotensive and preeclamptic patients. *Obstet. Gynecol.*, **82**, 334–7.

Zeeman, G. G., Hatab, M. and Twickler, D. M. (2002). Magnesium sulfate and cerebral blood flow in severe preeclampsia by MR evaluation. *Am. J. Obstet. Gynecol.*, **187**, S211.

Zeeman, G. G., Hatab, M. and Twickler, D. M. (2003). Maternal cerebral blood flow changes in pregnancy. *Am. J. Obstet. Gynecol.*, **189**(4), 968–72.

Zeeman, G. G., Fleckenstein, J. L., Twickler, D. M. and Cunningham, F. G. (2004a). Cerebral infarction in eclampsia. *Am. J. Obstet. Gynecol.*, **190**, 714–20.

Zeeman, G., Hatab, M. and Twickler, D. (2004b). Increased large vessel cerebral blood flow in severe preeclampsia by magnetic resonance evaluation. *Am. J. Obstet. Gynecol.*, **191**, 2148–53.

Zunker, P., Happe, S., Georgiadis, A. L., *et al.* (2001). Maternal cerebral hemodynamics in pregnancy-related hypertension. A prospective transcranial Doppler study. *Ultrasound Obstet. Gynecol.*, **16L**, 179–87.

Zunker, P., Georgiadis, A. L., Czech, N., Golombeck, K., Brossmann, J. and Deuschl, G. (2003). Impaired cerebral glucose metabolism in eclampsia: a new finding in two cases. *Fetal Diagn. Ther.*, **18**(1), 41–6.

29

Pathogenesis and treatment of eclampsia

Joong Shin Park, Michael A. Belfort and Errol R. Norwitz

Introduction

Eclampsia refers to the occurrence of one or more generalized convulsions and/or coma in the setting of pre-eclampsia and in the absence of other neurologic conditions. Pre-eclampsia is a multisystem disorder of pregnancy and the puerperium, complicating approximately 6–8% of all pregnancies (ACOG, 1996, 2002). Pre-eclampsia is characterized by new onset hypertension (sitting blood pressure ≥140/90), proteinuria (≥2+ in a random urine sample or ≥300 mg in a 24-h collection) with or without non-dependent edema after 20 weeks' gestation. Eclampsia was at one time thought to be the end result of pre-eclampsia, hence the nomenclature. It is now clear, however, that seizures are but one clinical manifestation of "severe" pre-eclampsia. Other manifestations include, among others, HELLP syndrome (Hemolysis, Elevated Liver enzymes and Low Platelets), disseminated intravascular coagulopathy (DIC), renal failure, hepatocellular damage, pancreatitis, congestive cardiac failure, pulmonary edema and fetal intrauterine growth restriction.

The pathophysiology of pre-eclampsia is poorly understood. It is a disease of human pregnancy; more precisely, it is a disease of the placenta since it is also described in pregnancies where there is trophoblast but no fetal tissue (complete molar pregnancies) (Goldstein and Berkowitz, 1994). The blueprint for the development of pre-eclampsia is laid down early in pregnancy. The pathologic hallmark of pre-eclampsia appears to be a failure of the second wave of trophoblast invasion from

8 to 18 weeks' gestation, a process that is responsible for destruction of the muscularis layer of the spiral arterioles and, as such, establishment of the definitive uteroplacental circulation (Brosens et al., 1972; Cross et al., 1994; Meekins et al., 1994). As the pregnancy progresses, the metabolic demands of the fetoplacental unit increases and – in the setting of shallow endovascular invasion – the spiral arterioles are unable to accommodate the increase in blood flow. This then leads to the development of – for the want of a more precise term – "placental dysfunction" which manifests clinically as pre-eclampsia. A recent publication suggested that soluble fms-like tyrosine kinase 1 (sFlt1), an antagonist of VEGF and placental growth factor, is the elusive "toxemia factor" released from the placenta and leading to widespread vasospasm and endothelial injury, which is the clinical hallmark of pre-eclampsia (Maynard et al., 2003). Although attractive, this hypothesis remains to be validated.

Scope of the problem

Despite recent advances in detection and management, pre-eclampsia remains the second most common cause of maternal death in the United States (after thromboembolism), accounting for approximately 15% of all maternal deaths (Rochat et al., 1988). It is estimated that eclampsia is a factor in up to 10% of all maternal deaths in developed countries, and probably accounts for around 50,000 maternal deaths per year worldwide (Duley, 1992).

In the United States and other developed countries, the incidence of eclampsia is relatively stable at around 4–5 per 10,000 live births (Douglas and Redman, 1994). In developing countries, however, the reported incidence varies widely from 6–7 to as high as 100 cases per 10,000 live births (WHO, 1988). Occurrence rates are highest amongst non-white nulliparous women from lower socioeconomic backgrounds. Peak incidence is in the teenage years and low twenties, but there is also an increased incidence in women over 35 years of age.

Natural history of eclampsia

Almost half of all cases of eclampsia occur preterm and over one-fifth occur before 31 weeks' gestation (Douglas and Redman, 1994). Of those occurring at term, the majority (approximately 75%) occur either intrapartum or within 48 h of delivery. Traditionally, convulsions occurring more than 48 h after delivery were not considered eclampsia. However, it is now clear that late postpartum eclampsia – i.e. seizures developing greater than 48 h but before 4 weeks' postpartum – does indeed exist and may account for up to 16% of all cases of eclampsia (Lubarsky et al., 1994). Eclampsia prior to 20 weeks' gestation is extremely rare and should raise the possibility of an underlying molar pregnancy.

Antepartum cases of eclampsia are often more dramatic with multiple seizures and maternal complication rates of up to 71%, including DIC, renal failure, hepatocellular injury, liver rupture, intracerebral hemorrhage, cardiorespiratory arrest, bronchial aspiration, acute pulmonary edema, and postpartum hemorrhage (López-Llera, 1992).

Prognosis of eclampsia

Factors affecting maternal outcome in eclampsia are summarized in Table 29.1. The reported maternal mortality associated with eclampsia varies between 0.4% and 13.9% (Douglas and Redman, 1994; López-Llera, 1992). In a retrospective analysis of 990 cases, López-Llera (1992) reported an overall maternal mortality rate of 13.9% (138/990). The highest maternal mortality rate (22.2% [12/54]) was seen in that subgroup of women with early eclampsia (i.e. ≤28 weeks' gestation). Maternal mortality and severe morbidity rates are lowest among women receiving regular prenatal care who are managed by experienced physicians in tertiary centers (Conde-Agudelo and Kafury-Goeta, 1997; Sibai, 1990).

Factors affecting fetal outcome in eclampsia are summarized in Table 29.2. The overall perinatal mortality for eclampsia is on the order of 9–23% (Douglas and Redman, 1994; López-Llera, 1992). As expected, perinatal mortality is closely related to gestational age, and may exceed 90% in pregnant women with eclampsia prior to 28 weeks' gestation (López-Llera, 1992). Fetal deaths result primarily from abruptio placenta, intrauterine asphyxia, and complications of prematurity.

Management

Can we predict an eclamptic seizure?

The relationship between hypertension, symptoms and signs of cortical irritability (headache, visual disturbances, nausea, vomiting, fever, hyperreflexia) and seizures remains unclear and unpredictable. That said, the majority of women do have one or more antecedent symptoms prior to an eclamptic seizure. In a retrospective analysis of 383 cases of eclampsia in the United Kingdom, Douglas and Redman (1994) reported that 59% (227/383) of eclamptic patients experienced either a prodromal headache, visual disturbance (scotomata, amaurosis, blurred vision, diplopia, homonymous hemianopsia) or epigastric pain. In 38% (146/383) of cases, however, eclampsia was the first manifestation of pregnancy-related hypertensive disease.

Although the magnitude of the blood pressure elevation correlates well with the incidence of

Table 29.3. Differential diagnosis of an eclamptic seizure

- Cerebrovascular accident (e.g. intracerebral hemorrhage, cerebral venous thrombosis)
- Hypertensive diseases (e.g. hypertensive encephalopathy, pheochromocytoma)
- Space-occupying lesions of the central nervous system (e.g. brain tumor, abscess)
- Metabolic disorders (e.g. hypoglycemia, uremia, inappropriate antidiuretic hormone secretion resulting in water intoxication)
- Infectious etiology (e.g. meningitis, encephalitis)
- Thrombotic thrombocytopenic purpura
- Idiopathic epilepsy

have a postpartum seizure, and those who develop localizing neurological signs should be evaluated further. The differential diagnosis for eclampsia is detailed in Table 29.3.

Although neuroimaging studies have not proven useful in the management of pre-eclampsia/eclampsia, such studies have provided an opportunity to investigate the nature of eclamptic seizures. Nearly half of eclamptic women will have transient abnormalities on head CT (Brown et al., 1988; Royburt et al., 1991), most commonly white matter hypodensities (Fredriksson et al., 1989). In an MRI study of 10 women with eclampsia, Digre et al. (1993) documented abnormal findings (either cortical edema and hemorrhage or increased signal at the gray–white matter junction on T2-weighted images suggestive of cortical edema) in 9 women. An autopsy study showed that more than 50% of women who died within 2 days of an eclamptic seizure had evidence of cerebral hemorrhage, primarily petechial cortical hemorrhages involving the occipital lobe (Sheehan and Lynch, 1973). These data have been confirmed by subsequent reports (Crawford et al., 1987; Dierckx and Appel, 1989). The question as to whether an eclamptic seizure is the cause or the consequence of an intracerebral hemorrhage remains unclear. The effect of

eclampsia on the subsequent risk for cerebrovascular accident has not been evaluated systematically. In one report (Salerni et al., 1988), an intracerebral hemorrhage developed in an area of "ischemic infarction" previously identified in an eclamptic patient, suggesting that the seizure predated the hemorrhage. Whether this is true of all such cases, however, is not known.

Results of invasive and functional imaging studies are conflicting. Some angiographic studies have reported widespread vasospasm of the intracranial vessels in patients with pre-eclampsia/eclampsia (Trommer et al., 1988; Will et al., 1987), whereas other studies have been unable to confirm this observation (Zunker et al., 2003). Several investigators have used SPECT (single photon emission CT) and/or PET (positron emission tomography) technology to investigate the neuropathophysiologic alterations in pre-eclampsia/eclampsia (Naidu et al., 1997; Schwartz et al., 1992; Zunker et al., 2003), but the data are similarly inconclusive.

Prevention of recurrent convulsions

Without treatment, approximately 10% of eclamptic women will have repeated seizures (Prichard et al., 1984). Although there is agreement that patients with eclampsia require anticonvulsant therapy to prevent further seizures, complications of repeated seizure activity (neuronal death, rhabdomyolysis, metabolic acidosis, aspiration pneumonitis, neurogenic pulmonary edema and respiratory failure, and possible cerebrovascular accident), the choice of agent has been controversial. Alternative therapeutic regimens for the management of eclampsia are detailed in Table 29.4.

Obstetricians have long favored magnesium sulfate as the drug of choice for the prevention and treatment of eclamptic seizures, whereas neurologists have favored more established anticonvulsants, such as phenytoin or diazepam. This dispute appears to have been resolved by a number of recent clinical studies. In 1995, the Eclampsia

Table 29.4. Prevention of recurrent seizures in patients with eclampsia

Drug	Loading dose	Maintenance dose	Therapeutic level
Magnesium sulphate	4–6 g over 10–20 min	2–3 g h^{-1} infusion	4–8 mEq l^{-1}*
Phenytoin	10 g (5 g into each buttock) 1–1.5 g over 1 h (depending on body weight)	5 g every 4 h Depending on serum level (usually 250–500 mg every 10–12 h IV or PO)	4–8 mEq l^{-1}* 10–20 μg ml^{-1}
Diazepam	–	10 mg h^{-1} infusion	–

*Not tested prospectively.

Trial Collaborative Group (1995) reported on a prospective trial in which 905 eclamptic women were randomized to receive either magnesium or diazepam, and 775 eclamptic women were randomized to receive either magnesium or phenytoin. Primary measures of outcome were recurrence of seizures and maternal death. Women allocated magnesium had a 52% lower incidence of recurrent convulsions as compared with those allocated diazepam (13.2% [60/453] vs. 27.9% [126/452], respectively). There was no significant difference in maternal or perinatal mortality and/or morbidity between the two groups. Similarly, women allocated magnesium had a 67% lower risk of recurrent seizures than those on phenytoin (5.7% [22/388] vs. 17.1% [66/387], respectively). In this arm of the study, the women who received magnesium were 8% less likely to be admitted to an intensive care facility, 8% less likely to require ventilatory support, and 5% less likely to develop pneumonia as compared with women who were given phenytoin. There was no significant difference in maternal mortality or in perinatal outcome. A 2001 Cochrane review also reported magnesium sulfate was safer and better than "lytic cocktail" (containing promethazine hydrochloride, chlorpromazine, and meperidine hydrochloride) for the prevention of repeat seizures in eclamptic women (Duley and Gulmezoglu, 2001).

Magnesium sulfate therapy has other advantages. It is cheaper and easier to administer than phenytoin (for which cardiac monitoring is required if given at an infusion rate of ≥50 mg min^{-1}), and it is less sedative than diazepam. Further, magnesium appears to selectively increase cerebral blood flow and oxygen consumption in patients with pre-eclampsia (Belfort and Moise, 1992), whereas this does not appear to be the case for phenytoin (Gerthoffer et al., 1987).

The most common magnesium sulfate regimen is a loading dose of 4–6 g administered intravenously over 20 min, followed by 2–3 g h^{-1} as a continuous infusion. The maintenance phase is given only if a patellar reflex is present (loss of deep tendon reflexes are the first manifestation of symptomatic hypermagnesemia), respirations are greater than 12 min^{-1}, and urine output is greater than 100 ml in 4 h. Following serum magnesium levels is not required if the woman's clinical status is closely monitored for evidence of potential magnesium toxicity. There also does not appear to be a clear threshold concentration for ensuring the prevention of convulsions, although a range of 4.8–8.4 mg dl^{-1} has been recommended (Sibai et al., 1981a). The dose should be adjusted according to the clinical response of individual patients.

Exactly how magnesium acts as an anticonvulsant in eclampsia is not known. Several mechanisms have been proposed, including selective vasodilatation of the cerebral vasculature (Belfort and Moise, 1992), protection of endothelial cells from damage by free radicals, prevention of calcium ion entry into ischemic cells, and/or as a competitive antagonist to the glutamate N-methyl-D-aspartate receptor (which is epileptogenic) (Roberts, 1995).

Control of blood pressure

Cerebral hemorrhage accounts for 15–20% of deaths from eclampsia and is often associated with significant elevation in blood pressure (≥170/120). For this reason, aggressive blood pressure control is recommended in all patients. However, blood pressure control alone does not appear to affect the natural course of the disease and does not prevent recurrent seizures. Pharmacologic treatment of mild hypertension is not recommended, because the use of antihypertensive agents to control mildly elevated blood pressure in the setting of pre-eclampsia has not been shown to alter the course of the disease nor to diminish perinatal morbidity or mortality (Magee et al., 1999; Sibai, 1996; von Dadelszen et al., 2000).

It is not clear whether there is a threshold pressure above which emergent therapy should be instituted (Lindenstrom et al., 1995). Most investigators recommend aggressive antihypertensive therapy for sustained diastolic pressures of ≥105–110 mmHg and systolic blood pressures of ≥160 mmHg to prevent cerebrovascular accident (National High Blood Pressure Program, 2000), although these thresholds have not been tested prospectively. Initial treatment options include hydralazine (5 mg IV push followed by 5–10 mg boluses as needed q 20 min) or labetalol (10–20 mg IV push, repeat q 10–20 min with doubling doses not to exceed 80 mg in any single dose for a maximum total cumulative dose of 300 mg). The cerebral vasculature of women with underlying chronic hypertension can probably tolerate higher systolic pressures without injury, while adolescents with normally low blood pressures may benefit from starting treatment at lower levels.

The risk of hemorrhagic stroke correlates directly with the degree of elevation in systolic blood pressure and is less related to, but not independent of, the diastolic pressure (Lindenstrom et al., 1995).

However, diastolic pressure may play a more important role in eclampsia through its effect on cerebral perfusion pressure, which is dependent on maternal mean and diastolic pressure and the mean and diastolic blood flow velocities of the middle cerebral artery measured by transcranial Doppler velocimetry (Belfort et al., 2001, 2002, 2003; Williams and Galerneau, 2003). It has been hypothesized that cerebral vasospasm and resultant ischemia are the predominant cause of eclampsia. However, a recent multicenter trial comparing magnesium sulfate and nimodipine for the prevention of eclampsia does not support this hypothesis (Belfort et al., 2003). If this were the case, nimodipine – a calcium-channel blocker that is a specific cerebral vasodilator (Belfort et al., 1994; van Gijn and Rinkel, 2001) – should have been as good if not better than magnesium sulfate in preventing eclampsia. However, the study by Belfort et al. (2003) showed that intravenous magnesium sulfate was significantly better than oral nimodipine at preventing eclamptic seizures in women with severe pre-eclampsia. Several recent reports on the cerebral hemodynamic changes in patients with pre-eclampsia may explain this result, since they suggest that the primary cause of cerebral injury in pre-eclampsia is elevated cerebral perfusion pressure (overperfusion), rather than vasospasm and a decrease in cerebral blood flow (Apollon et al., 2000; Belfort et al., 2002). Increased cerebral perfusion pressure, in turn, is believed to lead to cerebral "barotrauma" and vasogenic edema (Belfort et al., 2003). This may explain why eclampsia can occur also in the setting of low blood pressure. Women with severe pre-eclampsia are more likely to have high cerebral perfusion pressures than those with mild pre-eclampsia, and pre-eclamptic women with elevated cerebral perfusion pressures are more likely than those with normal cerebral perfusion pressures to be symptomatic (Belfort et al., 2002). Williams and Wilson (1999) have also demonstrated elevated cerebral perfusion pressures in women with eclampsia, thereby further supporting the cerebral barotrauma theory.

Considerations regarding delivery

The only effective treatment for pre-eclampsia/eclampsia is delivery. Immediate delivery does not necessarily imply Cesarean section. The decision of whether to proceed with Cesarean section or induction of labor and attempted vaginal delivery should be individualized based on such factors as parity, gestational age, cervical examination (Bishop score), maternal desire for vaginal delivery, and fetal status, and presentation. In general, less than one-third of women with severe pre-eclampsia remote from term (<32 weeks' gestation) with an unfavorable cervix will have a successful vaginal delivery (ACOG, 1999; Alexander et al., 1999; Nassar et al., 1998). Cervical ripening agents can be used to improve the Bishop score, but prolonged inductions should be avoided.

More recently there has been a trend toward expectant management of severe pre-eclampsia less than 32 weeks' gestation (Sibai et al., 1994). In this setting, the mother assumes the risk of continuing the pregnancy in the hope of increasing gestational age at the time of delivery and thereby improving neonatal outcome. However, even in such studies, eclampsia was considered an absolute contraindication to expectant management.

As regards anesthesia, neuraxial techniques (epidural, spinal) are preferred for women with pre-eclampsia/eclampsia so long as close attention is paid to volume expansion and anesthetic technique, and there is no thrombocytopenia (National High Blood Pressure Program, 2000). In one randomized study, 80 women with severe pre-eclampsia were given epidural, combined spinal–epidural, or general anesthesia with similar outcomes (Wallace et al., 1995). Hypotension is the major concern from regional anesthesia since pre-eclamptic women are total body fluid overloaded but have depleted intravascular volumes. Airway edema and exacerbation of hypertension with intubation are issues during general anesthesia.

Pre-eclampsia/eclampsia always resolves following delivery, although this may take a few days or even weeks. Diuresis ($>4 l\ d^{-1}$) is believed to be the most accurate clinical indicator of resolution, but is not a guarantee against the development of subsequent seizures (Miles et al., 1990).

Can initial eclamptic seizures be prevented?

Anticonvulsant therapy can be administered to prevent a first seizure in women with severe pre-eclampsia. Two large studies have demonstrated an advantage of magnesium sulfate over phenytoin for the prevention of eclampsia (Belfort et al., 2003; Coetzee et al., 1998; Lucas et al., 1995). The Parkland Hospital group, for example, randomly assigned 2138 pre-eclamptic women admitted to Labor and Delivery to receive either magnesium sulfate or phenytoin (Lucas et al., 1995). Eclamptic seizures developed in 10 of 1089 women assigned to phenytoin compared to none of 1049 women assigned to magnesium sulfate ($P = 0.004$). Maternal and neonatal outcomes were similar in both groups. These data are supported by a study performed in South Africa in which 685 women with severe pre-eclampsia were randomly assigned to seizure prophylaxis with magnesium sulfate therapy or placebo (Coetzee et al., 1998). Progression to eclampsia was much lower in the magnesium group (0.3% vs. 3.2% [$P = 0.003$]).

Anticonvulsant therapy is generally initiated during labor or while administering antenatal corticosteroid therapy or cervical ripening agents prior to planned delivery in women with severe pre-eclampsia. Seizure prophylaxis is generally continued until 24–48 h postpartum, when the risk of seizures is low.

It has long been debated whether all women with pre-eclampsia require seizure prophylaxis. The efficacy and safety of magnesium sulfate prophylaxis for prevention of eclampsia in women with any severity of pre-eclampsia was illustrated in the largest study ever performed on pre-eclamptic women: the Magpie Trial (2002) (magnesium sulfate for prevention of eclampsia trial). Over 10,000 women (pregnant or within 24 h of delivery) with blood pressure ≥140/90 mmHg on two occasions and proteinuria of at least +1 in whom the caregiver was uncertain about the benefit of starting magnesium sulfate therapy were randomly assigned to receive magnesium sulfate (4 g intravenous loading dose then $1\,g\,h^{-1}$ infusion or 5 g intramuscularly into each buttock followed by 5 g intramuscularly every 4 h) or placebo for 24 h. Approximately 25% of the patients met criteria for severe disease and 75% were given antihypertensive drugs. The major findings from this trial were that magnesium sulfate therapy:

- significantly reduced the risk of eclamptic convulsions (0.8% vs. 1.9%; RR 0.42, 95% CI, 0.29–0.60). To prevent one convulsion, 63 women with severe pre-eclampsia or 109 women with mild to moderate pre-eclampsia would need to be treated;
- showed a trend toward a reduced rate of maternal death (0.2% vs. 0.4%; RR 0.55, 95% CI, 0.26–1.14); and
- prevented convulsions regardless of severity of pre-eclampsia, gestational age, or parity.

Maternal morbidity, perinatal mortality, and neonatal morbidity were similar in both groups, except for a lower rate of abruption in treated women (2.0% vs. 3.2%) (Magpie Trial, 2002). Magnesium sulfate therapy should be considered for prevention of eclampsia in all women with pre-eclampsia (Magpie Trial, 2002; Roberts *et al.*, 2002; Sheth and Chalmers, 2002), including those with non-severe disease, although some authors have questioned the value of treating all pre-eclamptic women to prevent seizures in a small number of patients (0.6–3.2%) (Hall *et al.*, 2000). Approximately 10–15% of women in labor with mild pre-eclampsia will develop signs of severe pre-eclampsia (severe hypertension, headache, visual disturbance, epigastric pain, laboratory abnormalities) whether or not they receive magnesium therapy (Livingston *et al.*, 2003; Witlin and Sibai, 1998).

In summary, the World Health Organization, Federation Internationale de Gynecologie et d'Obstetrique, and the International Society for the Study of Hypertension in Pregnancy recommend magnesium sulfate therapy for prevention

and treatment of eclampsia (Roberts *et al.*, 2002). The American College of Obstetricians and Gynecologists recommends use of magnesium sulfate in women with severe pre-eclampsia and acknowledges the lack of consensus as to whether mildly pre-eclamptic women require such treatment to prevent seizures in a small number of patients (ACOG, 2002). The incidence of seizures is much lower in women with non-proteinuric hypertension (less than 0.1%) (Coetzee *et al.*, 1998). For this reason, it may be safe to withhold seizure prophylaxis in such women.

Subsequent management

Long-term outcome of women with eclampsia

The long-term prognosis for the mother is dependent largely upon the degree of injury sustained as a result of the disease. Hepatocellular damage, renal dysfunction, DIC, and hypertension all resolve following delivery. However, cerebrovascular accident may result in permanent neurologic sequelae.

HELLP syndrome complicates 4–14% of patients with severe pre-eclampsia/eclampsia, and has been associated with poor maternal and/or perinatal outcome (Sibai, 1990; Sibai *et al.*, 1986a, 1995). The incidence of this syndrome is higher in white, multiparous patients, especially those with delayed diagnosis of pre-eclampsia and/or delayed delivery. Overall perinatal mortality rates of up to 36.7% (41/112) have been reported (Sibai *et al.*, 1986a). In a cohort of 442 patients with severe pre-eclampsia and HELLP syndrome followed by Sibai *et al.* (1993b) there were 5 maternal deaths (1.1%) and significant maternal morbidity: DIC in 92 patients (21%), abruptio placenta in 69 patients (16%), acute renal failure in 33 patients (7.7%), 26 patients with pulmonary edema (6%), 4 patients with ruptured subcapsular liver hematomas (0.9%), 4 patients with retinal detachment (0.9%), and 3 patients with acute respiratory distress syndrome (1%). Of note, the incidence of maternal complications (specifically pulmonary edema and acute renal failure) appear to be higher if HELLP syndrome develops postpartum as compared with prior to delivery (Sibai *et al.*, 1993b). The recurrence rate of HELLP syndrome in subsequent pregnancies is approximately 2% (1/49) (Sibai *et al.*, 1986a).

Acute renal failure occurs in 1.8% of patients with severe pre-eclampsia/eclampsia (Sibai *et al.*, 1990), and is almost always secondary to acute tubular necrosis. It usually occurs in the setting of abruptio placenta and DIC, and is associated with poor maternal and/or perinatal outcome (including maternal and perinatal mortality rates of 10–13% and 34–41%, respectively) (Sibai and Ramadan, 1993; Sibai *et al.*, 1990). Approximately 30–50% of patients with acute renal failure will require dialysis during the current pregnancy for the management of azotemia and/or hyperkalemia. Long-term follow-up (average 4.0 ± 3.1 years) of 31 patients with severe pre-eclampsia/eclampsia complicated by renal failure demonstrated full recovery and normal renal function in all 16 surviving patients with pre-eclampsia. In patients with underlying parenchymal renal disease and/or chronic hypertension, 9 of the 11 surviving patients (82%) required long-term dialysis and 4 ultimately died of end-stage renal disease. The authors conclude that "proper management of acute renal failure in patients with pure pre-eclampsia–eclampsia does not result in residual function impairment" (Sibai *et al.*, 1990). In the absence of underlying renal disease, recurrence of acute renal failure in a subsequent pregnancy has yet to be described.

Pulmonary edema is a rare complication of severe pre-eclampsia/eclampsia with an incidence of approximately 2–3%. It appears to be more common in patients with underlying chronic hypertension as compared with previously normotensive patients (7.1% vs. 1.7%, respectively) (Sibai *et al.*, 1987). In a series of 37 consecutive cases, Sibai and colleagues (1987) reported 4 maternal deaths and significant maternal morbidity. The overall perinatal mortality in this series was 53%

(18/39). Of note, 70% (26/37) of these patients developed pulmonary edema after delivery with an average onset of 71 h postpartum. Almost all of the women had predisposing factors for pulmonary edema, including massive crystalloid and/or colloid infusions, surgical procedures, sepsis, or anemia.

Are women with pre-eclampsia/eclampsia at risk of chronic hypertension in later life?

In women with a history of pre-eclampsia/eclampsia, the reported risk for the development of chronic hypertension ranges from 0% to 78% (average 23.8%) (Chesley *et al.*, 1976; Sibai *et al.*, 1986b, 1991, 1992).The risk appears to be increased in that subgroup of women who have subsequent hypertensive pregnancies as well as in those with eclampsia remote from term (Chesley *et al.*, 1976; Sibai *et al.*, 1986b, 1992). The wide range in reported risk is due to the influence of variables such as maternal age and duration of follow-up (the increased risk of subsequent hypertension only becomes apparent after an average follow-up of ≥10 years) (Sibai *et al.*, 1986b).

In addition to hypertension, women with a history of pre-eclampsia/eclampsia are also at risk of developing diabetes. In one report, the incidence of diabetes in this cohort at an average follow-up of 25 years was 8.3%, which is 2.5-fold higher than expected (Chesley *et al.*, 1976). This is similar to the 5.6% incidence of subsequent diabetes reported by Sibai *et al.* (1986b) in women with severe pre-eclampsia/eclampsia followed for at least 10 years.

Conclusions

Eclampsia is an obstetrical emergency occurring in around 4–5 per 10,000 live births. Both the fetus and the mother are at immediate risk for death or life-long neurologic disability. The ultimate goals of management should be safety of the mother first, and then delivery of a live newborn in optimal condition. Delivery is the only effective treatment. With prompt and effective management and in the absence of cerebrovascular hemorrhage, maternal prognosis is good. Fetal prognosis is dependent largely on gestational age at delivery. The recurrence rate for pre-eclampsia in subsequent pregnancies is reported to be 12–68%, and approximately 10% of these women will experience an eclamptic seizure in a future pregnancy. Magnesium sulfate is the drug of choice for the prevention of the primary as well as recurrent eclamptic seizures.

REFERENCES

Alexander, J. M., Bloom, S. L., McIntire, D. D. and Leveno, K. J. (1999). Severe preeclampsia and the very low birth weight infant: is induction of labor harmful? *Obstet. Gynecol.*, **93**, 485–8.

American College of Obstetricians and Gynecologists. (1996). *Hypertension in Pregnancy*. Technical Bulletin No. 219. Washington, DC: ACOG.

American College of Obstetricians and Gynecologists. (2002). *Diagnosis and Management of Preeclampsia and Eclampsia*. Practice Bulletin No. 33. Washington, DC: ACOG.

American College of Obstetricians and Gynecologists. (1999). *Induction of Labor*. Practice Bulletin No. 10. Washington, DC: ACOG.

Apollon, K. M., Robinson, J. N., Schwartz, R. B. and Norwitz, E. R. (2000). Cortical blindness in severe preeclampsia: computed tomography, magnetic resonance imaging, and single-photon-emission computed tomography findings. *Obstet. Gynecol.*, **95**, 1017–19.

Belfort, M. A. and Moise, K. J. Jr. (1992). Effect of magnesium sulfate on maternal brain blood flow in preeclampsia: a randomized, placebo-controlled study. *Am. J. Obstet. Gynecol.*, **167**, 661–6.

Belfort, M. A., Saade, G. R., Moise, K. J. Jr., *et al.* (1994). Nimodipine in the management of preeclampsia: maternal and fetal effects. *Am. J. Obstet. Gynecol.*, **171**, 417–24.

Belfort, M. A., Tooke-Miller, C., Allen, J. C. Jr., *et al.* (2001). Changes in flow velocity, resistance indices, and cerebral perfusion pressure in the maternal middle cerebral artery distribution during normal pregnancy. *Acta Obstet. Gynecol. Scand.*, **80**, 104–12.

Belfort, M. A., Varner, M. W., Dizon-Townson, D. S., Grunewald, C. and Nisell, H. (2002). Cerebral perfusion pressure, and not cerebral blood flow, may be the critical determinant of intracranial injury in preeclampsia: a new hypothesis. *Am. J. Obstet. Gynecol.*, **187**, 626–34.

Belfort, M. A., Anthony, J., Saade, G. R., Allen, J. C. Jr., *et al.* for the Nimodipine Study Group. (2003). A comparison of magnesium sulfate and nimodipine for the prevention of eclampsia. *N. Engl. J. Med.*, **348**, 304–11.

Brosens, I. A., Robertson, W. B. and Dixon, H. G. (1972). The role of the spiral arteries in the pathogenesis of preeclampsia. *Obstet. Gynecol. Annu.*, **1**, 177–91.

Brown, C. E., Purdy, P. and Cunningham, F. G. (1988). Head computed tomographic scans in women with eclampsia. *Am. J. Obstet. Gynecol.*, **159**, 915–20.

Chesley, L. C., Annitto, J. E. and Cosgrove, R. A. (1976). The remote prognosis of eclamptic women. *Am. J. Obstet. Gynecol.*, **124**, 446–59.

Coetzee, E. J., Dommisse, J. and Anthony, J. (1998). A randomised controlled trial of intravenous magnesium sulphate versus placebo in the management of women with severe preeclampsia. *Br. J. Obstet. Gynaecol.*, **105**, 300–3.

Conde-Agudelo, A. and Kafury-Goeta, A. C. (1997). Case-control study of risk factors for complicated eclampsia. *Obstet. Gynecol.*, **90**, 172–5.

Crawford, S., Varner, M. W., Digre, K. B., Servais, G. and Corbett, J. J. (1987). Cranial magnetic resonance imaging in eclampsia. *Obstet. Gynecol.*, **70**, 474–7.

Cross, J. C., Werb, Z. and Fisher, S. J. (1994). Implantation and the placenta: key pieces of the development puzzle. *Science*, **266**, 1508–18.

Delgado-Escueta, A. V., Wasterlain, C., Treiman, D. M. and Porter, R. S. (1982). Current concepts in neurology: management of status epilepticus. *N. Engl. J. Med.*, **306**, 1337–40.

Dierckx, I. and Appel, B. (1989). MR findings in eclampsia. *Am. J. Neuroradiol.*, **10**, 445.

Digre, K. B., Varner, M. W., Osborn, A. G. and Crawford, S. (1993). Cranial magnetic resonance imaging in severe preeclampsia vs eclampsia. *Arch. Neurol.*, **50**, 399–406.

Douglas, K. A. and Redman, C. W. G. (1994). Eclampsia in the United Kingdom. *Br. Med. J.*, **309**, 1395–400.

Duley, L. (1992). Maternal mortality associated with hypertensive disorders of pregnancy in Africa, Asia,

Latin America and the Caribbean. *Br. J. Obstet. Gynaecol.*, **99**, 547–53.

Duley, L. and Gulmezoglu, A. M. (2001). Magnesium sulphate versus lytic cocktail for eclampsia (Cochrane Review). *Cochrane Database Syst. Rev.*, **1**, CD002960.

Fredriksson, K., Lindvall, O., Ingemarsson, I., Astedt, B., Cronqvist, S. and Holtas, S. (1989). Repeated cranial computed tomographic and magnetic resonance imaging scans in two cases of eclampsia. *Stroke*, **20**, 547–53.

Gerthoffer, W. T., Shafer, P. G. and Taylor, S. (1987). Selectivity of phenytoin and dihydropyridine calcium channel blockers for relaxation of the basilar artery. *J. Cardiovasc. Pharmacol.*, **10**, 9–15.

Goldstein, D. P. and Berkowitz, R. S. (1994). Current management of complete and partial molar pregnancy. *J. Reprod. Med.*, **39**, 139–46.

Hall, D. R., Odendaal, H. J. and Smith, M. (2000). Is the prophylactic administration of magnesium sulphate in women with pre-eclampsia indicated prior to labour? *Br. J. Obstet. Gynaecol.*, **107**, 903–8.

Lindenstrom, E., Boysen, G. and Nyboe, J. (1995). Influence of systolic and diastolic blood pressure on stroke risk: a prospective observational study. *Am. J. Epidemiol.*, **142**, 1279–90.

Livingston, J. C., Livingston, L. W., Ramsey, R., *et al.* (2003). Magnesium sulfate in women with mild preeclampsia: a randomized controlled trial. *Obstet. Gynecol.*, **101**, 217–20.

López-Llera, M. (1992). Main clinical types and subtypes of eclampsia. *Am. J. Obstet. Gynecol.*, **166**, 4–9.

Lubarsky, S. L., Barton, J. R., Friedman, S. A., Nasreddine, S., Ramadan, M. K. and Sibai, B. M. (1994). Late postpartum eclampsia revisited. *Obstet. Gynecol.*, **83**, 502–5.

Lucas, M. J., Leveno, K. J. and Cunningham, F. G. (1995). A comparison of magnesium sulphate with phenytoin for the prevention of eclampsia. *N. Engl. J. Med.*, **333**, 201–5.

Magee, L. A., Ornstein, M. P. and von Dadelszen, P. (1999). Fortnightly review: management of hypertension in pregnancy. *Br. Med. J.*, **318**, 1332–6.

Maynard, S. E., Min, J. Y., Merchan, J., *et al.* (2003). Excess placental soluble fms-like tyrosine kinase 1 (sFlt1) may contribute to endothelial dysfunction, hypertension, and proteinuria in preeclampsia. *J. Clin. Invest.*, **111**, 600–2.

Meekins, J. W., Pijnenborg, R., Hanssens, M., McFadyen, I. R. and van Asshe, A. (1994). A study of placental bed spiral arteries and trophoblast invasion in normal and severe pre-eclamptic pregnancies. *Br. J. Obstet. Gynaecol.*, **101**, 669–74.

Miles, J. F. Jr., Martin, J. N. Jr., Blake, P. G., *et al.* (1990). Postpartum eclampsia: a recurring perinatal dilemma. *Obstet. Gynecol.*, **76**, 328–31.

Moller, B. and Lindmark, G. (1986). Eclampsia in Sweden, 1976–1980. *Acta Obstet. Gynecol. Scand.*, **65**, 307–14.

Naidu, K., Moodley, J., Corr, P. and Hoffmann, M. (1997). Single photon emission and cerebral computerised tomographic scan and transcranial Doppler sonographic findings in eclampsia. *Br. J. Obstet. Gynaecol.*, **104**, 1165–72.

Nassar, A. H., Adra, A. M., Chakhtoura, N., *et al.* (1998). Severe preeclampsia remote from term: labor induction or elective Cesarean delivery? *Am. J. Obstet. Gynecol.*, **179**, 1210–13.

Paul, R. H., Koh, K. S. and Bernstein, S. G. (1978). Changes in fetal heart rate–uterine contraction patterns associated with eclampsia. *Am. J. Obstet. Gynecol.*, **130**, 165–9.

Prichard, J. A., Cunningham, F. G. and Prichard, S. A. (1984). The Parkland Memorial Hospital protocol for treatment of eclampsia: evaluation of 245 cases. *Am. J. Obstet. Gynecol.*, **148**, 951–63.

Report of the National High Blood Pressure Education Program Working Group on High Blood Pressure in Pregnancy. (2000). *Am. J. Obstet. Gynecol.*, **183**(Suppl.), 1–22.

Roberts, J. M. (1995). Magnesium for preeclampsia and eclampsia. *N. Engl. J. Med.*, **333**, 250–1.

Roberts, J. M., Villar, J. and Arulkumaran, S. (2002). Preventing and treating eclamptic seizures. *Br. Med. J.*, **325**, 609–10.

Rochat, R. W., Koonin, L. M., Atrash, H. F., Jewett, J. F. and the Maternal Mortality Collaborative Study Group. (1988). Maternal mortality in the United States: report from the Maternal Mortality Collaborative. *Obstet. Gynecol.*, **72**, 91–7.

Royburt, M., Seidman, D. S., Serr, D. M. and Mashiach, S. (1991). Neurologic involvement in hypertensive disease of pregnancy. *Obstet. Gynecol. Surv.*, **46**, 656–64.

Salerni, A., Wald, S. and Flanagan, M. (1988). Relationship among cortical ischemia, infarction, and hemorrhage in eclampsia. *Neurology*, **22**, 408–10.

Schwartz, R. B., Janes, K. M., Kalina, P., *et al.* (1992). Hypertensive encephalopathy: findings on CT., MR imaging, and SPECT imaging in 14 cases. *Am. J. Roentgenol.*, **159**, 379–83.

Sheehan, H. L. and Lynch, J. B. (1973). *Pathology of Toxemia of Pregnancy*. Baltimore: Williams & Wilkins.

Sheth, S. S. and Chalmers, I. (2002). Magnesium for preventing and treating eclampsia: time for international action. *Lancet*, **359**, 1872–3.

Sibai, B. M. (1990). Eclampsia. VI. Maternal-perinatal outcome in 254 consecutive cases. *Am. J. Obstet. Gynecol.*, **163**, 1049–54.

Sibai, B. M. (1996). Treatment of hypertension in pregnant women. *N. Engl. J. Med.*, **335**, 257–65.

Sibai, B. M., Lipshitz, J., Anderson, G. D. and Dilts, P. V. Jr. (1981a). Reassessment of intravenous MgSO$_4$ therapy in preeclampsia–eclampsia. *Obstet. Gynecol.*, **57**, 199–202.

Sibai, B. M., McCubbin, J. H., Anderson, G. D., Lipshitz, J. and Dilts, P. V. Jr. (1981b). Eclampsia. I. Observations from sixty-seven recent cases. *Obstet. Gynecol.*, **58**, 609–13.

Sibai, B. M., Taslimi, M. M., el-Nazer, A., Amon, E., Mabie, B. C. and Ryan, G. M. (1986a). Maternal–perinatal outcome associated with the syndrome of hemolysis, elevated liver enzymes, and low platelets in severe preeclampsia–eclampsia. *Am. J. Obstet. Gynecol.*, **155**, 501–9.

Sibai, B. M., el-Nazer, A. and Gonzalez-Ruiz, A. (1986b). Severe preeclampsia–eclampsia in young primigravid women: subsequent pregnancy outcome and remote prognosis. *Am. J. Obstet. Gynecol.*, **155**, 1011–16.

Sibai, B. M., Abdella, T. N., Spinnato, J. A., *et al.* (1986c). Eclampsia. V. The incidence of nonpreventable eclampsia. *Am. J. Obstet. Gynecol.*, **154**, 581–6.

Sibai, B. M., Mabie, B. C., Harvey, C. J. and Gonzalez, A. R. (1987). Pulmonary edema in severe preeclampsia–eclampsia: analysis of thirty-seven consecutive cases. *Am. J. Obstet. Gynecol.*, **156**, 1174–9.

Sibai, B. M., Villar, M. A. and Marbie, B. C. (1990). Acute renal failure in hypertensive disorders of pregnancy: pregnancy outcome and remote prognosis in thirty-one consecutive cases. *Am. J. Obstet. Gynecol.*, **162**, 777–83.

Sibai, B. M., Mercer, B. and Sarinoglu, C. (1991). Severe preeclampsia in the second trimester: recurrence risk and long-term prognosis. *Am. J. Obstet. Gynecol.*, **165**, 1408–12.

Sibai, B. M., Sarinoglu, C. and Mercer, B. M. (1992). Eclampsia. VII. Pregnancy outcome after eclampsia and long-term prognosis. *Am. J. Obstet. Gynecol.*, **166**, 1757–61.

Sibai, B. M. and Ramadan, M. K. (1993a). Acute renal failure in pregnancies complicated by hemolysis, elevated liver enzymes, and low platelets. *Am. J. Obstet. Gynecol.*, **168**, 1682–90.

Sibai, B. M., Mercer, B. M., Schiff, E. and Friedman, S. A. (1994). Aggressive versus expectant management of severe preeclampsia at 28 to 32 weeks' gestation: a randomized controlled trial. *Am. J. Obstet. Gynecol.*, **171**, 818–22.

Sibai, B. M., Ramadan, M. K., Usta, I., Salama, M., Mercer, B. M. and Friedman, S. A. (1993b). Maternal morbidity and mortality in 442 pregnancies with hemolysis, elevated liver enzymes, and low platelets (HELLP syndrome). *Am. J. Obstet. Gynecol.*, **169**, 1000–6.

Sibai, B. M., Ramadan, M. K., Chari, R. S. and Friedman, S. A. (1995). Pregnancies complicated by HELLP syndrome (hemolysis, elevated liver enzymes, and low platelets): subsequent pregnancy outcome and long-term prognosis. *Am. J. Obstet. Gynecol.*, **172**, 125–9.

The Eclampsia Trial Collaborative Group. (1995). Which anticonvulsant for women with eclampsia? Evidence from the Collaborative Eclampsia Trial. *Lancet*, **345**, 1455–63.

The Magpie Trial. (2002). Do women with pre-eclampsia, and their babies, benefit from magnesium sulphate? The Magpie Trial: a randomised placebo-controlled trial. *Lancet*, **359**, 1877–90.

Trommer, B. L., Homer, D. and Mikhael, M. A. (1988). Cerebral vasospasm and eclampsia. *Stroke*, **19**, 326–9.

van Gijn, J. and Rinkel, G. J. (2001). Subarachnoid haemorrhage: diagnosis, causes and management. *Brain*, **124**, 249–78.

von Dadelszen, P., Ornstein, M. P., Bull, S. B., Logan, A. G., Koren, G. and Magee, L. A. (2000). Fall in mean arterial pressure and fetal growth restriction in pregnancy hypertension: a meta-analysis. *Lancet*, **355**, 87–92.

Wallace, D. H., Leveno, K. J., Cunningham, F. G., *et al.* (1995). Randomized comparison of general and regional anesthesia for cesarean delivery in pregnancies complicated by severe preeclampsia. *Obstet. Gynecol.*, **86**, 193–9.

Will, A. D., Lewis, K. L., Hinshaw, D. B. Jr., *et al.* (1987). Cerebral vasoconstriction in toxemia. *Neurology*, **37**, 1555–7.

Williams, K. and Galerneau, F. (2003). Maternal transcranial Doppler in pre-eclampsia and eclampsia. *Ultrasound Obstet. Gynecol.*, **21**, 507–13.

Williams, K. P. and Wilson, S. (1999). Persistence of cerebral hemodynamic changes in patients with eclampsia: a report of three cases. *Am. J. Obstet. Gynecol.*, **181**, 1162–5.

Witlin, A. G. and Sibai, B. M. (1998). Magnesium sulfate therapy in preeclampsia and eclampsia. *Obstet. Gynecol.*, **92**, 883–9.

World Health Organization International Collaborative Study of Hypertensive Disorders of Pregnancy. (1988). Geographic variation in the incidence of hypertension in pregnancy. *Am. J. Obstet. Gynecol.*, **158**, 80–3.

Zunker, P., Georgiadis, A. L., Czech, N., Golombeck, K., Brossmann, J. and Deuschl, G. (2003). Impaired cerebral glucose metabolism in eclampsia: a new finding in two cases. *Fetal Diagn. Ther.*, **18**, 41–6.

30

Anesthesia for the pre-eclamptic patient

Jose M. Rivers and Maya S. Suresh

Hypertensive disease affects roughly 6–8% of all pregnancies and is the second leading cause of maternal morbidity and mortality. It accounts for almost 15% of pregnancy-related maternal deaths, and is a major risk factor for fetal morbidity and mortality (Berg *et al.*, 1996; Longo *et al.*, 2003); there is also a substantial contribution to stillbirths, neonatal morbidity and mortality as a result of premature deliveries.

Terminology and classification

Historically, there have been varied and diverse terminologies used to describe hypertension during pregnancy. Previous terminology such as *pregnancy-induced hypertension* has been abandoned. The Report of the National High Blood Pressure Education Program Working Group on High Blood Pressure in Pregnancy (2000) has attempted to standardize the classification.

The currently accepted classification is as follows:
- pre-eclampsia–eclampsia with or without HELLP (hemolysis, elevated liver enzymes, and low platelet count) syndrome;
- pre-eclampsia superimposed on chronic hypertension;
- chronic hypertension; and
- gestational hypertension.

Pre-eclampsia

Background

Unique to humans, pre-eclampsia is a multiorgan disease of unknown origin. Symptoms present themselves in a normotensive woman after the twentieth week of gestation. However, pre-eclampsia can occur in normotensive patients with trophoblastic disease (e.g. molar pregnancy) prior to the twentieth week (Ness and Roberts, 1996). The risk of developing pre-eclampsia is greater in women with pre-existing conditions such as chronic hypertension, diabetes, antiphospholipid syndrome and collagen vascular disease.

A detailed discussion of the etiology and pathogenesis of pre-eclampsia and eclampsia is beyond the scope of this chapter. Some of the etiologic factors include: (1) immunological factors (Lyall, 2003; Redman, 1991); (2) genetic factors (Dizon-Townson *et al.*, 1996); (3) coagulation factors (Scholtes *et al.*, 1983); (4) platelet factors (Kilby *et al.*, 1993); (5) endothelial factors (Dekker and Sibai, 1998; Rogers *et al.*, 1990); (6) metabolic fatty acids (Sattar *et al.*, 1996), and failure of second-wave invasion of the trophoblast (Matteo *et al.*, 1998; Zuspan, 1991). These subjects have been covered in detail in other sections of this book.

Criteria for diagnosis

- Hypertension, associated with hyperdynamic circulation and/or increased vascular resistance.
- Glomerulopathy with proteinuria.
  - Edema (edema is no longer a key criterion for diagnosis. The existence of hypertension and proteinuria are sufficient for a diagnosis of pre-eclampsia).

Pre-eclampsia can be mild or severe. Mild pre-eclampsia is characterized by a sustained systolic blood pressure equal to or greater than 140 mmHg, a diastolic blood pressure equal to or greater than 90 mmHg, and proteinuria of 300 mg in a 24-h urine collection. Pre-eclampsia is considered severe when systolic pressure is 160 mmHg or higher, diastolic pressure is 110 mmHg or higher, or there is a proteinuria of at least 5 g in a 24-h urine collection. Other manifestations of severe pre-eclampsia are oliguria (urine output <400 ml in 24 h), cerebral or visual disturbances, pulmonary edema, thrombocytopenia, and impaired liver function (Ramanathan, 2003).

Hemolysis, elevated liver enzymes and low platelet count (HELLP) syndrome is a disease of pre-eclamptic women (Weinstein, 1985). It is part of a continuum of a disease that includes severe pre-eclampsia (Martin *et al.*, 1991) and postpartum eclampsia (Stricker *et al.*, 1992).

Eclampsia is defined as the occurrence of a seizure in a parturient with pre-eclampsia that cannot be attributed to other causes.

Systemic effects of pre-eclampsia

Classic pre-eclampsia, a hypertensive disorder peculiar to pregnancy has diverse and widespread pathophysiology and has long been known to be associated with multi-organ involvement. Understanding the pathophysiology forms the basis for clinical and anesthetic management. The pre-eclamptic patient is a high-risk patient. Before administering an anesthetic to these patients, it is vitally important to consider, understand and evaluate the following areas:
- airway and respiratory system;
- hemodynamic profile;
- central nervous system;
- coagulation profile;
- renal function;
- hepatic function;
- fetal evaluation; and
- drug therapies and interactions.

Airway and respiratory system

Anatomic and physiological factors alter the airway during pregnancy, placing the parturient at risk for difficult intubation. An effect of hormones on the ground substance of connective tissue leads to an increase in interstitial water resulting in edema of the respiratory tract, including the oral and nasal pharynx, larynx, and trachea. These airway changes are further exacerbated in pre-eclampsia.

Pharyngolaryngeal and vocal cord edema of normal pregnancy can be aggravated in pre-eclampsia leading to total airway obstruction and may hinder the passage of a tracheal tube that would easily pass in a nonpregnant female (Heller *et al.*, 1983). The reduced plasma proteins and marked fluid retention, especially in the head and neck region, make the tongue larger and less mobile, causing identification of landmarks to be more difficult in a pre-eclamptic patient. There is no single reason for the high incidence of failed intubation in obstetrics particularly in pre-eclamptic patients. All of the following factors have been suggested as contributory: capillary engorgement and swelling of the nasopharyngeal mucosa and larynx; increase in body weight, total body water, and fat deposition; additional laryngeal edema in pre-eclampsia associated with decreased plasma proteins and water retention; enlarged breasts; decreased mobility of the floor of the mouth because of tongue engorgement; lead to exacerbated airway changes thus placing the pre-eclamptic patient at an added risk for difficult intubation (Brimacombe, 2003; Brock-Utne, 2003; Dobb, 1978; Ebert, 2003; Farcon *et al.*, 1994; Joupilla, 2003; Procter and White, 1983; Rocke and Scoones, 1992; Seager and Macdonald, 1980; Tillman Hein, 2003). A correlation between the excessive weight gain and an increase in the Mallampati score suggests that fluid retention causing pharyngeal edema is perhaps the underlying cause of difficult intubation (Pilkington, 2003). Furthermore, the course of labor and bearing down in labor has been shown to worsen the Mallampati score, thus requiring re-evaluation of the airway before induction of general anesthesia (Farcon *et al.*, 1994).

Significant weight gain during pre-eclampsia and the enlarged gravid uterus can result in decreased functional residual capacity. However, the lung volumes and capacities, and function are not significantly altered by pre-eclampsia (Rees *et al.*, 1990).

Another change in respiratory function includes increased oxygen consumption. The decrease in functional residual capacity and increase in oxygen consumption makes the pre-eclamptic patient more susceptible to rapid development of hypoxemia during periods of apnea or hypoventilation, especially if confronted with a difficult or failed intubation, or difficult mask ventilation.

Maternal carboxyhemoglobin levels increase (hemolysis and increased red cell catabolism) and 2,3-diphosphoglycerate decreases causing a leftward shift of the oxyhemoglobin dissociation curve (Kambam *et al.*, 1986) in pre-eclampsia. This results in less delivery of oxygen to the fetus (Kambam *et al.*, 1988a).

Solutions to minimize the hazards of difficult laryngoscopy in these patients include taping of breasts laterally and caudally, proper "sniff position" (head positioning) with blankets/ramp under the shoulders if necessary, use of a short laryngoscope handle, use of a pediatric laryngoscope handle with an adult blade, and insertion of the laryngoscope blade followed by attachment of the handle (Suresh, 2003). For these reasons, the American Society of Anesthesiologists (ASA) Practice Guidelines in Obstetric Anesthesia (2003) suggest that operating rooms and labor and delivery suites need to be equipped with difficult airway carts with different sizes and types of endotracheal tubes, laryngeal mask airways, fiberoptic bronchoscopes, and Combitube™ devices (American Society of Anesthesiologists, in press).

Hemodynamic profile

Women with pre-eclampsia may present with a wide spectrum of cardiovascular changes. Thus,

Table 30.1. Hemodynamic changes in nonpregnant and healthy term pregnant women

	Nonpregnant ($n = 10$)	Healthy pregnant ($n = 10$)
MAP (mmHg)	86 ± 7.5	90 ± 5.8
Heart rate (beat min^{-1})	$71 + 10$	$83 + 10$
Cardiac output (l min^{-1})	4.3 ± 0.9	6.2 ± 1.0
SVR (Dynes s^{-1} cm^{-5})	1530 ± 520	$1210 + 265$
PCWP (mmHg)	6.3 ± 2.1	7.5 ± 1.8
CVP (mmHg)	3.7 ± 2.6	3.6 ± 2.5
LVSWI (g mm^2)	41 ± 8	48 ± 6
COP (mmHg)	21 ± 1	18 ± 1.5

Data from Clark, S., Cotton, D. B. and Lee, W. (1989). Central hemodynamic assessment of normal term pregnancy. *Am. J. Obstet. Gynecol.*, **161**, 1439–42, with permission.

definition of their precise hemodynamic status prior to anesthetic intervention is important. The hemodynamic changes seen in normotensive term parturients, as compared with nonpregnant women, include: increases in heart rate (HR), stroke volume (SV) and cardiac output (CO), a decrease in systemic vascular resistance (SVR), and minimal if any change in pulmonary artery capillary wedge pressure (PCWP), central venous pressure (CVP), and left ventricular stroke work index (LVSWI) (Table 30.1) (Clark *et al.*, 1989).

The hemodynamic changes in pre-eclampsia are based on factors such as the duration and severity of pre-eclampsia, previous administration of intravenous fluids, use of antihypertensive drugs, stage of labor and co-morbidities such as chronic hypertension, diabetes, and peripartum cardiomyopathy. In severe pre-eclampsia, expansion of blood volume fails to occur. This results in decreased intravascular volume, generalized vasoconstriction, and hemoconcentration (Cotton *et al.*, 1988). In mild pre-eclampsia, plasma volume is 9% lower than normotensive pregnant individuals, while in severe pre-eclampsia the plasma

Table 30.2. Hemodynamic changes in severe pre-eclampsia

Hemodynamic variables	Untreated patients[a] (n = 87)	Treated patients[b] (n = 45)	Treated patients[c] (n = 41)	Pulmonary edema[c] (n = 8)
MAP (mmHg)	–	138 ± 3	130 ± 2	136 ± 3
CVP (mmHg)	2	4 ± 1	4.8 ± 0.4	11 ± 1
PCWP (mmHg)	7	10 ± 1	8.3 ± 0.3	18 ± 1
Cardiac index ($1\,min^{-1}\,m^{-2}$)	3.3	–	–	–
Cardiac output ($l\,min^{-1}$)		7.5 ± 0.2	8.4 ± 0.2	10.5 ± 0.6
SVR ($dynes\,s^{-1}\,cm^{-5}$)	3003	1496 ± 64	1226 ± 37	964 ± 50
PVR ($dynes\,s^{-1}\,cm^{-5}$)	131	70 ± 5	65 ± 3	71 ± 9
LVSWI ($g\,mm^2$)	–	81 ± 2	84 ± 4	87 ± 10

[a]Data from Wallenburg, H. C. S. (1988). Hemodynamics in hypertensive pregnancy. In *Handbook of Hypertension*, ed. P. C. Rubin. The Netherlands: Elsevier, pp. 66–101, with permission.
[b]Data from Cotton, D. B. *et al.* (1988). Hemodynamic profile of severe pregnancy-induced hypertension. *Am. J. Obstet. Gynecol.*, **158**, 9, with permission.
[c]Data from Mabie, W. C. *et al.* (1989). The central hemodynamic of severe pre-eclampsia. *Am. J. Obstet. Gynecol.*, **161**, 1443–8, with permission.
Modified table from Ramanthan, J. and Bennet, K. (2003). Anesthesiology. *Clin. N. Amer.*, **21**, 145–63, with permission.

volume is reduced by 30–40% (Cotton *et al.*, 1986). This hemoconcentration explains why hemoglobin and hematocrit are frequently noted to be elevated.

In untreated patients with severe pre-eclampsia, the hemodynamic findings are characterized by high systemic vascular resistance (SVR), low left and right ventricular filling pressures, low to normal cardiac index (CI) and a normal to high PCWP (Table 30.2). There are reports that pre-eclamptic patients develop hyperdynamic left ventricular function in early pregnancy and that this finding is a hallmark of the disease (Bolte *et al.*, 2001; Clark *et al.*, 1989; Cotton *et al.*, 1985; Mabie *et al.*, 1989; Young and Johanson, 2001). There is no doubt that in late-presenting severe disease the cardiac output is often decreased and there may be hypertensive cardiomyopathy. In those patients treated with intravenous fluids and/or antihypertensive agents, the findings may be quite different due to the effects of the therapy (Cotton *et al.*, 1986; Gambling, 2003a). The hemodynamic status in patients with severe pre-eclampsia varies from a hyperdynamic state to a low cardiac output/high peripheral vascular resistance state (Bolte *et al.*, 2001). These patients in particular will present with diminished

compliance of the left ventricle, and therefore reliance on central venous pressure alone for making therapeutic decisions regarding fluid loading and drug administration is not advised.

Pulmonary edema, both cardiogenic and non-cardiogenic, is a serious complication of severe pre-eclampsia with an incidence of approximately 3% (Mabie *et al.*, 1988). Cardiogenic pulmonary edema is due to impaired left ventricular systolic or diastolic function, and is more prevalent in patients with severe chronic hypertension, valvular heart disease or cardiomyopathy. Noncardiogenic pulmonary edema results from increased capillary permeability, iatrogenic fluid overload, an imbalance between colloid osmotic pressure and hydrostatic pressure, or a combination of all these factors (Young and Johanson, 2001).

Renal function

A characteristic renal lesion (which has been recently challenged) in pre-eclamptic patients is glomerular enlargement with ischemia (glomerular endotheliosis) (Morris *et al.*, 1964). The glomerular filtration rate (GFR) is 25% below that seen in normal pregnancy. This reduction in GFR is the result of decreased plasma volume, vasospasm and capillary endothelial swelling. The proteinuria is caused by glomerulopathy that leads to an increase in permeability of the glomerular membrane to large molecules. Serum creatinine and uric acid are elevated. Rapid deterioration of renal function is indicated by an elevation in serum creatinine and oliguria. Hemodynamic monitoring, either with echocardiography or with invasive catheters, is sometimes indicated in patents with oliguria especially when they are unresponsive to repetitive challenges with intravascular volume boluses. By defining the patient's hemodynamic profile, the most appropriate treatment to prevent acute renal failure can be instituted (Clark et al., 1986). In oliguric pre-eclamptic patients with the classic signs of hypovolemia, i.e. low filling pressures, elevated SVR and hyperdynamic cardiac function, treatment should be with intravenous fluid and volume expansion. In oliguric pre-eclamptic patients with normal or elevated filling pressures, elevated CO and high SVR, the preferred therapy would be vasodilator drugs and fluid restriction. Finally, the subset of oliguric pre-eclamptic patients with increased SVR and PCWP, and depressed cardiac function, will benefit from after-load reduction and inotropic support (Clark et al., 1986).

Coagulation profile

Thrombocytopenia and thromboastenia are frequently found in pre-eclampsia. The incidence of thrombocytopenia ranges from 15% to 20% and may be as high as 50% in severe pre-eclampsia (Burrows et al., 1987; Giles and Inglis, 1981; Kelton et al., 1985). The etiology is multifactorial. Thrombocytopenia is related to endothelial injury with increased activation and consumption of platelets or secondary to an autoimmune mechanism (Maynard et al., 1977; Ramanathan et al., 1989).

Platelets

Normally, the vascular endothelium actively prevents blood clot formation, platelet aggregation, and platelet thrombi formation. Pre-eclampsia, however, is accompanied by endothelial injury, increased microvascular platelet consumption, and excessive clotting activity (Freidman, 2003; Roberts et al., 1989; Taylor et al., 1991). This leads to a decreased circulating platelet count secondary to an increased consumption rate. Circulating platelets adhere to collagen exposed at the sites of damaged vascular endothelium.

Platelet aggregation, platelet activation and platelet thrombi formation

In pre-eclampsia, especially associated with HELLP syndrome platelet aggregation, platelet thrombi formation, and endothelial injury stem from defective production or increased destruction of vasodilator prostacyclin (PGI_2), and a relative increase in vasoconstrictor thromboxane (TxA_2) (Figure 30.1).

Endothelial cells interface between circulating blood products and vascular smooth muscle. Vascular endothelium is a complex and active monolayer in all blood vessels with metabolic, endocrine, and structural functions. Three functions relevant to pre-eclampsia are maintenance of vascular system integrity, modulation of vessel wall tone, and prevention of intravascular coagulation.

Pre-eclampsia demonstrates morphologic, functional, and biochemical evidence of endothelial injury. The morphologic changes reported in the kidneys (Spargo, 1976), spiral arteries (Arias and Mancilla-Jimenez, 1976; Robertson et al., 1975) and umbilical arteries (Dadak et al., 1984) all suggest underlying endothelial or vessel wall damage in pre-eclampsia. Direct functional evidence of altered endothelial cell permeability is the increased disappearance rate of Evans blue dye from the vascular compartment in pre-eclampsia (Brown et al., 1989; Campbell, 2003). Biochemical findings include an increased TxA_2/PGI_2 ratio (the major source of prostacyclin is endothelial cells); increased plasma level of substances normally located on the endothelial cell membrane, namely factor VIII antigen (Fournie et al., 1981),

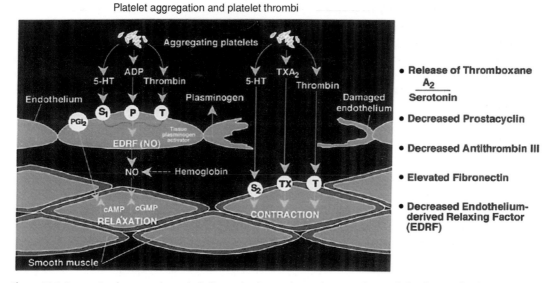

Platelet aggregation and platelet thrombi

Figure 30.1 Interaction between the endothelium, platelets and vascular smooth muscle leading to platelet aggregation and platelet thrombi formation.

and fibronectin (Lazarchick *et al.*, 1986; Rappaport *et al.*, 1990) several weeks or months before the appearance of clinical disease.

Poorly perfused trophoblasts elaborate a substance toxic to endothelial cells, and endothelial injury may antedate the clinical signs and symptoms associated with pre-eclampsia/HELLP syndrome. Another suggested mechanism of endothelial cell damage is antibody mediated. Pre-eclamptic women possess higher titers of autoantibodies directed against endothelial cells (Rappaport *et al.*, 1990).

The role of endothelium-derived relaxing factor (EDRF)/nitric oxide in the pathophysiology and management is not fully understood. Increasing evidence shows that EDRF/nitric oxide released from vascular endothelial cells induces smooth muscle relaxation by production of cyclic guanylate monophosphate acid (cGMP) (Vane *et al.*, 1990). EDRF is a potent inhibitor of platelet aggre-gation acting through cGMP (Busse, 1987). The antiag-gregatory property of EDRF is abolished when free hemoglobin is present. EDRF release is enhanced from isolated uterine arteries in normal pregnant

women compared to nonpregnant women (Nelson, 2003). It is not known whether EDRF/nitric oxide release from endothelial cells in pre-eclampsia HELLP syndrome is decreased or absent, and the role of EDRF/nitric oxide in the pathophysiology and management is not fully understood. However, clinically, the nitric oxide donor, *s*-nitroglutathione, a potent inhibitor of platelet activation, has been used in the management of pre-eclamptic patients with HELLP syndrome (de Belder *et al.*, 1995).

Elevated levels of platelet-associated immunoglobin G (IgG) in 35% of pre-eclamptic patients suggests that an immune mechanism is partly responsible for the thrombocytopenia (Burrows *et al.*, 1987). Platelet antiglobulin have been observed in significant numbers of pre-eclamptic women and their neonates (Samuels *et al.*, 1987).

Other evidence of platelet activation in women with pre-eclampsia includes the following: (1) an increase in beta-thromboglobuin release by platelets; (2) decreased platelet half-life as evidenced by shorter production time; and (3) presence of megathrombocytes (giant platelets) in the peripheral blood, indicating a younger platelet population (Inglis *et al.*, 1982).

Because of the on-going platelet activation, platelet aggregation and platelet abnormalities it is essential to assess the platelet function in addition to the platelet count prior to anesthetic involvement.

Platelet function

Platelet function tests include bleeding time, thromboelastography, and aggregometry. Even with an acceptable platelet count, a functional platelet abnormality and a prolonged bleeding time exist in some women with pre-eclampsia and HELLP syndrome (Kelton *et al.*, 1985; Ramanathan *et al.*, 1989). Ramanathan *et al.* (1989) correlated bleeding time and platelet counts in pre-eclamptic women undergoing Cesarean section. Platelet counts were significantly lower and bleeding times prolonged in pre-eclamptic compared to normal pregnant women. The investigators indicated that bleeding time is abnormal in some pre-eclamptics with a platelet count of 100,000 mm^{-3}.

Antiplatelet therapy such as low-dose aspirin has been suggested as prophylaxis to prevent pre-eclampsia and as a possible treatment for thrombocytopenia. Aspirin has also been used as a reversal strategy, as well as to prolong gestation in patients with HELLP syndrome (Dekker and Sibai, 1993; Sibai and Carbis, 1993). Low-dose aspirin inhibits platelet cyclooxygenase, thus reducing thromboxane production. This tilts the balance in favor of prostacyclin and leads to vasodilation and inhibition of platelet aggregation. The effect of aspirin on platelets is irreversible and persists for their life span of 7–10 days. Aspirin increases bleeding time. Epidural anesthesia may be potentially dangerous in HELLP syndrome patients with coagulopathy or those on aspirin therapy. Prolonged bleeding time places the patient at risk for development of epidural hematoma following regional anesthesia (Costabile, 2003; Locke *et al.*, 1976).

Table 30.3. Normal thromboelastography (TEG) values from pregnant and nonpregnant women

Subject	R (min)	K (min)	R + K (min)	MA (mm)
Nonpregnant	6–12	3–6	9–18	40–60
Pregnant	7.9 (0.9)	3.4 (0.7)	10.9 (1.1)	59.7 (3.5)

From Orlikowski, C. E., Payne, A. J., Moodley, J., *et al.* (1992). Thromboelastography after aspirin ingestion in pregnant and non-pregnant-subjects. *Br. J. Anaesth.*, **69**(2), 159–61, with permission.

Bleeding time is a well-established, simple bedside laboratory test that evaluates a combination of both the quality and quantity of the platelets. This test, however, is no longer considered useful to determine the safety of epidural catheter placement because it does not necessarily assess platelet function, predict hemorrhage in a wide range of clinical settings, or reflect the risk of bleeding at other sites (Channing-Rodgers, 2003; Lind, 1991; Orlikowski *et al.*, 1992).

A thromboelastogram (TEG), a whole blood viscoelastic coagulation screening test, can measure all phases of coagulation and fibrinolysis in a single sample of blood. The normal TEG values for nonpregnant and pregnant women are shown in Table 30.3. The TEG's sensitivity and specificity are affected by the quality and quantity of platelets. A decreased maximum amplitude (MA) suggests a functional platelet disorder. MA, a direct function of the maximum dynamic properties of fibrin and platelets, also determines the fibrin clot strength. The normal TEG variables and those indicating platelet and coagulation abnormalities are shown in (Figures 30.2 and 30.3). Abnormal TEG variable indicating platelets dysfunction or coagulation abnormality should discourage the use of epidural anesthesia. TEG parameters assessed in healthy laboring women and pre-eclampsia show that mild pre-eclamptic are hypercoagulable whereas those with severe disease are hypocoagulable (Chadwick *et al.*, 1993). While potentially useful, this test has yet to find its place in most obstetric anesthesia units and is not widely employed in pre-eclampsia patients.

Hypercoagulability

Hypercoagulability involving the extrinsic pathway, in pre-eclampsia, is evidenced by an accelerated prothrombin time (PT), increased activation of the common pathway (II, V, X), and decreased fibrinogen (Perry and Martin, 1992).

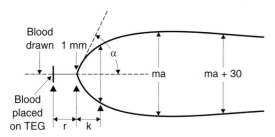

Figure 30.2 Thromboelastography (TEG). R time (min) = reaction time to initial fibrin formation; k time (min) = rapid fibrin build-up and crosslinking; ma (mm = maximum amplitude of the TEG trace – a measure of maximum clot strength and dependent on the concentration of fibrinogen, platelet numbers, and function: α = angle of divergence rate of clot formation; ma + 30 = clot retraction after 30 min.

An accelerated hypercoagulable state in pre-eclampsia is demonstrated by the presence of a red cell anomaly which alters the configuration of phospholipids within the cell membrane thus triggering thrombin formation (Grisaru *et al.*, 1997).

The end-point of the coagulation cascade is the formation of fibrin. The degradation of the fibrin polymer results in non-cross-linked fragments represented by stable dimeric fragments such as the D-dimer. Routine laboratory tests/assays measure fibrin/fibrinogen degradation products (FDP) in order to detect intravascular coagulation; however these assays cannot distinguish between the degradation products resulting from fibrinogen versus fibrin. The presence of D-dimer, indicates significant intravascular coagulation, fibrinolysis, and breakdown of fibrin (Trofatter *et al.*, 1989). The presence of thrombocytopenia (platelet count $< 100,000\,mm^{-3}$), positive D-dimer, and FDP correlated with significantly higher BP measurements, greater proteinuria, abnormal liver function tests, and higher creatinine and blood urea measurements (BUN). Therefore a pre-anesthetic coagulation profile evaluation in severe pre-eclamptic/ eclamptic patients should include testing of the prothrombin time (PT), the activated partial

Variable	Measures	Abnormality		Example
r reaction time	Thromboplastin generation via the intrinsic pathway	↑r	Factor deficiency Heparin Severe thrombocytopenia	Factor deficiency
α angle of divergence	Rate of clot formation	↓α	Hypofibrinogenemia Thrombocytopenia Thrombocytopathy	Hypofibrinogenemia
ma maximum amplitude	Maximum clot strength/elasticity	↓ma	Thrombocytopenia Thrombocytopathy Hypofibrinogenemia Factor XIII deficiency	Thrombocytopenia
ma + 30	Clot retraction after 30 minutes	↓ma + 30	Fibrinolysis	Fibrinolysis

Figure 30.3 Typical thromboelastogram (TEG) pattern and variables measured, normal values, and examples of some abnormal tracings; r = 21–30 mm (normal range, 3–6 min); α = 50–60°. ma = 50–60 mm; ma +30 = minimal reduction. (From Faust, 1994, with permission.)

thromboplastin time (PTT), the FDPs, and the D-dimer.

Central nervous system

The clinical manifestations of pre-eclampsia in the central nervous system include headache, visual disturbances and CNS hyperexcitability and hyper-reflexia. The occurrence of seizures indicates eclampsia until proven otherwise. Eclampsia is a serious condition and is associated with high maternal and fetal morbidity and mortality.

Severe hypertension can cause an increase in cerebral blood (CBF) flow velocity (Richards *et al.*, 1988) and a decrease in blood flow (Zunker *et al.*, 1995). A positive correlation exists between CBF velocity and systemic blood pressure. Persistent hypertension can cause overdistention of cerebral blood vessels, forced vasodilatation, loss of cerebral autoregulation, vasogenic cerebral edema and intracerebral bleeding. This has led to the belief that hypertensive encephalopathy is an important cause of eclampsia. This subject has been further dealt with in other chapters in this book.

Hepatic function

Major changes in the liver cause right upper-quadrant and/or epigastric pain plus abnormal liver enzyme elevation. The right upper-quadrant or epigastric pain is secondary to blood flow obstruction in the sinusoids, blocked by intravascular fibrin deposition.

The classic hepatic lesion in pre-eclampsia associated with HELLP syndrome is periportal necrosis. Immunofluorescence studies reveal fibrin microthrombin and fibrinogen deposits in the sinusoids (Aarnoudse *et al.*, 1986; Arias and Mancilla-Jimenez, 1976). Doppler velocimetry shows an enhancement of hepatic artery resistance to blood flow in postpartum pre-eclamptic patients with HELLP syndrome (Oosterhof *et al.*, 1994). In addition to the hepatic artery constriction there is also decreased portal venous blood flow (portal vein is responsible for 75% of hepatic blood flow) (Aarnoudse *et al.*, 1986; Arias and Mancilla-Jimenez, 1976). Although postpartum hepatic artery vasospasm is quickly reversed, the increased resistance to flow in the portal circulation as a result of fibrin deposition is more slowly reversed (Kurzel *et al.*, 1996). The implication is that this diminished portal blood flow primarily underlies the observed injury seen in severe pre-eclamptic patients with severe pre-eclampsia associated with HELLP syndrome (Kurzel *et al.*, 1996).

Epigastric or subcostal pain is an ominous symptom that is caused by subcapsular parenchymal bleeding. Rarely, severe hemorrhage disrupts the liver capsule and causes intraperitoneal bleeding (Manas *et al.*, 1985). Liver rupture occurs if the intrahepatic pressure exceeds the capacity of the Glisson's capsule to distend. Spontaneous rupture of the liver in severe pre-eclamptic patients with HELLP syndrome has a high rate of maternal and fetal mortality. Successful management of hepatic hemorrhage and rupture requires prompt recognition by the ultrasound or magnetic resonance imaging of the liver to confirm the diagnosis of subcapsular hematoma, hemorrhage, or rupture.

Serum transaminase and lactic dehydrogenase levels frequently increase in patients with pre-eclampsia. The extent of liver enzyme elevation in pre-eclamptic patients correlates with the disease severity. Plasma pseudo-cholinesterase activity is decreased in pre-eclamptic patients as compared with normal gravid women (Kambam *et al.*, 1987). This decrease is not due to the effect of magnesium used to treat the disorder (Kambam *et al.*, 1988b). Although plasma pseudo-cholinesterase levels are decreased, the duration of action of succinylcholine and ester local anesthetics is seldom affected (Kambam *et al.*, 1987).

Uteroplacental perfusion

During normal pregnancy, the uteroplacental bed constitutes a low resistance circuit with continuous diastolic flow (low systolic/diastolic ratio). Pre-eclamptic women have decreased uteroplacental perfusion leading to intra-uterine growth retardation (IUGR) of the fetus. In pre-eclampsia, downstream resistance increases, with a decrease in diastolic velocity and an increase in systolic/diastolic ratio (Trudinger and Cook, 1990). Pre-eclampsia can be categorized as severe if there is evidence of IUGR or oligohydramnios.

Treatment

Hospitalization and bed rest may provide effective treatment for women with mild pre-eclampsia. Initially the primary goals of management include: (1) prevention of convulsions; (2) control of hypertension; (3) stabilization of cardiovascular status and optimization of intravascular volume.

Prevention of convulsions

Initially, the primary therapeutic goal is to prevent convulsions. Magnesium sulfate (Mg^{2+}) remains the treatment of choice for seizure prophylaxis in North America and is gaining popularity in the United Kingdom. In North America magnesium sulfate is the drug of choice because it has several positive effects. Magnesium sulfate: (1) depresses both central and peripheral nervous systems. The mechanism of action of Mg^{2+} involves general-ized central nervous system (CNS) depression which is mediated by N-methyl-D-aspartate (NMDA) receptors; (2) reduces hyperreflexia; (3) acts at the neuromuscular junction by decreas-ing (i) the amount of acetylcholine liberated from the presynaptic junction, (ii) the sensitivity of the motor end plate to acetylcholine, and (iii) the excitability of muscle membrane; (4) produces mild to moderate vasodilation; (5) depresses uterine hyperactivity, to improve uterine blood flow; (6) suppresses cortical neuronal burst firing and electro-encephalographic spike generation; and (7) opposes Ca^{2+}-dependent arterial constriction and relieves vasospasm. Because Mg^{2+} impairs peripheral neuromuscular transmission at the neuromuscular junction, the intensity of the neuromuscular block following the administration of muscle relaxants during general anesthesia correlates with elevated serum magnesium and decreased serum calcium levels (Ramanathan et al., 1988a).

The other benefits of Mg^{2+} include:

(a) vasodilation in vascular beds (Sibai, 2003);
(b) mild antihypertensive effect;
(c) increased production of cGMP (Barton et al., 1992);
(d) inhibition of synthesis of TxA_2;
(e) attenuation of the vascular response to pressor substances;
(f) decreased levels of angiotensin-converting enzyme (ACE) (Sipes et al., 1989);
(g) lowering the plasma endothelin-1 levels;
(h) increased production of prostacyclin by endothelial cells (Watson et al., 1986). The results of a recent thromboelastographic study indicated that Mg^{2+} does not affect overall coagulation (Harnett et al., 2001).

Magnesium sulfate is administered by continu-ous intravenous infusion with a loading dose of 6 g over 15–20 min, followed by a maintenance dose of $2\,g\,h^{-1}$. This regimen gives adequate, therapeutic serum magnesium levels in the majority of patients. The therapeutic range is $5.0–7.0\,mg\,dl^{-1}$. Pulmonary function may be transiently affected even when magnesium level is in the therapeutic range. Toxic levels of magnesium result in accidental overdose or decreased elimination (Figure 30.4 and Table 30.4). The treatment is administration of calcium chloride to reverse the effects of Mg^{2+} and to provide cardio-respiratory support. Mg^{2+} is also used in the treatment of eclampsia in bolus dose of 4 g IV.

Control of hypertension

The second important goal is to control the patient's blood pressure. Most anesthesiologists use parenteral antihypertensive therapy for short-term blood pressure control in severe pre-eclampsia. The threshold for treatment is a diastolic blood pressure of 105–110 mmHg or a

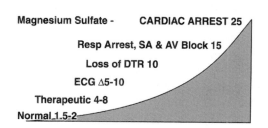

Figure 30.4 Magnesium sulfate therapy toxicity, and complications.

Table 30.4. Magnesium therapy and complication

Plasma levels (mg dl^{-1})	Effects
25	Cardiac arrest
15	Respiratory paralysis
15	Sinoatrial and atrioventricular block
10	Loss of deep rendon reflexes
5.0–10	Electrocardiographic
	– Changes (P–Q interval)
	– Widening of QRS complex
4.0–8.0	Therapeutic range
1.5–2.0	Normal plasma level

Effects of increasing levels of magnesium sulfate.

mean arterial pressure (MAP) of 125–126 mmHg. The aim of therapy is to maintain a diastolic blood pressure of 90–105 mmHg or a mean blood pressure (MAP) of 105–125 mmHg (Sibai, 1996). Afterload reduction with appropriate antihypertensive agents is important. Elevated systemic vascular resistance not only limits the cardiac output, but can also lead to endothelial cell damage and intravascular agglutination.

Hydralazine

In the past, hydralazine was the antihypertensive of choice for acute blood pressure control during pregnancy. Hydralazine is a direct vasodilator that lowers mean arterial pressure and systemic vascular resistance, increases cardiac output, stroke volume and heart rate without affecting pulmonary capillary wedge pressure (Cotton *et al.*, 1985). Hydralazine also increases renal blood flow. Hydralazine was thought to increase the placental blood flow (Jouppila *et al.*, 1985). However, studies have shown that it may decrease uterine blood flow by as much as 25% (Lipshitz *et al.*, 1987; Lunell *et al.*, 1983), and it may be associated with neonatal thrombocytopenia (Vink and Moodley, 1982). The dose is 5 mg intravenously every 20 min, as needed up to a cumulative dose of 20 mg. The onset of action is approximately 20 min (Sibai, 1996). The slow onset, delayed peak effect, and compensatory tachycardia make hydralazine a less than ideal agent to attenuate the hypertensive response to laryngoscopy and intubation during the administration of general anesthesia in pre-eclamptic women.

Labetalol

Labetalol is a combined alpha- and beta-adrenergic receptor antagonist (ratio 1:3 when given orally and 1:7 when given intravenously). When compared, labetalol is found to be as, if not more, effective than hydralazine (Mabie *et al.*, 1987). Labetalol decreases maternal systemic vascular resistance without increasing heart rate or decreasing cardiac index, uterine blood flow or fetal heart rate (Morgan *et al.*, 1993). The initial intravenous dose of labetalol is 10–20 mg and this can be doubled every 10 min to a maximum dose of 300 mg. Labetalol crosses the placental barrier, but neonatal hypoglycemia and hypotension, initially thought to be a theoretical concern, are rarely seen (Rogers *et al.*, 1990).

Sodium nitroprusside (SNP)

A powerful smooth muscle vasodilator, its use is limited to situations such as acute hypertensive crisis, severe intractable hypertension and occasionally blunting of the hypertensive response to tracheal intubation (Ellis *et al.*, 1982). Typically administered at an initial dose of $0.5 \, \mu g \, kg^{-1} \, min^{-1}$, the dose is increased gradually to control blood pressure. The major concern of SNP is the potential for fetal cyanide toxicity, but administration of low doses for short duration is deemed safe (Naulty, 2003).

Nitroglycerin (NTG)

Nitroglycerin is a venodilator, which by means of its intracellular degradation to nitric oxide stimulates guanalate cyclase resulting in an increase in cGMP production. NTG lowers MAP, PCWP, and CI, but has no effect on CVP, SV, and HR (Cotton et al., 1986). The indications for its use are similar to those of SNP. NTG initial dose is $0.5-1 \, \mu g \, kg^{-1} \, min^{-1}$ and may be increased gradually until a satisfactory response occurs.

Calcium-channel blocking agents

Nifedipine and nicardipine, inhibit the influx of extracellular calcium into smooth muscle cells through slow channels. The vascular effects predominate in arterial and arteriolar smooth muscle. Nifedipine, given orally, lowers MAP reliably and safely within 10–30 min (Abdelwahab et al., 1995). Nicardipine has less negative inotropic effects than nifedipine and has more selective action on peripheral vasculature. Both nifedipine and nicardipine may theoretically enhance the cardiotoxic effects of magnesium sulfate, but in practice, with therapeutic levels of magnesium and normal dosages of calcium channel blockers, hypotension and myocardial depression are very uncommon when these agents are used simultaneously. Nifedipine has been reported to potentiate and prolong the neuromuscular blocking effects of magnesium (Snyder and Cardwell, 1989).

Stabilization of cardiovascular status and optimization of intravascular volume

The third important goal of the team is to stabilize the patient's cardiovascular status. Stabilization includes: (1) appropriate hemodynamic monitoring, (2) adequate volume resuscitation, and (3) adequate perfusion status.

Evaluation of the patient's fluid balance must include a strict intake/output chart, placement of an indwelling urinary catheter and (if possible) an assessment of the patient's current weight. The goal of fluid therapy is to provide an ideal intravascular volume, to maintain a satisfactory urinary output, to have immediate intravenous access for the administration of therapeutic agents, and to compensate for any reduction in preload and after-load during the administration of epidural anesthesia.

There is a paucity of data regarding the ideal volume and type of intravenous fluid (crystalloid or colloid) for patients with pre-eclampsia. Pre-eclampsia is associated with a complex set of hemodynamic changes and it is very difficult to predict how patients will respond to fluid loading (Young et al., 2000). Excessive administration of crystalloid or colloid may result in pulmonary or cerebral edema. There is little evidence that colloid preloading prior to regional anesthesia is more beneficial than crystalloid solutions. Belfort (1995) demonstrated a beneficial effect of volume expansion with a colloid solution in patients with severe pre-eclampsia. Colloid infusion resulted in an increase in CO, a decrease in SVR, improved regional perfusion, and an increase in oxygen delivery. However, the use of certain colloids is debatable. The use of albumin for plasma volume expansion versus no albumin was studied in nonpregnant patients. The outcome study demonstrated that albumin increased the risk of death (Cochrane Injuries Group, 1998). Similarly, increased mortality was associated with the use of colloid for resuscitation when compared to crystalloid (Alderson et al., 2003). Currently, there is insufficient scientific evidence to make a recommendation to select colloid versus crystalloid in pre-eclamptic patients.

Patients with mild pre-eclampsia do not need any special monitoring and will usually tolerate prophylactic hydration.

The current consensus opinion is that invasive hemodynamic monitoring is not necessary for safe fluid management. In the few cases where an assessment of the intravascular status is needed echocardiographic evaluation is often all that is required. Occasionally, complicated patients with precarious hemodynamic or respiratory status will need minute-by-minute assessment of the central hemodynamics and in these patients a pulmonary artery catheter may be required.

Indications for invasive hemodynamic monitoring with a pulmonary artery catheter have traditionally been as follows:

(1) persistent oliguria unresponsive to fluid challenges;
(2) intractable severe hypertension unresponsive to antihypertensive therapy;
(3) clinical or radiological evidence of pulmonary edema;
(4) evidence of preexisting cardiovascular conditions.

Recently the American Society of Anesthesiologists (ASA) Task Force on Pulmonary Artery Catheterization published their Practice Guidelines for pulmonary artery (PA) catheterization (1993). The ASA established the task force on PA catheterization in 1991 to examine the evidence for benefits and risks from PA catheter use in settings encountered by anesthesiologists. By the time the ASA guidelines were adopted in 1992 and published in 1993 several groups had issued statements on the appropriate indications for PA catheter and on competency requirements for hemodynamic monitoring. In subsequent years, a variety of studies, most notably an investigation by Connors *et al.*, raised doubts about the effectiveness and safety of PA catheterization (1996).

Scientific outcome studies regarding the effectiveness of PA catheterization in obstetrics and gynecology is lacking. PA catheterization has been recommended for severe pre-eclampsia (Clark and Cotton, 1988), case reports have supported its value (Hjertberg *et al.*, 1991) and its use in critical illness seems common (Collop and Sahn, 1993) but controlled clinical outcome studies have not been reported. The authors believe that a severe pre-eclamptic patient who develops pulmonary edema and has persistent oliguria would benefit from hemodynamic monitoring with a PA catheter. Evidence regarding the adverse effects of PA catheter comes from studies that examined multiple complications (Boyd *et al.*, 1983; Davies *et al.*, 1982; De Lange *et al.*, 1979; Elliott *et al.*, 1979; Gill, 2003; Horst *et al.*, 1984; Katz *et al.*, 1977; Kelso, 1997; Nehme, 1980; Polanczyk *et al.*, 2001; Rosenwasser *et al.*, 1995; Shah *et al.*, 1984; Sise *et al.*, 1981) and from studies of specific complication. Technologies such as ultrasound guided venous cannulation are now available and may reduce the risk of catheter misplacement (Andropoulos *et al.*, 1999; Conway and Wadsworth, 1999; Denys *et al.*, 1991, 1993; Troianos *et al.*, 1996; Verghese *et al.*, 1999).

In pre-eclamptic patients with low urinary output who are unresponsive to multiple fluid challenges, patients with pulmonary edema, and in those with intractable hypertension invasive monitoring may become necessary (Young and Johanson, 2001).

Timing of delivery

The final and most important goal for the obstetrician is to time the delivery. After the patient is stabilized, timing of the delivery is important so that the mother and fetus tolerate the delivery process and the fetus receives the best chance of extrauterine survival.

Anesthetic management

Pre-anesthetic evaluation

It is important for the anesthesiologist to be involved early so as to help with control of the hypertension, stabilization of the hemodynamic status, and optimization of intravascular resuscitation. It is also prudent to have a well thought out,

Table 30.5. Assessment parameters to evaluate extent of disease process

Hematologic	Hematocrit
	Platelet count/platelet function
	Studies
	PT, PTT, fibrinogen, FDP
	Peripheral smear
Liver function	SGOT
	Serum glutamic pyruvic
	transaminase
	LDH
	Alkaline phosphatase
	Serum bilirubin (Indirect)
	Serum glucose
	Abdominal sonogram
	Magnetic resonance imaging
	(severe epigastric pain)
Renal function	Urine output
	Blood urea nitrogen
	Creatinine
	Uric acid
	Creatinine clearance
Pancreatic function	Serum amylase
(pancrease)	
Fetoplacental function	Fetal monitoring
	Fetal maturity

FDP = fibrin degradation products.

yet flexible, anesthetic plan, since the situation may change suddenly.

It is vital to assess the extent of the disease process in the mother and its effects on the fetus. Hematological studies and liver, renal, and, in some cases, pancreatic tests are indicated to assess the disease process in the patient. Fetal evaluation should be carried out expeditiously once maternal condition is stabilized. The various assessment parameters are outlined in Table 30.5.

Maternal monitoring

For patients with mild pre-eclampsia, routine monitoring with pulse oximeter and automatic blood pressure cuff are often sufficient. For those with severe pre-eclampsia, a radial arterial catheter is recommended for accurate monitoring of arterial blood pressure and for blood sampling (arterial blood gases, complete blood count with platelets, coagulation panel, renal and liver function tests, and appropriate drug levels).

Analgesia for labor and delivery

Clinical experience supported by the literature shows that the use of epidural analgesia is an acceptable and appropriate technique for pre-eclamptic patients in labor (Jouppila *et al.*, 1982). Significant thrombocytopenia and coagulopathy contraindicates regional anesthesia, and thrombocytopenia occurs in approximately 18% of women with pre-eclampsia. The occurrence may be as high as 50% in those with severe pre-eclampsia and eclampsia. The anesthesia literature indicates that the accepted platelet count for safe regional anesthesia is $100,000\,\mathrm{mm}^{-3}$. The minimum platelet count above which it is safe to place a regional anesthetic is unknown. Bromage (1993), has recommended against the use of an epidural anesthetic in patients whose platelet count is less than $100,000\,\mathrm{mm}^{-3}$. However, others have argued that it is safe to administer an epidural anesthetic when the platelet count is less than $100,000\,\mathrm{mm}^{-3}$ and this viewpoint is supported by the results of two retrospective studies (Rasmus *et al.*, 1989; Rolbin *et al.*, 1988). Recently, Beilin *et al.* reported the largest series of parturients in whom an epidural anesthetic had been placed without complications despite a platelet count of less than $100,000\,\mathrm{mm}^{-3}$. None of their patients had any documented postpartum neurological problems. If the decision is made to proceed with regional anesthesia in thrombocytopenic patients, Beilin *et al.* (1997) recommend:

(1) using the lowest concentration of local anesthetic necessary;
(2) examination every 1–2 h to assess the extent of the motor block – they state that excessive motor block that is out of proportion to what is

expected should warrant immediate computed tomography or magnetic resonance imaging; and

(3) taking the entire clinical presentation of the patient into account prior to performing an epidural anesthetic.

The risk–benefit ratio of epidural/spinal hematoma with regional anesthesia versus general anesthesia in the pre-eclamptic patient with a difficult airway should be evaluated carefully (Crosby, 1991; Hew-Wing et al., 1989; Voulgaropoulos and Palmer, 1993).

The authors utilize a thorough clinical history and physical examination to rule out evidence of easy bruising, bleeding gums, petechiae, the evolution of the thrombocytopenia, coagulation tests and the thromboelastograph (Orlikowski et al., 1996) before taking the decision to perform a neuraxial block in pre-eclamptic patients with thrombocytopenia. In our practice, we tend to rely on the TEG and have found that the TEG variables, K time and MA, have a strong correlation with platelet count, whereas the bleeding time has no correlation with the platelet count, as shown in (Figures 30.5 and 30.6). Further, TEG results demonstrate that an MA of 53 mm (the lower limit for normal pregnancy) correlates with a platelet count of 54,000 mm^{-3} and adequate clot function. Because a platelet count range of 40,000–75,000 mm^{-3} falls within the 95% confidence limits (Orlikowski et al., 1996), we recommend that patients diagnosed with pre-eclampsia/eclampsia and HELLP syndrome, and who have a platelet count of above 75,000 mm^{-3} (upper limit of 95% confidence limit) with normal hemostasis, should not be denied regional anesthesia. Large-scale studies are still required to confirm the applicability and reliability of TEG in pregnancy, and use of this methodology in pre-eclampsia should not be regarded as a standard of care.

The benefits of epidural labor analgesia include:
(a) complete pain relief during labor;
(b) attenuation of any exaggerated hypertensive response to pain;

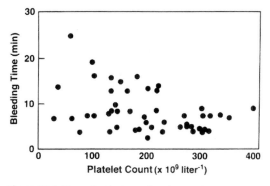

Figure 30.5 Thromboelastography changes in pre-eclampsia and eclampsia. Correction between bleeding time and platelet count. There was only a weak ($r = 0.41$, $P = 0.003$) correlation between the two variables. (From Orlikowski et al., 1996, with permission.)

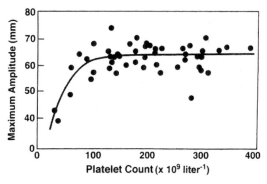

Figure 30.6 Thromboelastography changes in pre-eclampsia and eclampsia. Correction between TEG parameter; – maximum amplitude and platelet count. The equation MA = $63.9 \times (1 - \exp\{-0.033 \text{ platelets}\})$ represents a negative exponential curve of best fit which has been calculated using a non-linear regression procedure. (From Orlikowski et al., 1996, with permission.)

(c) the sympathetic block reduces the circulating levels of catecholamines and stress-related hormones, which facilitates blood pressure control;
(d) the vasodilation secondary to the sympathetic block improves the intervillous blood flow;

(e) it results in stable cardiac output; and

(f) the block can be extended to provide surgical anesthesia for instrumental or surgical delivery.

With judicious hydration and slow induction of the sympathetic block, hypotension can be minimized with minimal change in CVP, CI, and PCWP (Newsome *et al.*, 1986). If hypotension occurs, additional boluses of crystalloid should be administered and the patient should be placed in a full lateral position, preferably on her left side. Supplemental oxygen is indicated, and if these measures fail, a vasopressor such as ephedrine (5–10 mg) is administered to restore the maternal blood pressure.

Maintenance of analgesia throughout labor can be accomplished with the use of a continuous infusion or patient-controlled epidural analgesia (PCEA) device. The PCEA labor analgesia technique has the advantage of requiring less total drug (both bupivacaine and fentanyl) for the same level of analgesia (Gambling, 2003b). Currently a mixture of a low concentration of bupivacaine (0.0625%) and a lipid-soluble narcotic such as fentanyl (2 µg ml^{-1}) has been shown to provide excellent sensory analgesia with minimal or no motor block. Administration of 0.0625% or 0.125% bupivacaine with a lipid-soluble narcotic results in better analgesia than bupivacaine alone (Russell and Reynolds, 1996).

Other local anesthetics, such as ropivacaine and levobupicaine, may be used, but the superiority of these agents compared to bupivacaine is not established. The use of epinephrine should be avoided, because accidental intravascular injection into an epidural vessel can result in an exaggerated hypertensive response.

Combined-spinal epidural technique

Combined-spinal epidural regional anesthesia may be initiated using a needle-through-needle technique. In this technique a long fine-gauge spinal needle is placed through a properly sited epidural needle, and a small dose of lipid-soluble narcotic, such as fentanyl, or a combination of a small dose of local anesthetic and fentanyl, is injected through the spinal needle. The spinal needle is then removed, and an epidural catheter is placed through the epidural needle. The advantages of this technique are that it provides a rapid onset of spinal analgesia with sacral coverage for advanced labor and delivery, while the epidural catheter can be used for further maintenance of labor analgesia if the extent or duration of spinal analgesia is inadequate (Stacey *et al.*, 1993). This technique can be used safely to provide analgesia in patients with pre-eclampsia (Ramanathan *et al.*, 2001).

Anesthesia for Cesarean section

General considerations

There are several important general considerations in a pre-eclamptic patient scheduled for Cesarean section:

- meticulous examination of the airway;
- administration of aspiration prophylaxis;
- availability of blood products;
- pevention of aorto-caval compression;
- aministration of increased FiO$_2$ (face mask);
- etablishing a second peripheral IV;
- immediate access to a difficult airway cart;
- application of standard ASA monitoring;
- invasive hemodynamic monitoring if required; and
- monitoring of the fetal heart rate pattern until the beginning of the surgery.

Regional anesthesia

Regional anesthesia is the method of choice for Cesarean deliveries for the following reasons:

(1) lower maternal mortality as compared to general anesthesia (Hawkins *et al.*, 1997);

(2) better hemodynamic control;

(3) blunting of neuroendocrine stress response (Ramanathan *et al.*, 1991);

(4) mother is awake and is able to interact with her infant; and

(5) prevention of transient neonatal depression associated with general anesthesia.

Epidural anesthesia is the regional anesthesia technique most commonly used for pre-eclamptic patients. Hodgkinson *et al.* (1980) studied systemic and pulmonary artery pressures in severely pre-eclamptic patients undergoing Cesarean section. These investigators demonstrated a stable hemodynamic status with epidural anesthesia versus marked exacerbations in MAP and PCWP during induction, intubation and extubation with general anesthesia (Hodgkinson *et al.*, 1980).

The use of spinal anesthesia in patients with severe pre-eclampsia undergoing Cesarean section is controversial. In severely pre-eclamptic patients with decreased intravascular volume, some anesthesiologists argue that spinal anesthesia should be avoided because of the risk of severe hypotension following the sudden onset of sympathetic blockade. Recent evidence indicates that spinal anesthesia can be used in severely pre-eclamptic patients undergoing Cesarean section without any adverse maternal or fetal sequelae (Hood and Curry, 1999) and that the hemodynamic effects of spinal and epidural anesthesia are similar (Karinen *et al.*, 1996; Wallace *et al.*, 1995). A recent cohort prospective study compared the incidence and severity of spinal-associated hypotension in severely pre-eclamptic patients versus healthy normal parturients undergoing Cesarean section. This study demonstrated a lower incidence of hypotension, as defined by a 30% decrease in MAP in patients with severe pre-eclampsia undergoing Cesarean section under spinal anesthesia than in the healthy normal patients (Figure 30.7) (Aya *et al.*, 2003).

The use of the combined-spinal technique may also be considered in severe pre-eclampsia. Recent evidence indicates that hyperbaric bupivacaine in doses as low as 7.5 mg with 20 μg fentanyl provides adequate anesthesia for Cesarean section. Further, the presence of the epidural

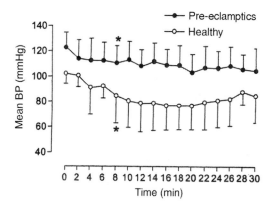

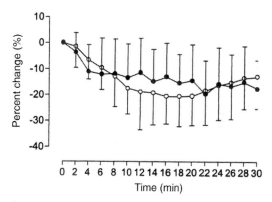

Figure 30.7 Changes in mean blood pressure (BP) after spinal anesthesia in pre-eclamptic and healthy parturients. The top panel shows raw data, whereas percentage changes are shown in the bottom panel. *Time point from which mean BP decreased significantly compared with the corresponding baseline value ($P < 0.05$). In both groups, mean BP decreased significantly from 8 min of the spinal injection until the end of the study period. (From Aya *et al.*, 2003, with permission.)

catheter provides the flexibility to extend the level and duration of the block (Ramanathan *et al.*, 2001).

Ideally, in pre-eclamptic patients undergoing urgent Cesarean section, a functioning epidural block should already be in place. The pre-existing block can be augmented with either 3% 2-chloroprocaine or pH-adjusted 2% lidocaine to rapidly provide surgical anesthesia. The fetal heart rate should be monitored in the operating room up until immediately prior to the preparation and initiation of surgery.

Published studies of spinal anesthesia in pre-eclamptics have largely excluded women with non-reassuring FHR (Wallace *et al.*, 1995). Until large randomized trials can determine the safety of spinal anesthesia in severely pre-eclamptic patients undergoing *urgent* Cesarean section for *non-reassuring* FHR, the use of a pre-established epidural block will continue to remain the preferred technique.

General anesthesia

General anesthesia is required in cases of non-reassuring FHR requiring emergency Cesarean section (no pre-existing epidural catheter), coagulopathy that precludes the use of regional anesthesia, and patient refusal of regional anesthesia.

The risks of general anesthesia in pre-eclamptic women include:

- difficult endotracheal intubation;
- the potential for aspiration of gastric contents;
- exacerbated hypertensive response to endotracheal intubation;
- impairment of intervillous blood flow; and
- drug interaction between magnesium and muscle relaxants.

Airway evaluation in pre-eclamptic patients undergoing general anesthesia is critical since endotracheal intubation in such patients may be difficult. Two of four maternal deaths in 442 cases reviewed by Sibai *et al.* (1993) resulted from cerebral hypoxia secondary to failed intubation. Airway evaluation is thus crucial, and a predicted difficult airway requires appropriate airway management preparation.

General anesthesia used in pre-eclamptic patients with hypertension causes exacerbation of blood pressure due to stimulation during laryngoscopy, tracheal intubation, and surgical incision. Any acute increase in blood pressure, particularly in the face of coagulopathy, places the patient at risk for intracranial hemorrhage. Other reasons to attenuate the hypertensive response

include a maternal risk of increased myocardial oxygen consumption leading to myocardial infarction, cardiac arrhythmias, and pulmonary edema. The fetus is also at risk from maternal hypertensive surges secondary to a significant reduction in uterine blood flow (Jouppila *et al.*, 1979).

Ramanathan *et al.* (1988b) prospectively evaluated the use of labetalol to attenuate the hypertensive response in pre-eclamptic women undergoing general anesthesia for Cesarean section. The labetalol group received 20 mg intravenously, followed by 10 mg increments (up to a maximum total dose of $1\,mg\,kg^{-1}$). The controls received no antihypertensive drug during induction of anesthesia. The increase in blood pressure response was less in the pre-eclamptic group.

Sodium nitroprusside (SNP) is particularly beneficial because it has an immediate onset of action and permits rapid control of blood pressure. The vasodilator action of sodium nitroprusside is thought to improve microvascular circulation and prevent worsening of the microangiopathy seen in pre-eclamptic patients with HELLP syndrome. Furthermore, nitroprusside antagonizes platelet aggregation and limits platelet consumption through its effects on cGMP (Busse, 1987). One of the negative aspects that should be considered when using SNP in the intrapartum period is the increased risk of cyanide toxicity for the mother and fetus if it is used in excess of the recommended clinical doses. The recommendation is to limit the use of SNP to a maximum of 30 min (Burke, 1991). The brief employment of SNP during induction of anesthesia should be considered safe when titrated with the use of invasive blood pressure monitoring.

Magnesium prolongs the action of muscle relaxants and therefore neuromuscular blockade should be monitored with a nerve stimulator (Ghoniem and Long, 1970) (Figure 30.8).

Postoperative care

After labor and delivery, all pre-eclamptic patients should be monitored in the recovery room or the

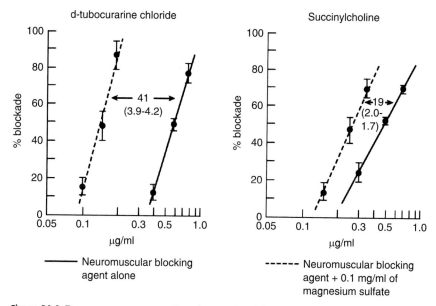

Figure 30.8 Dose—response curves of D-tubocurarine chloride and succinylcholine with and without added magnesium using a rat phrenic nerve preparation. Each point represents the mean of five observations with the standard error represented. Magnesium sulfate (0.1 mg ml^{-1}) is a subminimal dose. The magnitude of the potentiation by magnesium is shown between the curves with their fiducial limits. (From Ghoneim and Long, 1970, with permission.)

obstetric intensive care unit for the next 24 h or until adequate diuresis is established. The pre-eclamptic patient should not be discharged from the hospital until the hemodynamic and coagulation changes are corrected.

REFERENCE

Aarnoudse, J. G., Houthoff, H. J., Weits, J., Vellenga, E. and Huisjes, H. J. (1986). A syndrome of liver damage and intravascular coagulation in the last trimester of normotensive pregnancy. A clinical and histo-pathological study. *Br. J. Obstet. Gynaecol.*, **93**(2), 145–55.

Abdelwahab, W., Frishman, W. and Landau, A. (1995). Management of hypertensive urgencies and emergencies. *J. Clin. Pharmacol.*, **35**(8), 747–62.

Alderson, P, Schierhout, G. and Roberts, I. (2003). Colloids versus crystalloids for fluid resuscitation in critically ill patients. *The Cochrane Library Oxford: Update Software Issue*, **1**, 2003 (Cochrane review).

ASA. (1993). Practice guidelines for pulmonary artery catheterization. A report by the American Society of Anesthesiologists Task Force on Pulmonary Artery Catheterization. *Anesthesiology*, **78**(2), 380–94.

ASA. (in press). Practice Guidelines for Obstetrical Anesthesia. An updated report by the American Society of Anesthesiologists Task Force on Obstetrical Anesthesia. (Last amended 18 October 2006.)

Andropoulos, D. B., Stayer, S. A., Bent, S. T., *et al.* (1999). A controlled study of transesophageal echocardiography to guide central venous catheter placement in congenital heart surgery patients. *Anesth. Analg.*, **89**(1), 65–70.

Arias, F. and Mancilla-Jimenez, R. (1976). Hepatic fibrinogen deposits in pre-eclampsia. Immunofluorescent evidence. *N. Engl. J. Med.*, **295**(11), 578–82.

Aya, A. G., Mangin, R., Vialles, N., *et al.* (2003). Patients with severe preeclampsia experience less hypotension during spinal anesthesia for elective cesarean delivery than healthy parturients: a prospective cohort comparison. *Anesth. Analg.*, **97**(3), 867–72.

Barton, J. R., Sibai, B. M., Ahokas, R. A., Whybrew, W. D. and Mercer, B. M. (1992). Magnesium sulfate therapy in preeclampsia is associated with increased urinary cyclic guanosine monophosphate excretion. *Am. J. Obstet. Gynecol.*, **167**(4, Pt. 1), 931–4.

Beilin, Y., Zahn, J. and Comerford, M. (1997). Safe epidural analgesia in thirty parturients with platelet counts between 69,000 and 98,000 mm^{-3}. *Anesth. Analg.*, **85**(2), 385–8.

Belfort, M. A. (1995). Acute volume expansion with oxygen delivery and consumption but does not improve oxygen extraction in severe preeclapmsia. *J. Matern. Fetal Med.*, **4**, 57–64.

Berg, C. J., Atrash, H. K., Koonin, L. M. and Tucker, M. (1996). Pregnancy-related mortality in the United States, 1987–1990. *Obstet. Gynecol.*, **88**(2), 161–7.

Bolte, A. C., van Geijn, H. P. and Dekker, G. A. (2001). Management and monitoring of severe preeclampsia. *Eur. J. Obstet. Gynecol. Reprod. Biol.*, **96**(1), 8–20.

Boyd, K. D., Thomas, S. J., Gold, J. and Boyd, A. D. (1983). A prospective study of complications of pulmonary artery catheterizations in 500 consecutive patients. *Chest*, **84**(3), 245–9.

Brimacombe, J. (2003). Acute pharyngolaryngeal oedema and preclamptic toxaemia. *Anesth. Obstet.*, **20**, 97.

Brock-Utne, J. G. (2003). Laryngeal oedema associated with pre-eclamptic toxaemia. *Anaesthesia*, **32**, 556.

Bromage, P. R. (1993). Neurologic complications of regional anesthesia for obstetrics. *Anesth. Obstet.*, 443–4.

Brown, M. A., Zammit, V. C. and Lowe, S. A. (1989). Capillary permeability and extracellular fluid volumes in pregnancy-induced hypertension. *Clin. Sci. (Lond.)*, **77**(6), 599–604.

Burke, M. E. (1991). Hypertension in pregnancy. In: *Critical Care Obstetrics*, ed. C. Harvey. Gaithersburg, Aspen.

Burrows, R. F., Hunter, D. J., Andrew, M. and Kelton, J. G. (1987). A prospective study investigating the mechanism of thrombocytopenia in preeclampsia. *Obstet. Gynecol.*, **70**(3, Pt. 1), 334–8.

Busse, R. (1987). Endothelium-derived relaxant factor inhibits platelet activation. *Arch. Pharm.*, **366**(5), 566–71.

Campbell, D. M. (2003). Evans blue disappearance rate in normal and preeclamptic pregnancy. *Clin. Exp. Hypertens.*, **2**(1), 163–9.

Chadwick, H. D., Wall, M. H. and Chandler, W. (1993). Thromboelastography in mild and severe pre-eclampsia. *Anesthesiology*, **79**, A992. Ref. Type: Abstract.

Chang, A. B. (2004). Physiologic changes of pregnancy. In: *Obstetric Anesthesia, Principles and Practice* (3rd edn), ed. D. H. Chestnut. St Louis, Mosby.

Channing-Rodgers, R. P. (2003). A critical reappraisal of the bleeding time. *Semin. Thromb. Hemost.*, **16**(1), 1–20.

Clark, S. L. and Cotton, D. B. (1988). Clinical indications for pulmonary artery catheterization in the patient with severe preeclampsia. *Am. J. Obstet. Gynecol.*, **158**(3, Pt. 1), 453–8.

Clark, S. L., Greenspoon, J. S., Aldahl, D. and Phelan, J. P. (1986). Severe preeclampsia with persistent oliguria: management of hemodynamic subsets. *Am. J. Obstet. Gynecol.*, **154**(3), 490–4.

Clark, S. L., Cotton, D. B., Lee, W., *et al.* (1989). Central hemodynamic assessment of normal term pregnancy. *Am. J. Obstet. Gynecol.*, **161**(6, Pt. 1), 1439–42.

Cochrane Injuries Group Albumin Reviewers. (1998). Human albumin administration in critical patients: systemic review of randomized trials. *Br. J. Anaesth.*, **317**, 235–40.

Collop, N. A. and Sahn, S. A. (1993). Critical illness in pregnancy. An analysis of 20 patients admitted to a medical intensive care unit. *Chest*, **103**(5), 1548–52.

Connors, A. F. Jr., Speroff, T., Dawson, N. V., *et al.* (1996). The effectiveness of right heart catheterization in the initial care of critically ill patients. SUPPORT Investigators. *J. Am. Med. Ass.*, **276**(11), 889–97.

Conway, D. H. and Wadsworth, R. (1999). Portable ultrasound for central venous cannulation. *Br. J. Anaesth.*, **83**(6), 964.

Costabile, G. (2003). Spinal epidural hematoma. *Surg. Neurol.*, **21**, 489–92. Ref. Type: Abstract.

Cotton, D. B., Gonik, B. and Dorman, K. F. (1985). Cardiovascular alterations in severe pregnancy-induced hypertension seen with an intravenously given hydralazine bolus. *Surg. Gynecol. Obstet.*, **161**(3), 240–4.

Cotton, D. B., Longmire, S., Jones, M. M., Dorman, K. F., Tessem, J. and Joyce, T. H., III. (1986). Cardiovascular alterations in severe pregnancy-induced hypertension: effects of intravenous nitroglycerin coupled with blood volume expansion. *Am. J. Obstet. Gynecol.*, **154**(5), 1053–9.

Cotton, D. B., Lee, W., Huhta, J. C. and Dorman, K. F. (1988). Hemodynamic profile of severe pregnancy-induced hypertension. *Am. J. Obstet. Gynecol.*, **158**(3, Pt. 1), 523–9.

Crosby, E. T. (1991). Obstetrical anaesthesia for patients with the syndrome of haemolysis, elevated liver enzymes and low platelets. *Can. J. Anaesth.*, **38**(2), 227–33.

Dadak, C., Ulrich, W. and Sinzinger, H. (1984). Morphological changes in the umbilical arteries of babies born to pre-eclamptic mothers: an ultrastructural study. *Placenta*, **5**(5), 419–26.

Davies, M. J., Cronin, K. D. and Domaingue, C. M. (1982). Pulmonary artery catheterisation. An assessment of risks and benefits in 220 surgical patients. *Anaesth. Int. Care*, **10**(1), 9–14.

de Belder, A., Lees, C., Martin, J., Moncada, S. and Campbell, S. (1995). Treatment of HELLP syndrome with nitric oxide donor. *Lancet*, **345**(8942), 124–5.

Dekker, G. A. and Sibai, B. M. (1993). Low-dose aspirin in the prevention of preeclampsia and fetal growth retardation: rationale, mechanisms, and clinical trials. *Am. J. Obstet. Gynecol.*, **168**(1, Pt. 1), 214–27.

Dekker, G. A. and Sibai, B. M. (1998). Etiology and pathogenesis of preeclampsia: current concepts. *Am. J. Obstet. Gynecol.*, **179**(5), 1359–75.

De Lange, J. J., Stamenkovic, L. and den Otter, G. (1979). Pulmonary circulation pressures in surgical patients. The use of the Swan–Ganz catheter. *Arch. Chir. Neerl.*, **31**(1), 17–27.

Denys, B. G., Uretsky, B. F., Reddy, P. S., Ruffner, R. J., Sandhu, J. S. and Breishlatt, W. M. (1991). An ultrasound method for safe and rapid central venous access. *N. Engl. J. Med.*, **324**(8), 566.

Denys, B. G., Uretsky, B. F. and Reddy, P. S. (1993). Ultrasound-assisted cannulation of the internal jugular vein. A prospective comparison to the external landmark-guided technique. *Circulation*, **87**(5), 1557–62.

Dizon-Townson, D. S., Nelson, L. M., Easton, K. and Ward, K. (1996). The factor V Leiden mutation may predispose women to severe preeclampsia. *Am. J. Obstet. Gynecol.*, **175**(4, Pt. 1), 902–5.

Dobb, G. (1978). Laryngeal oedema complicating obstetric anaesthesia. *Anaesthesia*, **33**(9), 839–40.

Ebert, R. J. (2003). Post partum airway obstruction after vaginal delivery. *Anaesth. Int. Care*, **20**, 365.

Elliott, C. G., Zimmerman, G. A. and Clemmer, T. P. (1979). Complications of pulmonary artery catheterization in the care of critically ill patients. A prospective study. *Chest*, **76**(6), 647–52.

Ellis, S. C., Wheeler, A. S., James, F. M., III, *et al.* (1982). Fetal and maternal effects of sodium nitroprusside used to counteract hypertension in gravid ewes. *Am. J. Obstet. Gynecol.*, **143**(7), 766–70.

Farcon, E. L., Kim, M. H. and Marx, G. F. (1994). Changing Mallampati score during labour. *Can. J. Anaesth.*, **41**(1), 50–1.

Fournie, A., Monrozies, M., Pontonnier, G., Boneu, B. and Bierme, R. (1981). Factor VIII complex in normal pregnancy, pre-eclampsia and fetal growth retardation. *Br. J. Obstet. Gynaecol.*, **88**(3), 250–4.

Freidman, S. A. (2003). Pathophysiology of preeclampsia. *Clin. Perinatol.*, **18**(4), 661–82.

Gambling, D. R. (2003). Epidural infusion in labour should be abandoned in favour of patient-controlled epidural analgesia. *Int. J. Obstet. Gynecol.*, **5**, 59–63.

Gambling, D. R. (2004). Hypertensive disorder. In: *Obstetric Anesthesia, Principles and Practice* (3rd edn), ed. D. H. Chestnut. St Louis, Mosby.

Ghoneim, M. M. and Long, J. P. (1970). The interaction between magnesium and other neuromuscular blocking agents. *Anesthesiology*, **32**(1), 23–7.

Giles, C. and Inglis, T. C. (1981). Thrombocytopenia and macrothrombocytosis in gestational hypertension. *Br. J. Obstet. Gynaecol.*, **88**(11), 1115–19.

Gill, J. B. (2003). Prospective study of pulmonary artery balloon flotation catheter insertions. *J. Int. Care Med.*, **3**, 121–8.

Grisaru, D., Zwang, E., Peyser, M. R., Lessing, J. B. and Eldor, A. (1997). The procoagulant activity of red blood cells from patients with severe preeclampsia. *Am. J. Obstet. Gynecol.*, **177**(6), 1513–16.

Harnett, M. J., Datta, S. and Bhavani-Shankar, K. (2001). The effect of magnesium on coagulation in parturients with preeclampsia. *Anesth. Analg.*, **92**(5), 1257–60.

Hawkins, J. L., Koonin, L. M., Palmer, S. K. and Gibbs, C. P. (1997). Anesthesia-related deaths during obstetric delivery in the United States, 1979–1990. *Anesthesiology*, **86**(2), 277–84.

Heller, P. J., Scheider, E. P. and Marx, G. F. (1983). Pharyngolaryngeal edema as a presenting symptom in preeclampsia. *Obstet. Gynecol.*, **62**(4), 523–5.

Hew-Wing, P., Rolbin, S. H., Hew, E. and Amato, D. (1989). Epidural anaesthesia and thrombocytopenia. *Anaesthesia*, **44**(9), 775–7.

Hjertberg, R., Belfrage, P. and Hagnevik, K. (1991). Hemodynamic measurements with Swan-Ganz catheter in women with severe proteinuric gestational hypertension (pre-eclampsia). *Acta Obstet. Gynecol. Scand.*, **70**(3), 193–8.

Hodgkinson, R., Husain, F. J. and Hayashi, R. H. (1980). Systemic and pulmonary blood pressure during caesarean section in parturients with gestational hypertension. *Can. Anaesth. Soc. J.*, **27**(4), 389–94.

Hood, D. D. and Curry, R. (1999). Spinal versus epidural anesthesia for cesarean section in severely preeclamptic patients: a retrospective survey. *Anesthesiology*, **90**(5), 1276–82.

Horst, H. M., Obeid, F. N., Vij, D. and Bivins, B. A. (1984). The risks of pulmonary arterial catheterization. *Surg. Gynecol. Obstet.*, **159**(3), 229–32.

Inglis, T. C., Stuart, J., George, A. J. and Davies, A. J. (1982). Haemostatic and rheological changes in normal pregnancy and pre-eclampsia. *Br. J. Haematol.*, **50**(3), 461–5.

Joupilla, R. (2003). Laryngeal oedema as an obstetric anaesthesia complication. *Acta Anaesth. Scand.*, **24**, 97.

Jouppila, P., Kuikka, J., Jouppila, R. and Hollmen, A. (1979). Effect of induction of general anesthesia for cesarean section on intervillous blood flow. *Acta Obstet. Gynecol. Scand.*, **58**(3), 249–53.

Jouppila, P., Jouppila, R., Hollmen, A. and Koivula, A. (1982). Lumbar epidural analgesia to improve intervillous blood flow during labor in severe preeclampsia. *Obstet. Gynecol.*, **59**(2), 158–61.

Jouppila, P., Kirkinen, P., Koivula, A. and Ylikorkala, O. (1985). Effects of dihydralazine infusion on the fetoplacental blood flow and maternal prostanoids. *Obstet. Gynecol.*, **65**(1), 115–18.

Kambam, J. R., Handte, R. E., Brown, W. U. and Smith, B. E. (1986). Effect of normal and preeclamptic pregnancies on the oxyhemoglobin dissociation curve. *Anesthesiology*, **65**(4), 426–7.

Kambam, J. R., Mouton, S., Entman, S., Sastry, B. V. and Smith, B. E. (1987). Effect of pre-eclampsia on plasma cholinesterase activity. *Can. J. Anaesth.*, **34**(5), 509–11.

Kambam, J. R., Entman, S., Mouton, S. and Smith, B. E. (1988a). Effect of preeclampsia on carboxyhemoglobin levels: a mechanism for a decrease in P50. *Anesthesiology*, **68**(3), 433–4.

Kambam, J. R., Perry, S. M., Entman, S. and Smith, B. E. (1988b). Effect of magnesium on plasma cholinesterase activity. *Am. J. Obstet. Gynecol.*, **159**(2), 309–11.

Karinen, J., Rasanen, J., Alahuhta, S., Jouppila, R. and Jouppila, P. (1996). Maternal and uteroplacental haemodynamic state in pre-eclamptic patients during spinal anaesthesia for Caesarean section. *Br. J. Anaesth.*, **76**(5), 616–20.

Katz, J. D., Cronau, L. H., Barash, P. G. and Mandel, S. D. (1977). Pulmonary artery flow-guided catheters in the perioperative period. Indications and complications. *J. Am. Med. Ass.*, **237**(26), 2832–4.

Kelso, L. A. (1997). Complications associated with pulmonary artery catheterization. *New. Horiz.*, **5**(3), 259–63.

Kelton, J. G., Hunter, D. J. and Neame, P. B. (1985). A platelet function defect in preeclampsia. *Obstet. Gynecol.*, **65**(1), 107–9.

Kilby, M. D., Broughton, P. F. and Symonds, E. M. (1993). Changes in platelet intracellular free calcium in normal pregnancy. *Br. J. Obstet. Gynaecol.*, **100**(4), 375–9.

Kurzel, R. B., Au, A. H. and Rooholamini, S. A. (1996). Doppler velocimetry of hepatic blood flow in postpartum patients with HELLP syndrome (hemolysis, elevated liver enzymes, and low platelets). *Am. J. Obstet. Gynecol.*, **175**(6), 1677–8.

Lazarchick, J., Stubbs, T. M., Romein, L., Van Dorsten, J. P. and Loadholt, C. B. (1986). Predictive value of fibronectin levels in normotensive gravid women destined to become preeclamptic. *Am. J. Obstet. Gynecol.*, **154**(5), 1050–2.

Lind, S. E. (1991). The bleeding time does not predict surgical bleeding. *Blood*, **77**(12), 2547–52.

Lipshitz, J., Ahokas, R. A. and Reynolds, S. L. (1987). The effect of hydralazine on placental perfusion in the spontaneously hypertensive rat. *Am. J. Obstet. Gynecol.*, **156**(2), 356–9.

Locke, G. E., Giorgio, A. J., Biggers, S. L. Jr., Johnson, A. P. and Salem, F. (1976). Acute spinal epidural hematoma secondary to aspirin-induced prolonged bleeding. *Surg. Neurol.*, **5**(5), 293–6.

Longo, S. A., Dola, C. P. and Pridjian, G. (2003). Preeclampsia and eclampsia revisited. *South. Med. J.*, **96**(9), 891–9.

Lunell, N. O., Lewander, R., Nylund, L., Sarby, B. and Thornstrom, S. (1983). Acute effect of dihydralazine on uteroplacental blood flow in hypertension during pregnancy. *Gynecol. Obstet. Invest.*, **16**(5), 274–82.

Lyall, F. (2003). A multi-faceted vascular disorder of pregnancy. *J. Hypertens.*, **12**, 1339–45.

Mabie, W. C., Gonzalez, A. R., Sibai, B. M. and Amon, E. (1987). A comparative trial of labetalol and hydralazine in the acute management of severe hypertension complicating pregnancy. *Obstet. Gynecol.*, **70**(3, Pt. 1), 328–33.

Mabie, W. C., Ratts, T. E., Ramanathan, K. B. and Sibai, B. M. (1988). Circulatory congestion in obese hypertensive women: a subset of pulmonary edema in pregnancy. *Obstet. Gynecol.*, **72**(4), 553–8.

Mabie, W.C., Ratts, T.E. and Sibai, B.M. (1989). The central hemodynamics of severe preeclampsia. *Am. J. Obstet. Gynecol.*, **161**(6, Pt. 1), 1443–8.

Manas, K.J., Welsh, J.D., Rankin, R.A. and Miller, D.D. (1985). Hepatic hemorrhage without rupture in preeclampsia. *N. Engl. J. Med.*, **312**(7), 424–6.

Martin, J.N. Jr., Blake, P.G., Perry, K.G. Jr., McCaul, J.F., Hess, L.W. and Martin, R.W. (1991). The natural history of HELLP syndrome: patterns of disease progression and regression. *Am. J. Obstet. Gynecol.*, **164**(6, Pt. 1), 1500–9.

Matteo, R., Proverbio, T., Cordova, K., Proverbio, F. and Marin, R. (1998). Preeclampsia, lipid peroxidation, and calcium adenosine triphosphatase activity of red blood cell ghosts. *Am. J. Obstet. Gynecol.*, **178**(2), 402–8.

Maynard, J.R., Dreyer, B.E., Stemerman, M.B. and Pitlick, F.A. (1977). Tissue-factor coagulant activity of cultured human endothelial and smooth muscle cells and fibroblasts. *Blood*, **50**(3), 387–96.

Morgan, M.A., Silavin, S.L., Dormer, K.J., Fishburne, B.C. and Fishburne, J.I. Jr. (1993). Effects of labetalol on uterine blood flow and cardiovascular hemodynamics in the hypertensive gravid baboon. *Am. J. Obstet. Gynecol.*, **168**(5), 1574–9.

Morris, R.H., Vassalli, P., Beller, F.K. and McCluskey, R.T. (1964). Immunofluorescent studies of renal biopsies in the diagnosis of toxemia of pregnancy. *Obstet. Gynecol.*, **24**, 32–46.

Naulty, J. (2003). Fetal toxicity of nitroprusside in the pregnant. *Am. J. Obstet. Gynecol.*, **130**, 708–11.

Nehme, A.E. (1980). Swan–Ganz catheter: comparison of insertion techniques. *Arch. Surg.*, **115**(10), 1194–6.

Nelson, S.H. (2003). Endothelium-dependent increase in sensitivity to acetylcholine (ACH) in human uterine arteries during pregnancy. *Blood Vessels*, **24**, 218–19.

Ness, R.B. and Roberts, J.M. (1996). Heterogeneous causes constituting the single syndrome of preeclampsia: a hypothesis and its implications. *Am. J. Obstet. Gynecol.*, **175**(5), 1365–70.

Newsome, L.R., Bramwell, R.S. and Curling, P.E. (1986). Severe preeclampsia: hemodynamic effects of lumbar epidural anesthesia. *Anesth. Analg.*, **65**(1), 31–6.

Oosterhof, H., Voorhoeve, P.G. and Aarnoudse, J.G. (1994). Enhancement of hepatic artery resistance to blood flow in preeclampsia in presence or absence of HELLP syndrome (hemolysis, elevated liver enzymes, and low platelets). *Am. J. Obstet. Gynecol.*, **171**(2), 526–30.

Orlikowski, C.E., Payne, A.J., Moodley, J. and Rocke, D.A. (1992). Thromboelastography after aspirin ingestion in pregnant and non-pregnant subjects. *Br. J. Anaesth.*, **69**(2), 159–61.

Orlikowski, C.E., Rocke, D.A., Murray, W.B., *et al.* (1996). Thromboelastography changes in pre-eclampsia and eclampsia. *Br. J. Anaesth.*, **77**(2), 157–61.

Perry, K.G. Jr. and Martin, J.N. Jr. (1992). Abnormal hemostasis and coagulopathy in pre-eclampsia and eclampsia. *Clin. Obstet. Gynecol.*, **35**(2), 338–50.

Pilkington, S. (2003). Increase in Mallampati score during pregnancy. *Br. J. Anaesth.*, **74**, 638–42.

Polanczyk, C.A., Rohde, L.E., Goldman, L., *et al.* (2001). Right heart catheterization and cardiac complications in patients undergoing noncardiac surgery: an observational study. *J. Am. Med. Ass.*, **286**(3), 309–14.

Procter, A.J. and White, J.B. (1983). Laryngeal oedema in pregnancy. *Anaesthesia*, **38**(2), 167.

Ramanathan, J. (2003). Preeclampsia: fluids, drugs and anesthetic management. *Anesth. Clin. N. Amer.*, **21**, 145–63.

Ramanathan, J., Sibai, B.M., Pillai, R. and Angel, J.J. (1988a). Neuromuscular transmission studies in pre-eclamptic women receiving magnesium sulfate. *Am. J. Obstet. Gynecol.*, **158**(1), 40–6.

Ramanathan, J., Sibai, B.M., Mabie, W.C., Chauhan, D. and Ruiz, A.G. (1988b). The use of labetalol for attenuation of the hypertensive response to endotracheal intubation in preeclampsia. *Am. J. Obstet. Gynecol.*, **159**(3), 650–4.

Ramanathan, J., Sibai, B.M., Vu, T. and Chauhan, D. (1989). Correlation between bleeding times and platelet counts in women with preeclampsia undergoing cesarean section. *Anesthesiology*, **71**(2), 188–91.

Ramanathan, J., Coleman, P. and Sibai, B. (1991). Anesthetic modification of hemodynamic and neuroendocrine stress responses to cesarean delivery in women with severe preeclampsia. *Anesth. Analg.*, **73**(6), 772–9.

Ramanathan, J., Vaddadi, A.K. and Arheart, K.L. (2001). Combined spinal and epidural anesthesia with low doses of intrathecal bupivacaine in women with severe preeclampsia: a preliminary report. *Reg. Anesth. Pain. Med.*, **26**(1), 46–51.

Rappaport, V.J., Hirata, G., Yap, H.K. and Jordan, S.C. (1990). Anti-vascular endothelial cell antibodies in severe preeclampsia. *Am. J. Obstet. Gynecol.*, **162**(1), 138–46.

Rasmus, K. T., Rottman, R. L., Kotelko, D. M., Wright, W. C., Stone, J. J. and Rosenblatt, R. M. (1989). Unrecognized thrombocytopenia and regional anesthesia in parturients: a retrospective review. *Obstet. Gynecol.*, **73**(6), 943–6.

Redman, C. W. (1991). Immunology of preeclampsia. *Semin. Perinatol.*, **15**(3), 257–62.

Report of the National High Blood Pressure Education Program Working Group on High Blood Pressure in Pregnancy. (2000). *Am. J. Obstet. Gynecol.*, **183**(1), S1–22.

Rees, G. B., Pipkin, F. B., Symonds, E. M. and Patrick, J. M. (1990). A longitudinal study of respiratory changes in normal human pregnancy with cross-sectional data on subjects with pregnancy-induced hypertension. *Am. J. Obstet. Gynecol.*, **162**(3), 826–30.

Richards, A., Graham, D. and Bullock, R. (1988). Clinicopathological study of neurological complications due to hypertensive disorders of pregnancy. *J. Neurol. Neurosurg. Psychiatry*, **51**(3), 416–21.

Roberts, J. M., Taylor, R. N., Musci, T. J., Rodgers, G. M., Hubel, C. A. and McLaughlin, M. K. (1989). Preeclampsia: an endothelial cell disorder. *Am. J. Obstet. Gynecol.*, **161**(5), 1200–4.

Robertson, W. B., Brosens, I. and Dixon, G. (1975). Uteroplacental vascular pathology. *Eur. J. Obstet. Gynecol. Reprod. Biol.*, **5**(1–2), 47–65.

Rocke, D. A. and Scoones, G. P. (1992). Rapidly progressive laryngeal oedema associated with pregnancy-aggravated hypertension. *Anaesthesia*, **47**(2), 141–3.

Rogers, R. C., Sibai, B. M. and Whybrew, W. D. (1990). Labetalol pharmacokinetics in pregnancy-induced hypertension. *Am. J. Obstet. Gynecol.*, **162**(2), 362–6.

Rolbin, S. H., Abbott, D., Musclow, E., Papsin, F., Lie, L. M. and Freedman, J. (1988). Epidural anesthesia in pregnant patients with low platelet counts. *Obstet. Gynecol.*, **71**(6, Pt. 1), 918–20.

Rosenwasser, R. H., Jallo, J. I., Getch, C. C. and Liebman, K. E. (1995). Complications of Swan–Ganz catheterization for hemodynamic monitoring in patients with subarachnoid hemorrhage. *Neurosurgery*, **37**(5), 872–5.

Russell, R. and Reynolds, F. (1996). Epidural infusion of low-dose bupivacaine and opioid in labour. Does reducing motor block increase the spontaneous delivery rate? *Anaesthesia*, **51**(3), 266–73.

Samuels, P., Main, E. K., Tomaski, A., Mennuti, M. T., Gabbe, S. G. and Cines, D. B. (1987). Abnormalities in platelet antiglobulin tests in preeclamptic mothers and their neonates. *Am. J. Obstet. Gynecol.*, **157**(1), 109–13.

Sattar, N., Gaw, A., Packard, C. J. and Greer, I. A. (1996). Potential pathogenic roles of aberrant lipoprotein and fatty acid metabolism in pre-eclampsia. *Br. J. Obstet. Gynaecol.*, **103**(7), 614–20.

Scholtes, M. C., Gerretsen, G. and Haak, H. L. (1983). The factor VIII ratio in normal and pathological pregnancies. *Eur. J. Obstet. Gynecol. Reprod. Biol.*, **16**(2), 89–95.

Seager, S. J. and Macdonald, R. (1980). Laryngeal oedema and pre-eclampsia. *Anaesthesia*, **35**(4), 360–2.

Shah, K. B., Rao, T. L., Laughlin, S. and El Etr, A. A. (1984). A review of pulmonary artery catheterization in 6,245 patients. *Anesthesiology*, **61**(3), 271–5.

Sibai, B. M. (1996). Treatment of hypertension in pregnant women. *N. Engl. J. Med.*, **335**(4), 257–65.

Sibai, B. (2003). The case for magnesium sulfate in preclampsia–eclampsia. *Int. J. Obstet. Anaesth.*, **1**, 167–71.

Sibai, B. M. and Cartis, P. E. (1993). Prevention of preeclampsia: low dose aspirin in nulliparous women – a double-blind, placebo-controlled trial. *Am. J. Obstet.*, **168**, 286. Ref. Type: Abstract.

Sibai, B. M., Ramadan, M. K., Usta, I., Salama, M., Mercer, B. M. and Friedman, S. A. (1993). Maternal morbidity and mortality in 442 pregnancies with hemolysis, elevated liver enzymes, and low platelets (HELLP syndrome). *Am. J. Obstet. Gynecol.*, **169**(4), 1000–6.

Sipes, S. L., Weiner, C. P., Gellhaus, T. M. and Goodspeed, J. D. (1989). The plasma renin–angiotensin system in preeclampsia: effects of magnesium sulfate. *Obstet. Gynecol.*, **73**(6), 934–7.

Sise, M. J., Hollingsworth, P., Brimm, J. E., Peters, R. M., Virgilio, R. W. and Shackford, S. R. (1981). Complications of the flow-directed pulmonary artery catheter: a prospective analysis in 219 patients. *Crit. Care Med.*, **9**(4), 315–18.

Snyder, S. W. and Cardwell, M. S. (1989). Neuromuscular blockade with magnesium sulfate and nifedipine. *Am. J. Obstet. Gynecol.*, **161**(1), 35–6.

Spargo, G. H. (1976). The renal lesion in preeclampsia. In *Hypertension in Pregnancy*. New York: John Wiley & Sons, pp. 129–37.

Stacey, R. G., Watt, S., Kadim, M. Y. and Morgan, B. M. (1993). Single space combined spinal-extradural technique for analgesia in labour. *Br. J. Anaesth.*, **71**(4), 499–502.

Stricker, R. B., Main, E. K., Kronfield, J., *et al.* (1992). Severe post-partum eclampsia: response to plasma exchange. *J. Clin. Apheresis*, **7**(1), 1–3.

Suresh, M. S. (2003). Difficult airway in the parturient. In *Problems in Anesthesia*, ed. A. Ovassapian and D. W. Coalson. Philadelphia: Lippincott Williams & Wilkins, Inc., pp. 88–99.

Taylor, R. N., Casal, D. C., Jones, L. A., Varma, M., Martin, J. N. Jr. and Roberts, J. M. (1991). Selective effects of preeclamptic sera on human endothelial cell procoagulant protein expression. *Am. J. Obstet. Gynecol.*, **165**(6, Pt. 1), 1705–10.

Tillman Hein, H. A. (2003). Cardiorespiratory arrest with laryngeal oedema in pregnancy-induced hypertension. *Can. Anaesth. Soc. J.*, **31**, 210.

Trofatter, K. F. Jr., Howell, M. L., Greenberg, C. S. and Hage, M. L. (1989). Use of the fibrin D-dimer in screening for coagulation abnormalities in preeclampsia. *Obstet. Gynecol.*, **73**(3, Pt. 1), 435–40.

Troianos, C. A., Kuwik, R. J., Pasqual, J. R., Lim, A. J. and Odasso, D. P. (1996). Internal jugular vein and carotid artery anatomic relation as determined by ultrasonography. *Anesthesiology*, **85**(1), 43–8.

Trudinger, B. J. and Cook, C. M. (1990). Doppler umbilical and uterine flow waveforms in severe pregnancy hypertension. *Br. J. Obstet. Gynaecol.*, **97**(2), 142–8.

Vane, J. R., Anggard, E. E. and Botting, R. M. (1990). Regulatory functions of the vascular endothelium. *N. Engl. J. Med.*, **323**(1), 27–36.

Verghese, S. T., McGill, W. A., Patel, R. I., Sell, J. E., Midgley, F. M. and Ruttimann, U. E. (1999). Ultrasound-guided internal jugular venous cannulation in infants: a prospective comparison with the traditional palpation method. *Anesthesiology*, **91**(1), 71–7.

Vink, G. J. and Moodley, J. (1982). The effect of low-dose dihydralazine on the fetus in the emergency treatment of hypertension in pregnancy. *S. Afr. Med. J.*, **62**(14), 475–7.

Voulgaropoulos, D. S. and Palmer, C. M. (1993). Coagulation studies in the preeclamptic parturient: a survey. *J. Clin. Anesth.*, **5**(2), 99–104.

Wallace, D. H., Leveno, K. J., Cunningham, F. G., Giesecke, A. H., Shearer, V. E. and Sidawi, J. E. (1995). Randomized comparison of general and regional anesthesia for cesarean delivery in pregnancies complicated by severe preeclampsia. *Obstet. Gynecol.*, **86**(2), 193–9.

Watson, K. V., Moldow, C. F., Ogburn, P. L. and Jacob, H. S. (1986). Magnesium sulfate: rationale for its use in preeclampsia. *Proc. Natl Acad. Sci. U.S.A.*, **83**(4), 1075–8.

Weinstein, L. (1985). Preeclampsia/eclampsia with hemolysis, elevated liver enzymes, and thrombocytopenia. *Obstet. Gynecol.*, **66**(5), 657–60.

Young, P. and Johanson, R. (2001). Haemodynamic, invasive and echocardiographic monitoring in the hypertensive parturient. *Best Pract. Res. Clin. Obstet. Gynaecol.*, **15**(4), 605–22.

Young, P. F., Leighton, N. A., Jones, P. W., Anthony, J. and Johanson, R. B. (2000). Fluid management in severe preeclampsia (VESPA): survey of members of ISSHP. *Hypertens. Pregn.*, **19**(3), 249–59.

Zunker, P., Ley-Pozo, J., Louwen, F., Schuierer, G., Holzgreve, W. and Ringelstein, E. B. (1995). Cerebral hemodynamics in pre-eclampsia/eclampsia syndrome. *Ultrasound Obstet. Gynecol.*, **6**(6), 411–15.

Zuspan, F. P. (1991). New concepts in the understanding of hypertensive diseases during pregnancy. An overview. *Clin. Perinatol.*, **18**(4), 653–9.

31

Critical care management of severe pre-eclampsia

John Anthony

Pre-eclampsia remains one of the leading causes of maternal mortality in developing and industrialized societies and affects 2–6% of pregnant women (Duley, 1992; Hogberg *et al.*, 1994; WHO, 1988). Eclampsia with or without evidence of intracranial hemorrhage is the single most lethal complication of pre-eclampsia/eclampsia. Deaths have also been associated with pulmonary edema, HELLP syndrome, renal failure and the development of hypovolemia (commonly due to concurrent abruptio placentae). Some of the factors that predispose to a poor outcome include inadequate access to medical care resulting in delayed hospitalization and substandard care arising from inappropriate management. The provision of medical facilities is a socioeconomic priority that may not be easy to implement. The development of skills and knowledge necessary to care for critically ill pre-eclamptic women is a far more attainable goal and should be widely taught to all categories of medical staff.

Obstetric critical care is largely dependent on information derived from small (usually observational) studies, although there are now some randomized studies that inform clinical practice. The absence of an overwhelming burden of epidemiological evidence does not preclude the need for intervention and some of the principles of management, especially those based upon expert opinion alone, may change in time as further epidemiological data become available.

This chapter will briefly outline pathologic changes in the major organ systems affected in pre-eclampsia, discuss the role of monitoring in the intensive care unit, and will address the specific complications of severe pre-eclampsia that necessitate intensive care.

Neuropathology

The morbid anatomical changes associated with eclampsia are those of a swollen, pale brain together with evidence of petechial hemorrhage into the cortex, meninges and white matter. Histological findings are those of ring hemorrhages around small vessels, fibrinoid necrosis of arteriolar vessel walls as well as microhemorrhages and infarcts. These findings are consistent with ischemic damage to neuronal tissue and the vessel walls.

Radiological investigation using computerized tomography (CT) and magnetic resonance imaging (MRI) has contributed to our understanding of the pathogenesis of eclampsia by revealing a range of abnormalities that include cerebral edema and evidence of hemorrhage (Milliez *et al.*, 1990; Schwartz *et al.*, 1992). Cerebral edema typically affects the occipital lobes and the white matter but may occur in a "watershed" pattern. The latter picture represents the development of edema between the distribution territories of the major vessels supplying blood to the brain.

It has been debated whether eclamptic pathology is any different to hypertensive encephalopathy in nonpregnant patients (Donaldson, 1994). In the latter instance, the development of severe systemic hypertension exceeds the capacity of the cerebral vasculature to autoregulate flow. This results in high flow rates and barotrauma to the vessel walls. The alternative view proposed is that pre-eclamptic vasospasm alone may give rise to ischemic change.

The evidence favoring flow-related or vasogenic edema is based upon several observations. The most commonly observed changes occur in the posterior vertebro-basilar circulation, which has less sympathetic innervation and a lower autoregulatory blood pressure threshold (Schaefer et al., 1997). Single photon emission computed tomography (SPECT) and other studies have shown increased cerebral blood flow in eclamptic compared to pre-eclamptic patients (Schwartz et al., 1992; Williams and Wilson, 1995; Zunker et al., 1995). One publication establishes a positive correlation between cerebral blood flow and mean arterial pressure despite the majority of these patients having systemic mean arterial blood pressures of less than 150 mmHg. The authors conclude that the increased flow results from loss of normal endothelial homeostatic function rather than severe systemic hypertension overcoming the normal upper limit of cerebral autoregulation.

A number of investigators have argued against the notion of increased flow. Morriss et al. could find no evidence of either vasospasm or increased flow in a group of patients subject to phase-contrast MRI examination despite all eight of the eclamptic patients in this group having abnormal T2-weighted brain images (Morriss et al., 1997). However, the cohort investigated had all been treated with magnesium sulfate prior to investigation. Sibai (and others) have also pointed out that as many as 20% of women have seizure activity when their last measured diastolic blood pressures were below 90 mmHg (Sibai, 1990). They argue that blood pressure as low as this would render failure of the cerebral vascular autoregulatory function unlikely.

Despite these arguments against the likelihood of increased flow, the most recent evidence derived from Doppler ultrasound studies document increased cerebral flow rather than vasospasm. The only exception are reports concerning the ophthalmic vessels and central retinal vessels that exhibit increased pulsatility indices that decrease after the administration of vasodilators (Belfort, 1992; Belfort and Saade, 1993). Combined transcranial ultrasonography and MRI angiography have been used to document evidence of resolving postpartum vasospasm following eclampsia in individual case reports.

In summary, all the published studies may be flawed in one way or another. Most importantly, the influence of drugs such as magnesium sulfate and dihydralazine may confound the results of many studies. The use of dihydralazine is of particular concern because of evidence that it may diminish cerebral autoregulation and has been associated with increasing intracranial pressure when administered to nonpregnant neurosurgical patients with elevated intracranial pressure (Overgaard and Skinhoj, 1975).

It is therefore likely that both microcirculatory vasospasm as well as diminished autoregulation of cerebral blood flow are implicated in the pathogenesis of eclamptic seizures. In future, it may be possible to delineate different groups of patients with predominant vasogenic or cytotoxic edema and this may influence management significantly.

Cardiorespiratory pathology and pathophysiology

Patients with severe pre-eclampsia are predisposed to the development of pulmonary edema because of low oncotic pressure and altered capillary permeability with or without left ventricular dysfunction (systolic or diastolic) (Belfort et al., 1991; Visser and Wallenberg, 1991). Left ventricular diastolic dysfunction increases the risk of pulmonary edema following rapid plasma volume expansion; even small aliquots of intravenous fluids have been shown to cause a sharp rise in left-sided filling pressures, usually without any changes in central venous pressure. Iatrogenic fluid overload is consequently a frequent cause of pulmonary edema among these patients. Undiagnosed occult valvular disease may also increase the risk of pulmonary edema in hypertensive patients.

Other causes of respiratory distress include atelectasis and aspiration pneumonia. Atelectasis giving rise to respiratory distress may follow surgery and is also seen among patients with HELLP syndrome, who often splint the right hemi-diaphragm because of pain associated with hepatic ischemia. Aspiration pneumonia may develop as a result of eclampsia.

Adult respiratory distress syndrome (ARDS) is often cited as a complication of pre-eclampsia but is an unlikely primary complication of the disease although it may follow aspiration pneumonia or prolonged ventilation. Reporting the occurrence of ARDS in an obstetric intensive care unit, Mabie et al. found only 16 cases of respiratory distress attributable to ARDS over a 6-year period (Mabie et al., 1992). Only 4 of these 16 cases were linked to pre-eclampsia/eclampsia. Three of these four cases had additional complications that may have contributed to the development of ARDS (including aspiration pneumonia, lupus nephritis, sepsis and a ruptured liver hematoma with massive blood transfusion). The fourth case had pulmonary edema that developed into ARDS after the patient had a respiratory arrest. These observations are important because most cases of respiratory distress will have a cardiogenic component amenable to intervention. ARDS should never be accepted as a primary diagnosis in pre-eclampsia/eclampsia.

Renal pathology

Renal pathology is the result of anatomical changes within the glomerulus combined with changes in perfusion. The pathognomonic renal lesion of pre-eclampsia is that of glomerular capillary endotheliosus. These are glomeruli partially obstructed by lipid-laden mesangial cells giving rise to intrinsic ischemia aggravated by pre-renal vasospasm and a low cardiac output. Ischemia may result in acute tubular necrosis, although this occurs most commonly when a hypovolemic insult is superimposed upon pre-eclamptic

pathology. Hemoglobinuria from patients with the HELLP syndrome may also give rise to renal impairment.

Liver pathology

HELLP syndrome results from the development of hepatic ischemia in a periportal distribution. Examination of the liver surface will also show multiple areas of subcapsular petechial hemorrhage. Large subcapsular hematomas presumably develop from enlarging hemorrhages that become confluent. The histological findings are those of periportal hemorrhage and necrosis. The vasculature in the areas of ischemic change show evidence of fibrinoid necrosis. Microangiopathic changes result in platelet consumption and low-grade intravascular coagulation with consequent hemolysis.

Hemolysis and hemoglobinuria contribute to the development of renal failure and the characteristic passage of "Coke" colored urine.

Critical care and critical care monitoring

The philosophy of critical care is that of closely supervised individual care based upon the regular measurement of an extended range of biophysical variables with as little recourse to empirical therapy as possible.

In the context of pre-eclampsia as a hypertensive condition leading to multiorgan ischemia, the measurement of hemodynamic variables including cardiac output is critical. An adequate cardiac output is essential to deliver oxygenated blood to the peripheral tissues with a low output reflecting either hypovolemia or ventricular failure. Furthermore, knowledge of the cardiac output will determine management and will also allow calculation of other derived hemodynamic values, including vascular resistance, as well as oxygen delivery and consumption indices.

Cardiac output may be measured using the Fick principle, which states that the amount of a substance taken up by the body per unit time equals the difference between the arterial and venous levels multiplied by the blood flow. This principle has been modified to accommodate other markers including dye-dilution techniques and the thermodilution principle of the pulmonary artery catheter. In the latter case, iced water is the marker injected into the right atrium with a probe measuring the temperature of the blood flowing through the pulmonary artery, thus allowing the derivation of the cardiac output from the area under the curve. This technique is clinically robust and remains the cornerstone of hemodynamic monitoring in many intensive care units. However, alternative methods of monitoring have been developed in order to avoid the need to cannulate peripheral and central vessels. Ultrasound in the form of echocardiography allows estimation of cardiac output by measuring changes in left ventricular dimensions during systole measured in the plane below the level of the mitral valve. Doppler ultrasound has added to the utility of echocardiography by allowing an estimation of blood velocity. The combined use of Doppler with ultrasound to measure the diameter of the vessels containing the blood will allow calculation of cross-sectional area with subsequent derivation of stroke volume and cardiac output. The velocity of blood flow can also be related to the pressure gradient down which the blood is moving, providing a way of calculating intracardiac pressure gradients and pulmonary artery pressures. Other techniques of measuring cardiac output include impedance cardiography based upon changes in transthoracic electrical resistance associated with the ejection of blood into the pulmonary circulation. This technique has been shown to overestimate low cardiac output with the opposite error in high cardiac output states.

It is also important to be able to measure blood pressure accurately in women whose risk of complications, especially cerebrovascular hemorrhage, is directly related to their degree of hypertension. At Groote Schuur Hospital, two automated blood pressure monitors (the auscultatory WelchAllyn QuietTrak and the oscillometric SpaceLabs 90207) were compared to blood pressure measured by means of both sphygmomanometry and direct intra-arterial pressure readings in women with pre-eclampsia (Natarajan et al., 1999). Compared to mercury, the auscultatory QuietTrak consistently under-read systolic and diastolic blood pressure by 13 (±15) mmHg. The oscillometric 90207 also under-read systolic by 10 (±10) mmHg and diastolic pressure by 8 (±7) mmHg. Compared to intra-arterial readings, both monitors significantly under-read systolic and mean arterial pressure. These data have important implications for those involved in the care of women with severe pre-eclampsia. Automated blood pressure monitoring devices are generally inaccurate and blood pressure determination in the critically ill pre-eclamptic should take place by mercury sphygmomanometry or intra-arterial recording.

Clinical presentation of severe pre-eclampsia and the management of organ failure

Pre-eclampsia is a syndrome characterized by sustained hypertension (systolic pressure greater than 140 mmHg and/or diastolic pressure in excess of 90 mmHg) and proteinuria (more than 300 mg excreted per 24 h) during the latter half of pregnancy that always remits after delivery of the fetus (Davey and MacGillivray, 1988). Because the disease resolves after delivery, delivery of the baby is the most important intervention practised in the management of pre-eclampsia. Delivery may be precipitated by uncontrolled hypertension, organ dysfunction (renal, liver, neurological or cardiorespiratory), fetal distress, abruptio placentae or because the pregnancy has reached the point where the neonatal risks of prematurity are negligible.

Severe and resistant hypertension

Hypertension beyond a mean arterial pressure of 140 mmHg is associated with a risk of cerebrovascular hemorrhage. The mean arterial pressure (MAP) exact level at which the blood–brain barrier begins to break down in pre-eclampsia/eclampsia is unclear but we do know that cerebral autoregulation is affected in this condition and that brain overperfusion can occur at lower MAP levels than in non-pre-eclamptic patients (Belfort *et al.*, 1999a, b, 2000, 2001, 2002a). In practice, any blood pressure above 160/110 mmHg is usually regarded as an indication for aggressive antihypertensive therapy. The goal of antihypertensive therapy should be to maintain systemic MAP between 100 and 126 mmHg. Patients admitted to intensive care units and managed with the benefit of invasive hemodynamic monitoring should have vasodilator therapy titrated against both systemic blood pressure and derived parameters such as systemic vascular resistance (SVR). The SVR should be restored to normal levels (1000 and 1200 dyne.sec cm^{-5}), providing the MAP remains above 100 mmHg.

Plasma volume expansion is an essential adjunct to antihypertensive therapy. Diminishing peripheral perfusion may result from vasodilator therapy because of an excessive reduction in blood pressure but more commonly occurs because the necessary rise in cardiac output and stroke volume fails to occur. Many severe pre-eclamptic/eclamptic patients have a contracted intravascular blood volume, incompatible with a dilated vasculature. In these women, vasodilatation leads to falling venous return together with low preload and stroke volume. Clinically this may be evident when the pulse rate rises soon after commencing vasodilatation and typically leads to fetal distress and the development of oliguria. These adverse effects can be prevented by prior plasma volume expansion to increase ventricular preload. Plasma volume expansion on its own may have beneficial effects because it reduces vascular resistance, increases cardiac output and oxygen delivery to the peripheral tissues (Belfort *et al.*, 1991). Plasma volume expansion is probably a more important determinant of the efficacy and safety

of vasodilators than the specific characteristics of individual drugs themselves.

Plasma volume expansion, however, carries a risk of iatrogenic pulmonary edema. Patients with pre-eclampsia/eclampsia are susceptible to the development of pulmonary edema because left-sided ventricular filling pressures rise sharply in response to plasma volume expansion even when small volumes of fluid are infused (as little as 400–500 ml of intravenous fluid). Right-sided filling pressures (central venous pressure) are not similarly affected and do not change rapidly in response to volume expansion. These disparate effects are reflected when monitoring central venous pressure and pulmonary artery pressure measurements. Hemodynamic monitoring based upon the use of central venous pressure lines only may be misleading and is likely to increase the risk of iatrogenic pulmonary edema. Despite these difficulties, volume expansion should precede vasodilatation using small aliquots of fluid (400 ml) and may take place without invasive monitoring if only one or two challenges are to be given. Those requiring greater volumes of fluid intravenously or those in positive fluid balance are less likely to develop pulmonary edema if the clinician has knowledge of the pulmonary capillary wedge pressure.

Hypertension that fails to respond to standard vasodilator therapy has been cited as an indication for invasive hemodynamic monitoring, the purpose of this being to distinguish hypertension due to high cardiac output from that which arises from elevated systemic vascular resistance. Treatment aimed at reducing a high cardiac output may seem counter-intuitive but life-threatening hypertension due to this cause should be treated with drugs such as labetalol rather than the more traditionally used calcium channel blockers and direct-acting vasodilators such as hydralazine or dihydralazine.

Eclampsia

This is the occurrence of generalized tonic–clonic seizures in a pregnant patient with proteinuric hypertension. Most seizures occur prior to delivery although 40% of women will fit within 24 h of delivery. Eclampsia may be preceded by prodromal symptoms of headache and visual disturbances (blurred vision, photopsia, scotomata and diplopia) (Duncan *et al.*, 1989). The blood pressure at the time of seizure activity varies from levels that are mildly elevated or even normal although they more commonly have moderate to severe hypertension (Lindheimer, 1996). Seizure activity is, however, associated with a sharp increase in blood pressure and decreased peripheral oxygen saturation levels. This is important because severe hypertension has been linked to the risk of cerebrovascular hemorrhage.

The differential diagnosis of seizure activity in pregnancy is extensive and includes epilepsy, systemic lupus erythematosus, acute fatty liver of pregnancy (hepatic encephalopathy), thrombotic thrombocytopenic purpura, amniotic fluid embolus, cerebral venous thrombosis, herpes encephalitis, malaria and cocaine intoxication (Clark *et al.*, 1995; Hauser and Kurland, 1975; Towers *et al.*, 1993). Late postpartum eclampsia (seizures first developing between 48 h and 4 weeks after delivery) require neuroradiological investigation to exclude alternative diagnoses (Douglas and Redman, 1994; Lubarsky *et al.*, 1994; Tetzschner and Felding, 1994).

The critical care management of pre-eclampsia is centered on the prevention of recurrent seizures, control of the airway to prevent aspiration pneumonia, control of severe hypertension, management of other organ failure and termination of the pregnancy.

Seizure prophylaxis

Ongoing seizure activity should be treated with initial attention to airway management and standard emergency procedures. Magnesium sulfate is used as the agent of first choice in the USA to terminate eclampsia, while in other parts of the world intravenous benzodiazepines such as diazepam or clonazepam may be used as the first-line drug in an actively seizing patient. Once initial seizure activity has been controlled, attention should be paid to preventing recurrent seizures; magnesium sulfate is the drug of choice for this indication. Randomized evidence clearly demonstrates a significantly lower risk of recurrent seizures when magnesium sulfate is compared to phenytoin and fixed-dose benzodiazepines used for the same indication (Coetzee *et al.*, 1995; Collaborative Eclampsia Trial, 1995).

Magnesium sulfate is a weak calcium channel blocker that regulates intracellular calcium flux through the *N*-methyl-D-aspartate receptor in neuronal tissue and may inhibit ischemic neuronal damage brought about by anion flux through this receptor (Altura and Altura, 1984). Parenterally administered magnesium results in systemic vasodilatation and improved cardiac output as well as cerebral vasodilatation distal to the middle cerebral artery. Retinal artery vasospasm has been reversed by magnesium sulfate infusion (Belfort, 1992; Belfort and Moise, 1992; Belfort *et al.*, 1992). The myocardial effects of parenteral magnesium include slowing of the cardiac conduction times, and in high doses magnesium is significantly negatively inotropic (Arsenian, 1993). Intravenous magnesium sulfate reduces serum calcium levels possibly as a result of increased renal magnesium and calcium excretion (Arsenian, 1993). Falling serum calcium levels inhibits acetylcholine release at the motor endplate, the extent of which is directly related to the level of the serum magnesium and inversely proportional to the calcium concentration. This is the origin of magnesium sulfate toxicity leading to neuromuscular blockade and respiratory arrest (Cruikshank *et al.*, 1993; Ramanathan *et al.*, 1998; Richards *et al.*, 1985). Dosage regimens vary but the majority of women in the Collaborative Eclampsia Trial were treated with a 4 g intravenous loading dose followed by a constant infusion of $1 \, \mathrm{g \, h^{-1}}$. Magnesium sulfate is excreted by the kidney and impaired renal function may lead to toxicity, manifest as weakness, absent tendon reflexes and respiratory arrest. Patients with undiagnosed myasthenia gravis may have their disease unmasked by magnesium sulfate, even when the drug only reaches normal therapeutic levels (Bashuk and Krendel, 1990).

Patients who experience recurrent seizures in spite of magnesium sulfate are best managed by intubation and ventilation. Sedation using continuous high dose benzodiazepine or thiopental infusions will be necessary and will serve to prevent further convulsions. Following multiple seizures, these women are likely to have cerebral edema with raised intracranial pressure. Consequently care should be taken to maintain a mean arterial pressure in excess of 100 mmHg in order to preserve cerebral blood flow (Richards et al., 1986).

Patients who have their first convulsion after attaining therapeutic blood levels of magnesium sulfate, who continue to convulse after starting magnesium sulfate, who have lateralizing signs, who remain unconscious or have mental confusion after a seizure, have cortical blindness or who have a seizure postpartum should probably have some form of cerebral imaging such as an MRI/MRA or CT scan to exclude intracranial pathology.

Control of the airway

Clearing the airway is an important first-aid measure in any convulsing patient. This is most simply attained by suctioning and positioning the patient head-down, on her side. Endotracheal intubation is indicated in women with recurrent seizures, those who are inadequately oxygenated, and in circumstances where the patient remains persistently obtunded more than 30 min after the seizure. Ventilatory care should be maintained for a minimum of 24 h postpartum or until the patient is fully conscious and any upper airway edema has resolved.

Obstetric management

Vaginal delivery, if foreseeable within a short period, may be contemplated in the woman with no complicating features other than a single seizure. Induction of labor should not be protracted and an arbitrary time limit should be set as a goal for attaining a vaginal delivery. Cesarean delivery, when considered necessary, should follow after the mother has been stabilized (after the blood pressure has been controlled and seizure prophylaxis commenced).

Prevention of eclampsia

In cases of severe pre-eclampsia, the prevention of seizure activity is essential even though the incidence of seizure activity may be as low as 3–4%. Recent epidemiological evidence suggests that the drug of choice remains magnesium sulfate, although other drugs such as labetalol that lower the cerebral perfusion pressure are also under investigation.

The oliguric pre-eclamptic

The presentation of renal impairment is commonly that of oliguria (a urine output of less than $30 \, \text{ml h}^{-1}$ over several consecutive hours) with or without hematuria. Reduced intravascular volume, vasospasm and low cardiac output are the most likely cause. Providing the patient is not already in positive fluid balance, plasma volume expansion should be attempted, but if two fluid challenges (300 ml of colloidal solution) fail to improve the urinary output, no further fluid should be given without hemodynamic assessment. In some situations, if available, a single non-invasive echocardiographic assessment of the ejection fraction, cardiac output and status of filling of the inferior vena cava will be all that is required (Belfort et al., 1994, 1997). In such cases the patient may be shown to have a good ejection fraction, a low cardiac output and underfilling of the central veins. Usually fluid resuscitation is all that is needed and urine output will improve. If echocardiographic assessment is not available, or if the echo shows cardiac failure, overdistended central veins or poor ejection fraction, continuous invasive monitoring with a pulmonary artery catheter may be more appropriate.

Low dose dopamine may also be useful and should be commenced at an infusion rate of $1–5\,\mu g\,kg^{-1}\,mm^{-1}$. Low-dose dopamine is thought to act as a selective renal artery vasodilator and although of questionable benefit in general critical care, two randomized studies have demonstrated efficacy without adverse effects in the oliguric pre-eclamptic patient (Clark *et al.*, 1986; Mantel and Makin, 1997).

Patients who fail to respond to either of these measures may require more intensive monitoring. As outlined above, both echocardiography and pulmonary artery catheters are useful adjuncts in securing optimal left ventricular preload and afterload. The volume-replete vasodilated patient who fails to pass urine should be considered to have intrinsic renal pathology, namely acute tubular necrosis. A single large dose of furosemide (0.5–1 g intravenously) may convert these patients to high output renal failure. Should this measure also fail, care must be taken to avoid fluid overload and the patient should be prepared for dialysis.

Respiratory distress

Patients who present with respiratory distress are frequently a diagnostic challenge. Where the diagnosis remains in doubt after clinical examination and special investigation, echocardiography or pulmonary artery catheterization are indicated. The causes of respiratory distress include the development of upper airway edema, pulmonary edema, atelectasis and aspiration pneumonia. Patients with severe pre-eclampsia are predisposed to the development of pulmonary edema because of low oncotic pressure, leaky capillaries and left ventricular dysfunction. Diastolic dysfunction cannot be detected without invasive monitoring or access to echocardiography. Iatrogenic fluid overload (even with small amounts of fluid) is also a frequent cause of pulmonary edema. Both cardiomyopathy and valvular heart disease may be indistinguishable from other causes of pulmonary edema without echocardiography or invasive monitoring.

Pulmonary edema will need to be managed according to the hemodynamic findings. Elevated pulmonary capillary wedge pressure may result from high systemic vascular resistance, left ventricular failure or fluid overload. These complications may require vasodilatation, the use of diuretic drugs, or a combination of both. In the absence of iatrogenic fluid overload, afterload reduction may be the most important aspect of management.

The development of localized lung signs and purulent sputum should alert the clinician to the possibility of aspiration pneumonia. Radiological findings vary from normal lung fields to unilateral shadowing, atelectasis and collapse. Bronchoscopy may be necessary if aspiration of particulate matter is suspected. Treatment with broad-spectrum (including anerobic) antibiotic cover is required.

HELLP syndrome

This syndrome, a complication of pre-eclampsia, is due to hepatic ischemia giving rise to periportal hemorrhage and necrosis together with microangiopathic hemolytic anemia and thrombocytopenia (Weinstein, 1982). The mnemonic "HELLP" therefore stands for: Hemolysis, Elevated Liver enzymes and Low Platelets. These patients present with epigastric pain and in severe cases are usually obviously ill because of associated complications including renal failure (characterized by rising urea, creatinine and the passage of small quantities of bloodstained or "Coke" colored urine) and eclampsia. Many women with HELLP syndrome, however, seem to have unremarkable clinical disease.

Liver failure may arise from conditions that mimic pre-eclampsia such as thrombotic thrombocytopenic purpura and acute fatty liver of pregnancy (see below) (Atlas *et al.*, 1982; Kaplan, 1985). Obstetric cholestasis and viral hepatitis may also enter the differential diagnosis in milder cases of HELLP syndrome. Distinguishing between these conditions may be difficult but the hallmark of pre-eclamptic disease is that it resolves after delivery (Chandran et al., 1992).

Subcapsular liver hematoma is a rare complication of the HELLP syndrome. The surface of the liver is covered in petechial hemorrhages that may coalesce to form one large hematoma. Rupture of a hematoma is a life-threatening complication that presents with right-upper quadrant pain and sudden hypovolemia. Management is usually surgical and involves packing the abdomen to put pressure on the bleeding surface, drainage of the subdiaphragmatic spaces with wide bore drains, aggressive blood product replacement and careful attention to body temperature control. Cautery, resection and suturing of the liver are not recommended as methods of controlling the bleeding. Arterial embolization has been used and may be an option in selected cases. Recent use of Factor VII replacement in massive obstetric hemorrhage has been suggested and may also be an option (Bouwmeester et al., 2003; Danilos et al., 2003).

Coagulopathy is an uncommon feature of HELLP syndrome but thrombocytopenia and impaired platelet function both give rise to impaired coagulation. Prolonged partial thromboplastin times and INRs are more likely to occur in association with acute fatty liver than HELLP syndrome. Hypoglycemia may occur in some cases but is more characteristic of acute fatty liver of pregnancy.

The management of HELLP syndrome is delivery while the associated complications (renal failure, eclampsia and respiratory distress) may require critical care on their individual merits. Thrombocytopenia should reach a nadir within 72 h of delivery and if it is persistent beyond this point, a search for alternative diagnoses should commence (e.g. sepsis, folate deficiency, thrombotic thrombocytopenic purpura, systemic lupus erythematosus). Although steroids have been advocated as a means of accelerating the resolution of postpartum eclampsia, the studies involved are small and show no reduction in mortality.

Differential diagnosis of severe pre-eclampsia

Several conditions may mimic severe pre-eclampsia/eclampsia. Briefly, they include the following:

Anaphylactoid syndrome of pregnancy ("Amniotic Fluid Embolism")

This is a complication of labor or Cesarean delivery giving rise to peripartum collapse as a result of embolization of amniotic fluid and possibly fetal squamous cells into the maternal circulation. The syndrome may be rapidly lethal in women who develop severe pulmonary hypertension and cardiac arrest. Those who survive for longer periods develop an anaphylactoid type of response to the presence of amniotic fluid in the circulation (Clark et al., 1995).

The clinical syndrome is diagnosed every 1 in 8000 to 1 in 80,000 pregnancies. A national registry of cases that has been opened in the USA is currently the most authoritative source of information about this condition. The condition usually presents during labor but may occur at the time of Cesarean delivery or immediately after birth. There are no demographic predisposing factors and obstetric practices, such as prior amniotomy and oxytocin administration do not seem to influence the risk of developing amniotic fluid embolus. The onset of the condition is abrupt and *hypotension* is universally present. Most patients develop pulmonary edema with cyanosis and a profound coagulopathy which should immediately give rise to a suspicion of the diagnosis.

The single most common initial presenting symptom, however, in antenatal patients is seizure activity. This may lead to confusion with eclampsia, which is a far more frequent cause of seizures.

The patients who survive the initial embolus and who develop the anaphylactoid picture have markedly depressed left ventricular function. Cardiac electromechanical dissociation may develop and there is a high risk of cardiopulmonary arrest.

The prognosis is poor; in the American national registry, 61% of the patients died and only 15% survived neurologically intact. Diagnosis must be prompt and continuous vigorous resuscitation will be needed immediately. Intensive care is mandatory and inotropic support is necessary from the beginning. Hemorrhage should be anticipated and hypovolemia is also likely to be a problem as a result of postpartum hemorrhage or bleeding after Cesarean section. Continuous transfusion with blood and coagulation factors will be necessary and obstetric intervention in the form of oxytocic drugs and hysterectomy may be necessary to control bleeding. Although not currently studied or reported, in those cases with overwhelming coagulopathy treatment with recombinant activated Factor VII may be a last resort therapy (Bouwmeester *et al.*, 2003; Danilos *et al.*, 2003).

Intubation and mechanical ventilation along with pulmonary artery catheterization are likely adjuncts to intensive care management.

Thrombotic thrombocytopenic purpura (TTP)

TTP is one of a spectrum of microangiopathic hemolytic conditions that include pre-eclampsia, hemolytic uremic syndrome (HUS), acute fatty liver of pregnancy and autoimmune conditions such as systemic lupus erythematosus. TTP is a condition in which multimers of von Willebrand factor, derived from the endothelium, accumulate in the circulation due to lack (either functional or absolute) of a specific metalloproteinase enzyme that breaks down the multimers. Von Willebrand factor binds platelets to the endothelium and high concentrations are associated with peripheral platelet consumption and the formation of platelet microthrombi. Von Willebrand factor is usually broken down by a specific metalloproteinase but may accumulate if this enzyme is deficient or if endothelial damage provokes excessive release of von Willebrand factor. The metalloproteinase enzyme deficiency exists either as a hereditary condition or can be acquired as a consequence of autoimmune disease due to a specific IgG inhibitor of the enzyme. Many factors can precipitate both the congenital and acquired forms of TTP, including drugs, malignancy, bacterial infection, HIV and other viral infections. Pregnancy is the precipitating factor in 10–25% of cases (Chang and Kathula, 2002; Proia *et al.*, 2002).

TTP requires three major factors for the diagnosis: microangiopathic hemolytic anemia, thrombocytopenia, and some form of neurological involvement (which may be as mild as a slight headache or as severe as dense coma). TTP usually presents with a clinical pentad of features: microangiopathic hemolytic anemia, fever, neurological disturbance, renal impairment and thrombocytopenia. The neurological features of the syndrome may be transitory while mild hypertension and proteinuria may make the condition indistinguishable from HELLP syndrome. TTP does not, however, remit after delivery, whereas HELLP syndrome invariably resolves. Other diagnostic features that may help to distinguish between the two conditions include evidence of marked hemolysis on examination of the peripheral blood smear (this is more characteristic of TTP than HELLP). In most cases despite an extremely low platelet count, women with TTP will have a normal coagulogram (PT/PTT/Fibrinogen) and this may be useful in distinguishing TTP from HELLP syndrome, where the coagulogram is generally affected once the platelet count is less than $50,000 \, ml^{-1}$. Another useful pointer is the lactate dehydrogenase level, which, if greater than $20,000 \, IU$, should raise a concern for TTP as opposed to HELLP syndrome.

Without appropriate management TTP has a high mortality rate. Treatment consists of plasmaphoresis, infusion of fresh frozen plasma and high dose steroid therapy. Renal failure and the neurological manifestations may require appropriate intensive care management.

Acute fatty liver of pregnancy

Acute fatty liver of pregnancy (AFLP) is a condition characterized by microvesicular fatty infiltration of the liver, developing in the latter half of pregnancy. The incidence is approximately 1: 12,000 deliveries. Clinical disease severity varies with some patients having only mild right-upper quadrant discomfort associated with prodromal nausea and vomiting. Others develop fulminant liver failure leading to coma. A depressed level of consciousness may arise from either hypoglycemia or the onset of hepatic encephalopathy. Hypoglycemia is a common feature of AFLP and should alert the clinician to the possible diagnosis. More than 50% of affected patients will have mild hypertension and proteinuria, making the distinction from HELLP syndrome difficult. Jaundice is often present at the time of diagnosis. Liver enzymes are increased and transaminases may rise above $1000\,IU\,l^{-1}$ in severe cases. Liver failure leads to severe coagulopathy and a prolonged partial thromboplastin time and INR. Disseminated intravascular coagulation with microangiopathic hemolytic anemia develop together a mild neutrophil leucocytosis (Rahman and Wendon, 2002; Strauss et al., 1999).

Management principles include delivery of the fetus and treatment of the acute liver failure. Coagulopathy may complicate the delivery and must be corrected beforehand. Management of liver failure also includes maintenance of the blood glucose level, the use of lactulose to limit the effects of intestinal bacteria and administration of vitamin K to mother and baby. Intubation and ventilation may be necessary in the comatose mother who cannot protect her airway. Associated complications of renal failure and pancreatitis need to be managed individually.

Conclusion

The critical care management of severe preeclampsia is essentially quite simple, although these cases are probably better managed by clinicians and nursing staff familiar with this disease. Gratifyingly, women afflicted by preeclampsia usually make a complete recovery; on these grounds alone, there can be no better justification for investing resources and time in teaching and upgrading the standard of care provided to these unfortunate victims of a disease that has remained an enigma for years.

REFERENCES

Altura, B.T. and Altura, B.M. (1984). Interactions of Mg and K on cerebral vessels – aspects in view of stroke. Review of present status and new findings. Magnesium, 3(4–6), 195–211.
Arsenian, M.A. (1993). Magnesium and cardiovascular disease. Prog. Cardiovasc. Dis., 35(4), 271–310.
Atlas, M., Barkai, G., Menczer, J., Houlu, N. and Lieberman, P. (1982). Thrombotic thrombocytopenic purpura in pregnancy. Br. J. Obstet. Gynaecol., 89(6), 476–9.
Bashuk, R.G. and Krendel, D.A. (1990). Myasthenia gravis presenting as weakness after magnesium administration. Muscle Nerve, 13(8), 708–12.
Belfort, M.A. (1992). The effect of magnesium sulphate on blood flow velocity in the maternal retina in mild pre-eclampsia, a preliminary colour flow, Doppler study. Br. J. Obstet. Gynaecol., 99(8), 641–5.
Belfort, M.A. and Moise, K.J., Jr. (1992). Effect of magnesium sulfate on maternal brain blood flow in preeclampsia: a randomized, placebo-controlled study. Am. J. Obstet. Gynecol., 167(3), 661–6.
Belfort, M.A. and Saade, G.R. (1993). Retinal vasospasm associated with visual disturbance in preeclampsia: color flow Doppler findings. Am. J. Obstet. Gynecol., 169(3), 523–5.
Belfort, M.A., Anthony, J. and Kirshon, B. (1991). Respiratory function in severe gestational proteinuric hypertension: the effects of rapid volume expansion and subsequent vasodilatation with verapamil. Br. J. Obstet. Gynaecol., 98(10), 964–72.
Belfort, M.A., Saade, G.R. and Moise, K.J., Jr. (1992). The effect of magnesium sulfate on maternal retinal blood flow in preeclampsia: a randomized placebo-controlled study. Am. J. Obstet. Gynecol., 167(6), 1548–53.

Belfort, M. A., Rokey, R., Saade, G. R. and Moise, K. J. (1994). Rapid echocardiographic assessment of left and right heart hemodynamics in critically ill obstetric patients. *Am. J. Obstet. Gynecol.*, **171**(4), 884–92.

Belfort, M. A., Mares, A., Saade, G., Wen, T. S. and Rokey, R. (1997). Two-dimensional echocardiography and Doppler ultrasound in managing obstetric patients. *Obstet. Gynecol.*, **90**(3), 326–30.

Belfort, M. A., Grunewald, C., Saade, G. R. and Nissel, H. (1999a). Preeclampsia may cause both overperfusion and underperfusion of the brain: a cerebral perfusion pressure based model. *Acta Obstet. Gynecol. Scand.*, **78**(7), 586–91.

Belfort, M. A., Saade, G. R., Grunewald, C., Dildy, G. A., Varner, M. A. and Nisell, H. (1999b). Effect of blood pressure on orbital and middle cerebral artery resistance in healthy pregnant women and women with preeclampsia. *Am. J. Obstet. Gynecol.*, **180**, 601–7.

Belfort, M. A., Tooke-Miller, C., Varner, M., *et al.* (2000). Evaluation of a non-invasive transcranial Doppler and blood pressure bases method for the assessment of cerebral perfusion pressure in pregnant women. *Hypertens. Pregn.*, **19**(3), 331–40.

Belfort, M. A., Tooke-Miller, C., Allen, J. C., *et al.* (2001). Changes in flow velocity, resistance indices, and cerebral perfusion pressure in the maternal middle cerebral artery distribution during normal pregnancy. *Acta Obstet. Gynecol. Scand.*, **80**, 104–12.

Belfort, M. A., Varner, M. W., Dizon-Townson, D. S., Grunewald, C. and Nisell, H. (2002a). Cerebral perfusion pressure, and not cerebral blood flow, may be the critical determinant of intracranial injury in preeclampsia: a new hypothesis. *Am. J. Obstet. Gynecol.*, **187**, 626–34.

Belfort, M. A., Tooke-Miller, C., Allen, J. C., Dizon-Townson, D. and Varner, M. A. (2002b). Labetalol decreases cerebral perfusion pressure without negatively affecting cerebral blood flow in hypertensive gravidas. *Hypertens. Pregn.*, **21**(3), 185–97.

Bouwmeester, F. W., Jonkhoff, A. R., Verheijen, R. H. M. and van Geijn, H. P. (2003). Successful treatment of life–threatening postpartum hermorrhage with recombinant activated factor VII. *Obstet. Gynecol.*, **101**, 1174–6

Chandran, R., Serra-Serra, V. and Redman, C. W. (1992). Spontaneous resolution of pre-eclampsia-related thrombocytopenia. *Br. J. Obstet. Gynaecol.*, **99**(11), 887–90.

Chang, J. C. and Kathula, S. K. (2002). Various clinical manifestations in patients with thrombotic microangiopathy. *J. Investig. Med.*, **50**(3), 201–6.

Clark, S. L., Greenspoon, J. S., Aldahl, D. and Phelan, J. P. (1986). Severe preeclampsia with persistent oliguria: management of hemodynamic subsets. *Am. J. Obstet. Gynecol.*, **154**(3), 490–4.

Clark, S. L., Hankins, G. D., Dudley, D. A., Dildy, G. A. and Porter, T. F. (1995). Amniotic fluid embolism: analysis of the national registry. *Am. J. Obstet. Gynecol.*, **172**(4, Pt. 1), 1158–67.

Coetzee, E. J., Dommisse, J. and Anthony, J. (1998). A randomised controlled trial of intravenous magnesium sulphate versus placebo in the management of women with severe pre-eclampsia. *Br. J. Obstet. Gynaecol.*, **105**(3), 300–3.

Collaborative Eclampsia Trial. (1995). Which anticonvulsant for women with eclampsia? Evidence from the Collaborative Eclampsia Trial. *Lancet*, **345**(8963), 1455–63.

Cruikshank, D. P., Chan, G. M. and Doerrfeld, D. (1993). Alterations in vitamin D and calcium metabolism with magnesium sulfate treatment of preeclampsia. *Am. J. Obstet. Gynecol.*, **168**(4), 1170–6.

Danilos, J., Goral, A., Paluskiewicz, P., Przesmycki, K. and Kotarski, J. (2003). Successful treatment with recombinant factor VIIa for intractable bleeding at pelvic surgery. *Obstet. Gynecol.*, **101**, 1172–3

Davey, D. A. and MacGillivray, I. (1988). The classification and definition of the hypertensive disorders of pregnancy. *Am. J. Obstet. Gynecol.*, **158**(4), 892–8.

Donaldson, J. O. (1994). Eclampsia. *Adv. Neurol.*, **64**, 25–33.

Douglas, K. A. and Redman, C. W. (1994). Eclampsia in the United Kingdom. *Br. Med. J.*, **309**(6966), 1395–400.

Duley, L. (1992). Maternal mortality associated with hypertensive disorders of pregnancy in Africa, Asia, Latin America and the Caribbean. *Br. J. Obstet. Gynaecol.*, **99**(7), 547–53.

Duncan, R., Hadley, D., Bone, I., Symonds, E. M., Worthington, B. S. and Rubin, P. C. (1989). Blindness in eclampsia: CT and MR imaging. *J. Neurol. Neurosurg. Psychiatry.*, **52**(7), 899–902.

Hauser, W. A. and Kurland, L. T. (1975). The epidemiology of epilepsy in Rochester, Minnesota, 1935 through 1967. *Epilepsia.*, **16**(1), 1–66.

Hogberg, U., Innala, E. and Sandstrom, A. (1994). Maternal mortality in Sweden, 1980–1988. *Obstet. Gynecol.* **84**(2), 240–4.

Kaplan, M. M. (1985). Acute fatty liver of pregnancy. *N. Engl. J. Med.*, **313**(6), 367–70.

Lindheimer, M. D. (1996). Pre-eclampsia–eclampsia 1996: preventable? Have disputes on its treatment been resolved? *Curr. Opin. Nephrol. Hypertens.*, **5**(5), 452–8.

Lubarsky, S. L., Barton, J. R., Friedman, S. A., Nasreddine, S., Ramadan, M. K. and Sibai, B. M. (1994). Late postpartum eclampsia revisited. *Obstet. Gynecol.*, **83**(4), 502–5.

Mabie, W. C., Barton, J. R. and Sibai, B. M. (1992). Adult respiratory distress syndrome in pregnancy. *Am. J. Obstet. Gynecol.*, **167**(4, Pt. 1), 950–7.

Mantel, G. D. and Makin, J. D. (1997). Low dose dopamine in postpartum pre-eclamptic women with oliguria: a double-blind, placebo controlled, randomised trial. *Br. J. Obstet. Gynaecol.*, **104**(10), 1180–3.

Milliez, J., Dahoun, A. and Boudraa, M. (1990). Computed tomography of the brain in eclampsia. *Obstet. Gynecol.*, **75**(6), 975–80.

Morriss, M. C., Twickler, D. M., Hatab, M. R., Clarke, G. D., Peshock, R. M. and Cunningham, F. G. (1997). Cerebral blood flow and cranial magnetic resonance imaging in eclampsia and severe preeclampsia. *Obstet. Gynecol.*, **89**(4), 561–8.

Natarajan, P., Shennan, A. H., Penny, J., Halligan, A. W., de Swiet, M. and Anthony, J. (1999). Comparison of auscultatory and oscillometric automated blood pressure monitors in the setting of preeclampsia. *Am. J. Obstet. Gynecol.*, **181**(5, Pt. 1), 1203–10.

Overgaard, J. and Skinhoj, E. (1975). A paradoxical cerebral hemodynamic effect of hydralazine. *Stroke*, **6**(4), 402–10.

Proia, A., Paesano, R., Torcia, F., *et al.* (2002). Thrombotic thrombocytopenic purpura and pregnancy: a case report and a review of the literature. *Ann. Hematol.*, **81**(4), 210–11.

Rahman, T. M. and Wendon, J. (2002). Severe hepatic dysfunction in pregnancy. *Q. J. Med.*, **95**(6), 343–57.

Ramanathan, J., Sibai, B. M., Pillai, R. and Angel, J. J. (1988). Neuromuscular transmission studies in pre-eclamptic women receiving magnesium sulfate. *Am. J. Obstet. Gynecol.*, **158**(1), 40–6.

Richards, A., Stather-Dunn, L. and Moodley, J. (1985). Cardiopulmonary arrest after the administration of magnesium sulphate. A case report. *S. Afr. Med. J.*, **67**(4), 145.

Richards, A. M., Moodley, J., Graham, D. I. and Bullock, M. R. (1986). Active management of the unconscious eclamptic patient. *Br. J. Obstet. Gynaecol.*, **93**(6), 554–62.

Schaefer, P. W., Buonanno, F. S., Gonzalez, R. G. and Schwamm, L. H. (1997). Diffusion-weighted imaging discriminates between cytotoxic and vasogenic edema in a patient with eclampsia. *Stroke*, **28**(5), 1082–5.

Schwartz, R. B., Jones, K. M., Kalina, P., *et al.* (1992). Hypertensive encephalopathy: findings on CT, MR imaging, and SPECT imaging in 14 cases. *Am. J. Roentgenol.*, **159**(2), 379–83.

Sibai, B. M. (1990). Eclampsia. VI. Maternal–perinatal outcome in 254 consecutive cases. *Am. J. Obstet. Gynecol.*, **163**(3), 1049–54.

Strauss, A. W., Bennett, M. J., Rinaldo, P., *et al.* (1999). Inherited long-chain 3-hydroxyacyl-CoA dehydrogenase deficiency and a fetal–maternal interaction cause maternal liver disease and other pregnancy complications. *Semin. Perinatol.*, **23**(2), 100–12.

Tetzschner, T. and Felding, C. (1994). Postpartum eclampsia. Impossible to eradicate? *Clin. Exp. Obstet. Gynecol.*, **21**(2), 74–6.

Towers, C. V., Pircon, R. A., Nageotte, M. P., Porto, M. and Garite, T. J. (1993). Cocaine intoxication presenting as preeclampsia and eclampsia. *Obstet. Gynecol.*, **81**(4), 545–7.

Visser, W. and Wallenburg, H. C. (1991). Central hemodynamic observations in untreated preeclamptic patients. *Hypertension.*, **17**(6, Pt. 2), 1072–7.

Weinstein, L. (1982). Syndrome of hemolysis, elevated liver enzymes, and low platelet count: a severe consequence of hypertension in pregnancy. *Am. J. Obstet. Gynecol.*, **142**(2), 159–67.

Williams, K. P. and Wilson, S. (1995). Maternal cerebral blood flow changes associated with eclampsia. *Am. J. Perinatol.*, **12**(3), 189–91.

WHO. (1988). Geographic variation in the incidence of hypertension in pregnancy. World Health Organization International Collaborative Study of Hypertensive Disorders of Pregnancy. *Am. J. Obstet. Gynecol.*, **158**(1), 80–3.

Zunker, P., Ley-Pozo, J., Louwen, F., Schuierer, G., Holzgreve, W. and Ringelstein, E. B. (1995). Cerebral hemodynamics in pre-eclampsia/eclampsia syndrome. *Ultrasound Obstet. Gynecol.*, **6**(6), 411–15.

32

The role of maternal and fetal Doppler in pre-eclampsia

J. Hornbuckle and S. Robson

Introduction

Fitzgerald and Drumm (1997), using a combination of real-time imaging, pulsed wave and continuous wave Doppler, first reported the use of flow velocity waveforms (FVW) from the umbilical cord in 1977. Since then the value of umbilical artery (UA) Doppler to assess fetal wellbeing has been investigated extensively; indeed, no other tool in perinatal medicine has received such rigorous appraisal in the form of randomized controlled trials. Subsequent studies have investigated other fetal arterial and venous vessels and although a significant body of literature now exists, especially for the middle cerebral artery (MCA) and ductus venosus (DV), the absence of appropriately powered randomized trials makes the clinical utility of these investigations unclear.

Of all the clinical groups labeled as "high risk," women with pre-eclampsia and those at risk of developing the syndrome are probably those in which Doppler ultrasound has proven the greatest value. However, interpretation of the literature is often confounded by variations in the definition of the disorder. In this chapter we review the role of Doppler in screening and management of pre-eclampsia, focusing on uterine artery, UA, MCA and DV waveforms. Wherever possible an attempt will be made to distinguish between early onset (necessitating delivery before 34 weeks of gestation) and later disease.

Waveform acquisition and interpretation

Waveform indices

Measurement of absolute blood flow is dependent on multiple factors including angle of insonation, blood viscosity, and vessel diameter. The latter is difficult to measure and precludes accurate assessment of volume flow, especially in small fetal vessels. Instead, angle-independent non-dimensional analysis of the pulsatility of the flow velocity waveform (FVW) spectrum is used. The commonly used FVW indices are resistance index (RI), systolic/diastolic ratio (S/D or A/B) or pulsatility index (PI).

Uterine artery

Uteroplacental Doppler FVW can be recorded transabdominally from the main uterine artery proximally to the placental bed spiral arteries distally (Bower et al., 1992; Matijevic and Johnston, 1999). Color Doppler mapping allows accurate identification of the main uterine arteries at the site they "cross-over" the external iliac arteries (Bower et al., 1992). This is a convenient landmark for recording waveforms using pulsed Doppler from as early as 11–14 weeks of pregnancy (Martin et al., 2001). Uterine arteries can also be identified transvaginally lateral to the uterine cervix at the level of the internal cervical os.

Uterine artery RI and PI fall with gestational age and are lower on the placental side of the uterus compared with the non-placental side (Bower et al., 1992). Controversy exists as to whether the highest or lowest index should be used; latterly most authors have calculated the mean of the right and left uterine arteries with values >95th centile being regarded as abnormal. For studies performed between 20 and 24 weeks, this corresponds to a mean RI value > 0.57–0.65 and mean PI value > 1.45–1.6 (Papgeorghiou et al., 2002). The presence of an early diastolic notch, indicated by an upturn of the FVW at the beginning of diastole (Figure 32.1), is also predictive of subsequent adverse outcome (Bower et al., 1993). Interestingly, the prevalence of unilateral and bilateral notching at 18–23 weeks is lower in multiparous women (8.4% and 2.3%) than in nulliparous women (11.3% vs. 5.3%) (Prefumo et al., 2004). Most screening/intervention studies include women with unilateral or bilateral uterine artery notches within the screen positive group (Chappell et al., 1999).

Umbilical artery

Umbilical artery (UA) FVW are readily obtained transabdominally. Acquisition of waveforms, especially in the second trimester, is facilitated by color Doppler. Waveform indices are higher at the fetal than the placental end of the cord, and therefore the sample gate should be placed over a free loop of cord considered equidistant from the two insertion points (Arduini and Rizzo, 1990). All fetal Doppler measurements should be performed in the absence of fetal breathing and gross body movements and interpreted with care if the fetal heart rate is outside the normal range (110–160 bpm).

Umbilical artery PI falls with gestational age, although mean PI is relatively stable after 30 weeks gestation (Arduini and Rizzo, 1990). Values >95th centile are generally regarded as abnormal, equating to a PI > 1.4–1.5 during the third trimester (Arduini and Rizzo, 1990). While elevated indices are predictive of adverse outcome, absent or reversed end-diastolic velocities (AREDV)

(Figure 32.1) are of particular clinical significance (Karsdorp et al., 1994).

Middle cerebral artery

Middle cerebral artery (MCA) waveforms are easily obtained transabdominally; a transverse image of the fetal head is obtained at the level of the sphenoid bones. Color Doppler identifies the Circle of Willis and the MCA as the major lateral branch running along the greater wing of the sphenoid bone. Using a small sample gate, velocities are recorded ~ 1 cm distal to the origin from the internal carotid artery (Arduini and Rizzo, 1990) with minimal pressure, as compression of the fetal head alters waveform indices.

Mean MCA PI increases to approximately 28 weeks gestation and then falls to term (Arduini and Rizzo, 1990). Progressive hypoxemia results in a reduction in MCA PI (Figure 32.1) and therefore values <5th centile are regarded as abnormal. The ratio of UA/MCA PI has been widely used as an index of cerebral redistribution. Mean values fall from around 0.7 at 20 weeks to 0.5 at term, while the 95th centile falls from 1.1 to 0.9 (Arduini and Rizzo, 1990).

Ductus venosus

A number of sites have been used to assess venous return to the fetal heart. Waveform indices vary substantially in the inferior vena cava, depending on the sampling site, and the ductus venosus (DV) has emerged as the most clinically useful vessel. The DV originates from the intrahepatic portion of the umbilical vein (UV) and allows shunting of oxygenated blood to the left side of the heart via the foramen ovale. In an oblique transverse section of the fetal abdomen the DV can be identified readily using color Doppler. The higher velocities, due to the narrow lumen of the DV, frequently lead to aliasing, which facilitates identification. The sampling gate should be sufficiently wide to ensure peak velocities are captured but not confined to the proximal section of the DV where a right atrial

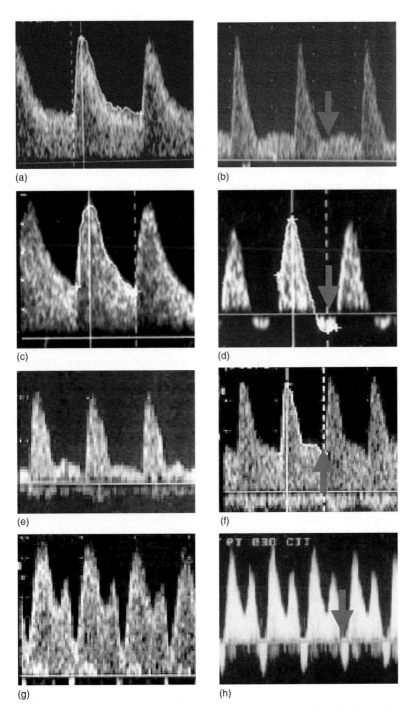

Figure 32.1 Uterine artery, fetal arterial and venous waveforms. Flow velocity waveforms from the uterine artery (a, b), umbilical artery (c, d), middle cerebral artery (e, f) and ductus venosus (g, h). Panel (a) illustrates a normal uterine artery waveform while Panel (b) shows an abnormal waveform with reduced end-diastolic velocities (EDV) and marked early diastolic notching (arrow). Panel (c) illustrates a normal umbilical artery Doppler waveform with high EDV. In contrast Panel (d) shows the most extreme abnormality with reversal of EDV (arrow). Panel (e) illustrates a normal middle cerebral artery Doppler waveform with relatively low EDV. An example of "brain sparing" is shown in Panel (f) with markedly elevated EDV (arrow). Panel (g) illustrates a normal biphasic waveform from the ductus venosus. A severely abnormal ductus waveform is shown in Panel (h) with reversal of the "a" wave (arrow).

pattern predominates. Care is also necessary to avoid nearby hepatic veins.

The DV FVW is biphasic with the first peak concomitant with ventricular systole and a second peak in late diastole concomitant with atrial systole (the "a" wave). Various indices have been used to describe venous waveforms but the pulsatility index for veins (PIV) is probably the most widely used. The PIV measures the degree of venous pulsatility, using the same ratio as PI in arterial vessels, but allows for reverse flow during diastole. The 95th centile for PIV falls from around 0.9 at 20 weeks to 0.7 at term, with values above this being regarded as abnormal (Hecher et al., 1994). As with the UA, absence or reversal of atrial systolic forward flow (Figure 32.1) are of particular clinical significance (Baschat et al., 2003).

Pathophysiological basis of abnormal Doppler waveforms

Relationship of uterine artery waveforms to placental bed morphology

During the first half of pregnancy, extravillous trophoblast (TB) cells invade the decidua and myometrium (interstitial TB) and the uterine spiral arteries (endovascular TB). Invasion results in "physiological transformation" of the spiral arteries characterized by a loss of normal musculo-elastic structure and replacement by amorphous fibrinoid material in which TB cells are embedded. In pre-eclampsia and FGR there is failure of TB invasion and consequent spiral artery trans-formation (Lyall and Robson, 2000).

Several studies have shown that uterine artery FVW indices are increased in women where there is failure of TB invasion on placental bed biopsy (Lin et al., 1995; Sagol et al., 1999). Between 73 and 90% of cases with a uterine artery systolic/diastolic (S/D) ratio $S/D \geq 2.5$ or an RI > 0.58 have absent TB migration into the myometrium (Lin et al., 1995; Sagol et al., 1999). Sagol et al. (1999) reported early diastolic notches in 57% of women with impaired

TB migration compared to 13% in those with normal migration. However, absence of physiolog-ical transformation of spiral arteries has also been reported in women with normal uterine artery Doppler FVW1 (Aardema et al., 2001).

Relationship of fetal Doppler indices to hypoxemia and acidemia

Data from direct animal experiments and indirect animal and human studies using Doppler techni-ques have demonstrated circulatory adaptations to impaired placental function and progressive hypoxemia (Hornbuckle and Thornton, 1998). Most of the human studies have been conducted on fetuses with fetal growth restriction (FGR) but are of direct relevance to pre-eclampsia, where FGR frequently coexists. An overview of Doppler changes is shown in Figure 32.2.

Under hypoxic conditions there is centralization of the fetal circulation with redistribution to preferentially supply the fetal brain, heart, spleen and adrenal glands. An increased amount of umbilical venous blood flow is also directed through the DV to maintain the oxygen tension in the left atrium (Edelstone, 1980). Doppler indices in fetal peripheral arteries are increased consistent with peripheral vasoconstriction. The ability to undergo these physiological adap-tations to hypoxemia is likely to be gestation-dependent.

Umbilical artery Doppler indices provide an indirect measure of downstream placental resis-tance; reduction of end-diastolic velocities (EDV) is associated with impaired placental villous devel-opment and a reduction in the number of small villous arteries and arterioles (Giles et al., 1985). Umbilical artery indices correlate with fetal pO_2 and pH at cordocentesis; 40–45% of fetuses with abnormal UA FVW but end-diastolic frequen-cies present are hypoxemic ($pO_2 > 2$ SD below mean for gestation) and 20–30% are acidemic (pH > 2 SD below mean for gestation) (Nicolaides et al., 1988; Nicolini et al., 1990; Yoon et al., 1994). In contrast, 80–90% of fetuses with absent

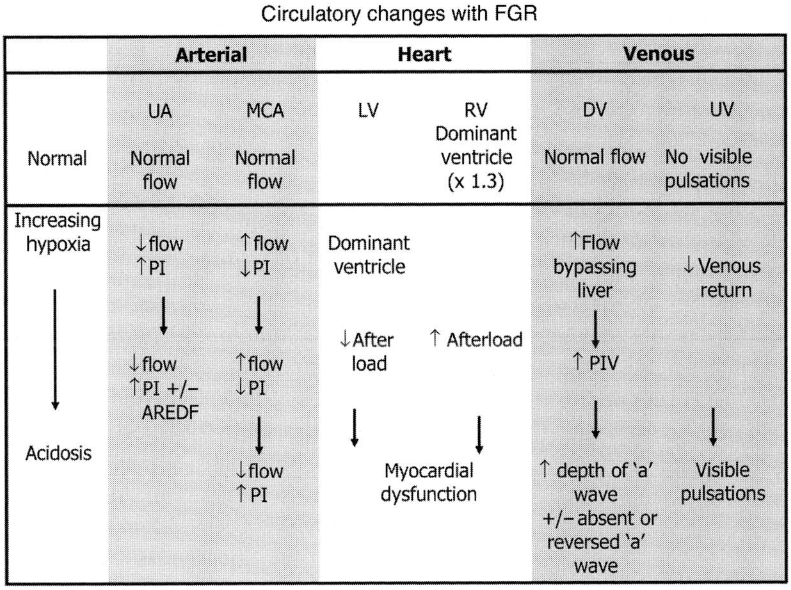

Circulatory changes with FGR

	Arterial		Heart		Venous	
	UA	MCA	LV	RV Dominant ventricle (x 1.3)	DV	UV
Normal	Normal flow	Normal flow			Normal flow	No visible pulsations
Increasing hypoxia ↓ Acidosis	↓flow ↑PI ↓flow ↑PI +/− AREDF	↑flow ↓PI ↑flow ↓PI ↓flow ↑PI	Dominant ventricle ↓After load	↑ Afterload Myocardial dysfunction	↑Flow bypassing liver ↑ PIV ↑ depth of 'a' wave +/−absent or reversed 'a' wave	↓Venous return Visible pulsations

Figure 32.2 Summary of circulatory changes in fetal growth retardation. Abbreviations: PI, pulsatility index; AREDF, absent/reversed end-diastolic frequencies; UA, umbilical artery; MCA, middle cerebral artery; LV, left ventricle; RV, right ventricle; DV, ductus venosus; UV, umbilical vein.

end-diastolic velocities are hypoxemic and 45–80% are acidemic (Nicolaides *et al.*, 1988; Nicolini *et al.*, 1990; Yoon *et al.*, 1994).

Hypoxemia leads to redistribution of left cardiac output with cerebral vasodilatation. This is reflected by a decrease in MCA PI values, maximal when fetal pO_2 is 2–4 SD below the mean for gestation (Vyas *et al.*, 1990). An increase in MCA PI (or an increase in UA/MCA PI ratio) is the earliest and most sensitive indicator of fetal hypoxemia (Rizzo *et al.*, 1995a). The reported rates of circulatory redistribution (MCA PI < 2 SD below mean for gestation) among growth restricted fetuses range from 20–76% and even with AREDV only 60–70% of fetuses show a reduction in MCA PI (Hornbuckle and Thornton, 1998). Importantly in some fetuses MCA PI subsequently normalizes (Konje *et al.*, 2001; Rowlands and Vyas, 1995). This "loss of brain sparing" is thought to represent a change in the vascular sensitivity to hypoxia and a decrease in left cardiac output.

With progressive hypoxemia/acidemia, systemic vascular resistance and afterload on the right heart increases, resulting in an increase, in the depth of the venous "a" wave. Changes in the DV PIV correlate closely with the presence or absence of acidemia (Rizzo *et al.*, 1995a). Reversal or absence of the "a" wave represents a near-terminal event (Baschat *et al.*, 2000; Muller *et al.*, 2002); in a study of 37 fetuses with UA AREDV increased PIV or reversed "a" wave in the DV was documented in 14/15 (93%) perinatal deaths (Hofstaetter *et al.*, 2002). With increasing cardiac dysfunction the abnormal venous pulsations are transmitted distally ultimately resulting in pulsations in the umbilical vein (UV). Pulsations may become evident prior to reversal of the DV "a" wave and are reported in 25–75% of fetuses with UA AREDV (Baschat *et al.*, 2003; Hofstaetter *et al.*, 2002). Rizzo *et al.* (1995b) reported that all fetuses with UV pulsations were hypoxemic and 91% acidemic, while their occurrence has a 71% sensitivity (and

95% specificity) for predicting perinatal death (Hofstaetter *et al.*, 2002). In a study of UA, DV and UV Doppler waveforms in 224 fetuses with FGR, Baschat *et al.* (2003) concluded that DV "a" wave reversal and UV pulsations offered the best prediction of acidemia and perinatal death, irrespective of the UA waveform.

With deterioration of the fetal arterial Doppler waveforms there is progressive change in fetal cardiac function. Longitudinal studies show that right heart diastolic function, as measured by DV and right E/A (ratio of early and active filling of the ventricle), is affected earlier and to a greater degree than systolic function and changes in the right heart precede those on the left (Figueras *et al.*, 2003).

Longitudinal changes in fetal Doppler indices and relationship to perinatal outcome

Middle cerebral artery

Several studies have reported that increased MCA PI precedes changes in other vessels (Arduini *et al.*, 1992; Ferrazzi *et al.*, 2002). While observational studies have shown a relationship between elevated MCA PI and perinatal morbidities (e.g. low Apgar scores and neonatal complications), positive predictive values are generally poor (Hornbuckle and Thornton, 1998). Fong *et al.* (1999) confirmed that UA PI was a better predictor of major adverse perinatal outcome (e.g. death, hypoxic-ischemic encephalopathy, grade 4 intraventricular hemorrhage [IVH], periventricular leukomalacia, necrotizing enterocolitis [NEC]), especially before 32 weeks, but reported that a normal MCA PI had a lower negative likelihood ratio (0.15 [0.04,0.59]) compared to a normal UA PI (0.51 [0.32,0.82]). Loss of "brain sparing," however, is associated with a major increase in perinatal morbidity and mortality (Konje *et al.*, 2001; Rowlands and Vyas, 1995). Thus while a normal MCA PI is reassuring, using an increase in MCA PI alone to time delivery is not appropriate because the time between the onset of cerebral

vasodilatation and terminal hypoxic events may be 2–3 weeks (Konje *et al.*, 2001; Rowlands and Vyas, 1995).

Umbilical artery

Significant increases in umbilical PI have been reported 2–3 weeks prior to development of pathological FHR changes (Arduini *et al.*, 1992; Ferrazzi *et al.*, 2002; Hecher *et al.*, 2001). The median time from detection of AEDF in the UA to late FHR decelerations has been reported to be 7 days but the range was wide (1–26 days) (Arduini *et al.*, 1993). Unsurprisingly the interval between the development of REDF and delivery is shorter, averaging 3 days (Zelop *et al.*, 1996). An increased UA PI has consistently been shown to predict adverse outcome but progression to AREDV confers much greater risk of morbidity and mortality. Outcome data from two large studies (GRIT Study Group, 2003; Karsdorp *et al.*, 1994) and our own center are shown in Table 32.1.

Ductus venosus

Abnormalities in DV and UV are late findings. Ferrazi *et al.* (2002) reported that changes in DV PIV and reversal of DV "a" wave followed early increases in MCA and UA PI; by the time of delivery, 40% of fetuses had an abnormal PIV and 20% a reversed "a" wave. For fetuses delivered after 28 weeks, perinatal mortality was 10% in those with early changes in MCA and UA PI alone and 57% in those with "late" venous and cardiac Doppler abnormalities prior to delivery. Baschat (2004) summarized the available studies and concluded that 43% of growth–restricted fetuses have an abnormal DV waveform within 1 week of delivery and this increases to 60% on the day of delivery.

A summary of perinatal outcome in 522 GR fetuses conducted by Baschat (2004) is shown in Figure 32.3. Overall perinatal mortality was 41% in those with abnormal DV Doppler compared with 2% in fetuses where DV PIV was normal (Baschat, 2004). Morbidities were also higher;

Table 32.1. Mortality and major morbidity by umbilical artery Doppler

	All cases		Actively managed cases		
Study	Karsdorp et al. (1991–1993)	Hornbuckle et al. (1994–2002)	Hornbuckle et al. (1994–2002)	GRIT Study (1996–2001)	
PIH/PE (%)	206/459 (45)	62/137 (45)	49/99 (49)	149/348 (43) AREDV PEDV 140/239 (59) 234/548 (43) Overall	
Mortality					
PEDV	8/214 (4)			17/346 (5)	
AEDV	73/178 (41)	22/92 (24)	6/77 (8)	41/206 (20)	
REDV	50/67 (75)	27/45 (60)	5/22 (23)	8/33 (24)	
AREDV	123/245 (50)	49/137 (36)	11/99 (11)	49/239 (21)	
Morbidity					
	AREDV		21/88 (24)	PEDV	AREDV
RDS/BPD	40/168 (24)		15/94 (16)	N/A	
IVH/VM	17/168 (10)		3/94 (3)	11/348 (3)	14/239 (6)
NEC	10/168 (6)		6/94 (6)	13/348 (4)	17/239 (7)
Dead or serious disability at 2 years				32/348 (9)	67/239 (28)

Figures are numbers (%).

Abbreviations: EDV, end-diastolic velocities; PIH, pregnancy-induced hypertension; PE, pre-eclampsia; PEDV, present end-diastolic velocities; AEDV, absent end-diastolic velocities; REDV, reversed end-diastolic velocities; AREDV absent or reversed end-diastolic velocities; RDS, respiratory distress syndrome; BPD, bronchopulmonary dysplasia; IVH, intraventricular hemorrhage; VM, ventriculomegaly; NEC, necrotizing enterocolitis.

RDS (85% vs. 43%), BPD (30% vs. 13%), NEC (13% vs. 9%) and IVH (21% vs. 7%). For severely compromised fetuses with AREDF of the UA reversed "a" wave in the DV was associated with an increased risk of stillbirth (24% vs. 6%) and neonatal death (29% vs. 12%) (Baschat, 2004).

In conclusion although the overall pattern of fetal Doppler changes in chronic placental insufficiency, indicative of progressive hypoxemia and acidemia, has been established, the rate of progression is variable. This is partly determined by the degree of placental vascular dysfunction, gestational age and the co-existence of maternal disease, particularly pre-eclampsia (Baschat, 2004).

Relationship between fetal Doppler indices and long-term outcome

There is a paucity of long-term neurological outcomes in high-risk pregnancies and few studies have looked at the predictive value of prenatal Doppler. Although abnormal UA Doppler waveforms are accurate predictors of adverse neonatal outcome, Wilson et al. (1992) found they were not predictive of long-term neurodevelopmental problems at 5 years of age. A larger study of women with severe pre-eclampsia also found no difference in Developmental Quotient at either 24 or 48 months in babies with normal or abnormal UA Doppler indices, although infants with AREDF in-utero scored lower in the performance subscale (Kirsten et al., 2000). Further follow-up is warranted to see whether this disadvantage persists. Unlike UA Doppler, fetal aortic waveforms have been shown to predict intellectual outcome at 2 years (Soothill et al., 1992) and impaired intellectual outcome at the age of 6–7 years (Ley et al., 1996).

With respect to the MCA, preterm fetuses with evidence of in-utero "brain sparing" have

Perinatal Mortality in relation to UA and DV Doppler

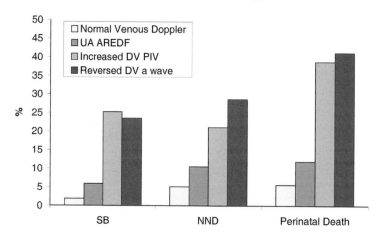

Perinatal Morbidity in relation to DV Doppler indices

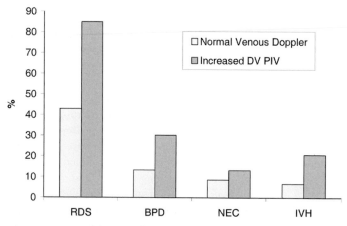

Figure 32.3 Perinatal mortality and morbidity in relation to ductus venous Doppler. Summary of outcome data from studies of ductus venosus Doppler. Reproduced from Baschat (2004), with permission. Abbreviations: UA, umbilical artery; DV, ductus venosus; AREDF, absent/reversed end-diastolic frequencies; PIV, pulsatility index for veins; RDS, respiratory distress syndrome; BPD, bronchopulmonary dysplasia; NEC, necrotizing enterocolitis; IVH, intraventricular hemorrhage.

accelerated neuronal maturation, as measured by visual evoked potentials, compared to gestation matched controls (Scherjon *et al.*, 1996). At 2 years, fetal brain sparing seems a beneficial adaptation for neurological outcome (Chan *et al.*, 1996; Scherjon *et al.*, 1998). However, by 5 years it is associated with a lower cognitive outcome as evidenced by a 10-point reduction in mean IQ (Scherjon *et al.*, 2000). No data are yet available on venous Doppler waveforms and long-term neurodevelopmental outcome.

Clinical application of uterine artery Doppler

Prediction of pre-eclampsia by uterine artery Doppler at 18–24 weeks' gestation

Low-risk pregnancies

Based on a review of 19 studies, Papageorghiou *et al.* (2002) found an overall sensitivity of uterine artery Doppler for predicting pre-eclampsia of 55% but this ranged from 24% to 89%. The pooled likelihood ratio (LR) for a positive result (LR+) was 5.90 (5.30, 6.52) while the pooled LR for a negative result was 0.55 (0.50, 0.60). Lees *et al.* (2001) subsequently showed that likelihood of severe adverse pregnancy outcome (fetal death, abruption

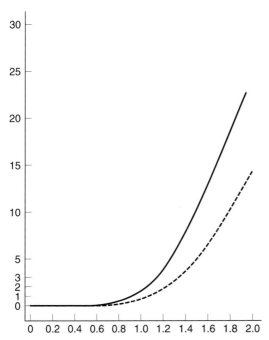

Figure 32.4 Prediction of adverse outcome by uterine artery Doppler at 23 weeks. Likelihood ratio (vertical axis) for severe adverse outcome (fetal death, pre-eclampsia before 34 weeks, small-for-gestational age fetus [<10th centile] before 34 weeks, placental abruption) relating to mean pulsatility index (horizontal axis). Smokers are represented by a thick block line, nonsmokers by a thin line. Reproduced from Lees *et al.* (2001), with permission.

and delivery before 34 weeks associated with pre-eclampsia and birthweight <10th centile) increased quadratically with mean uterine artery PI (Figure 32.4); the 95th centile for mean PI was 1.45 and at this level the LR for severe adverse outcome was 5 for nonsmokers and 10 for smokers.

The clinical usefulness of routine uterine artery screening in low-risk women is, however, debatable. Based on the overview of Chien *et al.* (2000) of 27 studies, uterine artery Doppler has not been recommended for inclusion in routine antenatal care in England (National Collaborating Centre for Women's and Children's Health, 2003). However, the benefit of screening is also influenced by the effectiveness of therapies to prevent or ameliorate pre-eclampsia in screen-positive women.

At present, Doppler screening of uterine arteries, with the aim of reducing pre-eclampsia in screen-positive women, cannot be recommended. If the greater therapeutic benefit of antioxidants (Chappell *et al.*, 1999) versus aspirin therapy is confirmed in large randomized trials this will need to be reviewed. With the current drive to reduce antenatal visits in "low-risk" women (National Collaborating Centre for Women's and Children's Health, 2003), the value of a normal uterine artery screen, also needs to be addressed.

High-risk pregnancies

The positive predictive value of uterine artery Doppler is greater in women at high risk of pre-eclampsia based on underlying maternal vascular disease, e.g. SLE, chronic hypertension or renal disease and also in women with previous severe pre-eclampsia. A recent detailed comparison of screening performance in high-risk women suggested that a mean RI > 0.69 performed as well as a mean PI > 1.51, irrespective of notch status (sensitivity 55%, PPV 72%, NPV 80%) (Friedman *et al.*, 1995).

Application of uterine Doppler in specific patient groups has generally confirmed these results. Recent studies of normotensive women with previous adverse pregnancy outcomes (previous pre-eclampsia, stillbirth, abruption, FGR) have generally reported sensitivities for pre-eclampsia of 78–95% with PPV 39–44% (Coleman et al., 2003; Harrington et al., 2004; Parretti et al., 2003). Studies in women with chronic hypertension have indicated slightly lower PPV (Harrington et al., 2004; Parretti et al., 2003). Perhaps more importantly in these high-risk groups, a normal uterine artery Doppler waveform confers a risk of adverse outcome similar to that of women with an uncomplicated obstetric history or normotension (Frusca et al., 1998; Harrington et al., 2004).

Prediction of pre-eclampsia by uterine artery Doppler prior to 16 weeks' gestation

Several studies have suggested that uterine artery Doppler screening before 16 weeks is also predictive of subsequent pre-eclampsia. Harrington et al. (1997), using a transvaginal approach at 12–16 weeks, reported promising results; if bilateral notches were present the risk of pre-eclampsia was markedly increased (OR 22 [7,74]). Martin et al. (2001) reported that the 95th centile for mean PI, obtained transabdominally, was 2.35 and was unchanged between 11 and 14 weeks. The sensitivity for predicting pre-eclampsia was, however, markedly reduced compared with 23 week screening, especially for early-onset pre-eclampsia. Whether earlier knowledge of an abnormal uterine artery Doppler result is of value remains to be determined and, as with later screening, this is currently not recommended in low-risk women.

Use of uterine artery Doppler after 24 weeks' gestation

The presence of abnormal uterine artery Doppler waveforms after 28 weeks of pregnancy has been associated with adverse pregnancy outcome in several studies, although predictive values for pre-eclampsia have generally been poor (Brown et al., 1990).

In women presenting with PIH uterine artery Doppler appears to identify those at greatest risk of adverse maternal and fetal outcome. Frusca et al.

(2003) undertook uterine artery Doppler assessment in 344 hypertensive pregnant women and concealed the results from clinicians. A uterine artery RI > 0.62 and/or bilateral diastolic notching was identified in 164/188 (87%) of women with pre-eclampsia and 71/158 (45%) with PIH and was associated with a greater incidence of FGR. In women with both pre-eclampsia and PIH, those with an abnormal Doppler were more likely to deliver <34 weeks (pre-eclampsia: 63% vs. 23%; PIH: 46% vs. 5%). Multivariate analysis of the severity of hypertension, presence of proteinuria, and uterine Doppler found that only abnormal uterine Doppler was associated with poor feto-maternal outcome [OR 13.2 (95% CI 7.1,24.5)]. Uterine artery Doppler also predicts adverse outcome in FGR; in pregnancies with a fetal abdominal circumference <10th centile after 34 weeks, 28% had bilateral notching and/or a mean RI > 0.58 (Frusca et al., 2003). Those with an abnormal uterine artery group are delivered earlier and have a higher incidence of NICU admission (35% vs. 11%), UA PI >95th centile (12% vs. 3%) and Cesarean section for non-reassuring fetal status (27% vs. 10%) (Vergani et al., 2002).

While the available evidence does not support third-trimester screening in low-risk women, assessment of uterine artery Doppler appears to be useful in women with previously abnormal waveforms and in those presenting with PIH/pre-eclampsia in order to stratify perinatal risk.

Clinical studies of umbilical and fetal Doppler in pre-eclampsia

The effects of abnormal placentation are frequently seen on both sides of the maternal–fetal unit. Frusca et al. (2003) found that 41% of women with pre-eclampsia and 22% with PIH developed abnormal UA Doppler waveforms. Further, in series with AREDF in the UA, the incidence of pre-eclampsia is between 33 and 47% and of PIH 6–15% (Hornbuckle *et al.*, 2003; Montenegro *et al.*, 1998).

Few studies have investigated the role of UA and fetal Doppler in pre-eclampsia pregnancies alone. One small study of 42 women with pre-eclampsia assessed UA Doppler and concealed results from clinicians (Eronen *et al.*, 1993). Those with abnormal UA Doppler were delivered at earlier gestations (mean 29.7 vs. 31.4 weeks) and 26% had serious morbidity compared with 5% with normal UA Doppler. Multiple regression analysis showed adverse outcome was significantly associated with both abnormal UA Doppler and GA at delivery. A larger study of 72 women with pre-eclampsia also investigated the association between abnormal UA Doppler and perinatal outcome (Yoon *et al.*, 1994). Doppler indices were again concealed from clinicians with monitoring undertaken by biophysical profile and FHR monitoring. Abnormal Doppler indices were found in 37/72 (51%) and were associated with earlier delivery (32 weeks vs. 38 weeks) and higher rates of adverse perinatal (86% vs. 11%) and neonatal (53% vs. 3%) outcome. All 13 perinatal deaths occurring in the abnormal UA Doppler group. Logistic regression identified GA at delivery, severity of pre-eclampsia and abnormal UA Doppler to be significantly related to adverse perinatal and neonatal outcome. Only abnormal UA Doppler remained a significant predictor for adverse outcome after adjusting for confounding variables, including GA at birth.

An elevated MCA PI or MCA/UA PI ratio has also been associated with adverse outcome in pre-eclampsia. Ozeren *et al.* (1999) compared UA and MCA Doppler in a group of women with pre-eclampsia ± FGR and normal controls. Significant differences were found in all mean Doppler indices. In keeping with other high-risk studies, UA PI had the highest sensitivity for adverse perinatal outcome and FGR (88%). Interestingly, those with pre-eclampsia and a normally grown fetus had a lower MCA PI and MCA/UA PI ratio than controls.

Toward a rational fetal monitoring strategy in pre-eclampsia

With improvements in neonatal management clinicians have been willing to deliver high-risk pregnancies at earlier gestations, particularly where there is evidence of both maternal and fetal compromise. Clinicians should avoid early delivery in the belief that in pre-eclampsia fetal maturation is accelerated; in a large cohort of preterm infants delivered to women with pre-eclampsia matched to preterm deliveries to normotensive mothers there were no differences in the rates of mortality, RDS, severe IVH and NEC between the groups, even at gestations less than 32 weeks (Friedman *et al.*, 1995). Trials of "aggressive versus expectant management" in severe pre-eclampsia show that expectant management is not detrimental to maternal outcome and improves neonatal outcome (Odendaal *et al.*, 1990; Sibai *et al.*, 1994). The latest trial of timed delivery for high-risk pregnancies, the GRIT study, also showed a trend toward improved perinatal and two-year outcomes with expectant management (The Grit Study Group, 2003) (Table 32.1).

Thus in pre-eclampsia prior to term, where maternal disease does not necessitate delivery, expectant management is justified in the interests of the fetus until the risks in-utero are greater than those from prematurity. In practice, delivery is usually undertaken when surveillance tests such as FHR monitoring, biophysical profile or venous Doppler are deemed to indicate a fetal decompensatory response to hypoxia or acidosis. Where pregnancies are complicated by both pre-eclampsia and FGR, similar surveillance tools should be utilized but with an increase in the frequency of monitoring. Even where there is no evidence of FGR, 30% of women with pre-eclampsia will require delivery within 24 h of previously reassuring monitoring (Chari *et al.*, 1995). The risk of abruption is high and in severe pre-eclampsia, 8-hourly fetal heart rate monitoring has been advocated (Odendaal *et al.*, 1998).

Management decisions and monitoring strategies vary with gestational age and the degree of maternal and fetal compromise. Integrated testing using a combination of utero-placental and fetal Doppler, biophysical parameters and FHR patterns is now recommended for FGR (Harman and Baschat, 2003). For women with pre-eclampsia, the addition of uterine artery Doppler may identify apparently normally grown fetuses who are at increased perinatal risk and for whom increased fetal surveillance is required.

The fetal monitoring strategy currently in use for women with pre-eclampsia at the Royal Victoria Infirmary, Newcastle is shown in Figure 32.5. This is based on the literature reviewed in

Sections 3 and 4. The basis of monitoring is UA Doppler; this is the only test for which we have evidence from randomized trials in high-risk pregnancies that inclusion improves perinatal outcome (Neilson and Alfirevic, 2000). Although the possible benefits of studying fetal arterial and venous circulations have been highlighted in observational studies, there are no randomized controlled trials. The frequency of repeat Doppler monitoring in fetuses with a normal UA PI is unclear. In small-for-gestational age fetuses, preliminary evidence suggests that twice-weekly testing is associated with a higher rate of induction of labor but no difference in neonatal morbidity compared with fortnightly testing

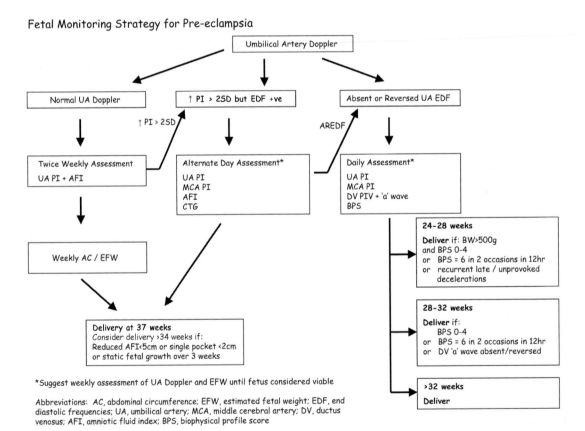

Figure 32.5 Guideline for fetal monitoring in pre-eclampsia.

(McCowan et al., 2000). However, <5% of the 167 women randomized in this trial had pre-eclampsia and most authorities would recommend at least weekly UA Doppler assessment in established pre-eclampsia.

Of far greater significance is how to monitor fetuses with an abnormal umbilical artery PI, especially those with AREDF. We would regard this finding alone as an indication for delivery >32 weeks. Below this gestation the options are daily FHR monitoring, biophysical profile scoring, venous Doppler or a combination. The recent study of Bilardo et al. (2004) suggests that DV Doppler is a better predictor of adverse perinatal outcome than FHR variability. Previously we have used the biophysical profile to time delivery in very preterm fetuses with AREDF (Hornbuckle et al., 2004). In our series of 137 non-anomalous fetuses with AREDF, 45% of which occurred in women with pre-eclampsia, the overall mortality in actively managed cases (i.e. those where delivery would have been undertaken in the fetal interests) was 11%. This compares favorably with the results of the large European experience of fetuses with AREDF (Karsdorp et al., 1994) and the GRIT study (Table 32.1). However, the accumulating evidence that venous Doppler, particularly DV, is a useful adjunct to help identify the decompensating fetus (Baschat, 2004) has led us to include absence or reversal of the DV "a" wave as an indication for delivery prior to 33 weeks gestation. In practice, we have found that this is often synchronous with deterioration in the biophysical profile.

Conclusion

The increasing technical capabilities of ultrasound machines allow specific interrogation of vessels from the placental and fetal circulation. Uterine and UA Doppler are important clinical utilities to identify high-risk pregnancies. Once identified as high-risk, women can be counseled about the need for enhanced fetal surveillance using UA Doppler. In women with pre-eclampsia, the loss or reversal of EDF in the UA signals the need for daily surveillance by experienced clinicians working in units capable of managing preterm growth-restricted neonates. As such it is a seminal finding.

Evidence from randomized trials, incorporating women with pre-eclampsia, suggest that early delivery of the very preterm fetus confers no advantage over expectant management where there is uncertainty regarding the timing of delivery. However, daily monitoring of maternal and fetal condition is vital. Doppler assessment of the fetal venous system to time delivery looks promising. However, concealing Doppler assessments from clinicians involved in the timing of delivery is increasingly difficult and the use of descriptive monitoring strategies for pregnancies with defined risk categories in the clinical trial setting is timely. Only well-designed trials of timed delivery, including long-term neurodevelopment as an outcome, will confirm the role of fetal Doppler in the management of high-risk pregnancy.

REFERENCES

Aardema, M. W., Oosterhof, H., Timmer, A., van Rooy, I. and Aarnoudse, J. G. (2001). Uterine artery Doppler flow and uteroplacental vascular pathology in normal pregnancies and pregnancies complicated by pre-eclampsia and small for gestational age fetuses. Placenta, 22, 405–11.

Arduini, D. and Rizzo, G. (1990). Normal values of Pulsatility Index from fetal vessels: a cross sectional study on 1556 healthy fetuses. J. Perinatal. Med., 18, 165–72.

Arduini, D., Rizzo, G. and Romanini, C. (1992). Changes of pulsatility index from fetal vessels preceding the onset of late decelerations in growth-retarded fetuses. Obstet. Gynecol., 79, 605–10.

Arduini, D., Rizzo, G. and Romanini, C. (1993). The development of abnormal heart rate patterns after absent end-diastolic velocity in umbilical artery: analysis of risk factors. Am. J. Obstet. Gynecol., 168, 43–50.

Baschat, A. A. (2004). Doppler application in the delivery timing of the preterm growth-restricted fetus: another step in the right direction. *Ultrasound Obstet. Gynecol.*, **23**, 111–18.

Baschat, A. A., Gembruch, U., Reiss, I., Gortner, L., Weiner, C. P. and Harman, C. R. (2000). Relationship between arterial and venous Doppler and perinatal outcome in fetal growth restriction. *Ultrasound Obstet. Gynecol.*, **16**, 407–13.

Baschat, A. A., Gembruch, U., Weiner, C. P. and Harman, C. R. (2003). Qualitative venous Doppler waveform analysis improves prediction of critical perinatal outcomes in premature growth-restricted fetuses. *Ultrasound Obstet. Gynecol.*, **22**, 240–5.

Bilardo, C. M., Wolk, H., Stigter, R. H., *et al.* (2004). Relationship between monitoring parameters and perinatal outcome in severe, early intrauterine growth restriction. *Ultrasound Obstet. Gynecol.*, **23**, 119–25.

Bower, S., Vyas, S., Campbell, S. and Nicolaides, K. H. (1992). Color Doppler imaging of the uterine artery in pregnancy: normal ranges of impedance to blood flow, mean velocity and volume of flow. *Ultrasound Obstet. Gynecol.*, **2**, 261–5.

Bower, S., Bewley, S. and Campbell, S. (1993). Improved prediction of preeclampsia by two-stage screening of uterine arteries using the early diastolic notch and color Doppler imaging. *Obstet. Gynecol.*, **82**, 78–83.

Brown, M. A., North, L. and Hargood, J. (1990). Uteroplacental Doppler ultrasound in routine antenatal care. *Aust. N.Z. J. Obstet. Gynaecol.*, **30**, 303–7.

Chan, F. Y., Pun, T. C., Lam, P., Lam, C., Lee, C. P. and Lam, Y. H. (1996). Fetal cerebral Doppler studies as a predictor of perinatal outcome and subsequent neurologic handicap. *Obstet. Gynecol.*, **87**, 981–8.

Chappell, L. C., Seed, P. T., Briley, A. L., *et al.* (1999). Effect of antioxidants on the occurrence of pre-eclampsia in women at increased risk: a randomised trial. *Lancet*, **354**, 810–16.

Chari, R. S., Friedman, S. A., O'Brien, J. M. and Sibai, B. M. (1995). Daily antenatal testing in women with severe preeclampsia. *Am. J. Obstet. Gynaecol.*, **173**, 1207–10.

Chien, P. W., Arnott, N., Gordon, A., Own, P. and Khan, K. (2000). How useful is uterine artery Doppler flow velocimetry in the prediction of pre-eclampsia, intrauterine growth retardation and perinatal death? An overview. *Br. J. Obstet. Gynaecol.*, **107**, 196–208.

Coleman, M. A. G., McCowan, L. M. E. and North, R. A. (2000). Mid-trimester uterine artery screening as a predictor of adverse pregnancy outcome in high risk women. *Ultrasound Obstet. Gynecol.*, **15**, 7–12.

Edelstone, D. I. (1980). Regulation of blood flow through the ductus venosus. *J. Dev. Physiol.*, **2**, 219–38.

Eronen, M., Kari, A., Pesonen, E., Kaaja, R., Wallgren, E. I. and Hallman, M. (1993). Value of absent or retrograde end-diastolic flow in fetal aorta and umbilical artery as a predictor of perinatal outcome in pregnancy-induced hypertension. *Acta Paediatr.*, **82**, 919–24.

Ferrazzi, E., Bozzo, M., Rigano, S., *et al.* (2002). Temporal sequence of abnormal Doppler changes in the peripheral and central circulatory systems of the severely growth-restricted fetus. *Ultrasound Obstet. Gynecol.*, **19**, 140–6.

Figueras, F., Puerto, B., Martinez, J. M., Cararach, V. and Vanrell, J. A. (2003). Cardiac function monitoring of fetuses with growth restriction. *Eur. J. Obstet. Gynecol. Reprod. Biol.*, **110**, 159–63.

FitzGerald, D. E. and Drumm, J. E. (1997). Non-invasive measurement of human fetal circulation using ultrasound: a new method. *Br. Med. J.*, **ii**, 1450–1.

Fong, W., Ohlsson, K., Arne, H. E., *et al.* (1999). Prediction of perinatal outcome in fetuses suspected to have intrauterine growth restriction: Doppler US study of fetal cerebral, renal, and umbilical arteries. *Radiology*, **213**, 681–9.

Friedman, S. A., Schiff, E., Kao, L. and Sibai, B. M. (1995). Neonatal outcome after preterm delivery for preeclampsia. *Am. J. Obstet. Gynecol.*, **172**, 1785–8.

Frusca, T., Soregaroli, M., Zanelli, S., Danti, L., Guandalini, F. and Valcamonico, A. (1998). Role of uterine artery Doppler investigation in pregnant women with chronic hypertension. *Eur. J. Obstet. Gynecol. Reprod. Biol.*, **79**, 47–50.

Frusca, T., Soregaroli, M., Platto, C., Enterri, L., Lojacono, A. and Valcamonico, A. (2003). Uterine artery velocimetry in patients with gestational hypertension. *Obstet. Gynecol.*, **102**, 136–40.

Giles, W. B., Trudinger, B. J. and Baird, P. J. (1985). Fetal umbilical artery flow velocity waveforms and placental resistance: pathological correlation. *Br. J. Obstet. Gynaecol.*, **92**, 31–8.

Harman, C. R. and Baschat, A. A. (2003). Arterial and venous Dopplers in IUGR. *Clin. Obstet. Gynecol.*, **46**, 931–46.

Harrington, K., Carpenter, R.G., Goldfrad, C. and Campbell, S. (1997). Transvaginal Doppler ultrasound of the uteroplacental circulation in the early prediction of pre-eclampsia and intrauterine growth retardation. *Br. J. Obstet. Gynaecol.*, **104**, 674–81.

Harrington, K., Fayyad, A., Thakur, V. and Aquilina, J. (2004). The value of uterine artery Doppler in the prediction of uteroplacental complications in multiparous women. *Ultrasound Obstet. Gynecol.*, **23**, 50–5.

Hecher, K., Campbell, S., Snijders, R. and Nicolaides, K. (1994). Reference ranges for fetal venous and atrioventricular blood flow parameters. *Ultrasound Obstet. Gynecol.*, **4**, 381–90.

Hecher, K., Bilardo, C.M., Stigter, R.H., *et al.* (2001). Monitoring of fetuses with intrauterine growth restriction: a longitudinal study. *Ultrasound Obstet. Gynecol.*, **18**, 564–70.

Hofstaetter, C., Gudmundsson, S. and Hansmann, M. (2002). Venous Doppler velocimetry in the surveillance of severely compromised fetuses. *Ultrasound Obstet. Gynecol.*, **20**, 233–9.

Hornbuckle, J. and Thornton, J.G. (1998). The fetal circulatory response to chronic placental insufficiency. and relation to pregnancy outcome. *Fetal. Mat. Med. Rev.*, **10**, 137–52.

Hornbuckle, J., Sturgiss, S.N. and Robson, S.C. (2003). Mangement of fetuses with absent and reversed end-diastolic frequencies (AREDF) in the umbilical artery; outcome of a policy of daily biophysical profile (BPP). *J. Obstet. Gynaecol.*, **23**(Suppl. 1), S35.

Karsdorp, V.H.M., van Vugt, J.M.G., van Geijn, H.P., *et al.* (1994). Clinical significance of absent or reversed end diastolic velocity waveforms in umbilical artery. *Lancet*, **344**, 1664–8.

Kirsten, G.F., Van Zyl, J.I., Van Zijl, F., Maritz, J.S. and Odendaal, H.J. (2000). Infants of women with severe early pre-eclampsia: the effect of absent end-diastolic umbilical artery Doppler flow velocities on neurodevelopmental outcome. *Acta Paediatr.*, **89**, 566–70.

Konje, J.C., Bell, S.C. and Taylor, D.J. (2001). Abnormal Doppler velocimetry and blood flow volume in the middle cerebral artery in very severe intrauterine growth restriction: is the occurrence of reversal of compensatory flow too late? *Br. J. Obstet. Gynaecol.*, **108**, 973–9.

Lees, C., Parra, M., Missfelder-Lobos, H., Morgans, A., Fletcher, O. and Nicolaides, K.H. (2001). Individualized risk assessment for adverse pregnancy outcome by uterine artery Doppler at 23 weeks. *Obstet. Gynecol.*, **98**, 369–73.

Ley, D., Tideman, E., Laurin, J., Bjerre, I. and Marsal, K. (1996). Abnormal fetal aortic velocity waveform and intellectual function at 7 years of age. *Ultrasound Obstet. Gynecol.*, **8**, 160–5.

Lin, S., Shimizu, I., Suehara, N., Nakayama, M. and Aono, T. (1995). Uterine artery Doppler velocimetry in relation to trophoblast invasion into the myometrium of the placental bed. *Obstet. Gynecol.*, **85**, 760–5.

Lyall, F, and Robson, S.C. (2000). Defective extravillous trophoblast function and pre-eclampsia. In *The Placenta: Basic Science and Clinical Practice*, ed. J. Kingdom, E. Jauniaux and S. O'Brien. London: RCOG Press, pp. 79–96.

Martin, A.M., Bindra, R., Curcio, P., Cicero, S. and Nicolaides, K.H. (2001). Screening for pre-eclampsia and fetal growth retardation by uterine artery Doppler at 11–14 weeks of gestation. *Ultrasound Obstet. Gynecol.*, **18**, 583–6.

Matijevic, R. and Johnston, T. (1999). In vivo assessment of failed trophoblastic invasion of the spiral arteries in pre-eclampsia. *Br. J. Obstet. Gynaecol.*, **106**, 78–92.

McCowan, L.M.E., Harding, J.E., Roberts, A.B., Barker, S.E., Ford, C. and Stewart, A.W. (2000). A pilot randomized controlled trial of two regimes of fetal surveillance for small-for-gestational age fetuses with normal results of umbilical artery Doppler velocimetry. *Am. J. Obstet. Gynecol.*, **182**, 81–6.

Montenegro, N., Santos, F., Tavares, E., Matias, A., Barros, H. and Leite, L.P. (1998). Outcome of 88 pregnancies with absent or reversed end-diastolic blood flow (ARED flow) in the umbilical arteries. *Eur. J. Obstet. Gynecol. Reprod. Biol.*, **79**, 43–6.

Muller, T., Nanan, R., Rehn, M., Kristen, P. and Dietl, J. (2002). Arterial and ductus venosus Doppler in fetuses with absent or reverse end-diastolic flow in the umbilical artery: correlation with short-term perinatal outcome. *Acta Obstet. Gynecol. Scand.*, **81**, 860–6.

National Collaborating Centre for Women's and Children's Health. (2003). Antenatal Care: Routine Care for the Healthy Pregnant Woman. London: RCOG Press, pp. 105–8.

Neilson, J.P. and Alfirevic, Z. (2000). Doppler ultrasound for fetal assessment in high risk pregnancies. *Cochrane Database Syst. Rev.*, (**2**): p. CD000073.

Nicolaides, K. H., Bilardo, C. M., Soothill, P. W. and Campbell, A. (1988). Absence of end-diastolic frequencies in umbilical artery: a sign of fetal hypoxia and acidosis. *Br. Med. J.*, **297**, 1026–7.

Nicolini, U., Nicolaidid, P., Fisk, N. M., *et al.* (1990). Limited role of fetal blood sampling in prediction of outcome in intrauterine growth retardation. *Lancet*, **336**, 768–72.

Odendaal, H. J., Pattinson, R. C., Bam, R., Grove, D. and Kotze, T. J. (1990). Aggressive or expectant management for patients with severe preeclampsia between 28–34 weeks' gestation: a randomized controlled trial. *Obstet. Gynecol.*, **76**, 1070–5.

Odendaal, H. J., Pattinson, R. C., du Toit, R. and Grove, D. (1998). Frequent fetal heart-rate monitoring for early detection of abruptio placentae in severe proteinuric hypertension. *S. Afr. Med. J.*, **74**, 19–21.

Ozeren, M., Dinc, H., Ekmen, U., Senekayli, C. and Aydemir, V. (1999). Umbilical and middle cerebral artery Doppler indices in patients with preeclampsia. *Eur. J. Obstet. Gynecol. Reprod. Biol.*, **82**, 11–16.

Papgeorghiou, A. T., Hu, C. K. H., Cicero, S., Bower, S. and Nicolaides, K. H. (2002). Second-trimester uterine artery Doppler screening in unselected populations: a review. *J. Mat. Fet. Neonatal. Med.*, **12**, 78–88.

Parretti, E., Mealli, F., Magrini, A., *et al.* (2003). Cross-sectional and longitudinal evaluation of uterine artery Doppler velocimetry for the prediction of pre-eclampsia in normotensive women with specific risk factors. *Ultrasound Obstet. Gynecol.*, **22**: 160–5.

Prefumo, F., Bhide, A., Sairam, S., Penna, L., Hollis, B. and Thilaganathan, B. (2004). Effect of parity on second-trimester uterine artery Doppler flow velocity and waveforms. *Ultrasound Obstet. Gynecol.*, **23**, 46–9.

Rizzo, G., Capponi, A., Arduini, D. and Romanini, C. (1995a). The value of fetal arterial, cardiac and venous flows in predicting pH and blood gases measured in umbilical blood at cordocentesis in growth retarded fetuses. *Br. J. Obstet. Gynaecol.*, **102**, 963–9.

Rizzo, G., Capponi, A., Soregaroli, M., Arduini, D. and Romanini, C. (1995b). Umbilical vein pulsations and acid-base status at cordocentesis in growth-retarded fetuses with absent end-diastolic velocity in umbilical artery. *Biol. Neonate*, **68**, 163–8.

Rowlands, D. J. and Vyas, S. K. (1995). Longitudinal study of fetal middle cerebral artery flow velocity waveforms

preceding fetal death. *Br. J. Obstet. Gynaecol.*, **102**, 888–90.

Sagol, S., Ozkinay, E., Oztekin, K. and Ozdemir, N. (1999). Comparison of uterine artery Doppler velocimetry with the histopathology of the placental bed. *Aust. N.Z. J. Obstet. Gynaecol.*, **39**, 324–9.

Scherjon, S. A., Oosting, H., de Visser, B. W., de Wilde, T., Zondervan, H. A. and Kok, J. H. (1996). Fetal brain sparing is associated with accelerated shortening of visual evoked potential latencies during early infancy. *Am. J. Obstet. Gynecol.*, **175**, 1569–75.

Scherjon, S. A., Oosting, H., Smolders-DeHaas, H., Zondervan, H. A. and Kok, J. H. (1998). Neurodevelopmental outcome at three years of age after fetal 'brain-sparing'. *Early Hum. Dev.*, **52**, 67–79.

Scherjon, S., Briet, J., Oosting, H. and Kok, J. (2000). The discrepancy between maturation of visual-evoked potentials and cognitive outcome at five years in very preterm infants with and without hemodynamic signs of fetal brain-sparing. *Pediatrics*, **105**, 385–91.

Sibai, B. M., Mercer, B. M., Schiff, E. and Friedman, S. A. (1994). Aggressive versus expectant management of severe preeclampsia at 28 to 32 weeks' gestation: a randomized controlled trial. *Am. J. Obstet. Gynecol.*, **171**, 818–22.

Soothill, P. W., Ajayi, R. A., Campbell, S., *et al.* (1992). Relationship between fetal acidemia at cordocentesis and subsequent neurodevelopment. *Ultrasound Obstet. Gynaecol.*, **2**, 80–3.

The GRIT Study Group (2003). A randomised trial of timed delivery for the compromised preterm fetus: short term outcomes and Bayesian interpretation. *Br. J. Obstet. Gynaecol.*, **110**, 27–32.

Vergani, P., Roncaglia, N., Andreotti, C., *et al.* (2002). Prognostic value of uterine artery Doppler velocimetry in growth-restricted fetuses delivered near term. *Am. J. Obstet. Gynecol.*, **187**, 932–6.

Vyas, S., Nicolaides, K. H., Bower, S. and Campbell, S. (1990). Middle cerebral artery flow velocity waveforms in fetal hypoxaemia. *Br. J. Obstet. Gynaecol.*, **97**, 797–803.

Wilson, D. C., Harper, A., McClure, G., Halliday, H. L. and Reid, M. (1992). Long term predictive value of Doppler studies in high risk fetuses. *Br. J. Obstet. Gynaecol.*, **99**, 575–8.

Yoon, B. H., Lee, C. M. and Kim, S. W. (1994). An abnormal umbilical artery waveform: a strong and independent predictor of adverse perinatal outcome in patients with preeclampsia. *Am. J. Obstet. Gynecol.*, **171**, 713–21.

Zelop, C. M., Richardson, D. K. and Heffner, L. J. (1996). Outcomes of severely abnormal umbilical artery Doppler velocimetry in structurally normal singleton fetuses. *Obstet. Gynecol.*, **87**, 434–8.

33

Pregnancy-induced hypertension – the effects on the newborn

Jonathan Coutts

Pregnancy-induced hypertension (PIH) is regarded as an obstetric complication of pregnancy. There are significant adverse maternal effects, some resulting in serious maternal morbidity or death. However, it must be remembered that placental abruption, acute renal failure, intracerebral hemorrhage and pulmonary edema will also have an adverse effect on the fetus. In addition, concern for the mother's safety may result in a plan to deliver the fetus early to avoid maternal ill health. Early delivery will result in the resolution of the maternal risk but will increase risk to the baby. The difficulty for the attending obstetrician is deciding whether continuing the pregnancy will result in harm to the mother and continued fetal compromise, or whether delivery will result in fetal morbidity or death.

Maternal reasons for delivery, such as the development of renal or hepatic dysfunction, may tax the skill of the fetal medicine specialist. When are proteinuria or elevated liver enzymes in a mother no longer tolerable; is the mother on the point of becoming significantly unwell with eclampsia or HELLP syndrome? Sometimes the risk to the mother is less immediate and the concern may be that continuing the pregnancy will result in fetal death. Worsening uteroplacental function will reduce the ability of the fetus to tolerate the in-utero environment. A biophysical profile may help in making the decision whether early delivery is indicated in the fetal interest. Oligohydramnios, non-reassuring electronic fetal heart rate monitoring or biophysical profile, reduced or absent end-diastolic umbilical arterial

Doppler velocity flow, and arrest of fetal growth are signs that the fetus is at risk.

Table 33.1 lists the early complications affecting the fetus and neonate in a PIH pregnancy. Table 33.2 lists complications that occur after the immediate newborn period. Many of these are complications of prematurity, rather than specific problems affecting newborns from PIH pregnancies. Prematurity from a neonatology perspective is effectively the period from 23 weeks to 35 weeks. Before 23 completed weeks the newborn is unlikely to survive. There are decreasing problems with advancing gestation and newborns at 36 weeks will often be able to be placed in the postnatal ward rather than the neonatal unit. Most complications occur in newborns of 32 weeks or below, with the highest risk of death or major handicap in children born before 28 weeks and in males (Larroque *et al.*, 2004).

Fetal medicine and neonatal intensive care specialists often concentrate on the initial problems a premature neonate faces, such as respiratory distress, and may forget that from a parent's and patient's perspective major problems such as learning difficulties will continue for many years.

- Early delivery in the maternal interest may not benefit the fetus.
- Many neonatal complications of PIH are due to prematurity.
- The highest risks occur in newborns less than 28 weeks.
- Long-term problems are often more significant than those occurring in the NICU.

Table 33.1. Fetal and early neonatal complications of PIH

Complications	Cause	Treatment
IUGR	Utero-placental insufficiency	Monitor for signs of maternal or fetal compromise Planned delivery if compromised
Perinatal asphyxia	Placental insufficiency Oligohydramnios Poor tolerance of labor and delivery	Monitor for signs of fetal compromise Planned delivery if compromised Neonatologist at delivery
Hypothermia	Prematurity with small size IUGR with reduced fat	Warm towels and incubators Occlusive dressing (polythene bag) at delivery
Hypoglycemia	IUGR with reduced energy store Labetalol (see below)	Prompt intravenous dextrose Early feeds if able to tolerate enteral feeds
Maternal drug effects	Hypotonia, apnea (magnesium sulfate) Hypoglycemia (Labetalol) Hypotension, renal failure (ACE inhibitors)	Avoid if possible Recognize and treat complication
Respiratory distress syndrome	Prematurity with surfactant deficiency Asphyxia with surfactant dysfunction	Antenatal steroids Exogenous surfactant Early CPAP Positive pressure ventilation
Sepsis	Neutropenia Decreased maternal immunoglobulin transfer Insertion of plastic cannulas and tubes	Infection control measures Early and appropriate antibiotics Fungal prophylaxis Colony-stimulating factors and immunoglobulin infusion
Necrotizing enterocolitis	Gut hypoxia in utero Persistent arterial duct post delivery Need for umbilical lines	Delay feeds in absent umbilical arterial flow Good general neonatal care Use breast milk Treat arterial duct

Early problems

Intra-uterine growth restriction

Intra-uterine growth restriction (IUGR) or small for gestational age (SGA) infants are born with a birthweight less than the tenth percentile for gestational age. It is essential to measure the child's length and head circumference (occipito-frontal circumference: OFC). IUGR will either be symmetrical (length and weight both decreased) or asymmetrical (length and OFC preserved).

Symmetrical IUGR is often familial (one or both parents are short) or a sign of an underlying fetal chromosomal abnormality. PIH causes asymmetrical IUGR with the fetal length and head (brain) growth preserved at the expense of fat and glycogen deposition. PIH stress imposed on the fetus causes an anti-insulin response probably regulated by increased levels of catecholamines. This results in a loss of fat and muscle mass and reduced glycogen stores. Blood flow to essential organs such as the brain, heart and adrenal glands

Table 33.2. Late neonatal complications of PIH

Problem	Cause	Treatment
Respiratory problems	CLD Increased problems from viral infections	Oxygen Nutrition to allow for growth Vaccinate (Flu and RSV)
Cerebral palsy	Periventricular hemorrhage Periventricular leukomalacia Perinatal asphyxia	May be antenatal in origin Good general care Neonatologist at delivery

Handicap and learning
  problems
	Cerebral palsy
	Deafness
	Retinopathy of prematurity
		Good general care and screening
		Neurodevelopmental follow-up
		Referral for therapist advice
		  problems detected

Visual problems	ROP PVH, PVL	Laser photocoagulation Visual aids
Hearing loss	PVH PVL Drug toxicity	Hearing aids Cochlear implants
Growth failure	IUGR Poor postnatal nutrition	Dietary supplements Human growth hormone

Increased adult-onset diseases
  (hypertension, diabetes, stroke)
	Prenatal programming
	  (Barker hypothesis)
		Prevent PIH

CLD, Chronic lung disease; PVH, periventricular hemorrhage; PVL, periventricular leukomalacia; ROP, retinopathy of prematurity.

is conserved. After birth examination shows a baby with a large head relative to body size. There is soft tissue wasting, reduced muscle bulk and large hands and feet. IUGR newborns are at risk of both early and late complications. Initial problems are an increased risk of perinatal asphyxia, polycythemia, hypoglycemia and hypothermia. The late complications of short stature and fetal programming of adult-onset disease will be discussed later in this chapter.

Perinatal asphyxia

IUGR often co-exists with oligohydramnios secondary to placental insufficiency. During labor, PIH infants are prone to hypoxemia from cord compression due to the oligohydramnios. This causes intermittent fetal hypoxemia, the results of which are more significant because of the background oxygen deficiency caused by uteroplacental

insufficiency in PIH. Stressed PIH infants may pass meconium in-utero with an increased risk of meconium aspiration. A neonatologist should attend all deliveries where there is a significant concern about fetal wellbeing.

Polycythemia

The normal hematocrit of a newborn is 65%. The need to transport oxygen in the hypoxic environment results in an increased red cell mass. This compensates for low hemoglobin saturation, resulting in increased oxygen delivery to the tissues. Following birth, when normal arterial oxygen saturations are achieved, this excess red cell mass can become problematic. All newborns have redundant red cells and the hemoglobin will drop in the first few weeks. The excess bilirubin produced from this, combined with immature enzyme systems in the liver, leads to the phenomenon of physiological jaundice. In an IUGR infant there is an increased bilirubin load from the extra red cells, often impaired liver function from in-utero hypoxemia, and the possibility of a compromised newborn. There is then concern that bilirubin levels will rise to harmful levels and phototherapy and exchange transfusion may be required to prevent kernicterus. The increased red cell mass may have other harmful effects relating to increased blood viscosity. These include hypoglycemia, hypocalcemia, decreased glomerular filtration, and decreased gastrointestinal perfusion leading to gut mucosal ischemia. The hematocrit can be lowered by a partial exchange transfusion using saline. There are risks from this procedure and in the author's experience this is rarely required. It is essential, however, that a venous hematocrit is checked, as capillary samples will often be falsely raised. Ensuring that the newborn is not dehydrated (by giving judicious intravenous fluids) and monitoring the blood glucose and calcium is usually sufficient to prevent complications.

Hypothermia

All low birthweight infants are at risk of hypothermia because of an increased surface area to body weight ratio. The risk increases in newborns with IUGR as they have little subcutaneous fat, have an increased head surface area to body weight, and are more likely to have neonatal complications predisposing to increased heat loss. Attention to maintaining a neutral thermal environment (NTE) is vital to such infants. The NTE is the environmental temperature in which a newborn is able to maintain a normal core temperature with minimal caloric expenditure, which varies with gestational age and weight. Traditionally, temperature control at delivery has been with the use of warm towels to dry the infant and radiant warmers on the resuscitaire. Recently, immediate placement of the newborn, without drying, into a plastic bag (either those specifically designed for use in a neonatal unit or freezer bags bought in the local supermarket) has been shown to be an effective means of temperature control. The technique is described by neonatologists working in Edinburgh, Scotland (Lyon and Stenson, 2004).

The baby is slid into the bag up to the neck while still wet. The head is covered with a hat. No blankets are used, allowing radiant heat to warm the infant through the bag. Clinical inspection and auscultation can be performed through the bag, and, if vascular access is needed, a small hole can be cut in the bag…On arrival in the unit, the baby is weighed and then placed in a warm humidified incubator before the bag is removed.

Hypoglycemia

Definitions of hypoglycemia have changed over the years and the acceptable level of blood sugar has risen in the last decade, driven in part by medico-legal concerns. The "paper that launched a thousand law suits" described changes in sensory-evoked brain stem potentials in neonates with blood sugars less than $2.6 \, micromol \, l^{-1}$ ($45 \, mg \, dl^{-1}$) (Koh et al., 1988). Because of this report most neonatalogists now treat any newborn that is shown to have a blood glucose level less than this. This leads, in many cases, to increased (and sometimes unnecessary) medical intervention in normal term breastfeeding newborns. In the case of an IUGR infant delivered from a pregnancy complicated by PIH (pre-eclampsia or superimposed pre-eclampsia) an aggressive approach is appropriate. Most neonatal units employ bedside capillary glucose monitors to screen for hypoglycemia. These are generally innacurate at the lower range of blood sugar recordings, which is the area of most interest to neonatologists and a confirmatory whole blood or plasma blood glucose (TBG) should be sent. Figure 33.1 defines an algorithm for monitoring and treating hypoglycemia in an IUGR infant.

Feeding

Breast milk is the best source of nutrition for term newborn infants. The long-chain fatty acids in

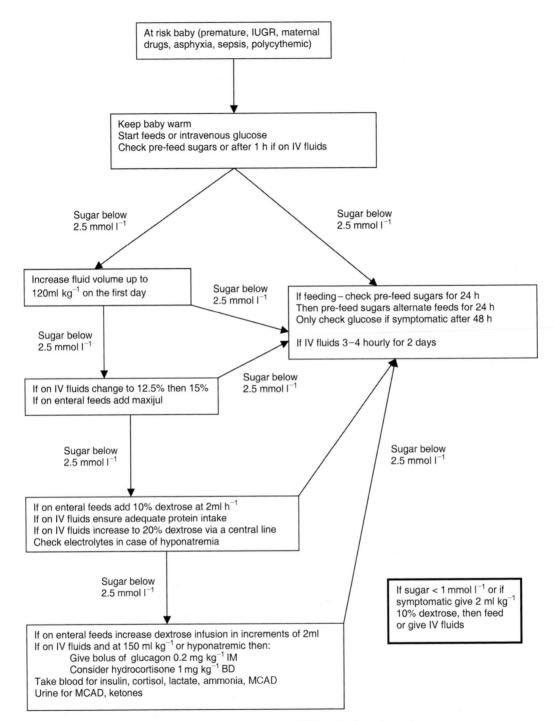

Figure 33.1 Stepwise approach to monitoring and treating a PIH baby for hypoglycemia.

breast milk are required for normal development of the central nervous system. Despite modification, formula feeds currently lack these fatty acids and therefore must be considered second choice. Breast milk also contains other non-nutritive substances such as immunoglobulins and hormones that are essential for the continued development of the gastrointestinal tract in the premature IUGR infant. Neonatal units should encourage mothers to start expressing breast milk, even if the mother plans to bottle feed. Some nurseries provide breast milk banks and consent for the use of donor breast milk should be sought for high-risk infants if the mother is unable to provide enough of her own milk. Unfortunately breast milk does not contain enough calories, protein or minerals for sustained growth in the very premature infant. Supplements either in the case of a mixture of breast milk and premature formula or breast milk plus HMF (human milk fortifiers) can be used. Both of these options will increase the osmolality of the feeds, leading to an increased risk of necrotizing enterocolitis (NEC) in infants with IUGR.

Maternal drugs

Drugs used in PIH can have detrimental effects on the fetus. Labetalol, in rare instances, may result in neonatal hypoglycemia, and an infant born to a mother prescribed labetalol should be monitored for hypoglycemia as outlined in Figure 33.1. Magnesium sulfate, when used in high doses, can cause hypotonia and apnea in the newborn. Angiotensin-converting enzyme inhibiting drugs (ACE inhibitors) can result in a dramatic decrease in renal function in both newborns and the fetus. In the neonatal intensive care unit this class of drugs would initially be introduced in a greatly reduced dose and slowly increased. Fetal and neonatal renal failure have been reported after prenatal use of ACE inhibitors.

- PIH pregnancies often result in asymmetric IUGR.
- Glucose must be kept above $2.5 \, \mathrm{mmol \, l^{-1}}$ $(45 \, \mathrm{mg \, dl^{-1}})$ in all newborns.

- Plastic freezer bags are a useful method of temperature control in small babies.
- Breast milk is best, but additives will be needed in most IUGR infants.
- Avoid ACE inhibitors in pregnancy.

Respiratory distress syndrome

Initial survival of premature newborns often depends on the degree of lung disease present. The lung bud in the fetus develops in stages. At approximately 24 weeks gestation gas exchange is possible since terminal branching of the airways has already taken place with the development of saccules and alveolar ducts. True alveolar formation does not start until 36 weeks when the lung surface area dramatically increases. This process continues for the first 2 years of life. Because of this ongoing pulmonary development there is great potential for lung growth and recovery in the post neonatal period.

By term sufficient surfactant has been produced to lower surface tension, maintain the functional residual capacity and improve lung compliance. The major constituent of surfactant, lecithin (phosphatidylcholine), first appears in significant quantities at about 24 weeks. In the past this was used to detect pulmonary maturity antenatally. A ratio of lecithin to sphingomyelin of 2:1 in amniotic fluid signifies reasonable pulmonary maturity and helped guide plans for delivery. In current perinatal management the L:S ratio is no longer universally used because of cost and time constraints, and newer tests such as the Fetal Lung Maturity (FLM) assay, or Lamellar Body Count are now more popular. Antenatal corticosteroid treatment is used routinely to accelerate surfactant production in babies delivered between 24 and 34 weeks (24 and 32 weeks in PPROM). Maternal steroid injection (usually betamethasone 12 mg IMI, two doses 12–24 h apart) is administered 12–48 h before birth in those cases where premature delivery can be anticipated.

Respiratory Distress Syndrome (RDS) is caused by a relative deficiency of active surfactant leading to alveolar collapse at the end of expiration. Respiratory failure occurs due to the atelectasis and presents as hypoxia with hypercapnia and acidosis. Without treatment, the shear forces acting on the fragile lung lead to capillary leak of a proteinaceous material noticeable on histology as a hyaline membrane. Because of antenatal steroids and postnatal surfactant treatment there has been a change in the pattern of respiratory distress seen in premature newborns. Frequently the premature neonate has minimal evidence of surfactant deficiency initially, although it may go on to develop significant respiratory problems.

Prompt resuscitation of at-risk infants to prevent hypoglycemia and cold injury, both of which inactivate surfactant, is vital. It is now accepted that exogenous surfactant should be administered early in high-risk infants rather than waiting until there is established atelectasis (Verder *et al.*, 1999). There is still debate as to whether this means elective intubation of every baby less than 29 weeks at birth, or if surfactant should be given only to those infants who truly require intubation at birth. There are two types of exogenous surfactant available for treatment. Natural surfactant harvested from pigs or cows (e.g. Curosurf, Survanta) contain varying amounts of the different surfactant proteins in comparison to artificial surfactant (e.g. Exosurf). The presence of these surfactant proteins is thought to explain the superior results seen with the administration of a natural surfactant (Halliday, 1996).

Supplemental inspired oxygen should be given to all infants who are hypoxemic. If the oxygen requirement is climbing, the pCO_2 is raised, or there is moderate respiratory distress, nasal continuous positive airway pressure (NCPAP) should be used. NCPAP recruits collapsed alveoli, increases the functional residual capacity and improves lung compliance, reversing the changes seen in RDS. A number of units around the world now use NCPAP electively in all of their premature newborns with the goal of prophylactically keeping the lungs inflated rather than delaying its use until the development of atelectasis. If NCPAP fails then the child needs intubation and positive pressure ventilation.

Positive end expiratory pressure (PEEP) will help keep alveoli from collapsing at the end of inspiration. A setting of 5 cm H_2O is usual. Lower settings may not be effective, while high settings can reduce venous return of blood to the heart. Peak pressures should be kept as low as possible to decrease the risk of lung injury due to excessive stretch of the alveoli. The inspiratory time should be set between 0.3 and 0.4 s. If the child is active then trigger ventilation is appropriate. Four-hourly blood gases (more frequent if unstable) should aim for pH 7.20–7.40, $PaCO_2$ 45–55 mmHg, and a saturation of 88–92% initially. It is now common practice to use more rapid rates with short inspiratory times rather than the longer inspiratory times used in the past. Newborns are more comfortable if they are not breathing against the ventilator.

High-frequency oscillation (HFO) is a method of ventilation which uses a high continuous distending pressure to open up the lungs. This provides the optimal surface area for gas exchange in a similar manner to surfactant resulting in a FiO_2 of <30%. Very fast ventilator breaths (typically 600 min^{-1}) using very small tidal volumes provide fresh gas for gas exchange with less traumatic stretching of fragile lungs compared to conventional tidal breathing ventilation. HFO is increasingly used as the initial form of ventilation in premature infants with hyaline membrane disease (Courtney *et al.*, 2002).

Nitric oxide (described by the journal *Science* as "Molecule of the Year" in 1982) is known to regulate pulmonary vessel smooth muscle. Initially introduced into neonatal practice as a treatment for term infants with persistent pulmonary hypertension of the newborn, it has also been used in premature infants with hypoxic respiratory failure. Initial studies suggested that there was an increase in intracerebral bleeds, though recently trials of inhaled NO have shown reduced incidence of death, chronic lung disease, and severe PVH/PVL (Schreiber *et al.*, 2003). At the present time it is prudent to restrict NO treatment in premature infants with hypoxic respiratory failure to those taking part in randomized clinical trials with appropriate informed consent (Martin, 2003).

- Antenatal steroids are the most important recent advance in neonatal respiratory therapy.
- Surfactant should be given early to premature infants.
- Early CPAP will keep a premature lung open and will reduce complications.
- High-frequency ventilation should be considered as routine ventilation for premature infants.
- Nitric oxide should only be prescribed to a premature infant as part of a randomized trial.

Infection

There have been advances in the development of antibiotic therapy, but neonatal sepsis is still a major problem. PIH pregnancies often result in the delivery of premature infants with IUGR requiring respiratory support and intravenous therapy. These infants are at high risk of neonatal sepsis and despite appropriate antibiotic therapy many still die due to deficiencies in their immune system responses. It has been recognized for some time that neutropenia often occurs in infants born to mothers with PIH. This is usually transient, but may persist for a month. The degree of neutropenia is more profound in the more premature or growth-restricted infants, and especially so in mothers with significant hypertension or HELLP syndrome. The etiology in PIH is thought to be reduced neutrophil production due to intrauterine hypoxia, possibly compounded by release of a specific inhibitor. This is made worse in premature infants since they have functionally immature neutrophils with reduced ability for neutrophil production. They also have less circulating immunoglobulin because of reduced maternal transfer of IgG, which mostly occurs after 32 weeks. Risks of infection are increased by procedures in the intensive care unit such as intubation and line insertion. Trials of colony stimulating factors

(G-CSF or GMCSF) either as prophylactic therapy in neutropenic infants, or when sepsis is suspected, have shown some improvement in survival in the latter group (Bernstein et al., 2001). In addition, intravenous immunoglobulin (IVIG) infusion has reduced mortality in septic newborns. IVIG provides IgG, which binds to cell surface receptors, promoting opsonization and activating complement. Currently a multicenter trial of IVIG in neonatal sepsis is underway (International Neonatal Immunotherapy Study).

In the last decade coagulase-negative staphylococcal infection has emerged as a common problem for premature infants. The NICHD experience (Stoll et al., 2002) (of nearly 7000 newborns) published in 2002 showed an increased risk of this infection if a central venous line or umbilical arterial line was in place, if parenteral nutrition was continued for longer than 7 days, and if the first feeds were delayed for more than 7 days. Early attainment of full feeds and regaining birthweight by day 7 were protective factors. Most of these findings can be explained by the need for intravenous cannulas. Coagulase-negative staphylococcus favors plastic cannulas and lines, which quickly become colonized. As early as the first days of life coagulase-negative staphylococcus should always be considered a likely pathogen and a clinical deterioration should prompt institution of vancomycin treatment. A monoclonal antibody has been developed (BSYX-A110) which is protective against both coagulase-negative staphylococcus and *Staphylococcus aureus*. This is still under investigation in humans; the company involved has obtained "orphan drug status" from the FDA allowing it to complete neonatal trials. Invasive fungal infections are common in this group as well following the use of broad-spectrum antibiotics. Prophylactic fluconazole (or nystatin) should be considered whenever antibiotics are used for the treatment of sepsis after the first week of life.

Nosocomial infections are usually caused by gut flora. We know that gut bacteria are of fundamental importance in the development of a premature newborn's immature immune system. One reason why breast milk is protective against infection is that it provides the nucleotides and immune cells needed for the modulation of the immune system in the gut. The initial bacteria to colonize the premature infant's gut have advantages compared to late arrivals. The normal gut flora of newborns initially consists of *E. coli* and *Enterococcus*, followed by *Bifidobacterium*, with heterogeneous bacterial flora becoming established by day 10. In breastfed newborns the benign bifidobacteria and lactobacilli predominate. In the neonatal intensive care unit a preterm baby will have delayed colonization with a limited bacterial species different to those described above. Coagulase-negative staphylococci, *Enterobacter cloacae* and *Klebsiella* predominate. There is a paucity of lactobacilli and bifidobacteria and increased candida colonization. Factors influencing this initial gut colonization are the (ab)use of broad-spectrum antibiotics, breast feeding versus use of formula, and the separation of mother and baby on the first night. Vaginal delivery is protective, as these babies will be exposed to the normal rectal flora of the mother during delivery. Babies born by Cesarean section have increased risk of sepsis, most likely due to the delay in colonization of their intestinal tract by non-pathogenic organisms. It has been suggested that smearing the faces of newborns delivered by Cesarian section with maternal feces would be an effective measure to reduce sepsis. This therapy is unlikely to elicit a favorable parental response.

Necrotizing enterocolitis (NEC) is a great concern in infants born after PIH pregnancies as they have many of the predisposing characteristics for infants at high risk of developing this complication. There is uncertainty about the timing of the introduction of feeding, and the rate of increase in these high-risk newborns. It is established that expressed breast milk is protective, and this is often the reason why some neonatal units have expressed breast milk banks available and will seek consent for the use of donor breast milk for high-risk infants when there is no maternal milk available. Unfortunately the needs of the IUGR infant from a PIH pregnancy means that additives

are required for normal growth. Both human milk fortifiers, and premature formula milk, increase the osmolality of the feed and increase the risk of NEC.

The promotion of normal GIT bacterial flora is also thought to be beneficial. The un-indicated use of enteral non-absorbable antibiotics such as vancomycin will promote the emergence of drug-resistant organisms and this practice should be discouraged.

- Neutropenia in PIH newborns is associated with increased sepsis.
- Colony stimulation and immunoglobulin infusions are useful adjunct therapies.
- Gut colonization with benign organisms is important in reducing nosocomial infection.
- Monoclonal antibodies may be the future treatment for sepsis.
- IUGR infants from PIH pregnancies are at increased risk of NEC.

Long-term complications

Respiratory problems

There has been a change in the pattern of long-term lung injury seen in modern neonatal units. The original description of Bronchopulmonary Dysplasia (BPD) by Northway *et al.* in 1967 remained relevant until the routine use of antenatal steroids and post-delivery surfactant in the mid 1990s. Technological advances have enabled neonatologists to measure tidal volumes, use trigger ventilation and oscillators and to reduce the degree of lung damage. We no longer usually see the marked overdistension, fibrosis and airway damage seen previously. However, the lungs of the smaller babies now rescued are easily damaged even if there is minimal initial RDS. Chronic Lung Disease (CLD) is now the preferred term for long-term lung damage rather than BPD, as there is less airway damage (Jobe and Bancalari, 2001). CLD is defined as oxygen dependency at 28 days, with clinical evidence of respiratory distress, and an abnormal CXR. CLD is a complication of any neonatal lung injury. This injury is caused virtually exclusively by prematurity combined with ventilator-induced lung damage from a high inspired oxygen concentration and over-distension in a surfactant-deficient lung. Infection, persistence of the ductus arteriosus, and the poorly developed antioxidant system of the premature infant, are all important contributing factors. Some severely affected infants behave in a fashion similar to "old-style" BPD infants where delivery was unexpected and there was no chance for the administration of antenatal steroids.

There is a lack of clear evidence regarding the preferred management of established CLD. The most important treatment is to ensure normal oxygen saturation. Untreated hypoxia will lead to pulmonary hypertension and death from cor pulmonale. With the ready availability of saturation monitors in modern neonatal practice this complication should no longer be seen. Unfortunately we do not know what the optimal saturation range is for a child with CLD (Saugstad, 2001). While it is known that normal children will have a saturation of 98–100% it is not clear what saturation level should trigger administration of additional oxygen. It is known that low oxygen saturations (in the 80s) are harmful and it is likely that growth and development is better with saturations >92%. In my practice at present I aim for a saturation of greater than 95% "most of the time". Another established treatment is to ensure normal growth as we hope the child will effectively outgrow their illness due to continued lung development, greatly increasing the surface area of the lung.

Apart from oxygen therapy and adequate nutrition, medical treatment is limited. Steroids have been shown to have short-term benefits such as expedited weaning from ventilation or decreased oxygen requirements, but these benefits are frequently at the expense of inducing a catabolic state with reduced growth. In addition, there are concerns about the long-term effects of steroids on neurodevelopment. Therefore steroids should be reserved for the most severely affected children with CLD who are at risk of dying from complications of long-term ventilation. Inhaled steroids do not generate the same concerns in terms of their long-term effects, but have not been shown to be an effective treatment. Diuretics have been shown to have short-term effects on lung function measurements, but do not improve long-term outcome and increase the risk of nephrocalcinosis. Bronchodilators (either inhaled or in the form of high-dose theophylline) have been advocated in children with CLD to treat bronchial smooth muscle hypertrophy and wheezing. There is, however, no convincing evidence for this practice and the wheezing is thought to be more likely due to an anatomically reduced airway diameter rather than pathologic bronchoconstriction.

In summary, optimal nutrition and adequate oxygenation are the most effective treatments for CLD. Most infants will outgrow their oxygen requirement before they are ready to be discharged. A small number will continue to need longer-term oxygen. A child who is stable, is sucking all feeds and is putting on weight should be discharged home with domiciliary oxygen. In the medium term, these children will have good respiratory function. Lung function testing in preadolescents shows desaturation with exercise (due to a lack of reserve from reduced lung surface area) but these children will have active, normal lives. In the first few years they are at risk for admission with lower respiratory tract infections, particularly Respiratory Syncytial virus (RSV). There is a monoclonal antibody that is active against RSV (palivizumab). It needs to be given on a monthly basis during the RSV season and it is effective in reducing admissions. Due to the high cost the use of palivizumab is often limited to the most premature infants. Children with CLD are often labeled as asthmatic, although many show an improvement in their respiratory symptoms as they become older. We are uncertain about the long-term effects of CLD as the oldest survivors are in their 30s. Prematurity and subsequent reduced lung volume, combined with the effects of smoking and aging, will lead to an increase in the natural age related decline in lung function. Whether or not we are producing a cohort of elderly respiratory cripples still remains to be seen.

- CLD is now the preferred term for the lung damage seen in ventilated newborns.
- Excess tidal volume damages lungs, not excess pressure from ventilators.
- The only effective treatments for CLD are time, growth, and oxygen.
- In the medium term, CLD does not produce severe handicap.
- We do not know the longer-term effects of CLD in an aging population.

Central nervous system problems

The fragile central nervous system of a premature infant is at risk of permanent damage. There is a high risk of periventricular hemorrhage (PVH) and periventricular leukomalacia (PVL), and sensory impairment such as deafness and blindness (Cioni *et al.*, 1997; Jacobson and Dutton, 2000; Larroque *et al.*, 2003) Unlike the long-term lung problems discussed above, which have potential to improve, injury to the central nervous system is permanent. The incidence of both PVH and PVL are increased in the newborns of mothers prematurely delivered because of pre-eclampsia.

Periventricular hemorrhage

PVH remains a significant cause of morbidity and mortality in premature infants despite recent advances in general neonatal care. PVH occurs in premature infants but not in those born at term because of a difference in the structure of the developing brain. A premature infant has a vascular area around the ventricles known as the subependymal germinal matrix. This is an area of neuronal proliferation and is present in the developing brain until about 32 weeks gestation. Bleeding in this area may occur in premature infants who have limited ability to control cerebral blood flow. Their lack of cerebral autoregulation, combined with

acute changes in cerebral blood flow from respiratory events such as pneumothorax, asynchrony between spontaneous and ventilator breaths, endotracheal suction, seizures, or rapid changes in pH, $PaCO_2$, or PaO_2, can lead to an acute intracranial bleed. This vascular area regresses in term infants, which explains the reduction in the incidence of PVH as infants become more mature. Head ultrasound examination is an excellent method for identifying PVH. There is an accepted grading system to describe the severity of PVH.

- Grade 1 – Germinal matrix bleed: Good outcome
- Grade 2 – Intraventricular bleed; no ventricular dilatation: Good outcome
- Grade 3 – Intraventricular bleed; ventricular dilatation: Less optimistic outcome (depends on degree of dilatation)
- Grade 4 – Intraventricular bleed; parenchymal bleed: Poor outcome

The major complications from PVH are due to either the destruction of cerebral parenchyma (porencephalic cyst) or to the development of post-hemorrhagic hydrocephalus.

Healing in areas of the brain that have been destroyed by PVH results in the formation of fluid-filled spaces. An area of the brain involved in a grade 4 hemorrhage becomes a porencephalic cyst. This will communicate with the adjoining ventricle, in contrast to the cysts of PVL (see below), which are adjacent to the ventricle. The pattern of injury depends on which area of the brain is involved. Motor handicap is common as the cortical spinal motor tracts are present in this region. If there is a large grade 4 hemorrhage, subsequent handicap will often be severe. Discussion with parents about discontinuing intensive care may be appropriate.

Blood present in the ventricle will not in and of itself cause any problem unless the blood volume loss is sufficient to cause hypotension. However, subsequent obstruction may lead to post-hemorrhagic hydrocephalus. Inflammation affecting the arachnoid villi and debris will obstruct drainage channels. Mild ventricular dilatation commonly occurs and probably has little effect on neurodevelopmental outcome. An increasing ventriculo-cerebral ratio as evident on serial U/S measurements with increasing OFC, separated sutures and tense fontanelle are indications for surgical intervention. Medical treatment with diuretics and acetazolamide are no longer considered beneficial. Experimental techniques using intraventricular catheters and irrigation over several days with artificial CSF (the DRIFT trial in Bristol, England) are available.

Periventricular leukomalacia

This is a significant cause of brain injury in premature infants. Hypotension results in poor cerebral perfusion in premature infants due to an inability to autoregulate the cerebral circulation. PVL may occur in utero if there is poor placental function or fetal blood loss, such as may result from antepartum hemorrhage. Antenatal chorioamnonitis has been shown to cause release of cytokines, which are known to damage the white matter of the premature brain. Post-natal events such as cerebral artery vasoconstriction secondary to hypocarbia from overventilation can decrease cerebral perfusion. A persistent ductus arteriosus can cause poor cerebral perfusion due to the "steal" of blood through the duct. The pattern of white matter injury in PVL is explained by the distribution of the watershed zones of the deep penetrating arteries of the middle cerebral artery. In keeping with a general hypoperfusion injury, PVL tends to be bilateral compared to the unilateral pattern of injury seen in PVH. In PVL ischemia damages the white matter containing descending corticospinal tract fibers. Visual and acoustic nerves may also be damaged.

The incidence of reported PVL ranges from 4 to 26%, and, in keeping with most neonatal complications, PVL occurs most commonly in infants less than 32 weeks' gestation. A head ultrasound initially shows white periventricular flare. In some infants this will fade but, with significant ischemia, a repeat ultrasound after 2–4 weeks will show cysts around but not communicating with the ventricle. Some infants may not develop cystic changes but

will have mild ventriculomegaly reflecting white matter loss. CT scan findings include ventriculomegaly and loss of white matter. In addition, MRI can show thinning of the posterior body and splenium of the corpus callosum with abnormal signal intensity of the deep white matter.

Most infants with PVL develop motor handicap and cerebral palsy. The commonest pattern is one of spastic diplegia, although if the injury is severe the child may have quadriplegia. There may be no intellectual impairment even in those with significant motor disability. Infants with PVL need input from a multidisciplinary team and careful assessment of vision and hearing. Subtle hearing and visual problems will significantly increase the functional disability experienced by a child.

- Neurological handicap is the most important sequelae from PIH.
- Experimental techniques for removing intraventricular blood are under research.
- PVL may cause motor handicap alone.
- PVL may be associated with visual and hearing handicap.

Follow-up of high-risk infants and long-term outcome

Neonatologists are faced with a dilemma as some complications arising during the neonatal period may not become apparent until the child is much older. All neonatal units must have a system to monitor neonatal unit graduates. Over a period either a problem will be identified and dealt with, or there will no longer be any significant risk of the problem occurring. In effect this means a follow-up program for 2 years as most children will be speaking and walking at this age. Without such follow-up it is difficult to be sure that any therapies used early in life are not harmful in the longer term. It can be argued that 2 years is not sufficiently long enough to identify problems such as learning difficulties. It is likely that large numbers of children born at the older gestations (32–34 weeks) will have problems at school. Criteria for initial follow-up will depend on the hospital but often will include ex-premature infants born less than 32 weeks, term infants who had either significant perinatal asphyxia or congenital malformation, and those with severe IUGR. Staff involved in the clinic should be part of a multidisciplinary team. The neonatologist functions as the general manager of the case. Ideally developmental therapists (physiotherapists, occupational therapists, speech and language therapists and psychologists), a dietician, social worker and community nurse should also be part of the team. Close links with a local child developmental clinic will provide a smooth transition for infants who require transferral to community care.

Cerebral palsy

Cerebral palsy is the end result of damage to the developing brain, resulting in problems with movement, tone and posture. Despite public misconception, intellect is often not affected. The major cause in premature infants is PVH and PVL. As noted below these complications can also affect sight and hearing. In most cases the newborn will leave the nursery with no apparent movement disorder. As the child becomes older and the nervous system matures, changes in tone become obvious. A picture of hemiplegia, diplegia or quadriplegia can be apparent, often with reduced truncal tone (causing problems with sitting) and dystonic movements. Early developmental physiotherapy is vital to encourage good posture to enable the child at risk to progress through each stage of normal development. The use of folded sheets as boundaries (similar to a nest), side lying to bring the newborn's hands together in the midline near the face are measures that should be routine in any nursery. In the clinic other measures such as educating parents to provide good truncal support when playing with their children and to discourage the use of "baby walkers" can be effective. Speech and language therapists can help with the feeding problems that these children may have, which can affect later speech development.

Occupational therapists can help provide aids for sitting, walking, etc. Many of the children will be able to go to mainstream school, but educational needs may favor placement in a special needs school.

Visual problems

Premature infants may develop visual problems secondary to damage to the retina, the visual pathways, or to the visual cortex. Retinopathy of prematurity (ROP) causes retinal damage either secondary to retinal detachment, or as a result of treatment which aims to prevent such detachment. It has been known for some time that hyperoxia is a risk factor for the development of ROP but, despite the reduction in indiscriminate oxygen therapy with strict monitoring of saturation levels, ROP remains a significant problem. It is likely that this is due to the increased survival of smaller babies who are more at risk of ROP. The blood vessels grow out of the optic disk to supply the retina. When a child is born prematurely the peripheral retina is still avascular. During the first few weeks of life the vessels will continue to grow and will, in most children, complete the normal supply to the whole retina. However, if this process is interrupted there is a risk that the avascular retina will produce an angiogenic substance. This causes abnormal vascular proliferation with an increased risk of bleeding and subsequent retinal detachment. The cause of ROP is multifactorial. Extreme prematurity, periods of both hypoxia and hyperoxia, and possible free radical damage are implicated in the development of significant retinopathy. Screening at 6 weeks of age by an experienced ophthalmologist will detect the earliest signs of ROP. A demarcation line between the vascular and avascular retina appears with subsequent ridge formation. Vascular tufts may then be seen and this "plus" sign is the signal for retinal ablation treatment. Initially cryotherapy, but more recently laser therapy, is used to destroy the peripheral avascular retina. This will prevent blindness from retinal detachment but there will be a loss of the peripheral retina and reduction in the visual field. The hope is that if the macula is preserved then visual function will be satisfactory.

The visual pathways and cortex can both be damaged by PVH and PVL and, even in the absence of significant ROP, visual function can be severely affected. Any concern about sight should prompt investigation with neurophysiological assessment of the visual pathway. Depending on the site of damage to the optic radiation in PVL, the child may seem to have good vision but could have significant problems. If the fibers from the upper retina are damaged then problems with the loss of the lower peripheral vision may be present. This may only be apparent, for example, when going downstairs causes a child to fall (the child is effectively stepping out into nothing) or the child may trample over his/her smaller siblings (they just don't see them). This may initially be thought to be due to a co-existing motor handicap or "clumsiness". Cortical damage can cause blindness in an extreme case, but may also cause "processing problems". A child may see single objects well but, as the amount of information received increases, the visual processing system "crashes". As a toddler they may have to pull all their toys out of the toybox and scatter them onto the floor to find their chosen toy. As an adult they may be unable to find a particular tin of soup on the shelves of a large busy supermarket. Therapists can provide coping mechanisms once a handicap is identified. For example, parents can ensure that toys are placed on plain backgrounds as opposed to patterned carpets. At school simple aids (such as using a ruler under the sentence while reading) can help the child from getting lost while reading a page of a book.

Hearing problems

Sensorineural hearing loss can occur due to damage from drugs (e.g. gentamicin), hypoxia, PVH and PVL. The cause in a single child is probably a combination of mechanisms. All neonatal unit graduates should be screened for hearing loss. Some hospitals may have a universal hearing screening program. The minimum should be to screen all children who have received aminoglycosides, all ventilated children, those born at less than 32 weeks, older asphyxiated children, plus any child with a family history of deafness or a congenital malformation which may cause deafness. In the neonatal unit there should be an effort to reduce the ambient noise levels. Simple measures to reduce noise include not placing objects onto the incubator roof (may result in a magnified thump if they fall onto the roof), not clicking the incubator door shut, and providing ear protection during episodes of predicted high noise such as helicopter transfer.

Short stature

Premature infants will mostly attain their expected adult height. PIH may cause asymmetric IUGR as discussed above. In comparison to symmetrical IUGR, which is often the result of an underlying genetic or teratogenic cause, these infants are able to show catch up growth during the first 1–2 years. This catch up growth will depend on adequate nutrition. Some of these infants remain small despite adequate calorie and protein intake. These children respond to human growth hormone treatment by increasing their height velocity (Czernichow, 1997). However, it is not yet clear if final adult height is affected, but even if adult height is not changed the increase in a child's height during school years will increase their confidence.

Learning problems

The graduates of the neonatal intensive care unit are at high risk of handicap in later life. This may be an obvious physical handicap such as cerebral palsy, but there is a "hidden" risk of learning problems, which often only becomes apparent as the children age and go to school. Some problems are a specific consequence of prematurity (e.g. visual problems from PVL) or severe IUGR (decreased number of brain cells). If a learning problem is identified early then successful intervention may be possible. The difficulty lies in identifying which children should be assessed. Children with cerebral palsy, hydrocephalus, retinopathy, etc., are obviously at increased risk for long-term problems. However, some less immature newborns and those who are initially assessed as "normal" at 2 years may subsequently develop significant long-term learning problems. One recent study showed an increase in the need for additional educational provision for these children from 15% at 8 years to 24% at 14–15 years (O'Brien *et al.*, 2004).

The Barker hypothesis (Barker, 2003)

The "thrifty phenotype" was popularized by Professor Barker in Southampton, England (Cheung *et al.*, 2004). From large epidemiological studies it has been recognized that IUGR children have an increased risk of developing some types of adult-onset disease. Diabetes, hypertension, myocardial events and stroke are all increased in IUGR infants when they become adults. The "Barker hypothesis" is that fetal programming in-utero, which leads to an IUGR infant, causes the resetting of normal physiological and biochemical development in the fetus as a survival technique. This is beneficial in the relatively hostile intra-uterine environment during pre-eclampsia, but becomes a problem when the child encounters different nutritional circumstances after birth. The concept of a "thrifty phenotype" child describes a child who will "hoard" fat when available in case of subsequent "famine". The initial observations by Barker were from data collected on English men born at the start of the twentieth century. As they became adults prosperity increased and nutrition improved. It could be that these later effects of IUGR are more apparent as a population moves from relative poverty to prosperity. Fetal growth restriction is often seen in the developing world secondary to small maternal size from previous poor nutrition. As countries such as India become more prosperous the Barker hypothesis suggests that the small children born at present (average birth weight in India is 2700 g) will become obese adults with increased risk of certain diseases. There has been an increase in the incidence of diseases such as type 2 diabetes in India. Better nutrition in childhood will counter the effect of maternal size causing small babies, but this will take one generation to take effect. In PIH maternal size is not an important factor in the development of IUGR. The reduced placental function causes IUGR as the fetus reacts with an anti-insulin response, and some of the long-term detrimental effects likely result from their increased insulin resistance in adult life. It has also been noted that in IUGR premature newborns there is increased arterial "stiffness" when measured at 8 years of age (Verder *et al.*, 1999). This is not present in appropriately grown premature infants, although it is not clear that this represents a definite risk for later development of hypertension.

- Long-term follow up is essential for high-risk newborns.
- Significant handicap can occur without cerebral palsy.
- Visual and hearing handicap must be screened for in children with PVH and PVL.
- Short stature resulting from IUGR is avoidable.
- Learning problems often only become apparent with increasing age.
- Fetal programming is now accepted as a cause of adult-onset disease.

REFERENCES

Barker, D. (2003). The midwife, the coincidence, and the hypothesis. *Br. Med. J.*, **327**, 1428–30.

Bernstein, H. M., Pollock, B. H., Calhoun, A. D. and Christensen, R. D. (2001). Administration of recombinant granulocyte colony-stimulating factor to neonates with septicemia: a meta-analysis. *J. Pediatr.*, **138**, 917–20.

Cheung, Y. F., Wong, K. Y., Lam, B. C. C. and Tsoi, N. S. (2004). Relation of arterial stiffness with gestational age and birth weight. *Arch. Dis. Child.*, **89**, 217–21.

Cioni, G., Fazzi, B., Coluccini, M., Bartalena, L., Boldrini, A. and van Hof-van Duin, J. (1997). Cerebral visual impairment in preterm infants with periventricular leukomalacia. *Pediatr. Neurol.*, **17**(4), 331–8.

Courtney, S. E., Durand, D. J., Asselin, J. M., Hudak, M. L., Aschner, J. L. and Shoemaker, C. T. for the Neonatal Ventilation Study Group. (2002). High-frequency oscillatory ventilation versus conventional mechanical ventilation for very-low-birth-weight infants. *N. Engl. J. Med.*, **347**, 643–52.

Czernichow, P. (1997). Growth hormone treatment of short children born small for gestational age. *Acta Paediatr. Suppl.*, **423**, 213–15.

Halliday, H. L. (1996). Natural vs synthetic surfactants in neonatal respiratory distress syndrome. *Drugs*, **51**(2), 226–37.

Jacobson, L. K. and Dutton, G. N. (2000). Periventricular leukomalacia: an important cause of visual and ocular motility dysfunction in children. *Surv. Ophthalmol.*, **45**(1), 1–13.

Jobe, A. H. and Bancalari, E. (2001). Bronchopulmonary dysplasia. *Am. J. Respir. Crit. Care Med.*, **163**(7), 1723–9.

Koh, T. H. H. G., Eyre, J. A. and Aynsley-Green, A. (1988). Neural dysfunction during hypoglycemia. *Arch. Dis. Child.*, **63**, 1353–8.

Larroque, B., Marret, S., Ancel, P. Y., *et al.* (2003). White matter damage and intraventricular hemorrhage in very preterm infants: the EPIPAGE study. *J. Pediatr.*, **143**(4), 477–83.

Larroque, B., Breart, G., Kaminski, M., *et al.* (2004). Survival of very preterm infants: Epipage, a population based cohort study. *Arch. Dis. Child. Fetal Neonatal Ed.*, **89**(2), F139–44.

Lyon, A. J. and Stenson, B. (2004). Cold comfort for babies. *Arch. Dis. Child. Fetal Neonatal Ed.*, **89**(1), F93–4.

Martin, R. J. (2003). Nitric oxide for preemies – not so fast. *N. Engl. J. Med.*, **349**, 2157–9.

Northway, W. H. Jr., Rosan, R. C. and Porter, D. Y. (1967). Pulmonary disease following respirator therapy of hyaline-membrane disease. Bronchopulmonary dysplasia. *N. Engl. J. Med.*, **276**(7), 357–68.

O'Brien, F., Roth, S., Stewart, A., Rifkin, L., Rushe, T. and Wyatt, J. (2004). The neurodevelopmental progress of infants less than 33 weeks into adolescence. *Arch. Dis. Child.*, **89**, 207–11.

Saugstad, O. D. (2001). Is oxygen more toxic than currently believed? *Pediatrics*, **108**(5), 1203–5.

Schreiber, M., Gin-Mestan, K., Marks, J. D., Huo, D., Lee, G. and Srisuparp, P. (2003). Inhaled nitric oxide in premature infants with the respiratory distress syndrome. *N. Engl. J. Med.*, **349**, 2099–107.

Stoll, B. J., Hansen, N., Fanaroff, A. A., *et al.* (2002). Late-onset sepsis in very low birth weight neonates: the experience of the NICHD neonatal research network. *Pediatrics*, **110**, 285–91.

Verder, H., Albertsen, P., Ebbesen, F., *et al.* (1999). Nasal continuous positive airway pressure and early surfactant therapy for respiratory distress syndrome in newborns of less than 30 weeks gestation. *Pediatrics*, **103**(2), E24.

34

Medico-legal implications of the diagnosis of pre-eclampsia

Jeffrey P. Phelan

Pre-eclampsia, with a reported incidence of 5–10% (Dildy, 2004), is not a stranger to the practising obstetrician. Infrequently, pre-eclampsia progresses to more severe forms marked by central nervous system changes, organ system dysfunction, and a greater degree of hypertension. Rarely, atypical presentations related to HELLP syndrome, thrombotic thrombocytopenic purpura (TTP), or hemolytic uremic syndrome (HUS), or an intracerebral hemorrhage may confuse the clinical picture (Sullivan and Martin, 2004). There is no question that there is potential for maternal and/or fetal or neonatal death or disability linked to a pregnancy complicated by pre-eclampsia (Table 34.1), and the underlying maternal vasospastic process. Not surprisingly, litigation as it relates to this hypertensive disorder is a frequent visitor.

Obstetric malpractice lawsuits whether the claims involve pre-eclampsia or not are, in general, more often related to the severity of the injury and the age of the patient and less often to issues of quality of care (Brennan et al., 1996). As such, the more severe the injury and the younger the patient, the greater the potential for damages or awards. Since obstetricians typically provide care to young women and their fetuses, death or disability to either the mother and/or her fetus(es) due to pre-eclampsia (or any other medical or obstetrical condition) has the potential for resulting in a large award or settlement. Since pre-eclampsia is frequently associated with the potential for liability, the purpose of this chapter is to familiarize

Table 34.1. Maternal or fetal death or disability and its link to pre-eclampsia

Maternal death or disability due to
Hemorrhage from
Hepatic rupture
Disseminated intravascular coagulation
Placental abruption (severe ≥50%)
Intracerebral hemorrhage
Hypertensive encephalopathy
Cardiopulmonary arrest
Fetal/neonatal death or disability due to
Maternal cardiopulmonary arrest
Recurrent seizures
Severe placental abruption (≥50%)
Preterm birth
Asphyxia

the reader with the concept of foreseeability of harm and its potential application to the care of the "pre-eclamptic patient." This chapter will also focus on a review of reported obstetrical malpractice cases involving pre-eclampsia. These cases were obtained from a search of Lexis–Nexis for the five-year period between 1 January 1998 and 31 December 2003. This chapter is intended to be used solely for educational purposes and is not designed to provide legal advice. Moreover, this chapter is one of many in the field of obstetrics, and does not necessarily represent the standard of care by the author or any other

Table 34.2. The difference in perspective between obstetricians and lawyers with respect to a fetal heart rate bradycardia

Professional	Event	Action
Obstetrician	FHR bradycardia	Prompt delivery
Lawyer	FHR bradycardia	Foreseeable?
		Avoidable?

obstetrical practitioner. It merely reflects a transmission of ideas that is hoped will result in an improvement in the perinatal outcome for pregnant women and their unborn children.

Foreseeability of harm

The concept of foreseeability of harm, first coined by Justice Benjamin Cardozo in 1916, is firmly entrenched in the US legal system and serves as a road map for any and all obstetrical malpractice litigation in the United States. This concept, which is taught to every aspiring lawyer in the US, has its roots in the case of *MacPherson v. Buick Motor Company* (1916). In that case, Justice Cardozo wrote that "because the danger is to be foreseen, there is a duty to avoid the injury … if [a person] is negligent where a danger is to be foreseen, a liability will follow" (*MacPherson v. Buick Motor Company*, 1916).

The simplest example for the application of this legal principle is the typical "stop sign case." Here, stop signs are positioned to protect drivers when entering and proceeding through intersections. If, for example, two cars enter the intersection simultaneously, it is foreseeable that an accident could result. Thus, stop signs impose an obligation on drivers entering that intersection to stop before proceeding through them. If a driver fails to stop, enters the intersection, and causes an accident, the driver could be held liable for any resultant injuries.

The application of this concept in the medical–legal setting demonstrates very quickly the differences in the training of physicians and lawyers (Table 34.2). In Table 34.2, the differing perspectives of these two professionals are illustrated with respect to a fetal heart rate (FHR) bradycardia. In the situation of a FHR bradycardia, the obstetrical provider reflexively responds by delivering the fetus in the most expeditious manner. The lawyer, on the other hand, asks whether the obstetrician/nurse should have predicted the FHR bradycardia and, thus, avoided it altogether. If an event is considered foreseeable or potentially avoidable such as the presence of repetitive severe variable FHR decelerations followed by a FHR bradycardia, the obstetrician/nurse is considered to be on notice. Notice means the circumstances in which a physician or nurse has sufficient time to identify the potential for acute fetal distress and an ample opportunity to correct or prevent the problem. Thus, the legal test becomes one based on "what a reasonably prudent obstetrician/nurse would do in light of that [information]" (Franklin and Rabin, 1983).

If we apply the principle of foreseeability of harm to a pre-eclamptic patient with a blood pressure (BP) reading of 225/150 mmHg and a severe headache, and who 6 h later has a massive intracerebral hemorrhage and dies, the lawyer will analyze and litigate this potential case using a two-step process (Figure 34.1). In the first step, the attorney will attempt to determine whether the physician or nurse were on notice or had sufficient warning of the potential for an intracerebral hemorrhage. In other words, should the physician or nurse have anticipated that an uncorrected BP elevation to that level (225/150 mmHg) in association with a severe headache would have resulted in an intracerebral hemorrhage. This means that during the course of a deposition or a trial of a case that involves a pregnant patient who died, for example, from an intracerebral hemorrhage, the initial focus will be on whether the intracerebral hemorrhage should have been anticipated. If, based on the facts, the intracerebral hemorrhage should have been anticipated, the primary focus will be on the obstetrician's and/or the nurse's efforts to prevent the patient from having the intracerebral hemorrhage. Once the intracerebral hemorrhage is manifested clinically, the focus of the litigation will shift to how the physician and/or nurse managed the patient's emergency.

The application of the foreseeability of harm principle is illustrated in Table 34.3. It is important to remember that the law evaluates conduct or what a physician or RN did or did not do under a given circumstance. To illustrate this, assume that the nurse has within the last few moments obtained a BP of 225/150 mm Hg and the complaint of a severe headache in a pregnant woman at 40 weeks gestation. As illustrated in this example, the usual course of events is that the nurse identifies an abnormality in the patient (in this case, an elevated BP and a severe headache). As soon as the nurse identifies the abnormality, the nurse is required to notify the physician, in most cases an obstetrician, to treat the maternal hypertension because the pregnant woman with a substantially elevated BP is at risk for an intracerebral hemorrhage. As such, the nurse would be expected to timely identify any change in maternal status and to promptly notify the patient's obstetrician. Therefore, once the nurse identifies the BP abnormality, she is on the clock to notify the obstetrician. Once the obstetrician is notified of the BP abnormality, the obstetrician is then on notice to timely respond to the clinical circumstance, and promptly evaluate and/or treat

the BP abnormality. If the physician does not respond, for whatever reason, the nurse has an independent duty to initiate the chain of command due to the lack of medical attention for purposes of obtaining care for the patient.

Therefore, once the obstetrician is notified, the obstetrician is obligated to respond in a timely manner and to evaluate the patient. To assist with physician documentation, a proposed model note is provided in Table 34.4. When documenting the timeliness of your response to the clinical circumstance, the same clock, such as your watch or the one on your beeper or mobile telephone, should be used. For the subsequent management of the patient, a single hospital clock such as the one on the fetal monitor should be used to time these clinical events. If there is a discrepancy in the times, the time discrepancy should be resolved when the patient is sufficiently stable, and the time

Table 34.3. The application of foreseeability of harm and the concept of notice as applied to the conduct of the obstetrician and/or nurse as measured by the time to respond to the clinical circumstances in a maternal death case due to an intracerebral hemorrhage. (BP, blood pressure)

BP/Headache abnormality	Abnormality identified
Abnormality identified	Physician notification
Physician notification	Physician evaluation
Physician evaluation	Physician decision
Physician decision	BP therapy
BP therapy	Therapeutic response

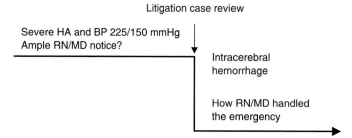

Figure 34.1 The two-step analytical process undertaken by an attorney in the evaluation of a medical malpractice case. (HA, headache; BP, blood pressure; mmHg, millimeters of mercury; RN, registered nurse; MD, medical doctor.)

Table 34.4. A sample note is provided to assist the obstetrician with documentation when contacted by the patient or nurse to come to the hospital to evaluate a patient

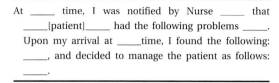

At _____ time, I was notified by Nurse _____ that _____[patient]_____ had the following problems _____. Upon my arrival at _____time, I found the following: _____, and decided to manage the patient as follows: _____.

difference recorded in the patient's medical records.

Once the physician evaluates the patient, the conduct issue becomes the duration of time required to establish a diagnosis and to decide on a course of therapy. Once the decision is made and an order given, the focus will be on the time required to administer the medication, an anti-hypertensive and/or $MgSO_4$ in this scenario. Once the medication is administered, how long did it take to obtain a therapeutic response? Often, this means that attention will be directed toward the need for any additional medical therapy to lower the BP.

Pre-eclampsia litigation

To identify the cases described in this section of the chapter, a search was done in Lexis-Nexis using the words pre-eclampsia, eclampsia, and pregnancy-induced hypertension for the period 1 January 1998 through 31 December 2003. The search identified 61 cases involving pre-eclampsia related to litigation. An overview of the maternal and perinatal outcomes for these 61 cases is listed in Table 34.5.

These cases support the observations of the Harvard Study (Brennan *et al.*, 1996) that law suits are often related to the severity of the injury and the age of the patient. For example, this group of patients were all young, in the reproductive age group, and had either a severe injury such as permanent brain damage or had died. As noted

Table 34.5. Maternal and perinatal outcome for 61 litigation cases reported in Lexis–Nexis for the years 1998–2003. [Perinatal outcome includes two sets of twins]

Maternal outcome ($N=61$)	
Death	15 (25%)
Brain damage	5 (8%)
Blind	1 (2%)
Normal	40 (65%)
Perinatal outcome ($N=63$)	
Brain damage	23 (37%)
Fetal death	19 (30%)
Neonatal death	2 (3%)
Leg amputation	1 (2%)
Unknown	3 (5%)
Normal	15 (23%)

in the Harvard study, the least reliable indicator of whether a law suit was brought was the quality of care. Whether quality of care was an issue in reported cases is less clear because there was not always sufficient information to draw an accurate conclusion.

The causes of maternal or perinatal death or disability are illustrated in Tables 34.6 and 34.7. As noted in Table 34.6, the leading cause of maternal death or permanent brain injury was intracerebral hemorrhage due, in most cases, to uncontrolled hypertension. However, what is less well known is how many of these pre-eclamptic patients who presented to a physician's office or hospital with the complaint of a severe headache in association with hypertension had already had a pre-existing intracerebral bleed. Not infrequently, the sole manifestation of a prior bleed is a slow maternal heart rate and a widened pulse pressure due, in part, to an increase in intracranial pressure. Under these circumstances, the cerebral vascular response is designed to limit and prevent further bleeding by localized cerebral artery spasm and thrombosis. When medical therapy with agents such as magnesium sulfate or hydralazine is administered, the physiologic impact of these agents is frequently directed at relieving central

Table 34.6. Identifiable causes of maternal death or permanent neurologic disability in 21 cases of pre-eclampsia reported in Lexis–Nexis for the years 1998–2003. [The remaining 40 women had apparently normal outcomes. BP, Blood pressure]

Intracerebral hemorrhage	9 (46%)
Postpartum hemorrhage	5 (24%)
Hepatic rupture	2 (10%)
Peripartum cardiomyopathy	1 (4%)
Pulmonary edema	1 (4%)
Amniotic fluid embolus	1 (4%)
Blind-uncontrolled BP	1 (4%)
Unknown	1 (4%)

Table 34.7. Identifiable causes of fetal or neonatal death or permanent brain damage in cases of pre-eclampsia reported in Lexis–Nexis for the years 1998–2003. [SRS, sudden, rapid, and sustained deceleration; SIDS, Sudden Infant Death Syndrome]

Fetal death [$N = 19$ (30%)]	
Abruption	9
SRS deceleration	2
Maternal death	4
Maternal seizures	1
Unknown	2
Cord accident	1
Brain damage [$N = 23$ (37%)]	
Preadmission	4
Hon pattern of asphyxia	1
Maternal arrest	1
SRS deceleration	3
Maternal seizures	1
Vacuum related	1
Intracerebral hemorrhage	3
Abruption	1
Unknown	8
Neonatal death [$N = 2$ (3%)]	
Pneumonia	1
SIDS	1
Normal outcome [$N = 19$ (30%)]	

or peripheral vasospasm. As such, the administration of these agents has the potential to negatively affect these protective mechanisms, and, to potentiate a pre-existing bleed.

The Bustamonte matter (*Bustamonte v. Granada Hills Community Hospital*, 2001) is an example of a patient who presented to the hospital with hypertension and widened pulse pressures of 201/92 mmHg and 191/100 mmHg. Around the time of delivery, the decedent's blood pressure was 224/106 mmHg and she complained of a severe headache. Whether the decedent had a slow heart rate during her time prior to the manifestation of her intracerebral bleed is unknown because that information was not included in the synopsis. But, the key to the Bustamonte matter is to recognize this physiologic pattern and to obtain immediate consultation with a specialist in maternal–fetal medicine, neurology, or internal medicine.

Table 34.7 illustrates the causes of fetal death or brain damage. Of note, placental abruption was responsible for the death or permanent brain damage of 10 (16%) fetuses. These findings support, in part, the relationship between maternal hypertensive disease and placental abruption. As previously demonstrated by Abdella *et al.* (1984), the incidence of placental abruption is directly related to the level of the maternal blood pressure.

This means that the higher the maternal BP the greater the risk of an abruption. While this relationship appears to exist, the harder question is to identify among those patients with an elevated blood pressure which person, if any, will have an abruption and when that patient will actually separate her placenta.

Nevertheless, the patient with a significant blood pressure elevation will require antihypertensive drug(s) to lower her blood pressure. The lowering of the maternal blood pressure should, theoretically, reduce the risk of placental abruption. In addition, in a patient with the diagnosis of pre-eclampsia and signs or symptoms of placental abruption, consideration should be given to delivery, as soon as it is technically feasible, rather than waiting for fetal signs of an abruption.

Induction of labor and intrapartum "fetal distress"

Many cases also arose in the context of induction of labor for pre-eclampsia with the subsequent development of intrapartum "fetal distress." The alleged "fetal distress" resulted in a brain-damaged infant or an intrapartum fetal death. When a decision is made to intervene by induction of labor for pre-eclampsia, each pregnancy should be assessed for the prospects of safe vaginal birth. If, for example, there is clinical evidence of intrauterine growth impairment and/or oligohydramnios, Cesarean may be the preferred route of delivery to avoid the downstream consequences of abruption and/or intrapartum fetal distress.

If induction of labor for pre-eclampsia is, nevertheless, undertaken, the fetus should be monitored during labor. As noted in these case summaries, 4 (17%) cases appeared to have preadmission fetal brain injury, 1 (4%) case described a FHR pattern consistent with the Hon pattern of intrapartum asphyxia, and several cases had a sudden, rapid and sustained deterioration of the fetal heart rate due to abruption or recurrent maternal seizures (Greenberg et al., 2001; Phelan and Ahn, 1994, 1998; Phelan and Kim, 2000; Phelan et al., 2001; Schifrin et al., 1994).

In *Dans v. Rappaport* (2000), for example, the gravida was being followed prenatally for suspected pregnancy-induced hypertension and possible pre-eclampsia. On the morning of delivery, she was 35 weeks gestation and she noted that her fetus did not move. That day, she was evaluated by her obstetrician. A nonstress test (NST) done during that visit was considered nonreactive. Later the same day, she was admitted to the hospital. At the hospital, the FHR pattern continued to be nonreactive. Approximately 6 h after the NST in the obstetrician's office the infant was delivered by Cesarean section. During this 6-hour period, the FHR, according to the facts, remained nonreactive with an absence of FHR accelerations, and a normal baseline rate of 120–130 bpm.

At birth, the infant had Apgars of 0 and 1 at one and five minutes, respectively, with an umbilical artery pH of 6.8. Additionally, an extremely elevated nucleated red blood cell count was noted in the neonate. An MRI taken at 7 years of age demonstrated white matter injury in the periventricular region. As of the time of the verdict, the child was permanently neurologically impaired.

This case manifests many of the findings in fetuses with a preadmission CNS insult. For example, the fetus did not move or had stopped moving prior to the maternal visit to the obstetrician's office. In the usual circumstance, the fetus that does not move is presumed to be dead. In this case, the fetus by virtue of a nonreactive FHR pattern was alive. The finding of decreased or absent fetal movement is in keeping with the observations of Schifrin et al. (1994) and Phelan and Kim (2000). These investigators found a significant increase in reduced or absent fetal activity among pregnancies complicated by a preadmission fetal brain injury.

Additionally, this fetus had a persistent nonreactive FHR pattern over a 6-hour period. This finding is also in keeping with the literature (Greenberg et al., 2001; Phelan, 1998; Phelan and Ahn, 1994; Phelan and Kim, 2000; Phelan et al., 2001). In the absence of a rising baseline FHR in association with repetitive FHR decelerations or a sudden, rapid and sustained deterioration in the FHR unresponsive to remedial measures that lasts until delivery, the fetal brain injury is probably consistent with a static encephalopathy (Greenberg et al., 2001; Phelan and Ahn, 1994, 1998; Phelan and Kim, 2000; Phelan et al., 2001).

While the case discussion provides solely that the NRBC values were "extremely elevated," fetuses with preadmission brain injury have been linked to elevated NRBC (Korst et al., 1996; Phelan et al., 1995, 2003). An association has been shown between elevated NRBC and persistent nonreactive FHR patterns intrapartum and with indirectly reduced or absent fetal movement. (Ghosh *et al.*, 2003; Korst *et al.*, 1996; Phelan *et al.*, 1995, 2003.)

Thus, the *Dans* matter, though decided in favor of the plaintiff, was consistent with a preadmission neurologic insult and inconsistent with an acute intrapartum insult because of the persistent nonreactive FHR pattern, the elevated NRBC, the neuroimaging showing white matter injury, and the absence of fetal movement (Phelan and Kim, 2000).

In the *Novell* case (*Novell v. Community Hospital of Central California*, 1999) of fetal brain damage due to an apparent Hon pattern of intrapartum asphyxia (Phelan and Kim, 2000; Phelan and Ahn, 1994, 1998), a 22-year-old gravida was admitted at 37 weeks gestation for induction of labor due to pre-eclampsia. After 22 h of oxytocin-induced labor, the certified nurse midwife consulted with the obstetrician about performing a Cesarean section. The OB decided to increase the oxytocin. By 7:00 A.M., the FHR had gradually increased to 180 bpm in association with a maternal fever. As a result of the fever, the mother was treated with antibiotics. At 7:50 A.M., the FHR fell to 60 bpm for longer than 6 min. The patient was scheduled for a Cesarean delivery. In the meantime, the patient was given terbutaline for intrauterine fetal resuscitation. The fetus recovered to a rate of 180 bpm. By 8:20 A.M., the FHR was now over 200 bpm; and, the fetal head was at a +2 station. The OB decided to have the mother push in an effort to deliver the fetus vaginally. At 9:30 A.M., the OB decided to do a vacuum delivery. At 9:45 A.M., the vacuum was applied. The fetal head delivered at 10:02 A.M. and the body followed at 10:05 A.M. During the vacuum delivery, variable decelerations were observed; and, these decelerations culminated in a terminal bradycardia. At birth, the infant had Apgars of 0, 0, and 0 at 1, 5, and 10 min, respectively; and, an umbilical arterial pH of 7.02. The long-term followup of the infant demonstrated profound brain damage with a feeding gastrostomy and a tracheostomy.

This case illustrates a probable Hon pattern of intrapartum asphyxia (Phelan and Ahn, 1994, 1998; Phelan and Kim, 2000). The characteristics of this pattern are illustrated in Figure 34.2. As noted in the *Novell* case (*Novell v. Community Hospital of Central California*, 1999), the maximum FHR was 200 bpm from a previously normal tracing. In a situation such as this, the obstetrician and nurse should be asking themselves why the fetal heart rate or fetal cardiac output has risen to such a level during labor. Could the entire change in FHR be attributed to the maternal fever or is the fetus becoming asphyxiated? In the end, the fetus appeared to be unable to maintain its cardiac output, resulting in a terminal bradycardia.

In the setting of a Hon pattern of intrapartum asphyxia and maternal pyrexia, antibiotics and antipyretics should be administered. If the fetus does not revert to a normal tracing, similar to the one seen on admission, within a reasonable period of time, delivery should be accomplished in the most expeditious manner.

Sentinel hypoxic events in some, but not all, of these pre-eclampsia cases arose in the context of a maternal arrest or an abruption (MacLennan, 1999). Intrapartum, these sentinel events appeared to produce a sudden, rapid, and sustained deterioration of the fetal heart rate lasting until delivery after an apparently normal initial tracing.

The key distinction among "acute fetal distress" cases relates to whether the condition singularly affects the fetus, such as an abruption, or is the "fetal distress" due to a maternal arrest. Under the circumstances of a maternal arrest, maternal health overrides fetal health. Thus, if a pregnant pre-eclamptic patient sustains a cardiopulmonary arrest, cardiopulmonary resuscitation (CPR) should be initiated immediately. For efficient CPR, the patient should be supine and the uterus displaced laterally to optimize maternal cardiac output. Once CPR is initiated, the timing of the Cesarean is critical to enhance maternal and fetal outcome. According to Katz and associates (1986), "Cesarean

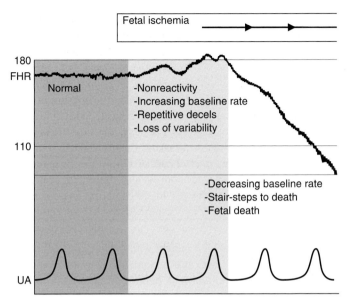

Figure 34.2 The characteristics of the Hon pattern of intrapartum asphyxia are represented. The pattern begins with a reactive admission fetal heart rate followed by nonreactivity, a progressive and substantial rise in the baseline rate to a level of tachycardia in association with repetitive decelerations and usually diminished variability.

delivery should be begun within 4 minutes, and the baby delivered within 5 minutes of maternal cardiac arrest." CPR should be continued throughout and after the delivery.

The fourth context in which fetal brain injury or death arose was in the eclamptic patient. As noted in the *Gold* matter (*Gold v. United Health Services Hospital*, 1998), the patient developed multiple seizures in association with FHR decelerations. Subsequently, the infant was delivered and later noted to be permanently neurologically impaired with spastic quadriplegia.

Maternal seizures are a well-known but infrequent sequel of pre-eclampsia. Maternal convulsions require prompt attention to prevent harm to both mother and fetus (Naidu *et al.*, 1996; Paul *et al.*, 1978; Pritchard *et al.*, 1984). During a seizure, the fetal response is usually manifested as an abrupt, prolonged FHR deceleration (Paul *et al.*, 1978). During the seizure, which generally lasts less than 1–2 min (Paul *et al.*, 1978), transient maternal hypoxia and uterine artery vasospasm occur and combine to produce a decline in uterine blood flow. In addition, uterine activity increases secondary to the release of norepinephrine, resulting in an additional reduction in uteroplacental perfusion. Ultimately, the reduction of uteroplacental perfusion causes the FHR deceleration. Such a deceleration may last up to 9 min (Paul *et al.*, 1978). Following the seizure and recovery from the FHR deceleration, a loss of variability and a compensatory rise in baseline FHR are characteristically seen. Transient late decelerations are not uncommon but resolve once maternal metabolic recovery is complete.

The cornerstone of patient management during an eclamptic seizure is to maintain adequate maternal oxygenation and to administer appropriate anticonvulsants. After a convulsion occurs, an adequate airway should be maintained and oxygen administered. To optimize uteroplacental perfusion, the mother should be repositioned onto her side. Anticonvulsant therapy with intravenous magnesium sulfate (Naidu *et al.*, 1996; Pritchard *et al.*, 1984) to prevent seizure recurrence is recommended. In spite of adequate magnesium sulfate therapy, adjunctive anticonvulsant therapy occasionally may be necessary (Pritchard *et al.*, 1984). In the event of persistent FHR decelerations, intrauterine resuscitation with a betamimimetic (Arias, 1978) or magnesium sulfate may be helpful in relieving eclampsia-induced uterine hypertonus. Continuous electronic fetal monitoring should be used to follow the fetal condition. It is also axiomatic in this circumstance of conflicting maternal and fetal interests that maternal interests take precedence over those of the fetus (Phelan, 1991). This means the first step is to stabilize the seizing pregnant woman. After the mother has been stabilized, and if the fetus continues to show signs of distress after a reasonable period of recovery, delivery in the most expeditious manner should be considered.

Outpatient vs. inpatient care

Medical–legal claims that arise in this setting revolve around "patient selection for outpatient management, documentation of instructions and patient options, and the failure to appreciate the clinical significance of patient complaints during telephone calls" (Sibai, 2003). As set forth by Sibai (2003), outpatient or home management should be reserved for patients satisfying the criteria in Table 34.8.

While many patients will satisfy the clinical requirements for outpatient management, many of these patients will not be able to satisfy the patient reliability requirements. The keeping of appointments and the patient's ability to follow instructions can help in providing an inference of reliability. But, if the patient does not have immediate transportation, telephone access, or family members readily available to help, she should be admitted to the hospital. Notwithstanding, worsening maternal and/or fetal condition mandates inpatient care (Sibai, 2003).

For example, the matter of *Anonymous Infant* (*Anonymous Infant v. Anonymous Midwife and Anonymous OB/Gyn*, 2000) involved the wrongful

Table 34.8. Criteria for outpatient management of mild pre-eclampsia

Systolic pressure ≤ 150 mmHg, or diastolic pressure ≤ 100 mmHg
Proteinuria ≤ 1000 mg 24 h^{-1}, or $\leq 2 +$ on dipstick
Highly reliable
Absence of labor
Absent cerebral signs and symptoms
Absent epigastric or upper quadrant pain
Ultrasound evidence of an appropriate for gestational age fetus
Normal fetal surveillance testing
Normal liver enzymes and platelet count

discharge of a patient with a falling platelet count. In that case, the patient had a prior history of abruption and fetal demise. In her eighth month, she was noted to have an elevated blood pressure, proteinuria, and a platelet count of 112,000 mm^{-3}. The lab tests were repeated the next day, and the platelet count had fallen to 95,000 mm^{-3}. Later the same day, she was discharged home for outpatient management.

A few days later, she was readmitted with severe abdominal pain and findings consistent with severe pre-eclampsia. At Cesarean, a placental abruption was confirmed. The infant was born with severe neonatal encephalopathy and has been diagnosed with spastic quadriplegia.

As noted in Table 34.8, this patient had a decreasing platelet count; and, as such, she was not a candidate for outpatient management. Her worsening condition probably was an indication for her to remain in the hospital.

In contrast, the *Galvez* matter (*Galvez v. The Thomas F. McCafferty Medical Center*, 2000) involved continued outpatient management in the face of a worsening maternal condition. In that case, the gravida had developed signs and symptoms suggestive of pre-eclampsia by 20 July 1998. Over the course of the next two visits on 6 and 13 August 1998, she continued to manifest excessive weight gain, proteinuria, and abnormally high blood pressures. By 19 August 1998, she developed head and abdominal pain in association with a significantly elevated BP. Subsequently, she sustained a massive intracerebral hemorrhage and died.

These two cases, *Anonymous Infant* (*Anonymous Infant v. Anonymous Midwife and Anonymous OB/ Gyn*, 2000) and *Galvez* (*Galvez v. The Thomas F. McCafferty Medical Center*, 2000), illustrate the concept of notice and foreseeability of harm. In *Anonymous Infant*, notice was the worsening maternal condition as evidenced by the decline in the maternal platelet count. Early warning or notice in the *Galvez* matter was the continual and substantial rise in maternal BP. As such, one patient should have remained in the hospital and the other should have been admitted to the hospital.

Telephone liability

The telephone is a major means by which obstetrician/gynecologists provide care to their patients (Phelan, 1998), and telephone calls account for approximately 20% of all encounters between obstetrician/gynecologists and their patients (Radecki *et al.*, 1989). Of these patient encounters, 70% of the calls are managed over the telephone without patient examination by the physician (Curtis and Talbot, 1981). With a greater emphasis on ambulatory services by managed care plans to reduce healthcare costs and the shifts in reimbursement, the telephone will play an even greater role in patient care.

The contemporary practice of obstetrics and gynecology has also witnessed a shift to ambulatory women's healthcare services. During the past several years the management of a variety of conditions including pre-eclampsia (Barton *et al.*, 1994) has been attempted in the outpatient setting through the use of the telephone.

With the increase in telephone use, the potential for telephone liability will necessarily rise. In evaluating one's risk of telephone liability, it is

Table 34.9. Allegations arising from the use of the telephone

Failure to diagnose
Delay in treatment
Improper treatment
Failure to follow-up
Poor telephone procedures
Breach of confidentiality
Inadequate documentation

important to understand that claims have arisen in a variety of clinical situations (Table 34.9).

Whenever there is a telephone contact, a thorough evaluation through questioning of the patient is necessary. To be certain of the details, the physician or a representative of the physician should carefully clarify the clinical issue. If the questioning does not provide a sufficient resolution to patient reports of symptoms, a clinical evaluation should be considered.

The *Doe v. Anonymous* matter (2000) illustrates the failure to diagnose, and the improper treatment relating to the telephone management of a pre-eclamptic woman. In that case, Jane Doe, a 34-year-old, was pregnant at 34 weeks gestation when she died at home. Two weeks prior to her death, she was noted to have an elevated BP. Over the next 2 weeks, she had a 13 pound weight gain, developed proteinuria, and exhibited significant BP elevation. Despite the period of worsening maternal condition, the pregnancy was allowed to continue. On the day prior to her death, she contacted her physician's office by telephone and complained of respiratory problems. Her physician instructed the nurse to call in a prescription for antibiotics. Jane Doe was neither examined nor hospitalized. The next day, she was found dead in her home.

The medical–legal issues in the *Doe* matter (*Doe v. Anonymous*, 2000) relate to the issue of notice and that the clinical exam was limited to a history. For example, Jane Doe's clinical condition appeared to worsen over a two-week period. During this time, she experienced signs and symptoms of worsening pre-eclampsia, weight gain, proteinuria, and an elevated BP. On the day prior to her death, she developed respiratory embarrassment. As such, the physician was on notice of her worsening condition and needed to evaluate and/or admit her to the hospital.

Additionally, improper treatment was rendered because the nurse rather than the physician took the call. The physician did not appear to have clarified Jane Doe's medical condition. Instead, the presumption was, based on the apparent representations made by the nurse, that Jane Doe appeared to have a respiratory infection. Under these circumstances, a good faith physical exam and pertinent laboratory studies may have identified her worsening pre-eclamptic condition prior to her death.

Timing of delivery

The expectant management of the pre-eclamptic patient is reserved for selected preterm pregnancies (Phelan, 1992). Once the pregnancy has advanced to a point when the fetus can be reasonably expected to live independent of its mother, as evidenced by fetal lung maturity or a gestational age ≥37 weeks gestation, the pre-eclamptic patient should be considered for delivery.

Medical–legal cases often arise in circumstances in which expectant management is continued in the presence of a term pregnancy (*Cartegna v. Leber*, 2002; Tri-Service Reference, 2000; *Vasquez v. Lin*, 1999). For example, fetal surveillance testing or delayed intervention was instituted at 37 weeks (*Cartegna v. Leber*, 2002), 38 weeks (*Vasquez v. Lin*, 1999) and 40 weeks (Tri-Service Reference, 2000) gestation. In the *Cartegna* matter (*Cartegna v. Leber*, 2002), for example, the patient had pre-existing essential hypertension and subsequently developed pre-eclampsia and diet-controlled diabetes mellitus. At 37 weeks gestation, she was referred for fetal surveillance testing. After the test was performed, she was sent home. Subsequently,

she had an intrauterine fetal death. At issue in the case was the proper performance and interpretation of the test prior to discharge.

In the *Vasquez* matter (*Vasquez v. Lin*, 1999), the patient was admitted to the hospital at 38 weeks gestation with the diagnosis of pre-eclampsia, early labor, and third-trimester bleeding due to a "low lying placenta." The treatment plan was expectant management. Three days after admission, she sustained a respiratory arrest. During the maternal arrest, the baby sustained acute asphyxia and permanent brain damage. The primary medical–legal issue was whether expectant management was appropriate rather than delivery in a 38 week pregnant pre-eclamptic. Delivery within 24 h of admission would, in all medical probability, have avoided the maternal arrest and fetal brain injury.

In the Tri-Service Reference case, the patient underwent fetal surveillance testing at 39 4/7 weeks gestation due to diet-controlled diabetes mellitus (DM). During the test, her BP was 158/90 mmHg. Throughout her pregnancy, she had periodic episodes of hypertension. Four days later at 40 1/7 weeks gestation she had an equivocal contraction stress test. After the equivocal test, the patient was sent home and requested to return four days later. Upon her return at 40 5/7 weeks gestation, the fetal monitoring strip was consistent with pre-existing fetal brain damage. Within a few hours of her arrival, she was delivered. According to the case summary, the child has persistent neurologic deficits.

These latter three cases of pre-eclampsia reinforce the concept of foreseeability of harm: *Cartegna* (*Cartegna v. Leber*, 2002) – intrauterine fetal death; *Vasquez* (*Vasquez v. Lin*, 1999) – maternal arrest with resultant fetal brain injury; and Tri-Service (Tri-Service Reference 2000) – continued expectant management beyond term in a diabetic with hypertension and resultant fetal brain damage. At the same time, these cases remind us of our goal to safely manage, when technically feasible, the pregnancy to the point that the fetus can survive independent of its mother. The case

Table 34.10. Clinical situations in which litigation arose in cases of pre-eclampsia

---

Induction of labor and intrapartum "fetal distress"
Outpatient vs. inpatient care
The use of the telephone
Timing of delivery

---

summaries suggest that had delivery been undertaken when the diagnosis of pre-eclampsia had been made, rather than continued expectant management, the maternal and fetal outcomes would, in all medical probability, have been improved.

Summary

Table 34.10 illustrates the litigation areas associated with the preeclamptic patient. Each issue identified in Table 34.10 is not a stranger to the practising clinician. But, whenever the clinician is confronted with a pre-eclamptic patient, the key ingredient to clinical management is whether the pregnancy can continue or is delivery warranted based on the circumstances and/or the gestational age of the pregnancy. When the decision to deliver has been made, the patient could be offered either a Cesarean delivery or a trial of labor depending on the circumstances. If the pre-eclamptic patient elects a trial of labor, vaginal birth should not be the goal. The goal is to deliver the pregnant woman and her fetus safely. This means that the Cesarean rate for this subpopulation of patients could rise.

REFERENCES

Abdella, T. N., Sibai, B. M., Hays, J. M. and Anderson, G. D. (1984). Relationship of hypertensive disease to abruption placentae. *Obstet. Gynecol.*, **63**, 365–70.

Anonymous Infant v. Anonymous Midwife and Anonymous OB/Gyn. (2000). Case No. Withheld, 7 November 2000. *The Massachusetts, Connecticut, Rhode Island Verdict Reporter.* JAS Publications 2001.

Arias, F. (1978). Intrauterine resuscitation with terbutaline: a method for the management of acute fetal distress. *Am. J. Obstet. Gynecol.*, **131**, 39–43.

Barton, J. R., Stanziano, G. J. and Sibai, B. M. (1994). Monitored outpatient management of mild gestational hypertension remote from term. *Am. J. Obstet. Gynecol.*, **170**, 765–9.

Brennan, T. A., Sox, C. M. and Burstin, H. R. (1996). Relation between negligent adverse events and the outcomes of medical-malpractice litigation. *N. Engl. J. Med.*, **335**, 1963–7.

Bustamonte v. Granada Hills Community Hospital. (2001). Case No. PC 026227X Superior Court California 13 November 2001. *Verdicts, Settlements & Tactics.*

Cartegna v. Leber, et al. (2002). Docket No. L-6057–99, Verdict Date February 2002 *New Jersey Jury Verdict Review & Analysis.* Jury Verdict Review Publications, Inc. March, 2002.

Curtis, P. and Talbot, A. (1981). The telephone in primary care. *J. Commun. Hlth.*, **6**, 194–8.

Dans v. Rappaport. (2000). *Jury Verdict Review Publications*, Inc. Index No. 1065–94. Jury Verdict 9 February 2000, published June 2000.

Dildy, G. A., III (2004). Complications of preeclampsia. In *Critical Care Obstetrics*, 4th edn, ed. G. A. Dildy, M. A. Belfort, G. R. Saade, J. P. Phelan, G. D. V. Hankins and S. L. Clark. Malden, MA: Blackwell Science, pp. 436–62.

Doe v. Anonymous. (2000). (Cuyahoga County Court of Common Pleas, Cleveland, Ohio June 2000) *West Group Verdicts, Settlements & Tactics* 2000.

Franklin, M. A. and Rabin, R. L. (1983). *Tort Law and Alternatives – Cases and Materials*, 3rd edn. Mineola, NY: The Foundation Press, Inc., p. 41.

Galvez v. The Thomas F. McCafferty Medical Center. (2000). Case No. 372797 13 April 2000 *West Group-Verdicts, Settlements & Tactics* 2000.

Ghosh, B., Mittal, S., Kumar, S. and Dadhwal, V. (2003). Prediction of perinatal asphyxia with nucleated red blood cells in cord blood of newborns. *Int. J. Gynecol. Obstet.*, **81**, 267–71.

Gold v. United Health Services Hospital Inc. (1998). No. 95–0177 Verdict Date 05/14/1998 *Verdict Search New York Reporter.*

Greenberg, J., Economy, K., Mark, A. and Ringer, S. (2001). In search of "true" birth asphyxia: labor characteristics associated with the asphyxiated term infant. *Am. J. Obstet. Gynecol.*, **185**, 554.

Katz, V. L., Dotters, D. J. and Droegemueller, W. (1986). Perimortem cesarean delivery. *Obstet. Gynecol.*, **68**, 571–6.

Korst, L. M., Phelan, J. P., Ahn, M. O. and Martin, G. I. (1996). Nucleated red blood cells: an update on the marker for fetal asphyxia. *Am. J. Obstet. Gynecol.*, **175**, 843–6.

MacLennan, A. (1999). A template for defining a causal relation between acute intrapartum events and cerebral palsy: international consensus statement. *Br. Med. J.*, **319**, 1054–9.

MacPherson v. Buick Motor Company. (1916). 217 N.Y. 382, 111 N.E. 1050.

Naidu, S., Payne, A. J., Moodley, J., *et al.* (1996). Randomized study assessing the effects of phenytoin and magnesium sulfate on maternal cerebral circulation in eclampsia using transcranial Doppler ultrasound. *Br. J. Obstet. Gynaecol.*, **103**, 111–16.

Novell v. Community Hospital of Central California. (1999). Case No. 608435–4 *Jury Verdicts Weekly* (California), 28 June 1999.

Paul, R. H., Koh, K. S. and Berstein, S. G. (1978). Change in fetal heart rate: uterine contraction patterns associated with eclampsia. *Am. J. Obstet. Gynecol.*, **130**, 165–9.

Phelan, J. P. (1991). The maternal abdominal wall: a fortress against fetal health care? *So. Cal. Law Rev.*, **65**, 461–90.

Phelan, J. P. (ed.) (1992). *Clinics in Perinatology.* Philadelphia, PA: W.B. Saunders Co., **19**(2), 449–59.

Phelan, J. P. and Ahn, M. O. (1994). Perinatal observations in forty-eight neurologically impaired term infants. *Am. J. Obstet. Gynecol.*, **171**, 424–31.

Phelan, J. P., Ahn, M. O., Korst, L. M. and Martin, G. I. (1995). Nucleated red blood cells: a marker for fetal asphyxia? *Am. J. Obstet. Gynecol.*, **173**, 1380–4.

Phelan, J. P. and Ahn, M. O. (1998). 300 term brain damaged infants: their FHR patterns. *Am. J. Obstet. Gynecol.*, **178**(2), S74.

Phelan, J. P. (1998). Ambulatory obstetrical care: strategies to reduce telephone liability. *Clin. Obstet. Gynecol.*, **41**, 640–6.

Phelan, J. P. and Kim, J. O. (2000). Fetal heart rate observations in the brain-damaged infant. *Semin. Perinatol.*, **24**, 221–9.

Phelan, J. P., Ahn, M. O. and Kirkendall, C. (2001). Fetal heart rate patterns in 423 brain damaged infants: an update. *Obstet. Gynecol.*, **97**(4), 34S.

Phelan, J. P., Kirkendall, C., Korst, L. and Martin, G. (2003). Nucleated red blood cells in fetal brain injury show a consistent relationship with the intrapartum FHR pattern. *Am. J. Obstet. Gynecol.*, **189**(6), S165.

Pritchard, J. A., Cunningham, F. G. and Pritchard, S. A. (1984). The Parkland Memorial Hospital protocol for treatment of eclampsia. Evaluation of 245 cases. *Am. J. Obstet. Gynecol.*, **148**, 951–63.

Radecki, S. E., Neville, R. E. and Girard, R. A. (1989). Telephone patient management by primary care physicians. *Med. Care.*, **27**, 817–22.

Schifrin, B. S., Hamilton-Rubinstein, T. and Shields, J. R. (1994). Fetal heart rate patterns and timing of injury. *J. Perinatol.*, **14**, 174–81.

Sibai, B. M. (2003). Cutting the legal risks of hypertension in pregnancy. *OBG Mgmt*, January, 44–64.

Sullivan, C. A. and Martin J. N. Jr. (2004). Thrombotic microangiopathies. In *Critical Care Obstetrics*, 4th edn, ed. G. A. Dildy, M. A. Belfort, G. R. Saade, J. P. Phelan, G. D. V. Hankins and S. L. Clark. Malden, MA: Blackwell Science, pp. 408–49.

Tri-Service Reference No. S00–10–11. Settlement Date: August 2000, Verdictum Jurics Press 2000.

Vasquez v. Lin (1999). Case No. BC 191 183 *Tri-Service Reference* No. 99–06–02 Verdict Date: January 21, 1999, Verdictum Juris Press 1999.

Subject Index